REVIEW
OF ORTHOPAEDIC
TRAUMA

SECOND EDITION

REVIEW OF ORTHOPAEDIC TRAUMA

Mark R. Brinker, MD

Director of Acute and Reconstructive Trauma

Texas Orthopedic Hospital and Fondren Orthopedic Group LLP

Houston, Texas

Clinical Professor of Orthopaedic Surgery

The University of Texas Health Science Center at Houston

Houston, Texas

Clinical Professor of Orthopaedic Surgery

Tulane University School of Medicine

New Orleans, Louisiana

Clinical Professor of Orthopedic Surgery

Baylor College of Medicine

Houston, Texas

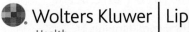

Wolters Kluwer | Lippincott Williams & Wilkins

Health

Philadelphia · Baltimore · New York · London
Buenos Aires · Hong Kong · Sydney · Tokyo

Acquisitions Editor: Brian Brown
Production Project Manager: David Orzechowski
Senior Product Manager: David Murphy
Design Manager: Terry Mallon
Manufacturing Manager: Benjamin Rivera
Marketing Manager: Lisa Lawrence
Compositor : S4Carlisle Publishing Services

351 West Camden Street
Baltimore, MD 21201

530 Walnut Street
Philadelphia, PA 19106

Printed in China

Library of Congress Cataloging-in-Publication Data

Review of orthopaedic trauma / [edited by] Mark R. Brinker. — Second Edition.
    p. ; cm.
 Includes bibliographical references and index.
 Summary: "The second edition of Review of Orthopaedic Trauma covers the entire
scope of adult and pediatric trauma care. Emphasis is placed on material likely to
appear on board and training exams. An easy-to-use outline is provided for rapid
access, exam preparation, or review of new and emerging topics. Information is
organized by anatomic region"—Provided by publisher.
 ISBN 978-1-58255-783-0
 I. Brinker, Mark R., editor of compilation.
 [DNLM: 1. Bone and Bones—injuries. 2. Joints—injuries. WE 200]

  617.4'71044—dc23

      2012049621

DISCLAIMER
Care has been taken to confirm the accuracy of the information present and to
describe generally accepted practices. However, the authors, editors, and publisher
are not responsible for errors or omissions or for any consequences from application
of the information in this book and make no warranty, expressed or implied, with
respect to the currency, completeness, or accuracy of the contents of the publication.
Application of this information in a particular situation remains the professional
responsibility of the practitioner; the clinical treatments described and recommended
may not be considered absolute and universal recommendations.

The authors, editors, and publisher have exerted every effort to ensure that drug selection and dosage set forth in this text are in accordance with the current recommendations
and practice at the time of publication. However, in view of ongoing research, changes
in government regulations, and the constant flow of information relating to drug therapy
and drug reactions, the reader is urged to check the package insert for each drug for any
change in indications and dosage and for added warnings and precautions. This is particularly important when the recommended agent is a new or infrequently employed drug.

Some drugs and medical devices presented in this publication have Food and Drug
Administration (FDA) clearance for limited use in restricted research settings. It is the
responsibility of the health care provider to ascertain the FDA status of each drug or
device planned for use in their clinical practice.

To purchase additional copies of this book, call our customer service department at (800)
638-3030 or fax orders to (301) 223-2320. International customers should call (301) 223-2300.

Visit Lippincott Williams & Wilkins on the Internet: http://www.lww.com. Lippincott
Williams & Wilkins customer service representatives are available from 8:30 am to
6:00 pm, EST.

10 9 8 7 6 5 4 3 2 1

To the three most amazing women on the planet: my mother Carole, my wife Newie, and my daughter Sloan. You gave me life, share my life, and make my life. In a world full of mangled extremities and infected nonunions, you are my shining lights of splendor.

CONTENTS

SECTION I: OVERVIEW

SECTION II: ADULT TRAUMA

PART I THE LOWER EXTREMITY 66

SECTION III: PEDIATRIC TRAUMA

CONTRIBUTORS

Daniel T. Altman, MD
Director of Orthopaedic Spine Trauma
Allegheny General Hospital
Associate Professor of Orthopaedic Surgery
Drexel University College of Medicine
Pittsburgh, Pennsylvania

Michael B. Banffy, MD
Orthopaedic Surgeon
Beach Cities Orthopedics & Sports Medicine
Manhattan Beach, California

O. Alton Barron, MD
Assistant Clinical Professor of Orthopaedics
Columbia College of Physicians and Surgeons
Senior Attending
St. Luke's-Roosevelt Hospital Center
New York, New York

James B. Bennett, MD
Clinical Professor
Department of Orthopedic Surgery and Division of
    Plastic Surgery
Baylor College of Medicine
Houston, Texas
Chief of Staff
Texas Orthopedic Hospital and Fondren
    Orthopedic Group LLP
Houston, Texas

Mark R. Brinker, MD
Director of Acute and Reconstructive Trauma
Texas Orthopedic Hospital and Fondren
    Orthopedic Group LLP
Houston, Texas
Clinical Professor of Orthopaedic Surgery
The University of Texas Health Science Center at
    Houston
Houston, Texas
Clinical Professor of Orthopaedic Surgery
Tulane University School of Medicine
New Orleans, Louisiana
Clinical Professor of Orthopedic Surgery
Baylor College of Medicine
Houston, Texas

Lisa K. Cannada, MD
Associate Professor
Orthopaedic Traumatology
Department of Orthopaedic Surgery
Saint Louis University School of Medicine
St. Louis, Missouri

Robert Victor Cantu, MD
Assistant Professor of Orthopaedic Surgery
Dartmouth-Hitchcock Medical Center
Lebanon, New Hampshire

Jens R. Chapman, MD
Professor
Department Chair
Director, Spine Service
Hansjöerg Wyss Endowed Chair
Department of Orthopaedics and Sports Medicine
University of Washington
Seattle, Washington

Luke S. Choi, MD
Director
Center for the Athlete's Shoulder and Elbow
Sports Medicine
Regeneration Orthopedics
St Louis, Missouri

C. Craig Crouch, MD
Orthopaedic Surgeon
Texas Orthopedic Hospital and Fondren
    Orthopedic Group LLP
Houston, Texas

Damien Davis, MD
Orthopaedic Surgery Resident
St. Luke's-Roosevelt Hospital Center
New York, New York

Kyle F. Dickson, MD, MBA
Professor of Orthopedic Surgery
Baylor College of Medicine
Houston, Texas

Gregory N. Drake, MD
Shoulder Fellow
Fondren Orthopedic Group LLP
Houston, Texas

T. Bradley Edwards, MD
Orthopaedic Surgeon
Texas Orthopedic Hospital and Fondren
 Orthopedic Group LLP
Houston, Texas

Howard R. Epps, MD
Medical Director
Pediatric Orthopaedics & Scoliosis
Texas Children's Hospital
Associate Professor
Department of Orthopaedic Surgery
Baylor College of Medicine
Houston, Texas

Michael Fehlings, MD, PHD, FRCSC
Director
Neural and Sensory Sciences Program
University Health Network
Toronto, Ontario

R. Jay French, MD
Orthopaedic Surgeon
Tennessee Orthopaedic Clinics
Oak Ridge, Tennessee

John T. Gorczyca, MD
Professor
Department of Orthopaedics
University of Rochester Medical Center
Rochester, New York

Frank A. Gottschalk, MD
Professor of Orthopaedic Surgery
UT Southwestern Medical Center
Dallas, Texas

Robert Greenleaf, MD
Reconstructive Orthopedics
Moorestown, New Jersey

Brian Edward Grottkau, MD
Chief
Pediatric Orthopaedic Service
Department of Orthopaedic Surgery
Massachusetts General Hospital
Pediatric Orthopaedic Surgeon
Assistant Professor of Orthopaedic
 Surgery
Harvard Medical School
Boston, Massachusetts

Joseph J. Gugenheim, MD
Associate Professor of Orthopedic Surgery
University of Texas Medical Branch
Galveston, Texas
Texas Orthopedic Hospital and Fondren
 Orthopedic Group LLP
Houston, Texas

David J. Hak, MD, MBA
Associate Professor
Denver Health
University of Colorado
Denver, Colorado

Mitchel B. Harris, MD
Professor
Department of Orthopaedic Surgery
Harvard Medical School
Chief
Orthopedic Trauma Service
Brigham and Women's Hospital
Boston, Massachusetts

Christopher C. Harrod, MD
Orthopaedic Surgeon
The Bone and Joint Clinic of Baton Rouge
Baton Rouge, Louisiana

Byron Hobby, MD
Orthopaedic Trauma Fellow
Department of Orthopaedics
UC Davis
Sacramento, California

Joseph R. Hsu, MD
Chief of Orthopaedic Trauma
Institute of Surgical Research
Assistant Program Director (Research)
Orthopaedic Surgery Residency
San Antonio Military Medical Center
Brook Army Medical Center
San Antonio, Texas

Catherine A. Humphrey, MD
Assistant Professor
Department of Orthopaedics
University of Rochester Medical Center
Rochester, New York

Kenneth J. Koval, MD
Director of Orthopaedic Research
Adult Orthopaedics
Orlando Health
Orlando, Florida

Steven C. Lochow, MD
Orthopaedic Surgeon
Scott Orthopedic Center
Huntington, West Virginia

Philip R. Lozman, MD
Orthopedic Surgeon
Orthopedic Specialists
Aventura, Florida

William C. McGarvey, MD
Associate Professor
Residency Program Director
Department of Orthopaedic Surgery
The University of Texas Health Science
    Center at Houston
Houston, Texas

Thomas L. Mehlhoff, MD
Orthopaedic Surgeon
Texas Orthopedic Hospital and Fondren
    Orthopedic Group LLP
Team Physician
Houston Astros
Houston, Texas

Umesh S. Metkar, MD
Consulting Spine Surgeon
Hartsville Orthopedics & Carolina Pines Regional
    Medical Center
Hartsville, South Carolina

Mark D. Miller, MD
S. Ward Casscells Professor of Orthopaedic Surgery
University of Virginia
Team Physician
James Madison University
JBJS Deputy Editor for Sports Medicine
Director
Miller Review Course
Charlottesville, Virginia

Sohail K. Mirza, MD, MPH
Chair
Department of Orthopaedics
Dartmouth Hitchcock Medical Center
Lebanon, New Hampshire

Kris Moore, MD
Orthopedic Surgeon
Providence Medical Group-Orthopedics
Newberg, Oregon

William D. Murrell, MD
Consultant Orthopaedic Sports Medicine
Dubai Bone & Joint Center
Dubai Healthcare City
Dubai, UAE

Sean E. Nork, MD
Associate Professor
Department of Orthopaedics and Sports Medicine
Harborview Medical Center
University of Washington
Seattle, Washington

Daniel P. O'Connor, PhD
Associate Professor
Department of Health and Human Performance
University of Houston
Houston, Texas

Steven A. Olson, MD
Professor of Orthopaedic Surgery
Department of Orthopaedic Surgery
Duke University School of Medicine
Durham, North Carolina

Nicolas Phan, MD, CM
Division of Neurosurgery and Spinal Program
Toronto Hospital and Univerity of Toronto Western
    Hospital
Toronto, Ontario

Robert A. Probe, MD
Chairman
Department of Orthopaedic Surgery
Scott & White Memorial Hospital
Temple, Texas

Jory D. Richman, MD
Clinical Assistant Professor of Orthopaedic Surgery
University of Pittsburgh
Pittsburgh, Pennsylvania

Dustin Richter, MD
Orthopaedic Surgeon
Department of Orthopaedics & Rehabilitation
University of New Mexico Medical School
Albuquerque, New Mexico

Scott B. Rosenfeld, MD
Assistant Professor of Orthopedic Surgery
Baylor College of Medicine
Pediatric Orthopedic Surgery
Texas Children's Hospital
Houston, Texas

Peter W. Ross, MD
Orthopaedic Surgeon
Kenai Peninsula Orthopaedics
Soldotna, Alaska

Robert C. Schenck, Jr., MD
Professor and Chair
Department of Orthopaedics
University of New Mexico
Albuquerque, New Mexico

Roman Schwartsman, MD
Orthopaedic Surgeon
Boise, Idaho

Milan K. Sen, MD
Assistant Professor
Department of Orthopaedic Surgery
The University of Texas Health
    Science Center at Houston
Houston, Texas

Jerry S. Sher, MD
Orthopedic Surgeon
Orthopedic Specialists
Aventura, Florida

Donald S. Stewart II, MD
Arlington Orthopedic Associates, P.A.
Mansfield, Texas

Marcus Timlin, MCh, FRCS (Tr&Orth)
Consultant Orthopaedic Surgeon
Mater Private Hospital
UPMC Beacon Hospital
Dublin, Ireland

Krishna Tripuraneni, MD
Orthopaedic Surgeon
New Mexico Orthopaedics
Albuquerque, New Mexico

Fredric H. Warren, MD
Director of Pediatric Orthopaedics
Ochsner Children's Health Center
New Orleans, Louisiana

Ian Whitney, MD
Resident
University of Texas Health Care
San Antonio, Texas

Michael W. Wolfe, MD
Assistant Professor
Department of Surgery
Virginia Tech Carilion School of Medicine
Roanoke, Virginia

I, and those who studied the first edition of Dr. Mark Brinker's *Review of Orthopaedic Trauma*, found it to be an extremely valuable textbook. Now Brinker gives us an equally comprehensive second edition with updated materials, new and expanded chapters, and hundreds of fresh and original illustrations.

The utility of this book is not achieved in spite of its purpose as a review text; rather, it is achieved because of it. While the more traditional fracture and trauma textbooks certainly still have their place, the reader is often overburdened with subtleties, nuances, and details concerning concepts and techniques that fall in and out of favor or are endorsed by one faction or institution. Furthermore, it is common to encounter lengthy discussions regarding the author's preferred methods and specific viewpoints that are not necessarily evidenced-based.

By contrast, in focusing on the review nature of this work, Brinker, acting as both the editor and an author, delivers an intellectually nourishing final product that distills out the important core knowledge of the subspecialty. At the same time, Brinker's work goes far beyond just the basics. *Review of Orthopaedic Trauma* provides an up-to-date, state-of-the-art approach to the essential issues of the multiply injured patient, damage control orthopedics, and long-bone and periarticular injuries, as well as covers the current clinical thought on specific musculoskeletal injuries in both adult and pediatric patients.

Mark Brinker has both selected and edited his colleagues well, using his highly developed educational skills to the fullest. The chapters on biomechanics and methodologies of deformity assessment and correction exemplify the focus and clarity of this text in organization, editing, and appropriateness. The reader's educational experience is further enhanced by the fact that each chapter is framed with an eye on commonly tested material encountered on In-Training Examinations, Self-Assessment Examinations, and ABOS Certification and Recertification Examinations.

Mark Brinker is widely known and highly respected as a gifted surgeon who routinely tackles the most difficult reconstructive challenges of our specialty. He brings the same energy and passion to *Review of Orthopaedic Trauma*, turning his talents to communicating the entire fund of knowledge of the specialty in one neat and tidy package. My advice is that residents and fellows read this book early on in their training; <u>AND</u>, that they read it again, near the end of their training. As a senior traumatologist, I found this book exceptionally valuable in filling in the gaps in my own knowledge base, and as a way to rapidly review the current thinking on the aspects of Orthopaedic Trauma that I don't encounter on a regular basis.

It's a real treat to be invited to write the Foreword to the second edition of *Review of Orthopaedic Trauma* and I am honored to have Mark as both a colleague and friend.

Andy R. Burgess, MD
Professor and Vice-Chairman
Chief, Division of Orthopaedic Trauma
Department of Orthopaedic Surgery
The University of Texas Health Science
Center at Houston

Why another text, one might ask. With the plethora of information now readily available, another text, another comprehensive "tome," especially on orthopaedic trauma, might be thought of as redundant. However, Mark Brinker and his colleagues are to be congratulated. They have identified an area, or niche, of need (i.e., a review text). Their target audience is obviously not those practicing as orthopaedic traumatologists, who want an in-depth analysis of the problem. Rather it is the general orthopaedic surgeon and/or resident looking for a concise review of the topic in an almost note-taking style and bolding of the key issues. In addition, the authors have provided ample diagrams, algorithms, and tables to review classification systems, treatment plans, and so forth. They also have provided the most significant references but not just as a list. Rather, they divide the bibliography into classic articles, recent articles, review articles, and textbooks, making it much easier for the reader to ascertain where to obtain specific further information.

Further, in their attempt to also make this a user-friendly text for those taking the OITE, ABOS Boards (certifying) or even recertifying examinations, the authors have listed which specific examinations and which specific questions are related to issues in each chapter. This is a useful tool for those in orthopaedic surgery who are in the examination review process.

Obviously, Dr. Mark Brinker did not achieve this on his own. He has elicited an array of experts who have written the many chapters. However, the style and theme remains consistent throughout, giving the book a specific feel and character. The text is broken up into three sections. Section I is an overview; Section II, Adult Trauma, is subdivided into the lower extremity, the pelvis and acetabulum, the upper extremity, and the spine. The final section deals with pediatric orthopaedic trauma.

This is clearly a very comprehensive review text of orthopaedic trauma. The style is concise, easy to read, and user friendly. Dr. Mark Brinker and his colleagues are to be congratulated for collating a prodigious amount of information and succeeding in achieving their goal, a real review text for orthopaedic trauma. My initial skepticism of another text has changed to enthusiasm after reading some of the chapters and realizing how this text differs. It is a very easy read, full of information, and well organized, and I can highly recommend Mark Brinker's *Review of Orthopaedic Trauma* for anyone, be it resident or general orthopaedic surgeon, but especially for those reviewing for OITE, ABOS Boards, or recertification examinations. In addition, this text would be applicable for nonorthopaedic surgeons (i.e., those involved in the management of trauma). As such, it would be a useful review text for emergency room residents and/or physicians and nurses and also as part of the general/trauma surgery curriculum for surgery residents for a quick and easy reference on the diagnosis and management of orthopaedic trauma.

David L. Helfet, MD
Director, Orthopaedic Trauma
Hospital for Special Surgery
New York, New York

FOREWORD TO THE FIRST EDITION

Someone recently referred to me as "The King of Orthopaedic Review Books." I accept this title with a sense of amusement, humility, and pride. It is now my honor and privilege to introduce *Review of Orthopaedic Trauma,* which is sure to find a prominent position in the Saunders royal lineage, not to mention your bookshelf. Dr. Mark Brinker has done an outstanding job of organizing, inviting the right authors, and editing this wonderful text. I have known Dr. Brinker as an associate and friend for 6 years. He was elected recently to the American Orthopaedic Association, one of its youngest inductees ever, has amassed significant clinical experience in the management of complex fractures, nonunions, and malunions; and is a well-known orthopaedic educator. These ample talents are evident throughout this book.

You may ask what are the advantages of this book over standard multivolume trauma texts. Very simply, I believe it is more user-friendly, easier to use, and more current than any other trauma text. Dr. Brinker organized this book to aid practicing orthopaedists, residents, and fellows, and I believe he has met his goal with regard to both audiences.

I know I will use it in my practice. In fact, I have already reserved a space for the book on my nightstand for those late-night calls!

Mark D. Miller, MD
Associate Professor
Department of Orthopaedics
University of Virginia
Charlottesville, Virginia

PREFACE TO THE
SECOND EDITION

There are more than 200 bones in the adult Homosa-pien skeleton; although extraordinarily well designed and constructed, each one is subject to cracking, splintering, and pulverization secondary to human mishap, aggression, and stupidity. We live in a world that is constantly moving faster, playing harder, and competing more fervently. It would, therefore, seem that so long as there are bones, there will likely be a need for those skilled in the art of mending them.

In the style of the first edition, this, the second edition of *Review of Orthopaedic Trauma* is organized in a pleasant outline format, empowering readers to rapidly access and absorb critical information essential to their studies and practice. Whether it is background epidemiologic statistics, diagnostic techniques, treatment options, or complications, the welcoming organization of the book allows facts and concepts to be quickly accessed and digested. The second edition significantly benefits from totally new and broadly updated chapters; the reconceived artwork heightens the educational impact, with over 200 all-new color illustrations crafted specifically for this textbook.

While the future of our specialty is undoubtedly bright, the world is changing at an ever-increasing rate. The introduction of the 80-hour work week for residents-in-training mandates the creation of more efficient educational tools. When I look on my bookshelf, I see multi-volume orthopedic trauma texts with pages numbering 3,000 or more. While these scholarly works are rich in clinical material, they are now simply too large to function as a first source for learning. Should we then simply throw these away? Of course not. But in addition to these reference texts, our specialty needs comprehensive source material with high-impact educational value that facilitates rapid assimilation of core knowledge by the reader. This is the mission of *Review of Orthopaedic Trauma*—to function as *the* first source for learning for medical students, residents, fellows, and practicing physicians interested in furthering their knowledge in the discipline of orthopedic traumatology.

Mark R. Brinker, MD

PREFACE TO THE

FIRST EDITION

Although orthopaedic surgery as a field continues to evolve into areas of subspecialty, musculoskeletal trauma remains an important focus for clinical practice and postgraduate education. Orthopaedic trauma is a vast subject matter and is somewhat unique in that it includes most of the body. Although several quality textbooks covering musculoskeletal trauma are available, none exists that reviews the essential knowledge of musculoskeletal trauma.

Review of Orthopaedic Trauma is a distillation of the core knowledge of musculoskeletal trauma. The contributors to the text are recognized experts in their field and were selected based on their unique talents and skills as writers and educators. The text includes material gathered from Orthopaedic In-Training Examinations and Self-Assessment Examinations; each contributor reviewed 5 years' worth of topic-specific examination questions during the preparation of his or her chapter. In addition, a variety of textbooks, journal articles, and board review course syllabi were reviewed during the preparation of the textbook.

The final product is a comprehensive textbook covering the important clinical and testable material in orthopaedic trauma. I hope that this textbook will aid practicing orthopaedic surgeons in the care of their patients and in successfully passing the board recertification examination. Furthermore, it is my hope that this textbooks will aid residents and fellows in their preparations for Orthopaedic In-Training Examinations and the American Board of Orthopaedic Surgery board certification examination.

ACKNOWLEDGMENTS
I gratefully acknowledge the generous contributions of the chapter authors, each a gifted writer and educator. I am indebted to the staff of the Joe W. King Orthopedic Institute of Texas Orthopedic Hospital (Lou Fincher, Rodney Baker, and Dan [the man] O'Connor) for their assistance in the preparation of the text and figures. I would also like to acknowledge Michael Cooley, a talented artist and illustrator, for the original artwork that appears in the textbook. Special thanks to Michele Clowers for her dedication and perseverance during my perfectionist moments. The author appreciates all of the individuals at Harcourt Health Sciences who worked so hard to bring the project to completion. I am particularly grateful to my Senior Medical Editor, Richard Lampert; my Project Specialist, Pat Joiner; my Project Manager, Carol Sullivan Weis; my Designer, Mark Oberkrom; and my Senior Editorial Assistant, Beth LoGiudice. Finally, I would like to acknowledge Dr. Mark Miller, who is a contributor to this textbook and is the originator of W.B. Saunders "Review of" series.

Mark R. Brinker, MD

ACKNOWLEDGMENTS

No project of this magnitude is possible without a dedicated team. The quality of this textbook begins and ends with the physician contributors whose tireless work on each chapter has resulted in a work of tremendous breadth and depth. To all contributors, I extend my most sincere appreciation for their willingness to share their experience and expertise with the reader. I would also like to thank my staff Nicole Wunderlich, MS, PA-C; Amy Shives, R.N.; and Glenda Adams for all of their assistance throughout the process. I am also extremely appreciative to the staff at my publisher, Lippincott Williams & Wilkins, for all of their hard work and attention to detail. I'd like to specifically thank Robert A. Hurley, Executive Editor; Brian Brown, Executive Editor; David Murphy, Senior Product Manager; David Orzechowski, Production Project Manager; Holly McLaughlin, Design Manager; Lisa Lawrence, Marketing Manager; Joel Jones Alexander, Project Manager; and Ben Rivera, Manufacturing Manager. I am also most grateful to Paul Schiffmacher, who has produced more than 200 original works of art for the second edition. Paul's images are not only beautiful, but they are rich in educational content. And finally, there is the hero of this tale, Eileen "Wolfie" Wolfberg. Eileen stepped in as a freelance Developmental Editor when the process needed supercharging and did a magnificent job functioning as a liaison/editor working with the contributors, publisher, illustrator, and yours truly. Without Wolfie's energy, unwavering commitment to excellence, and expertise, the quality (and perhaps existence) of this book might have been in question. Finally, I thank my family, friends, and partners at Fondren Orthopedic Group LLP for their continuous support. It takes a village!

Mark R. Brinker, MD

SECTION 1

Overview

CHAPTER 1

General Principles of Trauma

Joseph R. Hsu

I. Advanced Trauma Life Support—Initial assessment of an arriving trauma patient has several stages: Primary Survey, Resuscitation, Adjuncts to Primary Survey, Secondary Survey, Adjuncts to Secondary Survey, Reevaluation, and Definitive Care.

A. Primary Survey—The ABCDEs of trauma care are a way to systematically assess a patient's vital functions in a prioritized manner. Life-threatening conditions should be identified and managed simultaneously.

1. Airway maintenance with cervical spine precautions—Airway compromise in a trauma patient can be an imminently life-threatening condition. It must be evaluated and managed as the first priority. *A provider must assume that there is a cervical spine injury in order to protect the spinal cord until a more detailed assessment can be performed. This is especially a concern in patients with an altered level of consciousness and any blunt injury proximal to the clavicles*.

2. Breathing and ventilation—Adequate ventilation can be negatively impacted by conditions such as tension pneumothorax, flail chest with pulmonary contusion, massive hemothorax, and open pneumothorax. These disorders should be identified and managed during this stage.

3. Circulation with hemorrhage control—*Hemorrhage is the leading cause of preventable death after trauma. Hypotension in the setting of trauma must be considered hypovolemia until proven otherwise*. Clinical signs of hypovolemia include decreased level of consciousness, pale skin, and rapid, thready pulses. External hemorrhage should be identified and directly controlled during this stage.

4. Disability: Neurologic status—Rapid evaluation of potential neurologic injury should be performed to include level of consciousness,

pupillary size and reactivity, lateralizing signs, and spinal cord injury level (if present).

• Glasgow Coma Scale (GCS)—The GCS is a rapid method of determining the level of consciousness of a trauma patient and has prognostic value (Table 1-1). The GCS categorizes the neurologic status of a trauma patient by assessing eye opening response, motor response, and verbal response.

• Possible causes of decreased level of consciousness include hypoperfusion, direct

TABLE 1-1

Glasgow Coma Scale

Assessment Area	Score
Eye Opening (E)	
Spontaneous	4
To speech	3
To pain	2
None	1
BEST Motor Response (M)	
Obeys commands	6
Localizes pain	5
Normal flexion (withdrawal)	4
Abnormal flexion (decorticate)	3
Extension (decerebrate)	2
None (flaccid)	1
Verbal Response (V)	
Oriented	5
Confused conversation	4
Inappropriate words	3
Incomprehensible sounds	2
None	1

Adapted from American College of Surgeons. *Advanced Trauma Life Support For Doctors: Student Course Manual*. 7th ed. Chicago, IL: American College of Surgeons, 2004, with permission.

cerebral injury, hypoglycemia, and alcohol/drugs. Immediate reevaluation and correction of oxygenation, ventilation, and perfusion should be performed. Afterward, direct cerebral injury should be assumed until proven otherwise.

5. Exposure/environmental control: completely undress the patient, but prevent hypothermia—All garments must be removed from the trauma patient to ensure thorough evaluation. Once the evaluation is performed, *prevention of hypothermia is critical*. Blankets, external warming devices, a warm environment, and warmed intravenous fluids should be used to prevent hypothermia.

B. Resuscitation—In addition to airway and breathing priorities, circulatory resuscitation begins with control of hemorrhage. *Initial fluid resuscitation should consist of 2 to 3 L of Ringer's lactate solution*. All intravenous fluids should be warmed prior to or during infusion. If the patient is unresponsive to the fluid bolus, type-specific blood should be administered. O-negative blood may be used if type-specific blood is not immediately available. Insufficient fluid resuscitation may result in residual hypotension in a trauma patient, such as a patient with a pelvic fracture and multiple long bone fractures.

1. *Elevation of the serum lactate level (>2.5 mmol/L) is indicative of residual hypoperfusion*. Proceeding to definitive fixation of orthopaedic injuries in such a patient with occult hypoperfusion may result in significant perioperative morbidity such as adult respiratory distress syndrome.

C. Adjuncts to Primary Survey

1. ECG
2. Urinary and gastric catheters
3. Monitoring
   • Ventilatory rate; arterial blood gas (ABG)
   • Pulse oximetry
   • Blood pressure
4. X-rays and diagnostic studies
   • CXR
   • AP Pelvis
   • Lateral C-spine—This is a screening exam. It does not exclude a cervical spine injury.

D. Secondary Survey—The Secondary Survey is a head-to-toe examination that begins once the Primary Survey is complete and resuscitative efforts have demonstrated a stabilization of vital functions.

1. History
   • AMPLE—AMPLE is an acronym of the following categories that assist in collecting historical information from the patient, family, and/or prehospital personnel.
     (a) Allergies
     (b) Medications currently used
     (c) Past illnesses/Pregnancy
     (d) Last meal
     (e) Events/Environment related to the injury

2. Physical examination—The head-to-toe examination should occur at this point. The clinician must be sure to inspect the following body regions:
   • Head
   • Maxillofacial
   • Cervical spine and neck
   • Chest
   • Abdomen
   • Perineum/rectum/vagina
   • Musculoskeletal
   • Neurologic

E. Adjuncts to the Secondary Survey—At this point, specialized diagnostic tests can be performed. These tests may include radiographs of the extremities, CT scans of the head, chest, and abdomen. In addition, diagnostic procedures such as bronchoscopy, esophagoscopy, and angiography can be performed if the patient's hemodynamic status permits.

F. Reevaluation—Reevaluation is a continuous process during the evaluation and management of a trauma patient. Injuries may evolve in a life-threatening manner, and nonapparent injuries may be discovered.

G. Definitive Care—Definitive care for each injury occurs depending on the priority of the injury and the physiology of the patient. This requires coordinated multidisciplinary care.

II. Shock—Shock is an abnormality of the circulatory system that results in inadequate organ perfusion and tissue oxygenation. Manifestations of shock include tachycardia and narrow pulse pressure.

A. Hemorrhagic Shock—Hemorrhage is the acute loss of circulating blood volume. An element of hypovolemia is present in nearly all polytraumatized patients. *Hemorrhage is the most common cause of shock*.

1. Classes of hemorrhage
   • Class I hemorrhage is characterized by no measurable change in physiologic parameters (heart rate, blood pressure, urine output, etc.) with blood loss less than 15% (<750 mL).
   • Class II hemorrhage is characterized by mild tachycardia (>100 bpm), a moderate decrease in blood pressure and low normal

urine output (20 to 30 mL per hour). It represents a 15% to 30% blood loss (750 to 1,500 mL).

- Class III hemorrhage is characterized by moderate tachycardia (>120 bpm), a decrease in blood pressure, and a decrease in urine output (5 to 15 mL per hour). The patient is typically confused. It represents a 30% to 40% blood loss (1,500 to 2,000 mL).
- Class IV hemorrhage is characterized by a severe tachycardia (>140 bpm), decreased blood pressure, and negligible urine output. The patient is lethargic. It represents blood loss of over 40% (>2,000 mL).

2. Blood loss due to major fractures—Major fractures may result in blood loss into the site of the injury to such an extent that it may compromise the hemodynamic status of the patient.
- Tibia/humerus—As much as 750 mL (1.5 units) blood loss
- Femur—As much as 1,500 mL (3 units) blood loss
- Pelvic fracture—Several liters of blood may accumulate in the retroperitoneal space in association with a pelvic fracture. ***The greatest average transfusion requirement occurs with anteroposterior compression pelvic fractures.***

B. Nonhemorrhagic Shock
1. Neurogenic—Neurogenic shock can occur as a result of loss of sympathetic tone to the heart and peripheral vascular system in cases of cervical spinal cord injury. Loss of sympathetic tone to the extremities results in vasodilation, poor venous return, and hypotension. Because of unopposed vagal tone on the heart, tachycardia in response to hypotension is not

possible. The resultant clinical scenario, called neurogenic shock, is one of ***hypotension and bradycardia***. Assessment of the hemodynamic status may be aided by a Swan-Ganz catheter.

2. Cardiogenic—Cardiogenic shock is myocardial dysfunction that can result from blunt injury, tamponade, air embolism, or cardiac ischemia. Adjuncts such as ECG, ultrasound, and CVP monitoring may be useful in this setting.

3. Tension pneumothorax—Tension pneumothorax is the result of increasing pressure within the pleural space from a pneumothorax with a flap-valve phenomenon. As air enters the pleural space without the ability to escape, it causes a ***mediastinal shift*** with impairment of venous return and cardiac output. The clinical scenario involves decreased/absent breath sounds, subcutaneous emphysema, and tracheal deviation. ***Emergent decompression is warranted without the need for a diagnostic X-ray***.

4. Septic shock—Septic shock may occur as the result of an infection. In trauma, this would be more likely in a patient presenting late with penetrating abdominal injuries.

III. Associated Injuries
A. Head Injury—One of the guiding principles in managing a patient with a traumatic brain injury (TBI) is to prevent secondary brain injury from conditions such as hypoxemia and hypovolemia. Patients with head injury are at increased risk of developing heterotopic ossification (HO).
1. Glasgow Coma Scale (GCS)—The GCS (Table 1-1) is employed to stratify injury severity in patients with head injuries (TBI).

TABLE 1-2

Recommendations for Return to Play after Concussion

Grade	First Concussion	Second Concussion	Third Concussion
1	RTP if asymptomatic for 1 wk	RTP after 2 wk if asymptomatic for 1 wk	Terminate season. RTP next season if asymptomatic
2	RTP if asymptomatic for 1 wk	No RTP for 1 mo. May RTP after that if asymptomatic for 1 wk. Consider termination of the season	Terminate season. RTP next season if asymptomatic
3	No RTP for 1 mo. May RTP after that if asymptomatic for 1 wk. Consider termination of the season	Terminate season. RTP next season if asymptomatic	

RTP, return to play; "asymptomatic," no postconcussion syndrome (including retrograde or anterograde amnesia at rest or with exertion.

Adapted from Cantu RC. Posttraumatic retrograde and anterograde amnesia: pathophysiology and implications in grading and safe return to play. *J Athl Train.* 2001;36(3):244–248, with permission.

- Mild brain injury (GCS, 14 to 15)—Patients with a mild brain injury often have a brief loss of consciousness (LOC) and may have amnesia of the event. Most have an uneventful recovery, but approximately 3% will deteriorate unexpectedly. A CT of the head should be considered if the individual has lost consciousness for more than 5 minutes, has amnesia, severe headaches, GCS of less than 15, and/or a focal neurologic deficit.
  - (a) Concussion—The term "concussion" is often used to describe a mild TBI.
  - (b) Sports-related concussion—Return to athletic play after a concussion is guided by recommendations based on grading the concussion and the number of concussions that the individual has sustained (Table 1-2).
    - Grade 1 (mild): No LOC. Amnesia or symptoms for less than 30 minutes
    - Grade 2 (moderate): LOC for less than 1 minute. Amnesia or symptoms for 30 minutes to 24 hours.
    - Grade 3 (severe): LOC for more than 1 minute; amnesia for more than 24 hours; postconcussion symptoms for more than 7 days.
- Moderate brain injury (GCS, 9 to 13)—All of these patients require a CT of the head, baseline blood work, and admission to a facility with neurosurgical capability.
- Severe brain injury (GCS, 3 to 8)—Patients with severe TBI require a multidisciplinary approach to ensure adequate management and resuscitation of other life-threatening injuries and urgent neurosurgical care.

2. Anatomical types of brain injury (Figure 1-1)
- Diffuse brain injury—Diffuse brain injury can be a wide spectrum from mild TBI to a profound ischemic insult to the brain.
- Epidural hematoma—Epidural hematomas are located between the dura and the skull. They usually result from a tear of the middle meningeal artery secondary to a skull fracture.
- Subdural hematoma—Subdural hematomas are located beneath the dura as a result of injury to small surface vessels on the brain. They frequently result in a greater brain injury compared with epidural hematomas.
- Contusion and intracerebral hematoma—Contusion or hematoma within the brain can occur at any location, but they most frequently occur in the frontal or temporal

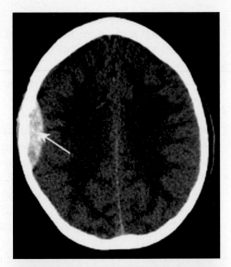

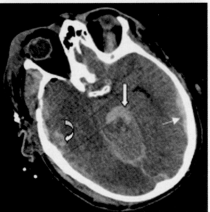

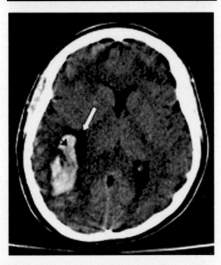

FIGURE 1-1 Computed tomography scans showing **(top)** epidural hematoma, **(center)** subdural hematoma (*right arrow*; this patient also has an intraparenchymal contusion at the *curved arrow* and a subarachnoid hemorrhage at the *center arrow*), and **(bottom)** intracerebral hemorrhage. (From Pascual JL, Gracias VH, LeRoux PD. Injury to the brain. In: Flint L, Meredith JW, Schwab CW, et al., eds. *Trauma: Contemporary Principles and Therapy*. Philadelphia, PA: Lippincott Williams & Wilkins, 2008, with permission.)

lobes. Contusions can evolve into intracerebral hematomas over time, which require emergent surgical evacuation.

3. Management of head injuries
    - Primary Survey—Includes an evaluation of airway, breathing, and circulation.
    - Neurologic examination.
    - Diagnostic procedures—Cervical spine radiograph series, computed tomography (CT) scan for intracranial conditions.
    - Intravenous fluids—Maintenance of normovolemia is important following head injury. Hypotonic fluids and glucose are no longer recommended, and hyponatremia can be a concern.
    - Hyperventilation—Hyperventilation may be used in select patients under close monitoring to decrease intracranial pressure by decreasing the partial pressure of carbon dioxide and increasing vasoconstriction.
    - Medications—A variety of adjunctive medications may be used, but should be administered under consultation with a neurologist.

B. Thoracic Trauma
    1. Tension pneumothorax—See description under nonhemorrhagic shock
    2. Open pneumothorax—Open pneumothorax is also called a "sucking chest wound." It occurs when there is a large chest wall defect. This external opening to the environment precludes the chest wall's ability to generate the negative pressure within the pleural space required to inflate the lung. Treatment is to close the defect with an occlusive dressing that is taped on three sides. This creates a valve that allows air to escape but not to enter the defect in the chest wall.
    3. Flail chest—Flail chest is a severe impairment of chest wall movement as a result of two or more rib fractures in two or more places, so that the segment has paradoxical movement during respiration. The underlying pulmonary contusion is the true challenge in this clinical scenario. The pulmonary contusion may cause severe impairment of oxygenation. Management involves ensuring adequate ventilation and appropriate fluid management to prevent fluid overload of the injured lung. Mechanical ventilation may be necessary.
    4. Massive hemothorax—Massive hemothorax occurs when large amounts of blood (>1,500 mL) accumulate within the pleural space. This results in lung compression and impairment of ventilation. Urgent, simultaneous restoration of blood volume and drainage of the chest are indicated. Thoracotomy may be required in cases of ongoing blood loss.
    5. Cardiac tamponade—Cardiac tamponade is due to fluid accumulation within the pericardial sac. Diagnosis has been described by Beck's triad: elevated venous pressure (distended neck veins), decreased arterial pressure, and muffled heart sounds. A focused assessment sonogram in trauma (FAST) or pericardiocentesis may be necessary to establish the diagnosis. The pericardiocentesis may be diagnostic and therapeutic.
    6. Simple pneumothorax—Simple pneumothorax may be associated with thoracic spine fractures and scapular fractures. Decreased breath sounds and hyperresonance upon percussion are present, and an upright expiratory chest radiograph may aid diagnosis. Treatment is with placement of a chest tube.
    7. Pulmonary contusion—Pulmonary contusion can lead to respiratory failure. Treatment includes intubation and assisted ventilation if the patient is hypoxemic.
    8. Blunt cardiac injury—Blunt injury to the heart can result in cardiac arrest ("commotio cordis"), cardiac contusion, valvular disruption, or rupture of a cardiac chamber.
    9. Aortic disruption—Aortic disruption usually occurs after a high-speed deceleration injury. Radiographic signs include a widened mediastinum, obliteration of the aortic knob, deviation of the trachea to the right, obliteration of the space between the pulmonary artery and aorta, depression of the left main stem bronchus, deviation of the esophagus to the right, widened paratracheal stripe, widened paraspinal interfaces, presence of a pleural or apical cap, hemothorax on the left side, and fractures of the first or second rib or scapula.
    10. Diaphragmatic injuries—Diaphragmatic injuries commonly occur on the left side and can be seen on chest radiographs.

C. Abdominal Trauma—Abdominal trauma can occur with varying degrees of frequency depending on whether the mechanism of injury was penetrating or blunt. Blunt injury to the abdomen may result in damage to the viscera by a crush or compression mechanism; **_the spleen is the most commonly injured organ_**, followed by the liver. Penetrating injuries such as stab wounds and gunshot wounds impart direct trauma to the viscera by laceration or perforation.

1. Blunt abdominal injuries
   - Diaphragm—Diaphragmatic rupture may be detected on the chest X-ray by elevation or blurring of the hemidiaphragm, an abnormal gas shadow, or nasogastric tube traveling into the chest.
   - Duodenum—Duodenal rupture may occur from a direct blow to the abdomen. Retroperitoneal air on CT may signal this injury.
   - Pancreas—A pancreatic injury should be suspected if a patient has a persistently elevated serum amylase level.
   - Genitourinary (GU)—A GU injury should be suspected with any hematuria. Associated injuries and the mechanism of injury may help in localization of the injury. Renal injuries tend to be associated with direct trauma to the flanks, while lower GU injuries such as urethral and bladder injuries are associated with anterior pelvic ring fractures.
   - Small bowel—Small bowel injury should be suspected in a patient with a "seat belt sign" across the abdomen or a flexion-distraction fracture or dislocation of the lumbar spine.
   - Solid organ—Traumatic lacerations to the liver, spleen, or kidney can be life threatening due to hemorrhage. Lesser injuries in stable patients may be observed. Urgent celiotomy is necessary in patients with a solid organ injury and evidence of ongoing hemorrhage.
2. Penetrating abdominal injuries—Emergent celiotomy is indicated in any patient with a penetrating abdominal injury with associated hypotension, peritonitis, and/or evisceration.
3. Assessment
   - History—Determining the type of accident is important. In automobile accidents, determine whether seat belts or other restraints were being used. In a penetrating injury, identifying the type of weapon used can be useful.
   - Signs—Involuntary muscle guarding, rebound tenderness, and free air under the diaphragm on chest radiograph suggest abdominal injury.
   - Tests
     (a) Diagnostic peritoneal lavage (DPL)—DPL is deemed positive if there are at least 100,000 red blood cells per cubic milliliter, at least 500 white blood cells per cubic milliliter, or a positive Gram's stain. Pelvic fractures can lead to false positive DPL, so DPL should be performed from a supraumbilical portal in these patients.
     (b) Ultrasound
     (c) CT scan
   D. Gastrointestinal—Range from ileus (treat with nasogastric tube and antacids) to upper GI bleeding. Postoperative ileus is more common in diabetics with neuropathy. Upper GI bleeding is more common in patients with a history of ulcers, use of NSAIDs, trauma, and smoking. Treatment of GI bleeding includes lavage, antacids, and H2-blockers. Vasopression (left gastric artery) may be required for more serious cases.
   E. Genitourinary
      1. Urinary tract infections (UTI)—***The most common nosocomial infection***, established UTIs should be treated before surgery. Perioperative catheter removed 24 hours after surgery may reduce the rate of postoperative UTI; prolonged catheterization increases incidence of UTI. UTI can increase risk of postoperative wound infection.
      2. Genitourinary injury—A retrograde urethrogram best evaluates lower genitourinary injuries in patients with displaced anterior pelvic fractures. The differential diagnoses after a direct blow to the scrotum are contusion, testicular rupture, epididymal rupture, and testicular torsion. Emergent urologic evaluation and consultation are required.
      3. Prostatic hypertrophy—Causes urinary retention; if the history, physical examination (prostate), and urine flow studies (<17 mL per second peak flow rate) are suggestive, urologic consultation should be obtained.
      4. Acute tubular necrosis—Can cause renal failure in trauma patients. Alkalinization of the urine is important during the early treatment of this disorder.
   F. Skin and Soft Tissue Injuries
      1. Thermal injuries
         - Burns
           (a) Assessment—Ruling out inhalation injury is imperative; signs of inhalation injury include facial burns, singeing of face and hair, carbon in the pharynx, and carbon in the sputum. Removing all clothing to stop the burning process is important.
           (b) Definitions
               - First-degree burn—Involves the epidermis
               - Second-degree burn—Involves the dermis
               - Third-degree burn—Involves the subcutaneous tissues
               - Fourth-degree burn—Involves the deep tissues

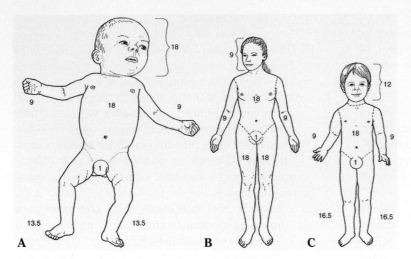

FIGURE 1-2 "Rule of nines" for **(A)** infant, **(B)** adult, and **(C)** child. (From Blinman TA, Nance ML. Special considerations in trauma in children. In: Flint L, Meredith JW, Schwab CW, et al., eds. *Trauma: Contemporary Principles and Therapy*. Philadelphia, PA: Lippincott Williams & Wilkins; 2008, with permission.)

(c) Calculation of burned body area—Involves the "rule of nines" (Fig. 1-2). This calculation is important for assessing fluid-replacement requirements.

(d) Fluid replacement—A total of 2 to 4 mL of lactated Ringer's solution per kg of body weight per percent of burned body area is administered in the first 24 hours for second- and third-degree burns. Half is given in the first 8 hours, and the remainder is given over the next 16 hours.

- Cold injuries
  (a) General—Injured tissues should be rapidly warmed in a water bath at 40° C (104° F). Local wound care and tetanus immunization should be administered. Cold injuries are the most common cause of bilateral upper and lower extremity amputations.
  (b) Frostbite—Results from tissue freezing caused by **intracellular formation of ice crystals** and the occlusion of the microcirculation. Treatment is via rapid warming in a 40° C water bath.
- Electrical injuries
  (a) Ignition—Involves a burn at the site of direct contact.
  (b) Conductant—Involves injury propagation along neurovascular structures.
  (c) Arc—Involves high-voltage currents propagating along flexor surfaces of joints and leads to contractures.
- Chemical burns—Severity of chemical burns depends on the amount and concentration of the agent, duration of contact, tissue penetrability of the agent, and the agent's mechanism of action. The most important aspect of treatment is copious irrigation.

TABLE 1-3

Abbreviated Injury Scale

AIS	Injury Description
1	Minor
2	Moderate
3	Serious
4	Severe
5	Critical
6	Unsurvivable

Adapted from Baker SP, O'Neill B, Haddon W Jr, et al. The injury severity score: a method for describing patients with multiple injuries and evaluating emergency care. *J Trauma*. 1974;14(3):187–196, with permission.

2. Injection injuries—Typically result from accidental high-pressure injection by paint or grease guns. These injuries may appear relatively benign but are surgical emergencies because these substances rapidly destroy soft tissues.

3. Wound healing—**Adequate soft-tissue healing after injury or surgery is promoted by a transcutaneous oxygen tension level higher than 30 mm Hg, an ischemic index (such as the ankle/brachial systolic index) of at least 0.45, an albumin level of at least 0.30 g/dL, and a total lymphocyte count higher than 1,500 cells/mm³.** These values may be improved by nutritional support, including oral hyperalimentation. Oxygenated blood is a prerequisite for wound healing. The ischemic index is the ratio of the Doppler pressure at the level being tested to the brachial systolic pressure; an index of 0.45 at the surgical level is generally accepted as the level to support wound healing. Values may be falsely elevated

and thereby misleading in patients with peripheral vascular disease due to noncompressibility and noncompliance of calcified arteries.

G. Pelvic Ring Injuries—*Hypotensive patients with evidence of a pelvic ring injury should have urgent placement of a pelvic binder or circumferential sheet*.

H. Injury Severity Score (ISS)—Injury Severity Score is a score utilized to stratify the severity of injury sustained by a polytrauma patient. In order to calculate the ISS, an Abbreviated Injury Score (AIS) must be assigned for each of the six body regions injured (head and neck, face, chest, abdomen, extremity, external). The AIS is scored from least severe to unsurvivable (Table 1-3). The highest AIS in each body region is used. The AIS scores from the three most severely injured body regions are squared and then summed together. This creates a score between 0 and 75. If any injury has an AIS score of 6 (unsurvivable), the ISS is automatically 75. Recent studies have demonstrated greater predictive value for the New Injury Severity Score (NISS) when compared with the ISS for outcomes such as sepsis, multiple organ failure, ICU days, and mortality.

IV. Other Trauma-Related Topics
A. Nutrition—Several indicators exist (e.g., anergy panels, albumin level, transferrin level); *measurement of arm muscle circumference is the best indicator of nutritional status*. Wound dehiscence and infection, pneumonia, and sepsis can result from poor nutrition. Lack of enteral feeding can lead to *atrophy of the intestinal mucosae, leading in turn to bacterial translocation*. Full enteral or parenteral nutrition (nitrogen 200 mg/kg per day) should be provided for patients who cannot tolerate normal intake. Early elemental feeding through a jejunostomy tube can decrease complications in the multiple-trauma patient. *Enteral protein supplements have proved effective in patients at risk of developing multiple organ system failure*.

B. Antibiotics—Antibiotics in orthopaedics may be used in prophylactic treatment to prevent postoperative sepsis (for clean surgical cases, administer 1 hour preoperatively and continue for 24 hours postoperatively), initial care after an open traumatic wound, and treatment of established infections. Types I and II open fractures require a first-generation cephalosporin (some authors have recently suggested the addition of an aminoglycoside or the use of a second-generation cephalosporin); type IIIA open fractures require a first-generation cephalosporin plus an aminoglycoside; penicillin is added for grossly contaminated (type IIIB) open fractures.

C. Overall, *Staphylococcus aureus* remains the leading cause of osteomyelitis and nongonococcal septic arthritis. In general, the virulence of *S. epidermidis* infections is closely related to orthopaedic hardware. *Clindamycin achieves the highest antibiotic concentrations in bone* (nearly equals serum concentrations after intravenous administration) *and is bacteriostatic*. To prevent the development of vancomycin-resistant strains, vancomycin should not be used in patients with a blood culture of coagulase-negative *S. aureus* that is not methicillin resistant.

D. Antibiotic-Resistant Bacteria—Two types of antibiotic resistance exist.
1. Intrinsic resistance—Inherent features of a cell that prevent antibiotics from acting on the cell (such as the absence of a metabolic pathway or enzyme). *MRSA has a gene (mecA) that produces penicillin-binding protein 2a (PBP2a), an enzyme that prevents the normal enzymatic acylation of antibiotics*.
2. Acquired resistance—A newly resistant strain emerges from a population that was previously sensitive (acquired resistance is mediated by plasmids [extrachromosomal genetic elements] and transposons).
3. Antibiotic indications and side effects (Table 1-4)
4. Mechanism of action of antibiotics (Table 1-5)
5. Alternate forms of antibiotic delivery
   • Antibiotic beads or spacers—polymethyl methacrylate (PMMA) impregnated with antibiotics (usually an aminoglycoside) can be useful when treating osteomyelitis with bony defects. Antibiotic powder is mixed with cement powder; the microorganism guides the antibiotic used, and the selected antibiotic and type of PMMA guide the dosage. Tobramycin, gentamicin, cefazolin (Ancef) and other cephalosporins, oxacillin, cloxacillin, methicillin, lincomycin, clindamycin, colistin, fucidin, neomycin, kanamycin, and ampicillin have been used with PMMA for infection. Chloramphenicol and tetracycline appear to be inactivated during polymerization. Antibiotics elute from PMMA beads, with an exponential decline over a 2-week period, and cease to be present locally at significant levels by 6 to 8 weeks. Much higher local tissue concentrations of antibiotic can be achieved than those obtained by systemic administration. Increased surface area of PMMA (e.g., with oval beads) enhances antibiotic elution.

TABLE 1-4

Antibiotic Indications and Side Effects

Antibiotics	Organisms	Complications/Other
Aminoglycosides	G−, PM	Auditory (most common) and vestibular toxicity is caused by destruction of the cochlear and vestibular sensory cells from drug accumulation in the perilymph and endolymph; renal toxicity; neuromuscular blockade
Amphotericin	Fungi	Nephrotoxic
Aztreonam	G−, no anaerobes	
Carbenicillin/ticarcillin/piperacillin	Better against G−	Bleeding diathesis (carbenicillin)
Cephalosporins		
First generation	Prophylaxis (surgical)	Cephazolin is the drug of choice
Second generation	Some G+/G−	
Third generation	G−, fewer G+	Hemolytic anemia (bleeding diathesis [moxalactam])
Chloramphenicol	*Haemophilus influenzae*, anaerobes	Bone marrow aplasia
Ciprofloxacin	G−, methicillin-resistant *S. aureus*	Tendon ruptures; cartilage erosion in children; antacids reduce absorption of ciprofloxacin; theophylline increases serum concentrations of ciprofloxacin
Clindamycin	G+, anaerobes	Pseudomembranous enterocolitis
Erythromycin	G+ (PCN allergy)	Ototoxic
Imipenem	G+, some G−	Resistance, seizure
Methicillin/oxacillin/nafcillin	Penicillinase resistant	Same as penicillin; nephritis (methicillin); subcutaneous skin slough (nafcillin)
Penicillin	Strep, G+	Hypersensitivity/resistance; hemolytic
Polymyxin/nystatin	GU	Nephrotoxic
Sulfonamides	GU	Hemolytic anemia
Tetracycline	G+ (PCN allergy)	Stains teeth/bone (up to age 8)
Vancomycin	Methicillin-resistant *S. aureus, C. difficile*	Ototoxic; erythema with rapid IV delivery

G+, gram positive; G−, gram negative; GU, genitourinary; IV, intravenous; PM, polymicrobial; PCN, penicillin; Strep, streptococcus.

Beads are inserted only after thorough debridement, and the beads should always be eventually removed. Antibiotic powder in doses of 2 g/40 g of powdered PMMA (simplex P) does not appreciably affect the compressive strength of PMMA, but higher concentrations (4 to 5 g antibiotic powder/40 g PMMA) significantly reduce the compressive strength.
- Osmotic pump—Delivers high concentrations of antibiotics locally. Used mainly for osteomyelitis.
- Home intravenous therapy—Cost-effective alternative for long-term intravenous antibiotics, facilitated by a Hickman or Broviac indwelling catheter.
- Immersion solution—Contaminated bone from an open fracture may be sterilized (100% effective) by immersion in a chlorhexidine gluconate scrub and an antibiotic solution.

E. Transfusion
  1. Transfusion reactions
     - Allergic reaction—Most common; occurs toward the end of transfusion and usually subsides spontaneously. Symptoms include chills, pruritus, erythema, and urticaria. Pretreatment with diphenhydramine (Benadryl)

TABLE 1-5

Mechanism of Action of Antibiotics

Class of Antibiotics	Examples	Mechanism of Action
β-lactam antibiotics	Penicillin Cephalosporins	Inhibit bacterial peptidoglycan synthesis (the mechanism is via binding to the penicillin-binding proteins on the surface of the bacterial cell membrane)
Aminoglycosides	Gentamicin Tobramycin	Inhibit protein synthesis (the mechanism is via binding to cytoplasmic ribosomal RNA)
Clindamycin and macrolides	Clindamycin Erythromycin Clarithromycin Azithromycin	Inhibit the dissociation of peptidyl-transfer RNA from ribosomes during translocation (the mechanism is via binding to 50S ribosomal subunits)
Tetracyclines		Inhibit protein synthesis (on 70S and 80S ribosomes)
Glycopeptides	Vancomycin Teicoplanin	Interfere with the insertion of glycan subunits into the cell wall
Rifampin		Inhibits RNA synthesis in bacteria
Quinolones	Ciprofloxacin Levofloxacin Ofloxacin	Inhibit DNA gyrase
Oxazolidinones	Linezolid	Inhibit protein synthesis (blocks formation of the 70S ribosomal translation complex)

and hydrocortisone may be appropriate in patients with a history of allergic reactions.

- Febrile reaction—Also common; occurs after the initial 100 to 300 mL of packed RBCs have been transfused. Chills and fever are caused by antibodies to foreign WBCs. Treatment consists of stopping the transfusion and giving antipyretics, as for an allergic reaction.
- Hemolytic reaction—Less common, but most serious. Occurs early in the transfusion, with symptoms that include chills, fever, tachycardia, chest tightness, and flank pain. Treatment consists of stopping the transfusion, administering intravenous fluids, performing appropriate laboratory studies, and monitoring the patient in an intensive care setting.

2. Transfusion risks—Include transmission of hepatitis (C [1 in 1,935,000 per unit transfused], B [1 in 205,000 per unit transfused]), cytomegalovirus (highest incidence, because over 70% of donors are positive, but not clinically important), human T-cell lymphotropic virus (HTLV-1) (1 in 2,993,000 per unit transfused), and HIV (1 in 1,125,000 per unit transfused).

F. Tetanus—*A potentially lethal neuroparalytic disease caused by an exotoxin of* **Clostridium**

tetani. Prophylaxis requires classifying the patient's wound (tetanus-prone or nontetanus-prone) and a complete immunization history. Tetanus-prone wounds are more than 6 hours old; are irregularly configured; are deeper than 1 cm or the result of a projectile injury, crush injury, burn, or frostbite; have devitalized tissue; and are grossly contaminated. Patients with tetanus-prone wounds who have an unknown tetanus status or have received fewer than three immunizations require tetanus and diphtheria toxoids and tetanus immune globulin (human). Fully immunized patients with tetanus-prone wounds do not require immune globulin, but tetanus toxoid should be administered if the wound is severe or over 24 hours old or if the patient has not received a booster within the past 5 years. A patient with a nontetanus-prone wound with an unknown immunization history or a history of fewer than three doses of tetanus immunization requires tetanus toxoid. Established tetanus is treated with diazepam to control the patient's muscle spasms. Initial antibiotic therapy includes penicillin G or doxycycline; alternative antibiotic therapy includes metronidazole.

G. Rabies—*An acute infection characterized by irritation of the CNS that may be followed by paralysis and death. The organism involved in rabies is a neurotropic virus that may be present in the saliva of rabid animals.* In dog or cat bites, healthy animals should be observed for 10 days; there is no need to start antirabies treatment. If the animal begins to experience symptoms, human rabies immune globulin with human diploid cell vaccine or rabies vaccine absorbed (inactivated) should be started. For bites from known rabid dogs and cats, vaccination of the patient should occur immediately. Skunks, raccoons, bats, foxes, and most carnivores should be considered rabid, and bitten patients immunized immediately. Mouse, rat, chipmunk, gerbil, guinea pig, hamster, squirrel, rabbit, and rodent bites rarely require antirabies treatment.

H. HIV Infection
 1. HIV primarily affects the lymphocyte and macrophage cell lines and **decreases the number of T-helper cells (formerly known as T4 lymphocytes but now known as CD4 cells)**.
 2. Diagnosis—**The diagnosis of AIDS requires an HIV-positive test plus one of the following two scenarios: (a) one of the opportunistic infections (such as pneumocystis) or (b) a CD4 count of less than 200 (normal CD4 count = 700 to 1,200).**
 3. Transmission—The risk of seroconversion from a contaminated needle stick is 0.3% (increases if the exposure involves a larger amount of blood); the risk of seroconversion from mucous membrane exposure is 0.09%. The risk of HIV transmission via a large, frozen bone allograft is 1 in 1 million; **donor screening is the most important factor in preventing viral transmission**.
 4. Associated risks—Even if asymptomatic, HIV-positive patients with traumatic orthopaedic injuries (especially open fractures) or undergoing certain orthopaedic surgical procedures appear to be at increased risk for wound infections and non–wound-related complications (e.g., UTI, pneumonia). Patients with HIV can develop secondary rheumatologic conditions such as Reiter syndrome.

I. Hepatitis
 1. Hepatitis A—Common in areas with poor sanitation and public health concerns, but not a major problem regarding surgical transmission.
 2. Hepatitis B—Approximately 200,000 people are infected with the hepatitis B virus each year, and there are currently more than 12 million carriers in the United States and 350 million carriers worldwide. Screening and vaccination have reduced the risk of transmission for health care workers. Immune globulin is administered after exposure in nonvaccinated persons.
 3. Hepatitis C—Recent advances in screening methods have decreased the risk of hepatitis C as a cause of transfusion-associated hepatitis (1 in 1,935,000 per unit transfused). **Hepatitis C is also related to intravenous drug abuse. PCR is the most sensitive method for early detection of infection**.

J. Hypothermia—Treatment of hypothermia (core body temperature $<35°$ C [$<95°$ F]) includes passive external warming with blankets, clothing, and warmed IV fluids, and active core rewarming with peritoneal lavage, and pleural lavage for severe cases. Hypothermia is life threatening and made worse by surgery and anesthesia; therefore, surgery should be delayed until the hypothermic state is corrected.

V. Orthopaedic Management in the Polytraumatized Patient
 A. Timing Definitive Procedures
  1. Stable patients—Patients who are hemodynamically stable can be treated for their injuries in a manner that is timely for those specific injuries. Since the stable patient does not have physiologic derangement, he or she may be able to undergo definitive reconstruction (e.g., intramedullary nailing of a femur fracture) at the discretion of the specialist.
  2. In extremis—A patient "in extremis" has a profound physiologic derangement. He/she can be hypotensive, coagulopathic, and hypothermic. These are life-threatening conditions. Such a patient requires urgent cessation and/or reversal of the cause of the derangement (e.g., hemorrhage) and adequate resuscitation. Restoration and stabilization of the patient's physiology takes priority over reconstruction of his/her non–life-threatening injuries.
  3. Borderline patients—**In patients with continued physiologic derangements after resuscitation, performance of "damage control orthopaedics" is prudent**. External fixation of long bone fractures rather than definitive fixation of these injuries is recommended in the borderline patient.
  4. Associated head injury—Orthopaedic interventions should be timed appropriately to minimize risk of detrimental neurologic effects. **Intraoperative hypotension adversely affects the long-term outcome of trauma patients with associated head injuries**.
 B. Inflammatory Mediators—Inflammatory mediators or cytokines are released into the bloodstream in

measurable levels as a response to trauma and tissue injury. Elevation of several of these mediators has been linked to the systemic inflammatory response to trauma. *IL-6 has been most closely associated with the magnitude of this systemic inflammatory response to trauma and with the development of multiple organ dysfunction syndrome.*

C. Open Fracture Management

1. Pre- and postdebridement cultures—The available evidence demonstrates a lack of utility for pre- and/or postdebridement wound cultures in open fractures. Ninety-two percent of infections are nosocomial. The wound cultures rarely identify the infecting organism and are often negative in fractures that become infected.

2. Antibiotics—Antibiotic use with open fractures decreases the risk of infection by 59%. Unfortunately, choice and duration of antibiotic are based largely on expert opinion. A recent evidence-based review by the Surgical Infection Society found sufficient evidence to support *the short duration use of a first generation cephalosporin (e.g., cefazolin) in open fractures.* This short duration can be as little as 24 hours. Although there is conflicting evidence on the effectiveness of extended coverage with an aminoglycoside, it is still the general recommendation to add an aminoglycoside to the first generation cephalosporin for type III open fractures. It is also recommended to add penicillin in farm or vascular injuries for activity against anaerobes.

3. Irrigation—High-volume irrigation (3 to 9 L) with sterile normal saline is recommended for open fractures. Additives to irrigation solutions include antiseptics, antibiotics, and soaps. Antiseptic additives are toxic to tissues. Antibiotics are of questionable value and have even shown higher wound complication rates than soap solutions. There are conflicting data on the use of soap solutions.

4. Timing of debridement—*Several recent publications have challenged the traditional "emergent" nature of debridement of open fractures within the first 6 hours.* Timely debridement (within 24 hours) remains the recommendation as long as other factors such as vascular injury and compartment syndrome are absent. Other orthopaedic emergencies such as a hip dislocation may now be prioritized ahead of open fracture debridement.

VI. Complications Associated with Trauma

A. Venous Thromboembolic Disease—Deep venous thrombosis (DVT) and pulmonary embolus (PE) may occur in the setting of trauma due to immobilization and endothelial injury. Approximately 700,000 people in the United States have an asymptomatic PE each year, of which 200,000 are fatal.

1. Deep venous thrombosis
   - Diagnosis—Clinical suspicion is often more helpful than physical examination (pain, swelling, Homans sign) for DVT. Useful studies include *venography (the "gold standard")*, which is 97% accurate (70% for iliac veins); ^{125}I-labeled fibrinogen (operative-site artifact causes false positives); impedance plethysmography (poor sensitivity); duplex ultrasonography (B-mode), which is 90% accurate for DVT proximal to the trifurcation vessels; and Doppler imaging (immediate bedside tool, often best first study). *Virchow's triad* of factors involved in venous thrombosis is venous stasis, hypercoagulability, and intimal injury.
   - Prophylaxis—DVT prophylaxis with mechanical, pharmacological, or both mechanisms is recommended. Immediate mechanical prophylaxis with delayed pharmacological prophylaxis in a study by Stannard et al. (2006) showed similar efficacy in DVT prevention. Retrievable inferior vena cava filters may also be considered in a patient with a contraindication to anticoagulation, although limited clinical data on efficacy and complication rate exists. *The anticoagulation effects of warfarin (Coumadin) result from the inhibition of hepatic enzymes, vitamin K epoxide, and perhaps vitamin K reductase. This inhibition results in decarboxylation of the vitamin K–dependent protein factors II (prothrombin), VII (the first to be affected), IX, and X. Warfarin inhibits posttranslational modification of vitamin K–dependent clotting factors.* Rifampin *and phenobarbital* are antagonists to warfarin.
   - Treatment—Treatment is recommended for all thigh DVTs; however, treatment of DVTs occurring below the popliteal fossa is controversial. *Preoperative identification of a DVT in a patient with lower extremity or pelvic trauma is an indication for placement of a vena cava filter.*

2. Pulmonary embolism
   - Diagnosis—PE should be suspected in patients with an acute onset of pleuritic pain, *tachypnea (90%)*, and tachycardia (60%). Initial workup includes an ECG (right bundle

branch block, right axis deviation in 25%; may also show ST depression or T-wave inversion in lead III), a chest radiograph (hyperlucency rare), and ABGs (normal pO_2 does not exclude PE). A nuclear medicine ventilation–perfusion scan may be helpful, but pulmonary angiography is considered the "gold standard" to make the diagnosis if there is any question.

- Treatment—The most important factor for survival is early diagnosis and prompt therapy initiation. Treatment may include heparin therapy (continuous intravenous infusion) and monitored by the partial thromboplastin time, thrombolytic agents, vena cava filter, or other surgical measures.

B. Compartment Syndrome—Compartment syndrome is increase in pressure within an osteofascial space to a level that compromises the perfusion within that space. When performing a four-compartment fasciotomy of the leg, injury to the superficial peroneal nerve can occur during release of the anterior and lateral compartments as it exits the fascia. Continuous traction during intramedullary nailing of tibia fractures has been found to contribute to the development of compartment syndrome.

C. Infection—Infection after orthopaedic trauma can occur most commonly in the setting of an open fracture. If an appropriate debridement of devitalized tissue and bone is not performed, a patient may develop a chronic infection. Treatment of chronic posttraumatic osteomyelitis requires excision of the sequestrum (necrotic bone) as well as an extensive debridement that may include removal of hardware.

1. Infection with flaps—***Infection rates and flap failure rates with open fractures requiring coverage are lowest if the flap is performed within 72 hours of the injury**.*

2. Cellulitis—Infection of the subcutaneous tissues, generally deeper and with less distinct margins than erysipelas. Clinical signs include erythema, tenderness, warmth, lymphangitis, and lymphadenopathy. Group A streptococcus is the most common organism, and *S. aureus* much less common. Initial antibiotic treatment is penicillinase-resistant synthetic penicillins (PRSPs [nafcillin or oxacillin]). Alternative therapies include erythromycin, first-generation cephalosporins, amoxicillin/clavulanate (Augmentin), azithromycin, clarithromycin, dithromycin, and tigecycline.

3. Erysipelas—Infection of the superficial tissues characterized by progressively enlarging, well-demarcated, red, raised, painful plaque, similar to cellulitis but more superficial. In diabetics, the most common organisms are group A Streptococcus, *Staphylococcus aureus*, Enterobacteriaceae, and Clostridia. Treatment of early or mild cases includes second- or third-generation cephalosporin or amoxicillin. Severe cases may require imipenem (Primaxin), meropenem, or trovafloxacin. Diabetics may require surgical debridement to rule out necrotizing fasciitis and obtain definitive cultures.

4. Necrotizing fasciitis—Infection of the muscle fascia that is aggressive and life threatening. It may be associated with an underlying vascular disease (particularly diabetes), and commonly occurs after surgery, trauma, or streptococcal skin infection. Many acute cases involve several organisms; groups A, C, and G streptococcus are the most commonly isolated. Clostridia or polymicrobial infections (aerobic plus anaerobic) are also seen, as well as methicillin-resistant *S. aureus* (MRSA). Treatment requires emergent, extensive surgical debridement involving the entire length of the overlying cellulitis and initial treatments with IV antibiotics: penicillin G for strep or clostridia; imipenem, cilastatin, or meropenem for polymicrobial infections; and vancomycin if MRSA is suspected.

5. Gas gangrene—Injuries contaminated with soil may result in anaerobic, Gram-positive, spore-forming rods producing exotoxins (classically Clostridium species) infections resulting in gas gangrene. Patients presenting with clinical sepsis and a limb infection with subcutaneous crepitus and visible gas on radiographs require an urgent surgical debridement, leaving the wound open, and intravenous antibiotics.

6. Toxic shock syndrome—TSS is a form of toxemia, not a septicemia. In orthopaedics, TSS is secondary to colonization of surgical or traumatic wounds (even after minor trauma).

- Staphylococcal—Presents with fever, hypotension, and erythematous macular rash with a serous exudate (Gram-positive cocci are present). The infected wound may look benign and may be misleading with regard to the seriousness of the underlying condition. Treatment is with irrigation and debridement and IV antibiotics with IV immune globulin. Initial antibiotic treatment is a PRSP (nafcillin or oxacillin), vancomycin if MRSA. Alternative therapies include first-generation cephalosporins. Patients may also require emergent fluid resuscitation.

TABLE 1-6

Bite Injuries

Source of Bite	Organism(s)	Primary Antimicrobial (or Drug) Regimen
Human	*Bacteroides* *Staphylococcus epidermidis* *Streptococcus viridans (100%)* *Corynebacterium* *S. aureus* *Peptostreptococcus* *Eikenella*	Early treatment (not yet infected): amoxicillin/clavulanate (Augmentin) With signs of infection: ampicillin/sulbactam (Unasyn), cefoxitin, ticarcillin/clavulanate (Timentin), or piperacillin-tazobactam Patients with penicillin allergy: clindamycin plus either ciprofloxacin or trimethoprim/sulfamethoxazole *Eikenella* is resistant to clindamycin, nafcillin/oxacillin, metronidazole, and possibly to first-generation cephalosporins and erythromycin; susceptible to fluoroquinolones and trimethoprim/sulfamethoxazole; treat with cefoxitin or ampicillin
Dog	*S. aureus* *Pasteurella multocida* *Bacteroides* *Fusobacterium* *Capnocytophaga*	Amoxicillin/clavulanate (Augmentin), clindamycin (adults), or clindamycin plus trimethoprim/sulfamethoxazole (children) Consider antirabies treatment Only 5% become infected
Cat	*P. multocida* *S. aureus* Possibly tularemia	Amoxicillin/clavulanate, cefuroxime axetil, or doxycycline
Rat	*S. moniliformis* *Spirillum minus*	Amoxicillin/clavulanate or doxycycline Antirabies treatment not indicated
Pig	Polymicrobial (aerobes and anaerobes)	Amoxicillin/clavulanate, third-generation cephalosporin, ticarcillin/clavulanate (Timentin), ampicillin/sulbactam, or imipenem–cilastatin
Skunk, raccoon, bat	Varies	Amoxicillin/clavulanate or doxycycline Antirabies treatment is indicated
Pit viper (snake)	*Pseudomonas* Enterobacteriaceae *S. epidermidis* *Clostridium*	Antivenom therapy Ceftriaxone Tetanus prophylaxis
Brown recluse spider	—	Dapsone
Catfish sting	Toxins (may become secondarily infected)	Amoxicillin/clavulanate

Adapted from Gilbert DN, Moellering RC, Eliopoulos GM, et al. *The Sanford Guide to Antimicrobial Therapy.* Hyde Park, VT: Antimicrobial Therapy, Inc.; 2006, p. 38, with permission.

- Streptococcal—Involves toxins from Group A, B, C, or G *Streptococcus pyogenes.* The clinical presentation is similar to staphylococcal TSS. Initial antibiotic treatment is clindamycin plus penicillin G and IV immune globulin. Alternative therapies include erythromycin, or ceftriaxone and clindamycin.

7. Surgical wound infections—Most commonly attributable to *S. aureus*, but Groups A, B, C, and G strep and Enterobacteriaceae are not uncommon. Methicillin-resistant *S. aureus* (MRSA) species infections are increasing, and vancomycin-methicillin–resistant *S. aureus* (VMRSA) has been reported. MRSA

species are best treated with vancomycin (alternatives to vancomycin for MRSA include teicoplanin, trimethoprim [Bactrim] plus sulfamethoxazole, quinupristin/dalfopristin, linezolid, daptomycin, dalbavancin, fusidic acid, fosfomycin, rifampin, and novobiocin).

8. VMRSA is treated with quinupristin/dalfopristin, linezolid, or daptomycin.

9. Bite injuries—See Table 1-6.

10. Puncture wounds of the foot—*The most characteristic organism resulting from a puncture wound from a nail through the sole of an athletic shoe is* P. aeruginosa (unless the host is immunocompromised or diabetic). *Pseudomonas* infections (Gram-negative rod) require aggressive debridement and appropriate antibiotics (often a two-antibiotic regimen). The initial antibiotic regimen for an established infection should include ceftazidime or cefepime; an alternative initial antibiotic regimen might include ciprofloxacin (except in children), imipenem, cilastatin, or a third-generation cephalosporin. The prophylactic antibiotic treatment for a recent (hours) puncture through the sole of an athletic shoe (without infection) remains controversial. *Osteomyelitis develops in 1% to 2% of children who sustain a puncture wound through the sole of an athletic shoe*.

11. Brackish water/shellfish exposure—A musculoskeletal injury involving brackish water (areas of mixing of fresh and sea water) or shellfish should include a third generation cephalosporin (e.g., ceftazadime). This will provide antibiotic coverage against *Vibrio vulnificus*, which, if untreated, can result in a life-threatening systemic infection.

D. Heterotopic Ossification—HO can result from traumatic injuries about the hip, knee, and elbow. *In the case of a traumatic amputation, performing the amputation through the zone of injury and blast mechanism are predictive of development of HO. Significant HO can even develop in the quadriceps from the use of distal femoral skeletal traction*. HO can also develop in the setting of a quadriceps contusion from trauma or athletics. *The treatment for a quadriceps contusion with early evidence of HO is rest and range-of-motion exercises*. It is also possible to develop HO in and around the knee as a result of a knee dislocation or retrograde nailing of the femur.

E. Nonunion—Nonunion is a common complication of orthopaedic trauma. *It is the most common complication after open reduction of a femoral neck fracture. Nonunion following intramedullary nail stabilization of femoral shaft fractures is associated with the use of nonsteroidal anti-inflammatory drugs*.

F. Occult Orthopaedic Injuries—Understanding patterns of injury and associated injuries may decrease the risk of missing an occult orthopaedic injury. The most common reason for missed fractures in a polytrauma patient is that the extremity was not properly imaged. *The most commonly missed component of a distal femur fracture is a coronal fracture of the lateral femoral condyle, which is best diagnosed by CT. The most common associated injury in a patient with a hip dislocation is an ipsilateral knee injury. Occult femoral neck fractures can be associated with femoral shaft fractures*. Diagnostic workup includes radiographs of the femoral neck.

G. Posttraumatic Stress Disorder (PTSD)—Posttraumatic stress disorder is common (51%) in orthopaedic trauma patients. The patient's feeling that their emotional problems caused by the injury have been more difficult to deal with than the physical problems is suggestive of PTSD.

VII. Miscellaneous Musculoskeletal Traumatic Injuries
A. Limb-Threatening Injuries—Recent publications have demonstrated similar outcomes with limb salvage and amputation in high-energy lower-extremity trauma (HELET) (Bosse et al., 2002; MacKenzie et al., 2005).

1. Limb Injury Severity Scores —Limb Iinjury Severity Scores such as the Mangled Extremity Severity Score (MESS); Limb Salvage Index (LSI); Predictive Salvage Index (PSI); the Nerve Injury, Ischemia, Soft-Tissue Injury, Skeletal Injury, Shock, and Age of Patient Score (NISSSA); and the Hannover Fracture Scale-97 (HFS-97) were not shown to have clinical utility in a prospective evaluation of more than 500 patients with HELET (Bosse et al., 2001).

2. Salvage versus amputation—Orthopaedic surgeons surveyed in the LEAP study identified limb injury characteristics as the most important factors in the decision to salvage or amputate the limb (MacKenzie et al., 2002). Severity of soft tissue injury and plantar sensation had the greatest impact on their decision. *The patient's overall ISS did not have an impact on their decision to attempt limb salvage*.

3. Plantar sensation—A lack of plantar sensation in a patient with a mangled lower extremity

has been a traditional indication for immediate amputation. A cohort of patients identified in the LEAP study had an "insensate foot" in association with their HELET. Of the 55 limbs that were insensate at presentation, 26 underwent amputation and 29 underwent salvage. At two years, there were no significant differences in the SIP scores or rates of return-to-work. *In the insensate salvage group, 55% had return of normal sensation by 2 years*. The others had some impairment of sensation with the exception of 1 limb that remained insensate. *In other words, the insensate foot in association with HELET likely represents a neuropraxia. It can be expected to recover to some degree at 2 years*.

4. Ischemic limbs—Muscle necrosis and secondary myoglobinemia and acidosis can result during the reperfusion phase after vascular reconstruction or replantation of an ischemic limb or traumatic amputation. *High-volume diuresis with alkalanization of the urine* will mitigate the impact of myoglobinemia due to ischemia-reperfusion injury.

B. Nerve Injuries—There are three types of traumatic nerve injury: neuropraxia, axonotmesis, and neurotmesis. Neuropraxia represents a temporary nerve injury from stretch or contusion that recovers in days to months. Axonotmesis is disruption of the axon itself with maintenance of the integrity of the nerve sheath (epineurium and perineurium). Recovery takes several weeks to several months, because the nerve must regenerate from proximal to distal. Neurotmesis is complete loss of the continuity of the nerve and its surrounding connective tissue layers. Surgical repair or reconstruction of the nerve is required in order to permit regeneration of the nerve to occur along the appropriate path. *The most important factor in determining recovery after surgical repair of a peripheral nerve injury is the age of the patient*.

C. Gunshot Fractures—Gunshot fractures represent a special type of open fracture. Uncomplicated, low-velocity gunshot fractures (pistol) can be generally treated in a similar fashion to closed injuries, while high-velocity gunshot fractures (hunting rifle, military, etc.) should be treated using open fracture principles of surgical debridement.

1. Low velocity—Low velocity is defined as less than 2,000 ft per second. Local wound care and a short course of oral antibiotics is appropriate for these low-velocity injuries.

2. High velocity—High velocity is defined as greater than 2,000 ft per second. Formal debridement and intravenous antibiotics are recommended.

3. Spine involvement—Gunshot injuries to the spine are generally mechanically stable. There is still some controversy over the necessity for surgical debridement of low-velocity gunshot injuries to the spine with involvement of an abdominal viscus. Current recommendations with a viscus injury are no debridement and 7 to 14 days of broad-spectrum intravenous antibiotics even when there is involvement of the spinal canal. Gunshot injuries to the cervical spine can be a life-threatening situation due to critical local anatomy such as the trachea and great vessels of the neck. With a gunshot injury to the cervical spine, ATLS principles are the priority: airway, breathing, and circulation.

VIII. Summary—General principles of orthopaedic trauma include prioritization of immediately life-threatening conditions through the employment of ATLS guidelines. Treatment of shock and associated injuries precedes orthopaedic intervention. The orthopaedic surgeon's role in the polytraumatized patient demands an understanding of the appropriate timing of intervention, damage control orthopaedics, and open fracture management. Throughout evaluation and management of a trauma patient, careful surveillance and prevention of complications are critical.

SUGGESTED READINGS

Classic Articles

Baker SP, O'Neill B, Haddon W Jr, et al. The injury severity score: a method for describing patients with multiple injuries and evaluating emergency care. *J Trauma.* 1994;14(3):187–196.

Born CT, Ross SE, Iannacone WM, et al. Delayed identification of skeletal injury in multisystem trauma: the 'missed' fracture. *J Trauma.* 1989;29(12):1643–1646.

Bosse MJ, MacKenzie EJ, Kellam JF, et al. A prospective evaluation of the clinical utility of the lower-extremity injury-severity scores. *J Bone Joint Surg Am.* 2001;83-A(1): 3–14.

Bosse MJ, MacKenzie EJ, Kellam JF, et al. An analysis of outcomes of reconstruction or amputation after leg-threatening injuries. *N Engl J Med.* 2002;347(24):1924–1931.

Bosse MJ, McCarthy ML, Jones AL, et al. The insensate foot following severe lower extremity trauma: an indication for amputation? *J Bone Joint Surg Am.* 2005;87(12):2601–2608.

Bottlang M, Krieg JC, Mohr M, et al. Emergent management of pelvic ring fractures with use of circumferential compression. *J Bone Joint Surg Am.* 2002;84-A(suppl 2):43–47.

Bottlang M, Simpson T, Sigg J, et al. Noninvasive reduction of open-book pelvic fractures by circumferential compression. *J Orthop Trauma.* 2002;16(6):367–373.

Brumback RJ, Uwagie-Ero S, Lakatos RP, et al. Intramedullary nailing of femoral shaft fractures. Part II: Fracture-healing with static interlocking fixation. *J Bone Joint Surg Am.* 1988;70(10):1453–1462.

Burd TA, Hughes MS, Anglen JO. Heterotopic ossification prophylaxis with indomethacin increases the risk of long-bone nonunion. *J Bone Joint Surg Br.* 2003;85(5):700–705.

Cantu RC. Posttraumatic retrograde and anterograde amnesia: pathophysiology and implications in grading and safe return to play. *J Athl Train.* 2001;36(3):244–248.

Carsenti-Etesse H, Doyon F, Desplaces N, et al. Epidemiology of bacterial infection during management of open leg fractures. *Eur J Clin Microbiol Infect Dis.* 1999;18(5):315–323.

Chesnut RM, Marshall LF, Klauber MR, et al. The role of secondary brain injury in determining outcome from severe head injury. *J Trauma.* 1993;34(2):216–222.

Crowl AC, Young JS, Kahler DM. Occult hypoperfusion is associated with increased morbidity in patients undergoing early femur fracture fixation. *J Trauma.* 2000;48(2):260–267.

Dalal SA, Burgess AR, Siegel JH, et al. Pelvic fracture in multiple trauma: classification by mechanism is key to pattern of organ injury, resuscitative requirements, and outcome. *J Trauma.* 1989;29(7):981–982.

Dellinger EP, Caplan ES, Weaver LD, Duration of preventive antibiotic administration for open extremity fractures. *Arch Surg.* 1988;123(3):333–339.

Dickson K, Watson TS, Haddad C, et al. Outpatient management of low-velocity gunshot-induced fractures. *Orthopedics.* 2001;24(10):951–954.

Giannoudis PV. When is the safest time to undertake secondary definitive fracture stabilization procedures in multiply injured patients who were initially managed using a strategy of primary temporary skeletal fixation. *J Trauma.* 2002;52(4):811–813.

Giannoudis PV, MacDonald DA, Matthews SJ. Nonunion of the femoral diaphysis. The influence of reaming and nonsteroidal anti-inflammatory drugs. *J Bone Joint Surg Br.* 2000;82(5):655–658.

Gillespie WJ. The incidence and pattern of knee injury associated with dislocation of the hip. *J Bone Joint Surg Br.* 1975;57(3):376–378.

Godina M. Early microsurgical reconstruction of complex trauma of the extremities. *Plast Reconstr Surg.* 1986;78(3):285–292.

Hadley M. Management of acute spinal cord injuries in an intensive care unit or other monitored setting. *Neurosurgery.* 2002;50(suppl 3):S51–S57.

Harley BJ, Beaupre LA, Jones CA. et al. The effect of time to definitive treatment on the rate of nonunion and infection in open fractures. *J Orthop Trauma.* 2002;16(7):484–490.

Hart GB, Lamb RC, Strauss MB. Gas gangrene. *J Trauma.* 1983;23(11):991–1000.

Horne LT, Blue BA. Intraarticular heterotopic ossification in the knee following intramedullary nailing of the fractured femur using a retrograde method. *J Orthop Trauma.* 1999;13(5):385–388.

Kaufman HH, Huchton JD, Patten BM, et al. Limb preservation for reimplantation. A review. *J Microsurg.* 1980;2(1):36–41.

Knapp TP, Patzakis MJ, Lee J, et al. Comparison of intravenous and oral antibiotic therapy in the treatment of fractures caused by low-velocity gunshots. A prospective, randomized study of infection rates. *J Bone Joint Surg Am.* 1996;78(8):1167–1171.

Kumar A, Wood GW II, Whittle AP. Low-velocity gunshot injuries of the spine with abdominal viscus trauma. *J Orthop Trauma.* 1998;12(7):514–517.

Lange RH, Bach AW, Hansen ST Jr, et al. Open tibial fractures with associated vascular injuries: prognosis for limb salvage. *J Trauma.* 1985;25(3):203–208.

Lee J. Efficacy of cultures in the management of open fractures. *Clin Orthop Relat Res.* 1997;(339):71–75.

Lew DP, Waldvogel FA. Osteomyelitis. *Lancet.* 2004;364 (9431):369–379.

Lipscomb AB, Thomas ED, Johnston RK. Treatment of myositis ossificans traumatica in athletes. *Am J Sports Med.* 1976;4(3):111–120.

Lu-Yao GL, Keller RB, Littenberg B, et al. Outcomes after displaced fractures of the femoral neck. A meta-analysis of one hundred and six published reports. *J Bone Joint Surg Am.* 1994;76(1):15–25.

MacKenzie EJ, Bosse MJ, Kellam JF, et al. Factors influencing the decision to amputate or reconstruct after high-energy lower extremity trauma. *J Trauma.* 2002;52(4):641–649.

MacKenzie EJ, Bosse MJ, Pollak AN, et al. Long-term persistence of disability following severe lower-limb trauma. Results of a seven-year follow-up. *J Bone Joint Surg Am.* 2005;87(8):1801–1819.

McQueen MM, Christie J, Court-Brown CM. Compartment pressures after intramedullary nailing of the tibia. *J Bone Joint Surg Br.* 1990;72(3):395–397.

Mills WJ, Tejwani N. Heterotopic ossification after knee dislocation: the predictive value of the injury severity score. *J Orthop Trauma.* 2003;17(5):338–345.

Pape HC, Hildebrand F, Pertschy S, et al. Changes in the management of femoral shaft fractures in polytrauma patients: from early total care to damage control orthopedic surgery. *J Trauma.* 2002;53(3):452–462.

Pape HC, van Griensven M, Rice J, et al. Major secondary surgery in blunt trauma patients and perioperative cytokine liberation: determination of the clinical relevance of biochemical markers. *J Trauma.* 2001;50(6):989–1000.

Partrick DA, Moore FA, Moore EE, et al. Barney Resident Research Award winner. The inflammatory profile of interleukin-6, interleukin-8, and soluble intercellular adhesion molecule-1 in postinjury multiple organ failure. *Am J Surg.* 1996;172(5):425–431.

Patzakis MJ, Harvey JP Jr, Ivler D. The role of antibiotics in the management of open fractures. *J Bone Joint Surg Am.* 1974;56(3):532–541.

Patzakis MJ, Wilkins J. Factors influencing infection rate in open fracture wounds. *Clin Orthop Relat Res.* 1989;(243): 36–40.

Peljovich AE, Patterson BM. Ipsilateral femoral neck and shaft fractures. *J Am Acad Orthop Surg.* 1998;6(2):106–113.

Pietropaoli JA, Rogers FB, Shackford SR, et al. The deleterious effects of intraoperative hypotension on outcome in patients with severe head injuries. *J Trauma.* 1992;33(3):403–407.

Porter JM, Ivatury RR. In search of the optimal end points of resuscitation in trauma patients: a review. *J Trauma.* 1998;44(5):908–914.

Riemer BL, Butterfield SL, Ray RL, et al. Clandestine femoral neck fractures with ipsilateral diaphyseal fractures. *J Orthop Trauma.* 1993;7(5):443–449.

Schmidt GL, Sciulli R, Altman GT. Knee injury in patients experiencing a high-energy traumatic ipsilateral hip dislocation. *J Bone Joint Surg Am.* 2005;87(6):1200–1204.

Shafi S, Kauder DR. Fluid resuscitation and blood replacement in patients with polytrauma. *Clin Orthop Relat Res.* 2004;(422):37–42.

Shakespeare DT, Henderson NJ. Compartmental pressure changes during calcaneal traction in tibial fractures. *J Bone Joint Surg Br.* 1982;64(4):498–499.

Simpson BM, Wilson RH, Grant RE. Antibiotic therapy in gunshot wound injuries. *Clin Orthop Relat Res.* 2003;(408):82–85.

Specht LM, Gupta S, Egol, KA, et al. Heterotopic ossification of the quadriceps following distal femoral traction: a report of three cases and a review of the literature. *J Orthop Trauma.* 2004;18(4):241–246.

Stannard JP, Wilson TC, Sheils TM, et al. Heterotopic ossification associated with knee dislocation. *Arthroscopy.* 2002;18(8):835–839.

Starr AJ, Smith WR, Frawley WH, et al. Symptoms of posttraumatic stress disorder after orthopaedic trauma. *J Bone Joint Surg Am.* 2004;86-A(6):1115–1121.

Tabuenca J, Truan JR. Knee injuries in traumatic hip dislocation. *Clin Orthop Relat Res.* 2000;(377):78–83.

Teasdale G, Jennett B. Assessment of coma and impaired consciousness. A practical scale. *Lancet.* 1974;2(7872):81–84.

Townsend RN, Lheureau T, Protech J, et al. Timing fracture repair in patients with severe brain injury (Glasgow Coma Scale score <9). *J Trauma.* 1998;44(6):977–982; discussion 982–983.

Valenziano CP, Chattar-Cora D, O'Neill A, et al. Efficacy of primary wound cultures in long bone open extremity fractures: are they of any value? *Arch Orthop Trauma Surg.* 2002;122(5):259–261.

Recent Articles

Anglen JO. Comparison of soap and antibiotic solutions for irrigation of lower-limb open fracture wounds. A prospective, randomized study. *J Bone Joint Surg Am.* 2005;87(7):1415–1422.

Apel PJ, Alton T, Northam C, et al. How age impairs the response of the neuromuscular junction to nerve transection and repair: an experimental study in rats. *J Orthop Res.* 2008.

Charalambous CP, Siddique I, Zenios M, et al. Early versus delayed surgical treatment of open tibial fractures: effect on the rates of infection and need of secondary surgical procedures to promote bone union. *Injury.* 2005;36(5):656–661.

Harwood PJ, Giannoudis PV, Probst C, et al. Which AIS based scoring system is the best predictor of outcome in orthopaedic blunt trauma patients? *J Trauma.* 2006;60(2):334–340.

Hauser CJ, Adams CA Jr, Eachempati SR. Surgical Infection Society guideline: prophylactic antibiotic use in open fractures: an evidence-based guideline. *Surg Infect (Larchmt).* 2006;7(4):379–405.

Hoff WS, Hoey BA, Wainwright GA, et al. Early experience with retrievable inferior vena cava filters in high-risk trauma patients. *J Am Coll Surg.* 2004;199(6):869–874.

Krieg JC, Mohr M, Ellis TJ, et al. Emergent stabilization of pelvic ring injuries by controlled circumferential compression: a clinical trial. *J Trauma.* 2005;59(3):659–664.

Nork SE, Segina DN, Aflatoon K, et al. The association between supracondylar-intercondylar distal femoral fractures and coronal plane fractures. *J Bone Joint Surg Am.* 2005;87(3):564–569.

Potter BK, Burns TC, Lacap AP, et al. Heterotopic ossification following traumatic and combat-related amputations. Prevalence, risk factors, and preliminary results of excision. *J Bone Joint Surg Am.* 2007;89(3):476–486.

Stannard JP, Lopez-Ben RR, Volgas DA, et al. Prophylaxis against deep-vein thrombosis following trauma: a prospective, randomized comparison of mechanical and pharmacologic prophylaxis. *J Bone Joint Surg Am.* 2006;88(2):261–266.

Review Articles

Anglen JO. Wound irrigation in musculoskeletal injury. *J Am Acad Orthop Surg.* 2001;9(4):219–226.

Beiner JM, Jokl P. Muscle contusion injuries: current treatment options. *J Am Acad Orthop Surg.* 2001;9(4):227–237.

Chiang SR, Chuang YC. Vibrio vulnificus infection: clinical manifestations, pathogenesis, and antimicrobial therapy. *J Microbiol Immunol Infect.* 2003;36(2):81–88.

Malinoski DJ, Slater MS, Mullins RJ. Crush injury and rhabdomyolysis. *Crit Care Clin.* 2004;20(1):171–192.

Olson SA, Glasgow RR. Acute compartment syndrome in lower extremity musculoskeletal trauma. *J Am Acad Orthop Surg.* 2005;13(7):436–444.

Parsons B, Strauss E. Surgical management of chronic osteomyelitis. *Am J Surg.* 2004;188(suppl 1A):57–66.

Turen CH, Dube MA, LeCroy MC. Approach to the polytraumatized patient with musculoskeletal injuries. *J Am Acad Orthop Surg.* 1999;7(3):154–165.

Werner CM, Pierpont Y, Pollak AN. The urgency of surgical debridement in the management of open fractures. *J Am Acad Orthop Surg.* 2008;16(7):369–375.

Whitesides TE, Heckman MM. Acute compartment syndrome: Update on diagnosis and treatment. *J Am Acad Orthop Surg.* 1996;4(4):209–218.

Wilkins J, Patzakis, M. Choice and duration of antibiotics in open fractures. *Orthop Clin North Am.* 1991;22(3):433–437.

Zalavras CG, Patzakis MJ. Open fractures: evaluation and management. *J Am Acad Orthop Surg.* 2003;11(3):212–219.

Zalavras CG, Patzakis MJ, Holtom PD, et al. Management of open fractures. *Infect Dis Clin North Am.* 2005;19(4):915–929.

Textbooks

American College of Surgeons. *Advanced Trauma Life Support For Doctors: Student Course Manual.* 7th ed. Chicago, IL: American College of Surgeons; 2004.

Gosselin RA, Roberts I, Gillespie WJ. Antibiotics for preventing infection in open limb fractures. *Cochrane Database Syst Rev.* 2004;(1):CD003764.

Roberts CS, Pape HC, Jones AL, et al. Damage control orthopaedics: evolving concepts in the treatment of patients who have sustained orthopaedic trauma. *Instr Course Lect.* 2005;54:447–462.

Vaccaro AR, An HS, Betz RR, et al. The management of acute spinal trauma: prehospital and in-hospital emergency care. *Instr Course Lect.* 1997;46:113–125.

CHAPTER 2

Principles of Fractures

Mark R. Brinker and Daniel P. O'Connor

I. Fracture Description
   A. Soft Tissues
   1. Closed fractures—The fracture is not exposed to the external environment. The soft-tissue injury ranges from minor to massive (e.g., crush injury). Closed soft-tissue injuries are commonly graded by the method of Tscherne.
      - *Grade 0* injuries have negligible soft-tissue injury.
      - *Grade 1* injuries have superficial abrasions or contusions of the soft tissues overlying the fracture.
      - *Grade 2* injuries have significant contusion to the muscle, contaminated skin abrasions, or both types of injury. The bony injury is usually severe in these injuries.
      - *Grade 3* injuries have a severe injury to the soft tissues, with significant degloving, crushing, compartment syndrome, or vascular injury.
   2. Open fractures—The fracture is exposed to the external environment. The amount of soft-tissue destruction is related to the level of energy imparted to the limb during the traumatic episode.
      - *Classification—Open fractures are commonly described using the Gustilo grading system*.
        (a) *Type I open fractures* have small (<1 cm), clean wounds; minimal injury to the musculature; and no significant stripping of periosteum from bone.
        (b) *Type II open fractures* have larger (>1 cm) wounds, but do not have significant soft-tissue damage, flaps, or avulsions.
        (c) *Type III open fractures* have larger wounds and are associated with extensive injury to the integument, muscle, periosteum, and bone. Gunshot injuries and open fractures caused by a farm injury are special categories of Type III open fractures.
        (d) *Type IIIa* injuries have extensive contamination and/or injury to the underlying soft tissues, but adequate viable soft tissue is present to cover the bone and neurovascular structures without a muscle transfer.
        (e) *Type IIIb* injuries have such an extensive injury to the soft tissues that a rotational or free muscle transfer is necessary to achieve coverage of the bone and neurovascular structures. These injuries usually have massive contamination.
        (f) *Type IIIc* injuries are any open fractures with an associated vascular injury that requires an arterial repair.

   Often, what appears to be a Type I or II open fracture on initial examination in the emergency room is noted to have significant periosteal stripping and muscle injury at the time of operative debridement, and may require muscle transfer for coverage after serial debridements. Thus, there is a tendency for the Gustilo classification type to increase with time.
      - Antibiotic prophylaxis for open fractures—Prophylactic antibiotics following an open fracture are given for 48 to 72 hours (as compared with only 24 hours in clean surgical cases). In patients returning to the operating room for serial debridement, most orthopedic surgeons continue the antibiotics for 48 hours following the final debridement. The regimen for prophylactic antibiotic coverage is dependent on the severity (Gustilo type) of the open fracture.
        (a) Gustilo Type I—First or second generation cephalosporin (most commonly, Ancef)

(b) Gustilo Type II—First or second generation cephalosporin (most commonly, Ancef)

(c) Gustilo Type IIIa—First or second generation cephalosporin plus an Aminoglycoside

(d) Gustilo Type IIIb and IIIc—First- or second-generation cephalosporin plus an Aminoglycoside plus Penicillin (additional antibiotic coverage with a third-generation cephalosporin should be considered for patients with open marine [such as swamp] injuries).

- Tetanus prophylaxis—See Chapter 1, General Principles of Trauma.
- Traumatic amputation—The recommended sequence of structural repair during replantation is skeletal stabilization, arterial repair, venous repair, nerve repair, and muscle suture.

3. Soft-tissue injuries
- Overview—The requirements for wound healing are oxygenation, functioning cellular mechanisms, and a clean wound without contamination or necrotic tissue. There are four phases of wound healing:
  (a) Coagulation phase (minutes)
  (b) Inflammatory phase (hours)
  (c) Granulation phase (days)
  (d) Scar formation phase (weeks)
- Specific issues
  (a) Skeletal muscle—Muscle injuries typically heal with dense scarring. Surgical repair of clean lacerations of skeletal muscle usually result in minimal regeneration of muscle fibers distally, scar formation at the laceration, and recovery of approximately 50% of muscle strength.
  (b) Tendons—Tendons are composed of fibroblasts arranged in parallel rows in fascicles. Two types of tendons exist:
    - Paratenon—Covered tendons (vascular tendons)—many vessels supply a rich capillary system.
    - Sheathed tendons—A mesotenon (vincula) carries a vessel that supplies only one segment of the tendon; avascular areas receive nutrition via diffusion from vascularized segments. Because of these differences in vascular supply, paratenon-covered tendons heal better than sheathed tendons.

  Tendinous healing in response to injury is initiated by fibroblasts that originate in the epitenon and macrophages that initiate healing and remodeling. Tendon repairs are weakest at 7 to 10 days; they regain most of their original strength at 21 to 28 days and achieve maximum strength at 6 months.

  (c) Ligaments—The ultrastructure of ligament is similar to that of tendons, but the fibers are more variable and have a higher elastin content. Unlike tendons, ligaments have a "uniform microvascularity," which receives its supply at the insertion site. Ligament healing benefits from normal stress and strain across the joint. Early ligament healing is with Type III collagen that is later converted to Type I collagen. Immobilization adversely affects the strength (elastic modulus decreases) of an intact ligament and of a ligament repair. *The most common mechanism of ligament failure is rupture of sequential series of collagen fiber bundles* distributed throughout the body of the ligament and not localized to one specific area. Ligaments do not plastically deform ("they break not bend"). *Midsubstance ligament tears are common in adults; avulsion injuries are more common in children*. Avulsion of ligaments typically occurs between the unmineralized and mineralized fibrocartilage layers.

- Management of soft-tissue injuries associated with fractures
  (a) Overview—The care of patients with soft-tissue injuries proceeds in an orderly fashion through three phases. *The acute phase* includes wound irrigation, wound debridement, skeletal stabilization, reconstruction of the soft tissues, and resumption of joint range of motion. *The reconstructive phase* deals with sequelae of the traumatic injury (delayed unions, nonunions, deformities, infections). *The rehabilitative phase* addresses the patients' psychological, social, and vocational recovery.
  (b) General principles of the acute phase treatment
    - Assess for the zone of soft-tissue injury—The soft-tissue zone of injury is generally much larger than the area of the fracture itself (Fig. 2-1).
    - Assess for associated vascular injuries (limb viability).
    - Assess for nerve injuries.
    - Pulsating irrigation in the operating room should be performed with copious isotonic solution, removing necrotic and foreign material.
    - Debridement (meticulous) of all foreign and necrotic material from the wound.

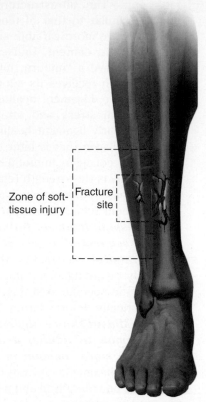

FIGURE 2-1 Diagrammatic representation of the zone of soft-tissue injury. Note that the area of soft-tissue injury is much greater than the area of the fracture site.

This should be performed every 24 to 48 hours until the wound is felt to be ready for closure or coverage.

- Open wounds should be extended using a scalpel to allow access to underlining tissues for assessment and debridement.
- Free bony ends should be delivered into the open wound; small devitalized pieces of cortical bone are removed. The intramedullary cavity is examined and cleaned.

(c) Types of wound closure or coverage
- Primary closure
- Delayed primary closure
- Healing by secondary intention
- Split-thickness skin grafts
- Random flaps—Such as a cross finger flap
- Vascularized pedicle flaps—Such as gastrocnemius flap
- Free flaps (Fig. 2-2)—These may be fasciocutaneous flaps or myocutaneous flaps.

(d) Timing of wound closure or coverage— Early wound closure or coverage (3 to 5 days) is associated with improved outcomes.

FIGURE 2-2 Topical atlas of the most commonly used donor sites for free tissue transfer.

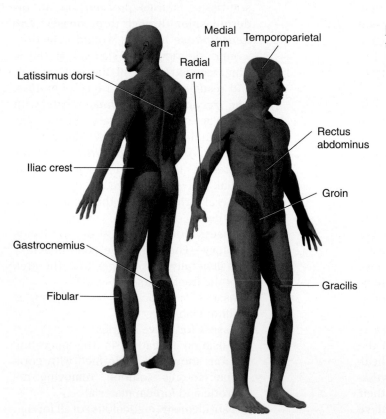

B. Bone
   1. Anatomic location—Name of bone(s) involved
   2. Regional location
      • Diaphysis
      • Metaphysis
      • Epiphysis
         (a) Extra-articular
         (b) Intra-articular
      • Physis (in skeletally immature individuals)
   3. Direction of fracture lines
      • Transverse—The loading mode resulting in fracture is tension
      • Oblique—The loading mode resulting in fracture is compression
      • Spiral—The loading mode resulting in fracture is torsion
   4. Condition of bone (Fig. 2-3)
      • Comminution—A comminuted fracture is one with three or more bony fragments.

Comminuted fractures generally result from high-energy injuries.
   • Pathologic fracture—A fracture through an area of pre-existing disease with weakened bone (primary bone tumors, metastases to bone, bone infections, osteoporosis, metabolic bone disease, and others).
   • Incomplete fracture—One in which the bone is not broken into separate fragments.
   • Segmental fracture—One in which there is a middle fragment of bone surrounded by a proximal and a distal segment. The middle fragment usually has an impaired blood supply. These injuries are typically high-energy injuries with soft-tissue stripping (muscle and periosteum) from bone, and are therefore prone to poor healing (delayed union or nonunion).
   • Fracture with bone loss—This may be caused by an open fracture where bone is left at

FIGURE 2-3   Condition of the bone in fractures.

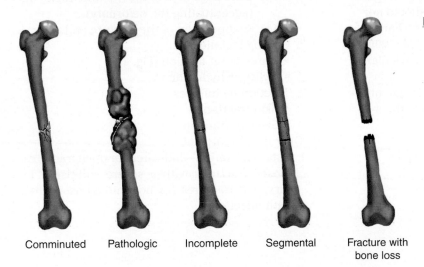

Comminuted   Pathologic   Incomplete   Segmental   Fracture with bone loss

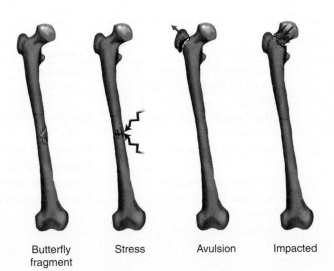

Butterfly fragment   Stress   Avulsion   Impacted

the scene of the injury (a high-energy open injury) or is devitalized by the injury and requires debridement, or a closed fracture where a segment is comminuted so severely that from a practical standpoint there is a "missing" segment of bone.

- Fracture with a butterfly fragment—This is similar to a segmental fracture except that the butterfly segment does not span the entire cross-section of the bone. The loading mode resulting in fracture is bending.
- Stress fracture—A fracture caused by repeated loading such as in military recruits (who march all day) or ballet dancers. Amenorrheic female runners are also prone to stress fractures. Common sites of stress fractures include the metatarsals, calcaneus, and tibia (other sites are possible).
- Avulsion fracture—Caused by the pull of a tendon or ligament at its site of bony insertion. Acute avulsion fractures display irregular borders on radiography. These should not be confused with sesamoid bones (hands, foot, others) or an unfused center of ossification (bipartite patella, accessory navicular, os trigonum).
- Impacted fracture—The fracture fragments are compressed together (generally the result of an axial load).

5. Type of bone involved (Table 2-1)
6. Deformities—See Chapter 3, Principles of Deformities
   - Length—Describes shortening or overlengthening
   - Angulation—Describes the direction (frontal, sagittal, oblique) in which the apex of the angulation points
   - Rotation—Describes the turning of fracture fragments (or healed bony segments) along the long axis of a bone
   - Translation—Describes anteroposterior and medial-lateral displacement of fracture fragments such that the fragments remain parallel to their initial position or each other

II. Fracture Management
   A. Nonoperative Treatment—It is best used in patients with lower-energy injuries or with patients who are not candidates for operative treatment because of systemic or local factors.
      1. Reduction via manipulation
         - Three steps
            (a) Longitudinal traction
            (b) Disengagement of the fracture fragments (accentuating the deformity)
            (c) Reapposition of the fracture ends
      2. Casting techniques
         - Three-point fixation (Fig. 2-4)
         - Cylinder hydraulics
      3. Traction techniques
         - Skin traction
         - Skeletal traction
   B. Operative Treatment
      1. External fixation—Indicated for open fractures, closed fractures with a severe soft-tissue injury, and fractures (or nonunions) associated with infection.

TABLE 2-1

Types of Bone

Microscopic Appearance	Subtypes	Characteristics	Examples
Lamellar	Cortical	Structure is oriented along lines of stress Strong	Femoral shaft
	Cancellous	More elastic than cortical bone	Distal femoral metaphysis
Woven	Immature	Not stress oriented	Embryonic skeleton Fracture callus
	Pathologic	Random organization Increased turnover Weak Flexible	Osteogenic sarcoma Fibrous dysplasia

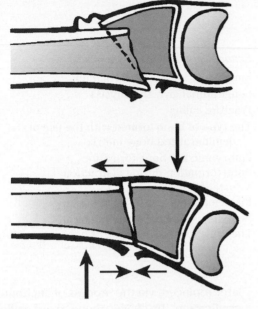

FIGURE 2-4 Three-point fixation casting technique. A three-point cast or splint can hold a fracture reduced by keeping the soft tissues hinge under tension. (From Court-Brown CM. Principles of nonoperative fracture treatment. In: Bucholz RW, Court-Brown CM, Heckman JD, et al., eds. *Rockwood and Green's Fractures in Adults.* 7th ed. Philadelphia, PA: Lippincott William & Wilkins, 2010, with permission.)

2. Internal fixation
   - Arbeitsgemeinschaft für Osteosynthesefragen (AO) Principles of Fracture Care (Table 2-2)
   - Interfragmentary compression
     (a) Static—Such as with a lag screw
     (b) Dynamic—Such as an intramedullary nail that is not locked, a sliding hip screw, or a tension band.
   - Splintage—A construct which allows sliding between the implant and the bone, such as occurs with intramedullary nail fixation
   - Bridging—Implants bridge an area of comminution
3. ***Indirect reduction*** is a technique in which distraction is performed across an area of comminution so that the fracture fragments are reduced by the tension generated in their soft-tissue attachments. The distraction force may be generated using a femoral distractor, an external fixator, an AO articulating tension device, or a lamina spreader. ***Ligamentotaxis*** is a method by which intra-articular fracture fragments may be reduced by applying traction to the ligamentous and capsular structures surrounding the joint.

TABLE 2-2

The Evolution of the AO Principles of Fracture Care

AO Principle	Original Concept	Current Concept
The first AO principle: anatomic reduction of the fracture fragments	Perfect anatomic reduction of all fracture fragments of the epiphysis, metaphysis, and diaphysis	*Epiphysis*—perfect anatomic reduction of articular fragments *Diaphysis*—restoration of length, alignment, and rotation *Metaphysis*—restoration of length, alignment, and rotation with bone grafting of bony defects
The second AO principle: stable internal fixation	Absolute rigid fixation of all fracture fragments of the epiphysis, metaphysis, and diaphysis	*Epiphysis*—rigid internal fixation *Diaphysis and Metaphysis*—relative stability (enough to allow bony union)
The third AO principle: preservation of blood supply	Atraumatic surgical techniques	Closed and indirect reduction techniques; implant constructs that are biologically sparing of the blood supply to bone and the soft tissues
The fourth AO principle: early active pain-free mobilization	Early joint range of motion exercises	Early joint range of motion exercises

TABLE 2-3

Types of Bone Formation

Type of Ossification	Mechanism	Examples of Normal Mechanisms
Enchondral	Bone replaces a cartilage model	Embryonic long bone formation Longitudinal growth (physis) Fracture callus The type of bone formed with the use of demineralized bone matrix
Intramembranous	Aggregates of undifferentiated mesenchymal cells differentiate into osteoblasts which form bone	Embryonic flat bone formation Bone formation during distraction osteogenesis Blastema bone
Appositional	Osteoblasts lay down new bone on existing bone	Periosteal bone enlargement (width) The bone formation phase of bone remodeling

III. The Biology of Bone Formation and Fracture Healing

A. *Overview*—Fracture healing involves a series of cellular events including inflammation, fibrous tissue and cartilage formation, and enchondral bone formation. The cellular events of fracture healing are influenced by undifferentiated cells in the area of the fracture and osteoinductive growth factors released into the fracture environment.

B. *Types of Bone Formation* (Table 2-3)

C. *Fracture Repair*—The response of bone to injury can be thought of as a continuum of histological processes, beginning with *inflammation*, proceeding through *repair* (soft callus followed by hard callus), and finally ending in *remodeling. Fracture repair is unique in that healing is completed without the formation of a scar*. Fracture healing may be influenced by a variety of biological and mechanical factors (Table 2-4).

1. Stages of fracture repair

   • *Inflammation*—Bleeding from the fracture site and surrounding soft tissues creates a hematoma (fibrin clot), which provides a source of hematopoietic cells capable of secreting growth factors. Subsequently, fibroblasts, mesenchymal cells, and osteoprogenitor cells are present at the fracture site, and fibrovascular tissue forms around the fracture ends. Osteoblasts, from surrounding osteogenic precursor cells and/or fibroblasts proliferate.

   • *Repair*—Primary callus response occurs within 2 weeks. If the bone ends are not in continuity, *bridging (soft) callus* occurs (fibrocartilage develops and stabilizes the bone ends). The soft callus (fibrocartilage) is later replaced, via the process of enchondral ossification, by woven bone (hard callus). Another type of callus, *medullary callus*, supplements the bridging callus, although it forms more slowly and occurs later. The amount of callus formation is related to

TABLE 2-4

Biological and Mechanical Factors Influencing Fracture Healing

Biological Factors	Mechanical Factors
Patient age	Soft-tissue attachments to bone
Metabolic bone disease	
Comorbid medical conditions	Stability (extent of immobilization)
Functional level	Anatomic location
Nutritional status (1,500 mg of elemental calcium/day recommended in patients with fractures)	Level of energy imparted
	Extent of bone loss
Nerve function	
Vascular injury	
Hormones	
Growth factors	
Health of the soft-tissue envelope	
Sterility (in open fractures)	
Cigarette smoke	
Medications	
Local pathologic conditions	
Level of energy imparted	
Type of bone affected	
Extent of bone loss	

TABLE 2-5

Type of Fracture Healing Based on Type of Stabilization

Type of Immobilization	Predominant Type of Healing	Comments
Cast (closed treatment)	Periosteal bridging callus	Enchondral ossification
Compression plate	Primary cortical healing (Remodeling)	Cutting cone type remodeling
Intramedullary nail	Early-periosteal bridging callus	Enchondral ossification and
	Late-medullary callus	intramembranous ossification
External fixator	Dependent of extent of rigidity	
	Less rigid—periosteal bridging callus	
	More rigid—primary cortical healing	
Inadequate	Hypertrophic nonunion	Failed enchondral ossification. Type II collage predominates

the amount of immobilization of the fracture. Primary cortical healing, which resembles normal remodeling, occurs with rigid immobilization and anatomic (or near-anatomic) reduction (bone ends are in continuity). Fracture healing varies with the method of treatment (Table 2-5). With closed treatment, "enchondral healing" with periosteal bridging callus occurs. With rigidly fixed fractures (such as with a compression plate), direct osteonal or primary bone healing occurs without visible callus. ***Intramedullary nailing results in repair through both intramembranous ossification and enchondral ossification***.

- ***Remodeling***—This process begins during the middle of the repair phase and continues long after the fracture has clinically healed (up to 7 years). Remodeling allows the bone to assume its normal configuration and shape based on the stresses to which it is exposed (Wolff's law). Throughout the process, woven bone formed during the repair phase is replaced with lamellar bone. Fracture healing is complete when there is repopulation of the marrow space.

2. Biochemistry of fracture healing—Four biochemical steps of fracture healing have been described (Table 2-6).

D. Growth Factors of Bone

1. Bone morphogeneticic proteins (BMPs)—Osteoinductive; induces metaplasia of plueuripotential stem cells into osteoblasts; up to 20 different BMPs have been described. ***The target cell for BMPs is the undifferentiated perivascular mesenchymal cell***. BMPs stimulate bone formation and their actions are inhibited

by noggin and chordin; balance between these agonists and antagonists appears to be important in fracture healing. ***Activation of a transmembrane serine/threonine kinase receptor leads to activation of intracellular proteins called SMADs, the signaling mediator for BMPs***. BMP 2, 6, and 9 appear most important for osteoblast differentiation of mesenchymal stem cells, whereas most BMPs appear to induce osteogenesis in mature osteoblasts.

2. Transforming growth factor–beta (TGF-β)—Induces mesenchymal cells to produce Type II collagen and proteoglycans. Also induces osteoblasts to synthesize collagen. TGF-β is found in fracture hematomas and is believed to ***regulate cartilage and bone formation in fracture callus***. Chondrocytes and osteoblasts synthesize TGF-β. The largest source of TGF-β is the extracellular matrix of bone.

3. Insulin-like growth factor II (IGF-II)—Stimulate Type I collagen, cellular proliferation, and cartilage matrix synthesis, and bone formation.

4. Platelet-derived growth factor (PDGF)—Released from platelets following fracture; it attracts inflammatory cells and osteoprogenitor cells to the fracture site (chemotactic).

TABLE 2-6

Biochemical Steps of Fracture Healing

Step	Predominate Collagen Type(s)
Mesenchymal	I, II, (III, V)
Chondroid	II, IX
Chondroid-osteoid	I, II, X
Osteogenic	I

5. Growth hormone–insulin-like growth factor I-Produces *proliferation without maturation of the growth plate,* resulting in *linear bone growth*.

E. Effects of Hormones on Fracture Healing (Table 2-7)

F. Ultrasound and Fracture Healing

1. Clinical studies show that low-intensity pulsed ultrasound accelerates fracture healing and increases the mechanical strength of callus including torque and stiffness.

2. The postulated mechanism of action is that the cells responsible for fracture healing respond in a favorable manner to the mechanical energy transmitted by the ultrasound signal.

G. Electricity and Fracture Healing

1. Definitions
   - Stress-generated potentials—Serve as signals that modulate cellular activity. Piezoelectric effect and streaming potentials are examples of stress-generated potentials.
   - Piezoelectric effect—Charges in tissues are displaced secondary to mechanical forces.
   - Streaming potentials—Occur when electrically charged fluid is forced over a tissue (cell membrane) with a fixed charge.
   - Transmembrane potentials—Generated by cellular metabolism.

2. Fracture healing—Electrical properties of cartilage and bone are dependent on their charged molecules. Devices intended to stimulate fracture repair by altering a variety of cellular activities have been introduced.

3. Types of electrical stimulation
   - Direct current (DC)—Stimulates an inflammatory-like response.
   - Alternating current (AC)—"capacity coupled generators." Affects cyclic AMP, collagen synthesis, and calcification during the repair stage.

- Pulsed electromagnetic fields (PEMF)—Initiate calcification of fibrocartilage (cannot induce calcification of fibrous tissue), upregulate BMPs and TGF-β.

H. Effect of Radiation on Bone

1. Long-term changes of bone injury following high dose irradiation are the result of changes in the Haversian system and a decrease in overall cellularity.

2. High dose irradiation (90 kGy, the dose needed for viral inactivation) of allograft bone significantly reduces its structural integrity.

IV. Bone Grafts

A. Overview—Bone grafts are an important adjunct in the treatment of fractures, delayed unions, and nonunions. Bone grafts have four important properties.

B. Graft Properties (Table 2-8)

1. Osteoconductive matrix—Acts as a scaffold or framework into which bone growth occurs.

2. Osteoinductive factors—Growth factors such as BMP and TGF-β promote bone formation.

3. Osteogenic cells—Include primitive mesenchymal cells, osteoblasts, and osteocytes.

4. Structural integrity

C. Specific Bone Graft Types

1. Type of graft
   - Cortical grafts—Incorporate through slow remodeling of existing Haversian systems via a process of resorption (which weakens the graft) followed by deposition of the new bone (restoring its strength). Resorption is confined to the osteon borders, and interstitial lamellae are preserved. Cortical bone is slower to turn over compared with cancellous bone, and it is used for structural defects.
   - Cancellous grafts—Cancellous bone is commonly used for grafting nonunions or cavitary defects because it is quickly remodeled and incorporated (via creeping substitution). Cancellous bone is rapidly revascularized; osteoblasts lay down new bone on old trabeculae, which are later remodeled ("creeping substitution").
   - Vascularized bone grafts—Although technically difficult, they allow more rapid union with preservation of most cells. Vascularized grafts are best employed for irradiated tissues or when large tissue defects exist. (However, there may be donor site morbidity with vascularized grafts [i.e., fibula]).
   - Osteoarticular (osteochondral) allografts—These are being used with increasing frequency for tumor surgery. These grafts are

TABLE 2-7

Effects of Hormones on Fracture Healing

Hormone	Effect	Mechanism
Growth hormone	Positive	Increased callus volume
Thyroid hormone	Positive	Bone remodeling
Parathyroid hormone	Positive	Bone remodeling
Calcitonin	Positive?	Unknown
Cortisone	Negative	Decreased callus proliferation

TABLE 2-8

Bone Graft Properties

Graft	Osteoconduction	Osteoinduction	Osteogenic Cells	Structural Integrity	Other Properties
Cancellous autograft	Excellent	Good	Excellent	Poor	Rapid incorporation
Cortical autograft	Fair	Fair	Fair	Excellent	Slow incorporation
Allograft	Fair	Fair	None	Good	***Fresh*** has the highest immunogenicity. ***Freeze dried*** is the least immunogenic but has the least structural integrity (weakest). ***Fresh frozen*** preserves bone morphogenic proteins (BMP)
Ceramics	Fair	None	None	Fair	
Demineralized bone matrix (DBM)	Fair	Good	None	Poor	
Bone marrow	Poor	Poor	Good	Poor	

Source: Modified from Brinker MR, Miller MD. *Fundamentals of Orthopaedics*. Philadelphia, PA: WB Saunders; 1999:7, with permission.

immunogenic (cartilage is vulnerable to inflammatory mediators of immune response [cytotoxic injury from antibodies and lymphocytes]); the articular cartilage is preserved with glycerol or dimethyl sulfoxide treatment; ***cryogenically preserved grafts leave few viable chondrocytes***. Tissue-matched fresh osteochondral grafts produce minimal immunogenic effect and incorporate well.

- ***Demineralized bone matrix (Grafton)—It is both osteoconductive and osteoinductive***.
- Bone marrow cells

2. Source of Graft
   - Autograft—Bone is harvested from the same person.
   - Allograft—Bone is harvested from a cadaveric donor. All allografts must be harvested with sterile technique, and donors must be screened for potential transmissible diseases.
   - Synthetic grafts—Composed of calcium, silicon, or aluminum.
     (a) Silicate-based grafts—These incorporate the element silicon (Si) in the form of silicate (silicon dioxide).
        - Bioactive glasses
        - Glass-ionomer cement
     (b) Calcium phosphate-based grafts—These grafts are capable of osseoconduction and osseointegration. ***These materials biodegrade at a very slow rate***. Many are prepared as ceramics (apatite crystals are heated to fuse the crystals [sintered]).
        - Tricalcium phosphate
        - Hydroxyapatite (e.g., Collagraft Bone Graft Matrix [Zimmer, Inc., Warsaw, IN, USA]; purified bovine dermal fibrillar collagen plus ceramic hydroxyapatite granules and β-tricalcium phosphate granules).
     (c) Calcium sulfate—Osteoconductive (e.g., OsteoSet [Wright Medical Technology Inc., Arlington, TN, USA]).
     (d) Calcium carbonate (chemically unaltered marine coral)—It is resorbed and replaced by bone (osteoconductive) (e.g., Biocora; Inoteb, France).
     (e) Corralline hydroxyapatite—Calcium carbonate skeleton is converted to calcium phosphate via a thermoexchange process (e.g., Interpore 200 and 500; Interpore Orthopaedics, Irvine, CA, USA).
     (f) Other materials
        - Aluminum oxide—Alumina ceramic bonds to bone in response to stress and strain between implant and bone.
        - Hard tissue—A replacement polymer is used.

D. Graft Preparation—Allograft bone can be prepared using a variety of methods.
   1. Fresh (increased antigenicity due to **cell surface glycoproteins**)
   2. Fresh frozen—Less immunogenic than fresh. Fresh frozen allograft bone preserves bone morphogenetic proteins (BMPs). The marrow cells of a bone allograft incite the greatest immunogenic response as compared with other constituents.
   3. Freeze-dried (lyophilized)—Loses structural integrity and depletes BMPs. Freeze-dried allograft bone is **least immunogenic and purely osteoconductive and lowest likelihood of viral transmission,** commonly known as "croutons."
   4. Bone matrix gelatin is the digested source of BMPs.

V. Distraction Osteogenesis (Fig. 2-5)
   A. Definition—The use of distraction to stimulate the formation of bone.
   B. Clinical Applications
      1. Limb lengthening
      2. Hypertrophic nonunions
      3. Deformity correction (via differential lengthening)
      4. Segmental bone loss (via bone transport)

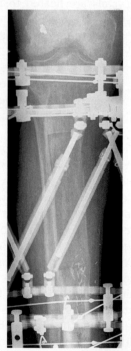

FIGURE 2-5 Radiograph of a patient who has undergone bone transport for a large distal tibial segmental defect. This AP radiograph of the proximal tibia shows the regenerate of distraction osteogenesis; bone formation is via intramembranous ossification.

C. Biology
   1. Under optimal stable conditions, **bone is formed via intramembranous ossification**.
   2. In an unstable environment, bone forms via enchondral ossification or, in an extremely unstable environment, a pseudoarthrosis may occur.
D. Histological Phases
   1. Latency phase (5–7 days)
   2. Distraction phase (typically 1 mm per day, approximately 1 inch per month)
   3. Consolidation phase (typically twice as long as the distraction phase)
E. Conditions That Promote Optimal Bone Formation During Distraction Osteogenis
   1. Low energy corticotomy or osteotomy
   2. Minimal soft-tissue stripping at the corticotomy site (preserving the blood supply)
   3. Stable external fixation to eliminate torsion, shear, and bending moments
   4. Latency period (no lengthening) of 5 to 7 days
   5. Distraction at 0.25 mm three to four times per day (0.75 to 1.0 mm per day)
   6. Neutral fixation interval (no distraction) during consolidation
   7. Normal physiologic use of the extremity, including weight bearing

VI. Imaging
   A. Nuclear Medicine
      1. Bone scan—**Technetium 99m-phosphate complexes reflect increased blood flow and metabolism and are absorbed onto the hydroxyapatite crystals of bone in areas of infection, trauma, neoplasia, and so forth.** Whole-body views and more detailed (pin-hole) views can be obtained. It is particularly useful for the diagnosis of subtle fracture, avascular necrosis (hypoperfused [diminished blood flow] early, increased uptake during the reparative phase), and osteomyelitis (especially when a triple-phase study is performed in conjunction with a gallium or indium scan). Three-phase (or even four-phase) studies may be helpful for evaluating diseases such as complex regional pain syndrome and osteomyelitis. The three phases of a triple phase bone scan are as follows:
         • **First phase (blood flow, immediate)**— This phase displays blood flow through the arterial system.
         • **Second phase (blood pool, 30 minutes)**— This phase displays equilibrium of tracer throughout the intravascular volume.

- **Third phase (delayed, 4 hours)**—This phase displays the sites at which the tracer accumulates.
2. Gallium scan—**Gallium 67 citrate localizes in sites of inflammation and neoplasia probably because of exudation of labeled serum proteins**. Delayed imaging (usually 24–48 hours or more) is required. Gallium scan is frequently used in conjunction with a bone scan—A "double tracer" technique. Gallium is less dependent on vascular flow than technetium and may identify foci that would otherwise be missed. It is difficult to differentiate cellulitis from osteomyelitis on a gallium scan.
3. Indium scan—**Indium 111-labeled WBC's (leukocytes) accumulate in areas of inflammation and do not collect in areas of neoplasia**. Indium scan is useful for evaluation of **acute infections** (such as osteomyelitis).
4. Technetium-Labeled WBC Scan—Similar to indium scan.

B. Magnetic Resonance Imaging
1. Overview—Magnetic resonance imaging (MRI) is an excellent study to evaluate the soft tissues and bone marrow. It is used frequently to evaluate osteonecrosis, neoplasms, infection, and trauma. MRI allows both axial and sagittal representations. It is contraindicated in patients with pacemakers, cerebral aneurysm clips, or shrapnel or hardware in certain locations.
2. Specific applications of MRI
   - Osteonecrosis—**MRI is the most sensitive method for early detection of osteonecrosis** (detects early marrow necrosis and ingrowth of vascularized mesenchymal tissue) (tomography is the best method for **staging** ON [of the hip]). MRI is highly specific (98%) and reliable for estimating age and extent of disease. T_1 images demonstrate diseased marrow as dark. MRI allows direct assessment of overlying cartilage.
   - Infection and trauma—MRI has excellent sensitivity to the increases in free water and demonstrates areas of infection and fresh hemorrhage (dark on T_1, and bright on T_2 studies; **postgadolinium T1-weighted image with fat suppression showing a bright bone marrow signal relative to the surrounding fat suggests osteomyelitis). MRI is an excellent (accurate and sensitive) method for evaluating occult fractures (particularly in the elderly hip)**.

C. Computed Tomography (CT)—It continues to be important for evaluating many orthopaedic areas. **CT demonstrates bony anatomy better than any other study**. CT best demonstrates joint incongruity following closed reduction of a dislocated hip. More recent **Multidetector CT (MDCT) uses more of the x-ray beams to produce a much higher resolution image**.

D. Measurement of Bone Density (Noninvasive Methods)—Several methods are available for measuring bone density and assessing the risk of fracture. These methods may be particularly useful in geriatric patients with fractures related to decreased bone density.
1. Single photon absorptiometry—The basic principle of this technique is that the density of the cortical bone being tested is inversely proportional to the quantity of photons passing through it. The best use of single photon absorptiometry is the appendicular skeleton (radius-diaphysis or distal metaphysis); the test cannot be reliably used for the axial skeleton (due to alterations caused by the depth of the soft tissues).
2. Dual photon absorptiometry—Similar to single photon absorptiometry, dual photon absorptiometry is an isotope-based means of measuring bone density. Dual photon absorptiometry, however, allows for measurement of the axial skeleton and the femoral neck (the method accounts for the attenuation of the signal which is caused by the soft tissues overlying the spine and the hip).
3. Quantitative computed tomography—Allows preferential measurement of trabecular bone density (the bone which is at the greatest risk of early metabolic changes). The technique involves the simultaneous scanning of phantoms of known density in order to create a standard calibration curve. Precision is excellent; accuracy is within 5% to 10%.
4. Dual-Energy X-ray absorptiometry (DEXA)—DEXA measures **bone mineral content and soft-tissue composition** by emitting X-ray beams at two different energy levels, which are differentially absorbed by different tissues. By evaluating the difference in the aborbances of the two beams, the presence and density of target tissues, such as bone, can be quantified. **DEXA is the most reliable and accurate method of predicting fracture risk, and has a lower radiation dose than quantitative CT**.

VII. Complications of Fractures
   A. Delayed Union—Represents a fracture that has failed to unite in the anticipated time frame but continues to show some biologic activity.
   B. Nonunion (Fig. 2-6)—Represents a fracture without clinical or radiographic evidence of healing (and without evidence of the ability for progression to healing).
      1. Atrophic nonunion—These nonunions are *avascular and lack the biological capacity to heal*. The ends of the bone are typically narrowed (such as a pencil point) and are avascular. The treatment of an atrophic nonunion is stimulation of the local biological activity (such as with a bone graft or a corticotomy for bone transport).
      2. Hypertrophic nonunions—These nonunions are *hypervascular and possess the biological capacity to heal but lack mechanical stability*. The ends of the bone are typically hypertrophied, and they give the appearance that the fracture has "attempted to heal." The treatment of a hypertrophic nonunion is to add further mechanical stability (such as with plate and screw fixation); bone grafting is not needed. *The initial biological response of a hypertrophic nonunion to plate stabilization is mineralization of fibrocartilage*.
      3. Oligotrophic nonunions—Have an adequate blood supply but little or no callus formation. Oligotrophic nonunions arise from inadequate reduction with displacement at the fracture site. The treatment of an oligotrophic nonunion is reduction to obtain contact between bone ends and mechanical stability.
      4. Infected nonunions—Nonunions associated with a chronic infection of bone. The treatment of an infected nonunion focuses first on eliminating the infection and then on healing the bone.
   C. Malunion (see Chapter 3, Principles of Deformities)
   D. Bone Infections
      1. Introduction—Osteomyelitis is an infection of bone and bone marrow which may be caused by direct inoculation of an open traumatic wound or by blood borne organisms (hematogenous). *It is not possible to predict the microscopic organism that is causing osteomyelitis based on the clinical picture and the age of the patient; therefore, a specific microbiologic diagnosis via deep cultures with sampling from multiple foci is essential (organisms isolated from sinus tract drainage typically do not accurately reflect the organisms present deep within the wound and within bone)*.
      2. Acute hematogenous osteomyelitis—Bone and bone marrow infection caused by blood borne organisms. Children are commonly affected (boys are more commonly affected than girls). In children, the infection is most common in the metaphysis or epiphysis of the long bones and is more common in the lower extremity than in the upper extremity. Radiographic changes of acute hematogenous osteomyelitis include soft-tissue swelling (early), bone demineralization (10–14 days), and *sequestra* (dead bone with surround granulation tissue) and *involucrum* (periosteal new bone) later.
         • Adults, 21 years of age or older—The most common organism is *Staphylococcus aureus,* but a wide variety of other organisms have been isolated. Initial empiric therapy includes nafcillin, oxacillin, or cefazolin; vancomycin can be used as an alternative initial therapy.
         • Sickle cell anemia—*Salmonella* is a characteristic organism. The primary treatment is with one of the fluoroquinolones (only in adults); alternative treatment is with a third generation Cephalosporin.
         • Hemodialysis patients and intravenous drug abusers—*S. aureus, S. epidermidis,* and *Pseudomonas aeruginosa* are common organisms. The treatment of choice is one of the penicillinase-resistant semisynthetic penicillins (PRSPs) plus Ciprofloxacin; an alternative treatment is vancomycin with Ciprofloxacin.
      3. Acute osteomyelitis (following open fracture or following open reduction with internal fixation)—Clinical findings may be similar to that of acute hematogenous osteomyelitis. Treatment includes radical irrigation and debridement with removal of orthopaedic hardware as necessary. Open wounds may require rotational or free flaps. The most common offending organisms are *S. aureus, P. aeruginosa*, and coliforms. Empiric therapy prior to definitive cultures is Nafcillin with Ciprofloxacin; alternative therapy is Vancomycin with a third generation Cephalosporin. Patients with acute osteomyelitis and vascular insufficiency and those who are immunocompromised generally show a polymicrobic picture.
      4. Chronic osteomyelitis—May arise as a result of an inappropriately treated acute osteomyelitis, trauma, or soft-tissue spread, especially

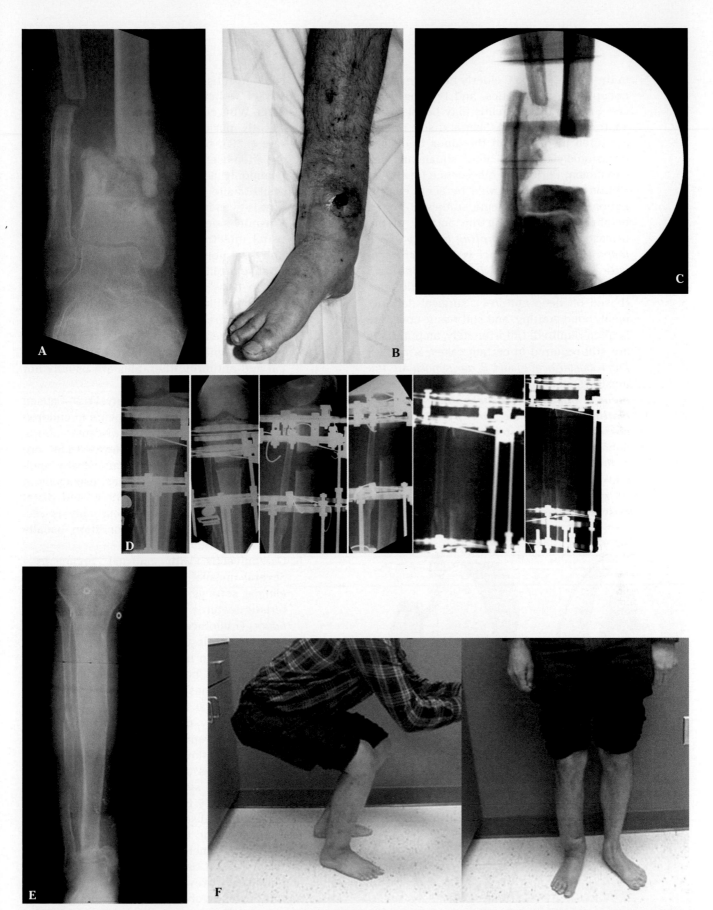

FIGURE 2-6 **A.** AP radiograph and **(B)** clinical photograph of a 59-year-old man with a grossly infected nonunion of the right distal tibia. **C.** Intraoperative radiograph following segmental bony resection of infected and necrotic bone.
D. Sequence of radiographs during proximal-to-distal bone transport. **E.** Final radiograph showing solid bony union.
F. Clinical photographs showing full weightbearing and excellent range of knee and ankle motion.

33

in the Cierney Type C elderly host, the immunosuppressed, diabetics, and IV drug abusers. Chronic osteomyelitis may be classified anatomically (Fig. 2-7). Skin and soft tissues are often involved and the sinus tract may occasionally develop into squamous cell carcinoma. Periods of quiescence (of the infection) are often followed by acute exacerbations. Nuclear medicine studies are often helpful for determining the activity of the disease. *Operative sampling of deep specimens from multiple foci is the most accurate means of identifying the pathologic organisms*. A combination of IV antibiotics (based on deep cultures), surgical debridement, bone grafting, and soft-tissue coverage is often required. Unfortunately, amputations are still required in certain cases. *S. aureus, Enterobacteriaceae*, and *P. aeruginosa* are the most frequent offending organisms. *Treatment is based on cultures and sensitivity testing and empiric therapy is not indicated in chronic osteomyelitis*.

5. Subacute osteomyelitis—Usually discovered radiologically in a patient with a painful limp and no systemic (and often no local) signs or symptoms. Subacute osteomyelitis may arise secondary to a partially treated acute osteomyelitis or may occasionally develop in a fracture hematoma. Unlike acute osteomyelitis, WBC count and blood cultures are frequently normal. Erythrocyte sedimentation rate (ESR), bone cultures, and radiographs are often useful. Subacute osteomyelitis most commonly affects the femur and tibia; and unlike acute osteomyelitis, it can cross the physis even in older children.

6. Chronic sclerosing osteomyelitis—An unusual infection that involves primarily diaphyseal bones of adolescents. Typified by intense proliferation of the periosteum leading to bony deposition, it may be caused by anaerobic organisms. Insidious onset, dense progressive sclerosis on radiographs, and localized pain and tenderness are common. Malignancy must be ruled out. Surgical and antibiotic therapies are usually not curative.

7. Chronic multifocal osteomyelitis—Caused by an infectious agent, it appears in children without systemic symptoms. Normal laboratory values, except for an elevated ESR, are common. Radiographs demonstrate multiple metaphyseal lytic lesions, especially in the medial clavicle, distal tibia, and distal femur. Symptomatic treatment only is recommended because this condition usually resolves spontaneously.

8. Osteomyelitis with unusual organisms—Several unusual organisms occur in certain clinical settings. Radiographs show characteristic features in syphilis (*Treponema pallidum*) (radiolucency in the metaphysis from granulation tissue) and tuberculosis (joint destruction on both sides of a joint). Histology can also be helpful (e.g., tuberculosis with granulomas).

E. Complex Regional Pain Syndrome—A disorder characterized by pain, hyperesthesia, tenderness of the extremity, as well as local irregularities in blood flow, sweating, and edema. The disorder involves an abnormality of the autonomic nervous system, commonly following trauma or surgery. Early clinical findings include burning pain, and sensitivity, which is out of the proportion to the traumatic or surgical insult. Later changes include dystrophic changes to the skin and soft tissues, which are progressive and ultimately irreversible. Radiographic examination of the involved extremity shows diffuse osteopenia. Treatment is with early recognition, aggressive physical therapy, and consideration of sympathetic blockade.

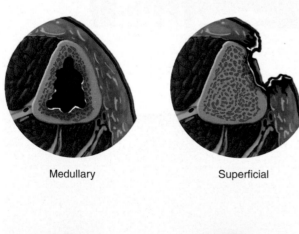

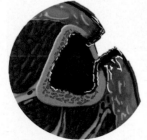

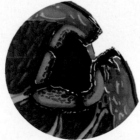

Medullary   Superficial

Localized   Diffuse

FIGURE 2-7 Cierny's anatomic classification of adult chronic osteomyelitis.

F. Heterotopic Ossification (HO)—Ectopic bone forms in the soft tissues, most commonly in response to an injury or a surgical dissection. Myositis ossificans (MO) is a form of HO that occurs specifically when the ossification is in muscle. Patients with traumatic brain injuries are particularly prone to developing HO and recurrence following operative resection is likely if the neurologic compromise is severe. Common sites of posttraumatic HO include the elbow, hip, and thigh; *Injury Severity Score is correlated with formation of HO following knee dislocation*. Irradiation (usually in doses of 700 rad) prevents proliferation and differentiation of primordial mesenchymal cells into osteoprogenitor cells that can form osteoblastic tissue. Oral diphosphonates inhibit mineralization of osteoid, but do not prevent the formation of osteoid matrix; when the oral diphosphonate therapy is discontinued, mineralization with formation of HO may occur.

G. Compartment Syndrome (see Chapter 1, General Principles of Trauma)

H. Neurovascular Injuries—Vary based on anatomic location (See specific chapters). Neurovascular injuries may arise as a result of the traumatic injury itself, or the surgical procedure involved in treating the injury.

I. Avascular Necrosis—Incidence varies by injury type and anatomic location (See specific chapters).

SUGGESTED READINGS

Classic Articles

Amadio PC. Pain dysfunction syndromes. *J Bone Joint Surg.* 1988;70A:944–949.

Burchardt H. The biology of bone graft repair. *Clin Orthop.* 1983;174:28–42.

Christian EP, Bosse MJ, Robb G. Reconstruction of large diaphyseal defects without free fibular transfer, in Grade-IIIB tibial fractures. *J Bone Joint Surg.* 1989;71A:994–1004.

Cierny G III, Byrd HS, Jones RE. Primary versus delayed soft tissue coverage for severe open tibial fractures: a comparison of results. *Clin Orthop.* 1983;178:54–63.

Gustilo RB, Gruninger RP, Davis T. Classification of type III (severe) open fractures relative to treatment and results. *Orthopedics.* 1987;10:1781–1788.

Gustilo RB, Mendoza RM, Williams DN. Problems in the management of type III (severe) open fractures: a new classification of type III open fractures. *J Trauma.* 1984;24:742–746.

Gustilo RB, Merkow RL, Templeman D. The management of open fractures: current concepts. *J Bone Joint Surg.* 1990;72A:299–304.

Kessler SB, Hallfeldt KKJ, Perren SM, et al. The effects of reaming and intramedullary nailing on fracture healing. *Clin Orthop.* 1986;212:18–25.

Lane JM, Suda M, von der Mark K, et al. Immunofluorescent localization of structural collagen types in endochondral fracture repair. *J Orthop Res.* 1986;4:318–329.

Neale HW, Stern PJ, Kreilein JG, et al. Complications of muscle-flap transposition for traumatic defects of the leg. *Plast Reconstr Surg.* 1983;72:512–517.

Nelson CL, Green TG, Porter RA, et al. One day versus seven days of preventive antibiotic therapy in orthopaedic surgery. *Clin Orthop.* 1983;176:258–263.

Panjabi MM, Walter SD, Karuda M, et al. Correlation of radiographic analysis of healing fractures with strength: a statistical analysis of experimental osteotomies. *J Orthop Res.* 1985;3:212–218.

Patzakis MJ, Wilkins J. Factors influencing infection rate in open fracture wounds. *Clin Orthop.* 1989;343:36–40.

Seale KS. Reflex sympathetic dystrophy of the lower extremity. *Clin Orthop Relat Res.* 1989;243:80–85.

Urist MR. Bone: formation by autoinduction. *Science.* 1965;150:893–899.

Van de Putte KA, Urist MR. Osteogenesis in the interior of intramuscular implants of decalcified bone matrix. *Clin Orthop Relat Res.* 1965;43:257–240.

Wahlig H, Dingeldein E, Bergmann R, et al. The release of gentamycin from polymethylmethacrylate beads: an experimental and pharmacokinetic study. *J Bone Joint Surg.* 1978;60B:270.

Waters RL, Campbell JM, Perry J. Energy cost of three-point crutch ambulation in fracture patients. *J Orthop Trauma.* 1987;1:170–173.

Wood MB, Cooney WP III. Above elbow limp replantation: functional results. *J Hand Surg.* 1986;11A:682–687.

Wood MB, Cooney WP, Irons GB. Lower extremity salvage and reconstruction by free-tissue transfer: analysis of results. *Clin Orthop.* 1985;201:151–161.

Recent Articles

Brinker MR, O'Connor DP, Monla YT, et al. Metabolic and endocrine abnormalities in patients with nonunions. *J Orthop Trauma.* 2007;21:557–570.

Cheng H, Jiang W, Phillips FM, et al. Osteogenic activity of the fourteen types of human bone morphogenetic proteins (BMPs). *J Bone Joint Surg.* 2003;85-A:1544–1552.

Clowes JA, Peel NF, Eastell R. Device-specific thresholds to diagnose osteoporosis at the proximal femur: an Approach to interpreting peripheral bone measurements in clinical practice. *Osteoporos Int.* 2006;17:1293–1302.

Engelke K, Libanati C, Liu Y, et al. Quantitative computed tomography (QCT) of the forearm using general purpose spiral whole-body CT scanners: accuracy, precision and comparison with dual-energy X-ray absorptiometry (DXA). *Bone.* 2009;45:110–118.

Gocke DJ. Tissue donor selection and safety. *Clin Orthop Relat Res.* 2005;435:17–21.

Holtom PD. Antibiotic prophylaxis: current recommendations. *J Am Acad Orthop Surg.* 2006;14:S98–S100.

Kanakaris NK, Calori GM, Verdonk R, et al. Application of BMP-7 to tibial non-unions: a 3-year multicenter experience. *Injury.* 2008;39(suppl 2):S83–S90.

Mills WJ, Tejwani N. Heterotopic ossification after knee dislocation: the predictive value of the injury severity score. *J Orthop Trauma.* 2003;17:338–345.

Mroz TE, Joyce MJ, Lieberman IH, et al. The use of allograft bone in spine surgery: is it safe? *Spine J.* 2009;9:303–308.

Allograft Safety and Ethical Considerations. Proceedings of the fourth symposium sponsored by the musculoskeletal transplant foundation. September 2003. Edinburgh, Scotland, United Kingdom. *Clin Orthop Relat Res.* 2005;435:2–117.

Patzakis MJ, Bains RS, Lee J, et al. Prospective, randomized, double-blind study comparing single-agent antibiotic therapy, ciprofloxacin, to combination antibiotic therapy in open fracture wounds. *J Orthop Trauma.* 2000;14:529–533.

Slongo T, Audigé L, Clavert JM, et al. The AO comprehensive classification of pediatric long-bone fractures: a web-based multicenter agreement study. *J Pediatr Orthop.* 2007;27:171–180.

Tielinen L, Lindahl JE, Tukiainen EJ. Acute unreamed intramedullary nailing and soft tissue reconstruction with muscle flaps for the treatment of severe open tibial shaft fractures. *Injury.* 2007;38:906–912.

Vercillo M, Patzakis MJ, Holtom P, et al. Linezolid in the treatment of implant-related chronic osteomyelitis. *Clin Orthop Relat Res.* 2007;461:40–43.

Wang J, Zhou J, Cheng CM, et al. Evidence supporting dual, IGF-I-independent and IGF-I-dependent, roles for GH in promoting longitudinal bone growth. *Endocrinol.* 2004;180:247–255.

Webb LX, Bosse MJ, Castillo RC, et al. Analysis of surgeon-controlled variables in the treatment of limb-threatening type-III open tibial diaphyseal fractures. *J Bone Joint Surg Am.* 2007;89:923–928.

Zalavras CG, Patzakis MJ, Holtom P. Local antibiotic therapy in the treatment of open fractures and osteomyelitis. *Clin Orthop Relat Res.* 2004;427:86–93.

Review Articles

De Long WG Jr, Einhorn TA, Koval K, et al. Bone grafts and bone graft substitutes in orthopaedic trauma surgery. A critical analysis. *J Bone Joint Surg Am.* 2007;89:649–658.

Fulkerson EW, Egol KA. Timing issues in fracture management: a review of current concepts. *Bull NYU Hosp Jt Dis.* 2009;67:58–67.

Gosselin RA, Roberts I, Gillespie WJ. Antibiotics for preventing infection in open limb fractures. *Cochrane Database Syst Rev.* 2004;1:CD003764. doi: 10.1002/14651858.CD003764.pub2.

Hannouche D, Petite H, Sedel L. Current trends in the enhancement of fracture healing. *J Bone Joint Surg Br.* 2001;83:157–164.

Khan Y, Yaszemski MJ, Mikos AG, et al. Tissue engineering of bone: material and matrix considerations. *J Bone Joint Surg Am.* 2008;90(suppl 1):36–42.

Koman LA, Smith BP, Ekman EF, et al. Complex regional pain syndrome. *Instr Course Lect.* 2005;54:11–20.

Kwong FNK, Harris MB. Recent developments in the biology of fracture repair. *J Am Acad Orthop Surg.* 2008;16:619–625.

Lieberman J, Daluiski A, Einhorn TA. The role of growth factors in the repair of bone: biology and clinical applications. *J Bone Joint Surg Am.* 2002;84:1032–1044.

Nelson FR, Brighton CT, Ryaby J. Use of physical forces in bone healing. *J Am Acad Orthop Surg.* 2003;11:344–354.

Textbooks

Brinker MR, O'Connor DP. Basic sciences. In: Miller MD, ed. *Review of Orthopaedics.* 5th ed. Philadelphia, PA: WB Saunders; 2008.

Brinker MR, O'Connor DP. Nonunions: evaluation and treatment. In: Browner BD, Jupiter JB, Levine AM, Trafton PG, eds. *Skeletal Trauma: Basic Science, Management, and Reconstruction.* 4th ed. Philadelphia, PA: WB Saunders; 2009:615–708.

Calhoun JH, Mader J, eds. *Musculoskeletal Infections.* New York, NY: Taylor & Francis; 2003.

Dabov G. Osteomyelitis. In: Canale ST, ed. *Campbell's Operative Orthopaedics.* 10th ed. Philadelphia, PA: Mosby; 2003:661–683.

Einhorn TA, O'Keefe RJ, Buckwalter JA, eds. *Orthopaedic Basic Science: Foundations of Clinical Practice.* 3rd ed. Rosemont, IL: American Academy of Orthopaedic Surgeons; 2000.

Kakar S, Einhorn TA. Biology and enhancement of skeletal repair. In: Browner BD, Jupiter JB, Levine AM, et al., eds. *Skeletal Trauma: Basic Science, Management, and Reconstruction.* Vol 1. 4th ed. Philadelphia, PA: WB Saunders, 2009:33–50.

Lieberman JR, Friedlaender GE, eds. *Bone Regeneration and Repair: Biology and Clinical Applications.* New York, NY: Springer-Verlag; 2004.

Mow VC, Huiskes R, eds. *Basic Orthopaedic Biomechanics and Mechano-Biology.* 3rd ed. Philadelphia, PA: Lippincott, Williams, and Wilkins; 2004.

Sirkin M, Liporace F, Behrens FF. Fractures with soft tissue injuries. In: Browner BD, Jupiter JB, Levine AM, et al., eds. *Skeletal Trauma: Basic Science, Management, and Reconstruction.* Vol 1. 4th ed. Philadelphia, PA: WB Saunders; 2009:367–396.

CHAPTER 3

Principles of Deformities

Joseph J. Gugenheim Jr.

I. Consequences of Lower Extremity Deformity
  A. Although degenerative arthritis has multiple etiologies, limb deformity may be one etiology due to:
    1. Eccentric stress on joint
    2. Shear stress on joint
  B. Limb length inequality may cause:
    1. Increased energy consumption with gait
    2. Possible detrimental effect on hip and spine (controversial)

II. Skeletal Deformity Is a Vector
  A. Like all vectors, a deformity has three components:
    1. Magnitude—The magnitude of a skeletal deformity has six components.
      • Three angulations—In a xyz three-dimensional coordinate system:
        (a) Angulation in the xy (anteroposterior [AP]) plane is:
          • Varus
          • Valgus
        (b) Angulation in the yz (lateral) plane is:
          • Apex anterior
          • Apex posterior
        (c) Angulation in the xz plane is:
          • Internal rotation
          • External rotation
      • Three translations—By convention in orthopedics, the direction of translation of the distal segment of the extremity with respect to the proximal segment determines the direction.
        (a) Translation on the x-axis (AP plane)
          • Medial translation
          • Lateral translation
        (b) Translation on the y-axis
          • Lengthening
          • Shortening
        (c) Translation on the z-axis (lateral plane)
          • Anterior translation
          • Posterior translation
      • A deformity may consist of a component in one, two, or three planes.
        (a) A deformity with a component in more than one plane is not a biplanar or triplanar deformity; it is an *oblique plane deformity*.
        (b) The magnitude of the oblique plane deformity is greater than the component of greatest magnitude in any of the three orthogonal planes.
    2. Direction (or orientation)
    3. Location
  B. Standardized radiographic techniques are necessary to measure the magnitude, direction, and location of the deformity.
  C. These three components can be used to accurately describe a deformity due to:
    1. Malunion
    2. Acute fracture
    3. Developmental and congenital disorders

III. For accurate deformity correction, it is both necessary and sufficient to correct:
  A. AP Mechanical Axis of the Extremity
  B. Joint Orientation Angles in all Three Orthogonal Planes
  C. Limb length inequality

IV. Mechanical Axis of the Lower Extremity
  A. The mechanical axis of the lower extremity is a straight line from the center of the hip to the center of the ankle on the AP radiograph (Fig. 3-1).
  B. In a normal lower extremity, the mechanical axis line intersects the knee at the center of the tibial spines or a maximum of 10 mm medial to the center of the spines.
  C. The distance in millimeters from the center of the tibial spines to the mechanical axis is mechanical axis deviation (MAD) (Fig. 3-2).
    1. Medial MAD is varus.
    2. Lateral MAD is valgus.

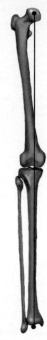

FIGURE 3-1 Mechanical axis of the lower extremity, which normally lies 0 to 10 mm medial to the knee joint center. (Adapted with permission from Brinker MR, O'Connor DP. Principles of malunions. In: Bucholz, RW, Court-Brown CM, Heckman JD, et al., eds. *Rockwood and Green's Fractures in Adults*. 7th ed. Philadelphia, PA: Lippincott Williams & Wilkins; 2010.)

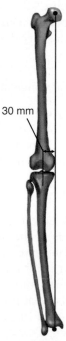

30 mm

FIGURE 3-2 Medial mechanical axis deviation. (Reprinted with permission from Brinker MR, O'Connor DP. Principles of malunions. In: Bucholz, RW, Court-Brown CM, Heckman JD, et al., eds. *Rockwood and Green's Fractures in Adults*. 7th ed. Philadelphia, PA: Lippincott Williams & Wilkins, 2010.)

D. Standardized radiographic imaging technique to insure accuracy and reproducibility requires:
1. A 51- × 14-in cassette with a variable grid to visualize the hip, knee, and ankle joints
2. A distance of 10 ft from the beam source to the film to minimize magnification and distortion, with the beam centered at the knee
3. Patient weight bearing, with weight equally distributed on both feet (Fig. 3-3)
   - Patellas straightforward.
   - Knees fully extended.
   - If there is a limb length discrepancy, a block should be placed under the shorter extremity to level the pelvis and to keep the knees extended with weight evenly distributed.
4. Magnification can be calculated precisely by affixing a 30-mm ball bearing at the level of

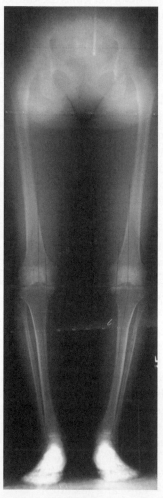

FIGURE 3-3 Bilateral weight-bearing 51-in AP alignment radiograph. (Reprinted with permission from Brinker MR, O'Connor DP. Principles of malunions. In: Bucholz, RW, Court-Brown CM, Heckman JD, et al., eds. *Rockwood and Green's Fractures in Adults*. 7th ed. Philadelphia, PA: Lippincott Williams & Wilkins, 2010.)

the bone and measuring the image of the ball bearing with calipers. Placing the ball bearing or a ruler with radiopaque graduations on the cassette will not facilitate measurement of magnification because they are closer to the film than the bone.

E. There is no similarly defined mechanical axis of the lower extremity in the sagittal plane (lateral view) because the knee flexes and extends during the gait cycle. However, the following technique is used to obtain an image orthogonal to the AP view (Fig. 3-4).

1. The patella is directed lateral, 90° to the position on the AP view.
2. Only one extremity can be imaged on a 51- × 14-in film.

3. The pelvis is rotated slightly to avoid superimposing both lower extremities.
4. The imaged knee is in maximum extension.

V. Axes of the Femur and Tibia

A. AP Mechanical Axes of the Femur and Tibia—In addition to the mechanical axis of the lower extremity, there are mechanical axes of the femur and the tibia. In the normal lower extremity, the mechanical axis of the femur and the mechanical axis of the tibia coincide with the mechanical axis of the lower extremity. Just as normal mechanical axis of the lower extremity (colinearity of the hip, knee, and ankle) is necessary but not sufficient for accurate deformity correction, superimposable mechanical axes of the femur and tibia with the mechanical axis of the lower extremity are necessary but not sufficient for accurate deformity correction.

1. The AP mechanical axis of the femur is a straight line from the center of the hip to the center of the knee (Fig. 3-5).

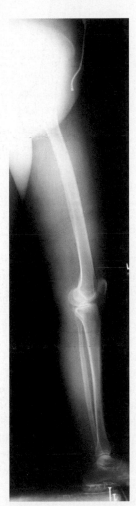

FIGURE 3-4   51-in lateral alignment radiograph. (Reprinted with permission from Brinker MR, O'Connor DP. Principles of malunions. In: Bucholz, RW, Court-Brown CM, Heckman JD, et al., eds. *Rockwood and Green's Fractures in Adults*. 7th ed. Philadelphia, PA: Lippincott Williams & Wilkins, 2010.)

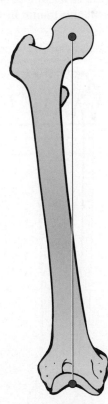

FIGURE 3-5   The mechanical axis of a long bone is defined as the line that passes through the joint centers of the proximal and distal joints. The mechanical axis of the femur is shown here. (Reprinted with permission from Brinker MR, O'Connor DP. Principles of malunions. In: Bucholz, RW, Court-Brown CM, Heckman JD, et al., eds. *Rockwood and Green's Fractures in Adults*. 7th ed. Philadelphia, PA: Lippincott Williams & Wilkins, 2010.)

2. The AP mechanical axis of the tibia is a straight line from the center of the knee to the center of the ankle (Fig. 3-6).

B. Anatomic Axes of the Femur and Tibia—The anatomic axis of any long bone is a line formed by a series of mid-diaphyseal points. It is the site of a straight intramedullary nail.

1. AP femoral anatomic axis—The AP femoral anatomic axis is a straight line from the piriformis fossa, extending distally in the diaphysis to a point approximately 10 mm medial to the center of the knee in an average adult (approximately, the intersection of the concave intercondylar notch with the convex medial femoral condyle) (Fig. 3-7).

2. AP tibial anatomic axis—The AP tibial anatomic axis is a straight line formed by a series of mid-diaphyseal points. It is parallel to the lateral tibial cortex, approximately, 2 to 5 mm medial to the mechanical axis. Because the AP tibial mechanical and AP tibial anatomic axes are so close, they can be considered identical (Fig. 3-8).

3. Lateral femoral anatomic axis—Because of the normal bow of the femur in the lateral plane,

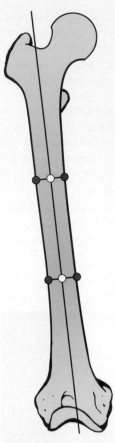

FIGURE 3-7 AP Anatomic axis of the femur. (Reprinted with permission from Brinker MR, O'Connor DP. Principles of malunions. In: Bucholz, RW, Court-Brown CM, Heckman JD, et al., eds. *Rockwood and Green's Fractures in Adults*. 7th ed. Philadelphia, PA: Lippincott Williams & Wilkins, 2010.)

a series of mid-diaphyseal points will not define a straight line. For deformity analysis, a best-fit straight line can be drawn for the proximal or distal segment of the femur. The intersection of the proximal and distal segments forms a 10° angle, apex anterior.

4. Lateral tibial anatomic axis—The lateral tibial anatomic axis is a series of mid-diaphyseal points parallel to the anterior cortex of the tibia. The lateral tibial mechanical and anatomic axes can be considered identical.

C. It is only necessary to differentiate between the AP anatomic femoral axis and the AP mechanical femoral axis. For deformity analysis, the lateral femoral axis, AP tibial axis, and lateral tibial axis can be considered to be a straight line formed by a series of mid-diaphyseal points, without differentiating between anatomic and mechanical methods.

VI. Joint Orientation—Normal joint orientation, as measured by the joint orientation angle, is also necessary but not sufficient for correction of deformity.

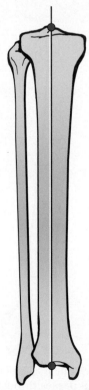

FIGURE 3-6 The mechanical axis of the tibia. (Reprinted with permission from Brinker MR, O'Connor DP. Principles of malunions. In: Bucholz, RW, Court-Brown CM, Heckman JD, et al., eds. *Rockwood and Green's Fractures in Adults*. 7th ed. Philadelphia, PA: Lippincott Williams & Wilkins, 2010.)

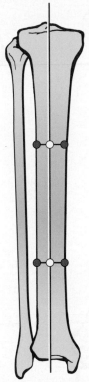

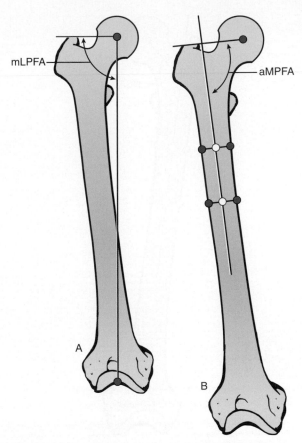

FIGURE 3-8   AP Anatomic axis of the tibia. (Reprinted with permission from Brinker MR, O'Connor DP. Principles of malunions. In: Bucholz, RW, Court-Brown CM, Heckman JD, et al., eds. *Rockwood and Green's Fractures in Adults*. 7th ed. Philadelphia, PA: Lippincott Williams & Wilkins, 2010.)

FIGURE 3-9   **A.** The joint orientation line from the tip of the greater trochanter to the center of the femoral head and the mechanical axis of the femur describe the mechanical Lateral Proximal Femoral Angle. **B.** The joint orientation line from the tip of the greater trochanter to the center of the femoral head and the anatomic axis of the femur describe the anatomic Medial Proximal Femoral Angle. (Reprinted with permission from Brinker MR, O'Connor DP. Principles of malunions. In: Bucholz, RW, Court-Brown CM, Heckman JD, et al., eds. *Rockwood and Green's Fractures in Adults*. 7th ed. Philadelphia, PA: Lippincott Williams & Wilkins, 2010.)

The joint orientation angle is the angle formed by the intersection of the joint orientation line with the axis (either anatomical or mechanical) of the respective bone.

A. Joint Orientation Lines
  1. AP plane
    • Proximal femur
      (a) Tip of the greater trochanter to the center of the femoral head (Fig. 3-9), or
      (b) Longitudinal axis of the femoral neck (Fig. 3-10)
    • Distal femur—A straight line tangential to the femoral condyles (Fig. 3-11)
    • Proximal tibia—A straight line from the medial corner to the lateral corner of the tibial plateau (Fig. 3-12)
    • Distal tibia—A line across the subchondral bone of the ankle mortise (Fig. 3-13)
  2. Lateral plane
    • Proximal femur—Neck–shaft angle is rarely used in the lateral plane.
    • Distal femur—A line connecting the anterior and posterior extent of the distal femoral physis or the site of the closed physis (Fig. 3-14)

    • Proximal tibia—A line across the subchondral bone of the tibial plateau (Fig. 3-15)
    • Distal tibia—A line between the anterior and posterior corners of the distal tibia (Fig. 3-16)
B. Joint Orientation Angles
  1. The angles are abbreviated by five letters:
    • The first letter is a lower case *a* or *m*, which designates *anatomic* or *mechanical*.
    • The second letter is *M* (medial), *L* (lateral), *A* (anterior), or *P* (posterior), which designates the location of the angle with respect to the axis of the bone so that the normal value of the joint orientation angle is 90° or less. This nomenclature is not used for the femoral neck–shaft angle because of the

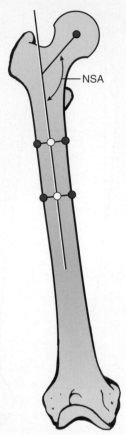

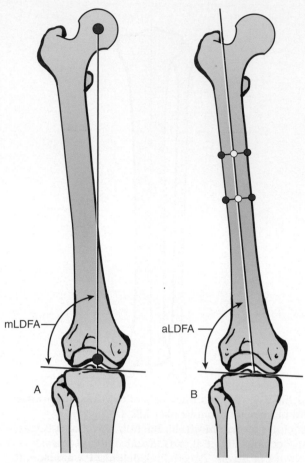

FIGURE 3-10 The longitudinal axis of the femoral neck and the anatomic axis of the femur describe the medial neck–shaft angle. (Reprinted with permission from Brinker MR, O'Connor DP. Principles of malunions. In: Bucholz, RW, Court-Brown CM, Heckman JD, et al., eds. *Rockwood and Green's Fractures in Adults*. 7th ed. Philadelphia, PA: Lippincott Williams & Wilkins, 2010.)

FIGURE 3-11 **A.** The distal femoral joint orientation line and the mechanical axis of the femur describe the mechanical Lateral Distal Femoral Angle. **B.** The distal femoral joint orientation line and the anatomic axis of the femur describe the anatomic Lateral Distal Femoral Angle. (Reprinted with permission from Brinker MR, O'Connor DP. Principles of malunions. In: Bucholz, RW, Court-Brown CM, Heckman JD, et al., eds. *Rockwood and Green's Fractures in Adults*. 7th ed. Philadelphia, PA: Lippincott Williams & Wilkins, 2010.)

longstanding traditional method of measuring the relationship between the femoral neck and shaft as the larger of the two supplementary angles at this site.
- The third letter is *P* (proximal) or *D* (distal).
- The fourth letter is *F* (femur) or *T* (tibia).
- The final letter is *A*, the abbreviation for angle.
- Usually *a* (anatomic) or *m* (mechanical) is only used at the distal femur in which the aLDFA and mLDFA differ by 7°.

2. The normal values and ranges of normal are:
- AP plane (mechanical)
   (a) Lateral proximal femoral angle (mLPFA) = 90° (range, 85° to 95°) (Fig. 3-9)
   (b) Mechanical lateral distal femoral angle (mLDFA) = 88° (range, 85° to 90°) (Fig. 3-11)
   (c) Medial proximal tibial angle (MPTA) = 87° (range, 85° to 90°) (Fig. 3-12)

(d) Lateral distal tibial angle (LDTA) = 89° (range, 86° to 92°) (Fig. 3-13)
- AP plane (anatomic)
   (a) Medial neck–shaft angle (NSA) = 130° (range, 124° to 136°) (Fig. 3-10)
   (b) Medial proximal femoral angle (aMPFA) = 84° (range, 80° to 89°) (Fig. 3-9)
   (c) Anatomic lateral distal femoral angle (aLDFA) = 81° (range, 79° to 83°) (Fig. 3-11)
   (d) In the tibia, the anatomic and mechanical joint orientation angles can be considered identical.
- Sagittal plane
   (a) The proximal femoral joint orientation angle is rarely used.

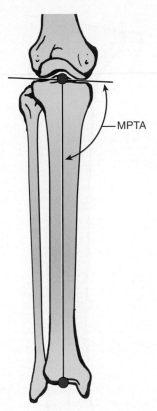

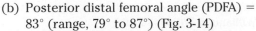

FIGURE 3-12 The proximal tibial joint orientation line and the mechanical axis of the tibia describe the Medial Proximal Tibial Angle. (Reprinted with permission from Brinker MR, O'Connor DP. Principles of malunions. In: Bucholz, RW, Court-Brown CM, Heckman JD, et al., eds. *Rockwood and Green's Fractures in Adults*. 7th ed. Philadelphia, PA: Lippincott Williams & Wilkins, 2010.)

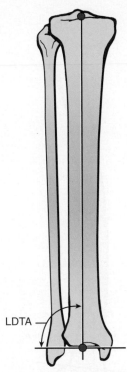

FIGURE 3-13 The distal tibial joint orientation line and the mechanical axis of the tibia describe the Lateral Distal Tibial Angle. (Reprinted with permission from Brinker MR, O'Connor DP. Principles of malunions. In: Bucholz, RW, Court-Brown CM, Heckman JD, et al., eds. *Rockwood and Green's Fractures in Adults*. 7th ed. Philadelphia, PA: Lippincott Williams & Wilkins, 2010.)

    (b) Posterior distal femoral angle (PDFA) = 83° (range, 79° to 87°) (Fig. 3-14)
- Although this angle is formed by the intersection of the anatomic axis of the femur with the distal femoral joint orientation line, it is not preceded by *a* (anatomic) because the mechanical posterior distal femoral angle is never used.
- Normally, the anatomic axis intersects the distal femoral joint orientation line at a point posterior to the anterior cortex by one third the distance between the anterior and posterior cortices at the distal femoral joint orientation line (Fig. 3-14).
- Posterior proximal tibial angle (PPTA) = 81° (range, 77° to 84°) (Fig. 3-15).
Normally, the anatomic axis intersects the proximal tibial joint orientation line posterior to the anterior cortex by one-fifth the distance between the anterior and posterior cortices at the proximal tibial joint orientation line (Fig. 3-15).
- Anterior distal tibial angle (ADTA) = 80° (range, 78° to 82°) Fig. 3-16)
Normally, the anatomic axis intersects the distal tibial joint orientation angle at a line midway between the anterior and posterior cortices at the distal tibial joint orientation line (Fig. 3-16).

    C. Other Considerations
      1. AP plane—The femoral and tibial joint orientation lines should be parallel or intersect laterally (valgus) at an angle of 2° or less (joint convergence angle [JCA]) (Fig. 3-17).
      2. Lateral plane—With the knee in maximum extension, the axis of the femur (or distal extension of the anterior cortex) and the axis of the tibia (or proximal extension of the anterior cortex) should form an angle of 0° (lateral femoral–tibial angle [LFTA]).

VII. Identification of the Presence of Lower Extremity Skeletal Deformity—The following sequence is

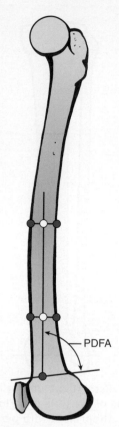

FIGURE 3-14 The lateral view distal femoral joint orientation line and the anatomic axis of the femur describe the Posterior Distal Femoral Angle. (Reprinted with permission from Brinker MR, O'Connor DP. Principles of malunions. In: Bucholz, RW, Court-Brown CM, Heckman JD, et al., eds. *Rockwood and Green's Fractures in Adults*. 7th ed. Philadelphia, PA: Lippincott Williams & Wilkins, 2010.)

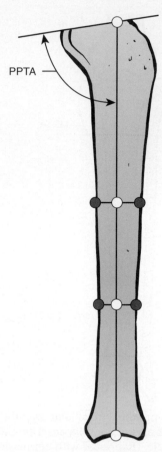

FIGURE 3-15 The lateral view proximal tibial joint orientation line and the anatomic axis of the femur describe the Posterior Proximal Tibial Angle. (Reprinted with permission from Brinker MR, O'Connor DP. Principles of malunions. In: Bucholz, RW, Court-Brown CM, Heckman JD, et al., eds. *Rockwood and Green's Fractures in Adults*. 7th ed. Philadelphia, PA: Lippincott Williams & Wilkins, 2010.)

recommended to identify the presence of skeletal deformity:

A. On the 51- × 14-in AP radiograph, draw the mechanical axis of the lower extremity from the center of the femoral head to the center of the ankle mortise.

B. Measure the MAD, the distance between the center of the knee and the mechanical axis at the level of the knee.
  1. MAD indicates presence of deformity.
  2. Absence of MAD does not indicate absence of deformity. The mechanical axis may be normal in the presence of:
     • Joint malorientation (abnormal joint orientation angles) at the hip, knee, or ankle
     • Compensatory angular deformities

C. On the AP radiograph, draw the mechanical axis of the femur, the anatomic axis of the femur, and the axis of the tibia.

D. Draw the joint orientation lines.
  1. Proximal femur
     • Tip of greater trochanter to center of femoral head
     • Axis of femoral neck
  2. Distal femur
  3. Proximal tibia
  4. Distal tibia

E. Measure the AP joint orientation angles and the AP joint convergence angles.
  1. NSA, mLPFA, aMPFA
  2. aLDFA and mLDFA
  3. MPTA
  4. LDTA
  5. JCA

F. Measure the effective total length discrepancy by measuring the vertical distance between the horizontal lines drawn perpendicular to the film edge to an easily visualized landmark on both

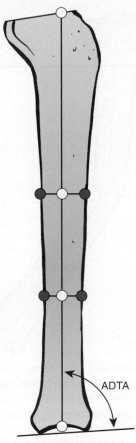

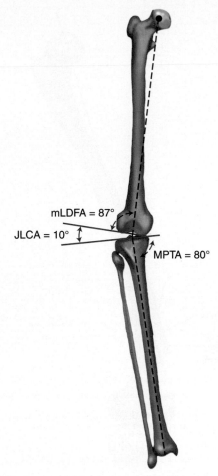

FIGURE 3-16 The lateral view distal tibial joint orientation line and the anatomic axis of the tibia describe the Anterior Distal Tibial Angle. (Reprinted with permission from Brinker MR, O'Connor DP. Principles of malunions. In: Bucholz, RW, Court-Brown CM, Heckman JD, et al., eds. *Rockwood and Green's Fractures in Adults.* 7th ed. Philadelphia, PA: Lippincott Williams & Wilkins, 2010.)

FIGURE 3-17 In this pathologic case, the joint line convergence angle is 10° medial (normal ≤2° lateral).

extremities (femoral head, sacroiliac joint, or iliac crest).

G. Measure the length of the femur from the superior aspect of the femoral head to the distal femoral joint orientation line.

H. Measure the length of the tibia from the center of the tibial spines to the center of the ankle mortise.

I. On the lateral radiograph, draw the axes of the femur and tibia.

J. On the lateral radiograph, draw the joint orientation lines.

K. Measure the lateral joint orientation angles.
   1. PDFA
   2. PPTA
   3. ADTA

L. Measure the LFTA.

M. Deformity is present if there is any of the following:
   1. MAD lateral to or more than 10 mm medial to the center of the knee
   2. Abnormal joint orientation angle(s)
   3. Abnormal JCA
   4. Abnormal LFTA

VIII. Measurement of Angular Deformity: Magnitude, Location, and the Concept of CORA

A. The deformity resolution point for an angular deformity is called the center of rotation of angulation (CORA).
   1. The CORA and apex of the deformity may not be identical (Fig. 3-18).
   2. The CORA differs from the apex if there is translation and/or more than one angular deformity.

B. The CORA is the intersection of the proximal axis with the distal axis of a deformed bone (Fig. 3-19).

C. The angle formed by the intersection of the proximal and distal axes is the magnitude of

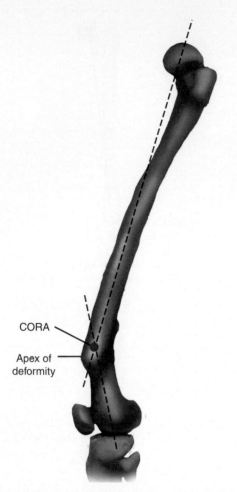

FIGURE 3-18   Apex of the deformity and CORA are different in this case, due to posterior translation of the distal fragment.

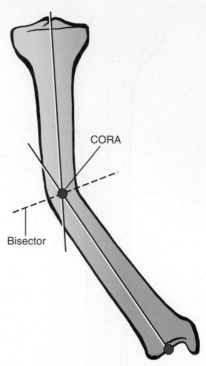

FIGURE 3-19   CORA and bisector for a varus angulation deformity of the tibia. (Reprinted with permission from Brinker MR, O'Connor DP. Principles of malunions. In: Bucholz, RW, Court-Brown CM, Heckman JD, et al., eds. *Rockwood and Green's Fractures in Adults.* 7th ed. Philadelphia, PA: Lippincott Williams & Wilkins, 2010.)

the angular deformity in the plane in which the deformity is being measured.

D. The level at which the axes intersect at the CORA is the level or location of the deformity.

E. The three angular components in the three orthogonal planes determine the magnitude of the resultant angle in an oblique plane, which differs from the orthogonal planes.

F. There is an infinite number of CORAs for an angular deformity. Any point on the bisector line of the supplementary angle to the angle of deformity is a CORA (Fig. 3-19).
   1. Points on the concavity of the deformity are shortening CORAs.
   2. Points on the convexity of the deformity are lengthening CORAs.
   3. A mid-diaphyseal CORA is a neutral CORA.

G. A line perpendicular to the plane of the deformity, passing through the CORA, is called the axis of correction of angulation (ACA). When using a hinged external fixator to correct angulation, the ACA is the axis of the hinge (Fig. 3-20).

IX. Measurement of AP Plane Angular Deformity

A. Femur—In the AP plane, either the mechanical or anatomic axis planning method may be used. Theoretically, the two methods should yield identical results for the magnitude and level of the deformity. The two methods must not be mixed for measuring the AP femoral angulation, that is, using the distal femoral mechanical axis with the proximal femoral anatomic axis or vice versa. Since one of the two goals (see III. A and B) of deformity correction is to restore the mechanical axis, it is preferable to use the mechanical axis method if possible. If portable intraoperative radiographs do not include the entire femur or if the deformity is purely diaphyseal, such as a diaphyseal malunion, the anatomic axis method may be used.
   1. AP femur—mechanical axis method
      • Draw the proximal femoral axis.
         (a) If the contralateral femur is normal, draw a line from the center of the femoral head extending distally to form a LPFA equal to the LPFA of the normal femur.
         (b) If the contralateral femur is abnormal, draw a line from the center of the femoral head extending distally to form

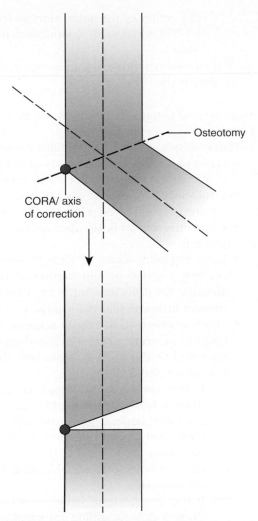

CORA/ axis
of correction

Osteotomy

FIGURE 3-20 When the ACA passes through the opening wedge CORA on the convex cortex, an opening wedge angulation results. (Reprinted with permission from Brinker MR, O'Connor DP. Principles of malunions. In: Bucholz, RW, Court-Brown CM, Heckman JD, et al., eds. *Rockwood and Green's Fractures in Adults*. 7th ed. Philadelphia, PA: Lippincott Williams & Wilkins, 2010.)

a LPFA equal to 90° (population normal value).

(c) If the femoral head and/or neck is abnormal or the patient is skeletally immature with incomplete ossification of the greater trochanter, draw a line through the center of the femoral head, extending distally parallel to the anatomic axis. Then draw a line through the center of the head lateral to the first line drawn through the center of the head to form an angle of 7° (the difference between the anatomic distal joint orientation angle and the mechanical distal joint orientation angle). The latter line represents the proximal femoral mechanical axis.

• Draw the distal femoral mechanical axis.
(a) If the ipsilateral tibia is normal, extend the tibial mechanical axis proximally.
(b) If the ipsilateral tibia is abnormal and the contralateral femur is normal, draw a line extending proximally from the center of the intercondylar notch to form a mLDFA equal to the contralateral extremity.
(c) If the ipsilateral tibia and contralateral femur are abnormal, draw a line extending proximally from the center of the intercondylar notch to form a mLDFA equal to 88° (population normal value).
• The intersection point of the proximal and distal axes is the CORA. The angle formed by the intersection of the axes defines the magnitude of the angular deformity. The level of the intersection of the axes identifies the location.

2. AP femur—anatomic axis method.
• Draw the proximal anatomic axis.
(a) Long segment—Draw a straight line connecting a series of mid-diaphyseal points.
(b) Short segment—If the proximal femur (head, neck, and greater trochanter) is normal, the following method is used:
  • If the contralateral femur is normal, draw a line extending distally from the proximal femoral joint orientation line to form an aMPTA equal to the contralateral femur.
  • If the contralateral femur is abnormal, draw a line extending distally from the proximal femoral joint orientation line to form an aMPFA equal to 84° (population normal).
  • If the proximal segment is too short to draw a mid-diaphyseal line and the proximal femur is abnormal, use the mechanical axis method.
• Draw the distal anatomic axis.
(a) Long segment—Draw a line connecting a series of mid-diaphyseal points. Measure aLDFA to identify any hidden additional juxtaarticular deformity.
(b) Short segment—If the distal segment is too short to draw a straight line connecting a series of mid-diaphyseal points and/or the aLDFA is abnormal, the following method is used:
  • If the contralateral femur is normal, draw a line extending proximally from the distal femoral joint orientation line, starting at a point medial to

the center of the intercondylar notch identical to the contralateral femur to form an aLDFA identical to the contralateral femur.

- If the contralateral femur is abnormal, draw a line extending proximally from the distal femoral joint orientation line starting at a point 1 cm medial to the center of the intercondylar notch to form an aLDFA equal to 81° (population normal value).
- The intersection point of the proximal and distal axes is the CORA.

B. Tibia—Since the mechanical and anatomic axes of the tibia are essentially identical, it is not necessary to describe two different methods.

1. Draw the proximal axis.
   - Long segment—Draw a line connecting a series of mid-diaphyseal points. Measure the MPTA at the knee to identify any hidden additional juxtaarticular deformity.
   - Short segment—If the proximal segment is too short to draw a straight line connecting a series of mid-diaphyseal points and/or the MPTA is abnormal, the following method is used:
     (a) If the ipsilateral femur is normal, extend the distal femoral mechanical axis distally through the proximal tibia.
     (b) If the ipsilateral femur is abnormal and the contralateral tibia is normal, draw a line extending distally from the center of the tibial spines to form a MPTA equal to the contralateral side.
     (c) If the ipsilateral femur is abnormal and the contralateral tibia is abnormal, draw a line from the center of the tibial spine extending distally to form a MPTA equal to 87° (population normal value).

2. Draw the distal axis.
   - Long segment—Draw a straight line connecting a series of mid-diaphyseal points. Measure the LDTA at the ankle joint to identify any hidden additional juxtaarticular deformity.
   - Short segment—If the distal segment is too short to draw a straight line connecting a series of mid-diaphyseal points and/or the LDTA is abnormal, the following method is used:
     (a) If the contralateral tibia is normal, draw a line extending proximally from the center of the ankle mortise to form a LDTA equal to the opposite side.
     (b) If the contralateral tibia is abnormal, draw a line extending proximally from

the center of the ankle mortise to form a LDTA equal to 89° (population normal value).

3. The intersection point of the proximal and distal axes is the CORA.

X. Measurement of Lateral Plane Angular Deformity.
A. Femur
1. Proximal axis—Draw a straight line connecting a series of mid-diaphyseal points of the proximal and distal segments. Because there is a normal femoral bow in the sagittal plane, these lines are drawn as best fit lines. The normal angle of intersection is 10° apex anterior.
2. Distal axis
   - Long segment—Draw a straight line connecting a series of mid-diaphyseal points. Measure the PDFA to identify any hidden additional juxtaarticular deformity.
   - Short segment—If the distal segment is too short to measure a series of mid-diaphyseal lines and/or the PDFA is abnormal, the following method is used:
     (a) If the contralateral femur is normal, draw a line extending proximally from the distal femoral joint orientation line, starting at a point one-third the width of the femur at the level of the joint orientation line to form a PDFA equal to the opposite side.
     (b) If the contralateral femur is abnormal, draw a line extending proximally from the joint orientation line as described above to form a PDFA equal to 83° (population normal value).
3. The intersection point of the proximal and distal axes is the CORA.
B. Tibia
1. Proximal axis
   - Long segment—Draw a straight line connecting a series of mid-diaphyseal points. Measure the PPTA at the knee to identify the presence of any hidden additional juxtaarticular deformity.
   - Short segment—If the proximal segment is too short to draw a mid-diaphyseal line and/or the PPTA is abnormal, the following method is used:
     (a) If the contralateral tibia is normal, draw a line extending distally from the proximal tibial joint orientation line starting at a point one-fifth the width of the tibial plateau at the joint orientation line to form a PPTA identical to the opposite side.

(b) If the contralateral tibia is abnormal, draw a line extending distally as described above from the proximal joint orientation line to form a PPTA equal to 81° (population normal value).

2. Distal axis
   • Long segment—Draw a straight line connecting a series of mid-diaphyseal points. Measure the ADTA to identify the presence of any hidden additional juxtaarticular deformity.
   • Short segment—If the distal segment is too short to draw a line connecting a series of mid-diaphyseal points and/or the ADTA is abnormal, the following method is used:
     (a) If the contralateral tibia is normal, draw a line extending proximally from the distal tibial joint orientation line starting at a midway between the anterior and posterior corners of the distal tibia at the distal joint orientation angle to form an ADTA equal to the opposite tibia.
     (b) If the contralateral tibia is abnormal, draw a line extending proximally from the distal tibial joint orientation, starting at a point midway between the anterior and posterior corners of the distal tibia on the distal joint orientation line to form an ADTA equal to 80° (population normal value).

3. The intersection point of the proximal and distal axes is the CORA.

XI. Measurement of Horizontal Plane Angular Deformity (Axial Rotation)
   A. Radiographic Methods—computerized tomography
   B. Clinical Methods—physical examination
      1. Femur
         • Measure hip rotation with the hip extended and the patient prone.
         • In the normal adult, internal and external rotations are approximately equal.
         • Half the difference between internal and external rotation is an approximation of femoral axial rotation.
         • The accuracy of this method can be affected by intraarticular hip pathology or juxtaarticular distal femoral or proximal tibial angular deformity.
      2. Tibia—The foot–thigh angle (as viewed from above with the patient prone and the knee flexed 90°) is an estimate of tibial rotation.

XII. Measurement of Translation
   A. The magnitude of translation in millimeters is the length of the line drawn perpendicular from

the axis (either mechanical or anatomic) of one segment to a point on the axis of the other segment (Fig. 3-21).
   1. In a fracture, the point from which the perpendicular line is drawn on the first fragment is usually the proximal end of the distal fragment since, by convention, orthopedic deformities are described as the distal fragment with respect to the proximal (reference) fragment.
   2. Translation can also be measured as the perpendicular distance from a point on the proximal fragment to the axis of the distal (reference) fragment.
   B. If angulation is also present, the magnitude of translation will vary, depending on the choice of the reference fragment or the location at which it is measured. The choice of the reference fragment and the effect on the magnitude of translation is relevant when using a hexapod external fixator (Taylor Spatial Frame).

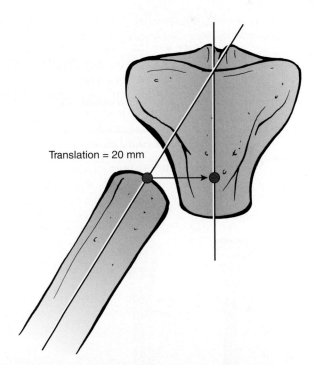

Translation = 20 mm

FIGURE 3-21 Method for measuring the magnitude of translational deformities. In this example, with both angulation and translation, the magnitude of the translational deformity is the horizontal distance from the proximal segment's anatomic axis to the distal segment's anatomic axis at the level of the proximal end of the distal segment. (Reprinted with permission from Brinker MR, O'Connor DP. Principles of malunions. In: Bucholz, RW, Court-Brown CM, Heckman JD, et al., eds. *Rockwood and Green's Fractures in Adults*. 7th ed. Philadelphia, PA: Lippincott Williams & Wilkins, 2010.)

XIII. Measurement of Orientation of Deformity: Oblique Plane Deformity

If an angular and/or translation deformity exists in the AP (*xy*) plane and lateral (*yz*) plane, the deformity is an oblique plane deformity, not a biplanar deformity. The deformity is in a single plane; it is just not in the AP or lateral plane. The plane of the deformity is the plane in which the deformity is a maximum. This oblique plane determines the orientation of the deformity, as measured by the angle between this oblique plane and the AP (*xy*) plane. There is a plane orthogonal (perpendicular) to this oblique plane of maximum deformity where there is no deformity.

A. Oblique Plane Angular Deformity
  1. Magnitude
    • Magnitude of the oblique plane angular deformity can be determined by either the graphic or the trigonometric method.
      (a) Graphic method
        • Based on the Pythagorean theorem

$$\theta = \sqrt{\theta_{AP}^2 + \theta_{lat}^2}$$

        where $\theta =$ the magnitude of true or resultant angle in the oblique plane
        $\theta_{AP} =$ the magnitude of the angular deformity AP plane
        $\theta_{lat} =$ the magnitude of the angular deformity lateral plane

        • Using the graphic method, θ can be measured without any calculation

by drawing two perpendicular lines. The length of the horizontal line represents the magnitude of the AP angular deformity. The length of the vertical line represents the magnitude of the lateral angular deformity. The magnitude of the oblique plane angular deformity is the length of the resultant line, the diagonal of the rectangle formed by the two perpendicular lines (Fig. 3-22 and 3-23).
      (b) Trigonometric method
        • Yields the exact magnitude of the angular deformity in the oblique plane.
        • Calculated from the equation

$$\theta = \tan^{-1} \sqrt{\tan^2\theta_{AP} + \tan^2\theta_{lat}}$$

        where $\tan^{-1} =$ arc tangent
        $\tan =$ the tangent of the angle of deformity in the AP and lateral planes
        • The graphic method is easier and yields an approximation that is usually within two degrees of the true deformity for physiologic angular deformities.
  2. Orientation—The oblique plane (the plane of maximum angulation) can be determined by either the graphic or trigonometric method.
    • Graphic method—Similar to the magnitude of the oblique plane angulation, the orientation calculated by the graphic method is only an approximation but is quite

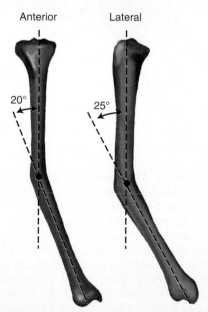

FIGURE 3-22 Graphic method for determining deformity magnitude.

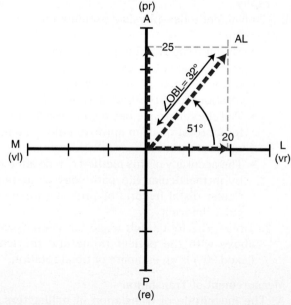

FIGURE 3-23 Graphic method for determining deformity orientation.

accurate within the range of physiologic deformities.

   (a) Similar to the method discussed earlier for measuring θ, α can be measured using the graphic method without any calculation by drawing two perpendicular lines. The angle between the resultant diagonal line and the horizontal line is the orientation of the oblique plane deformity (Fig. 3-23).

- Trigonometric method—Yields the exact orientation in the oblique plane.

The equation for calculating the plane of the deformity is

$$\alpha = \tan^{-1} \frac{\tan \theta_{lat}}{\tan \theta_{AP}}$$

B. Oblique Plane Translation Deformities
  1. Magnitude of translation deformities
- If a translation deformity is visualized on both the AP and lateral radiographs, there is a translation deformity in an oblique plane of maximum translation. There is a plane at 90° to this plane with no translation.
- Unlike oblique plane angular deformity calculations, the graphic method for oblique plane translation deformity is not an approximation but yields the exact magnitude.
- The graphic method equation is based on the Pythagorean theorem

$$t = \sqrt{t_{AP}^2 + t_{lat}^2}$$

where t = true translation in mm
t_{AP} = the translation in mm on the AP view
t_{lat} = the translation in mm on the lateral view

- Using the graphic method, t can be measured without any calculation by drawing two perpendicular lines. The length of the horizontal line represents the magnitude of the translation. The length of the vertical line represents the lateral translation. The magnitude of the oblique plane translation is the length of the resultant line, the diagonal of the rectangle formed by the two lines.
  2. Orientation of oblique plane translation
- Can be calculated from the formula:

$$\beta = \tan^{-1} \frac{\tan_{lat}}{\tan_{AP}}$$

where β = the orientation of the oblique plane of the translation deformity, the angle between the oblique plane and the AP plane

- The angle β can be measured without any calculations by drawing two perpendicular lines as described in the last bullet of section XIII.B.1. The angle β is the angle between this resultant diagonal line and the horizontal line.
- Oblique plane angular deformity may exist with or without oblique plane translation deformity, and vice versa.
- The orientation of the oblique plane angular deformity α and the orientation of the oblique plane translation deformity β may differ, especially in high-energy trauma.

XIV. Deformity Correction Truisms
A. Any angular deformity (with or without translation) can be accurately corrected by rotating around the ACA through the CORA.
  1. An osteotomy at the level of the CORA needs only to be angulated, not translated.
  2. An osteotomy performed at a level other than the CORA and rotated around the ACA at the osteotomy site must be angulated and translated at the osteotomy site to achieve accurate correction. This level of osteotomy at a level other than the CORA may be desirable due to:
- Soft tissue pathology at the CORA
- Hardware considerations of external fixation equipment or internal fixation implants
  3. As the distance between the osteotomy and CORA increases, increasing amounts of translation must be performed.
  4. The amount of translation can be calculated

$$t = \frac{2\pi r \theta}{360}$$

where r = the distance from the CORA to the osteotomy
θ = the magnitude of angulation
The equation can be simplified to $t = 0.017 r\theta$.

  5. If an osteotomy is performed at the CORA but rotated around an axis not at the CORA (i.e., an axis that is not the ACA), iatrogenic secondary translation will occur.
B. If the CORA does not "make sense," there is:
  1. Translation in addition to angulation
  2. More than one angular deformity

3. Both 1 and 2
4. Examples of a deformity that does not "make sense" include:
   - The CORA is at different levels on the AP and lateral radiographs.
   - The CORA is not at the apex of the angular deformity.
   - The CORA is in the diaphysis when there is no diaphyseal angulation.
   - The CORA is proximal or distal to the bone.

C. Any translation deformity can be resolved into two angular deformities (Fig. 3-24).
D. Any angular deformity (with or without translation) can be resolved into two or more angular deformities.
   1. One or more additional axis lines can be drawn to intersect the proximal or distal axes to form two or more angular deformities.
   2. The placement of the additional line(s) is chosen by its intersections with the proximal and distal axes where an osteotomy is to be performed.
   3. Useful when correcting bowing or multiapical deformities.
E. Translation Deformities
   1. Only present in deformities due to trauma (fractures or malunions) or previous surgery.
   2. Not seen in developmental or congenital deformities.

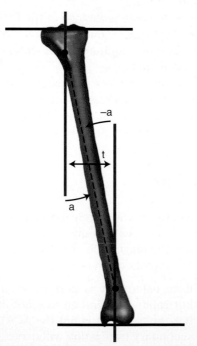

FIGURE 3-24   Two equal but opposite angular deformities (*a*) in the same plane have the same effect as one translational deformity (*t*).

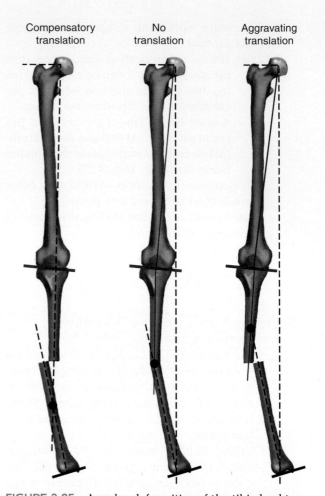

| Compensatory translation | No translation | Aggravating translation |

FIGURE 3-25   Angular deformities of the tibia lead to varying degrees of mechanical axis deviation, depending on the degree of angulation, the level of malunion, and the magnitude and direction of any associated translational deformity. These three varus deformities differ only in the magnitude and direction of the translational component of the deformitiy. The center example has pure angulation without translation of the bone ends. The example to the left of center has the same degree of angulation combined with translation toward the convexity of the deformity. The example to the right of center has the same degree of angulation combined with translation toward the concavity of the deformity. Notice the amount of mechanical axis deviation in all three examples. The mechanical axis deviation is decreased when the translation is toward the convexity and increased when it is aggravating translation. Notice the point of intersection of the mechanical axis lines of the proximal and distal tibia. When there is no translation, the intersection is at the level of the deformitiy. When there is a compensatory translation the intersection point is distal to the deformitiy. When there is aggravating translation the intersection point in proximal to the deformitiy. The intersection point is considered to be the true apex of the angulation/translation deformity, while the deformitiy is considered to be the apparent apex. (Adapted from Paley D, Tetsworth KD. Deformity correction by the Ilizarov technique. In: Chapman MW, ed. *Operative Orthopaedics*. 2nd ed. Philadelphia, PA: J.B. Lippincott Company; 1993, with permission.)

3. An angular deformity or a translation deformity may be present by itself or they may coexist.

4. The orientation of the angular deformity and translation deformity may be present in the same or different planes, the latter occurring in high-energy trauma.

5. When angulation and translation coexist, the direction of translation may increase or decrease the effect on the MAD (Fig. 3-25).

F. The magnitude of the angle of the deformity at the CORA is the angle of the wedge that must be removed for a closing wedge osteotomy or must be generated when performing distraction osteogenesis. The magnitude of the angular deformity is NOT the number of degrees the joint orientation angle differs from the normal value.

G. The location (level) of the CORA determines the effect on the joint orientation angle and the MAD, with deformities close to the knee (distal femur or proximal tibia) having greater effect than deformities farther from the knee in the proximal femur or distal tibia. If there is both translation and angulation, the direction of translation will also affect the MAD.

SUGGESTED READINGS

Classic Articles

Chao EYS, Neluheni EVD, Hsu RWW, et al. Biomechanics of malalignment. *Orthop Clin North Am.* 1994;25:379−386.

Cooke TD, Pichora D, Siu D, et al. Surgical implications of varus deformity of the knee with obliquity of joint surfaces. *J Bone Joint Surg.* 1989;71B:560−565.

Coventry MB. Proximal tibial varus osteotomy for osteoarthritis of the lateral compartment of the knee. *J Bone Joint Surg.* 1987;69A:32−38.

Hsu RW, Himeno S, Coventry MB, et al. Normal axial alignment of the lower extremity and the load-bearing distribution at the knee. *Clin Orthop Relat Res.* 1990;255:215−227.

Kettelkamp DB, Hillburg BM, Murrish DE, et al. Degenerative arthritis of the knee secondary to fracture malunion. *Clin Orthop Relat Res.* 1988;234:159−169.

Krackow KA. Approaches to planning lower extremity alignment for total knee arthroplasty and osteotomy about the knee. *Adv Orthop Surg.* 1983;7:69−88.

McKellop HA, Llinas A, Sarmiento A. Effects of tibial malalignment on the knee and ankle. *Orthop Clin North Am.* 1994;25:415−423.

Moreland JR, Bassett LW, Hanker GJ. Radiographic analysis of the axial alignment of the lower extremity. *J Bone Joint Surg Am.* 1987;69A:745−749.

Murphy SB. Tibial osteotomy for genu varum. *Orthop Clin North Am.* 1994;25:477−482.

O'Driscoll SW, Bell DF, Morrey BF. Posterolateral rotatory instability of the elbow. *J Bone Joint Surg Am.* 1991;73A:440−446.

Paley D, Herzenberg JE, Tetsworth K, et al. Deformity planning for frontal and sagittal plane corrective osteotomies. *Orthop Clin North Am.* 1994;25:425−465.

Paley D, Tetsworth K. Mechanical axis deviation of the lower limbs: preoperative planning of multiapical frontal plane angular and bowing deformities of the femur and tibia. *Clin Orthop.* 1992;280:65−71.

Potter C, Frost HM. Determining alignment of the knee. *Clin Orthop.* 1974;103:32.

Tetsworth K, Paley D. Malalignment and degenerative arthropathy. *Orthop Clin North Am.* 1994;25:367−377.

Wright JG, Treble N, Feinstein AR. Measurement of lower limb alignment using long radiographs. *J Bone Joint Surg.* 1991;73B:721−723.

Wu DD, Burr DB, Boyd RD, et al. Bone and cartilage changes following experimental varus or valgus tibial angulation. *J Orthop Res.* 1990;8:572–585.

Recent Articles

Brouwer GM, van Tol AW, Bergink AP, et al. Association between valgus and varus alignment and the development and progression of radiographic osteoarthritis of the knee. *Arthritis Rheum.* 2007;56:1204–1211.

Green SA, Gibbs P. The relationship of angulation to translation in fracture deformities. *J Bone Joint Surg.* 1994;76A:390–397.

Green SA, Green HD. The influence of radiographic projection on the appearance of deformities. *Orthop Clin North Am.* 1994;25:467–475.

Gugenheim JJ, Brinker MR. Bone realignment with use of temporary external fixation for distal femoral valgus and varus deformities. *J Bone Joint Surg.* 2003;85A:1229–1237.

Gugenheim JJ, Probe RA, Brinker MR. The effects of femoral shaft malrotation on lower extremity anatomy. *J Orthop Trauma.* 2004;18:658–664.

Heller MO, Taylor WR, Perka C, et al. The influence of alignment on the musculoskeletal loading conditions at the knee. *Langenbecks Arch Surg.* 2003;12:291–297.

Kaufman KR, Miller LS, Sutherland DH. Gait asymmetry in patients with limb-length inequality. *J Pediatr Orthop.* 1996;16:144–150.

Mahboubi S, Horstman S. Femoral torsion: CT measurement. *Radiology.* 1986;160:843–844.

Price CT, Izuka B. Osteotomy planning using the anatomic method: a simple method for lower extremity deformity analysis. *Orthopedics.* 2005;28:20–25.

Sharma L, Song J, Felson DT, et al. The role of knee alignment and disease progression and functional decline in knee osteoarthritis. *J Am Med Assoc.* 2001;286:188–195.

Song KM, Halliday SE, Little DG. The effect of limb-length discrepancy in gait. *J Bone Joint Surg.* 1997;79A:1690–1697.

Review Article

Probe RA. Lower extremity angular malunion: evaluation and surgical correction. *J Am Acad Orthop Surg.* 2003;11:302–311.

Textbooks

Brinker MR, O'Connor DP. Principles of malunions. In: *Rockwood and Green's Fractures in Adults.* Philadelphia, PA: Lippincott Williams & Wilkins; 2010.

Ilizarov GA. *Transosseous Osteosynthesis.* Berlin, Germany: Springer-Verlag; 1992.

Marti RK, van Heerwarden RJ, eds. *Osteotomies for Posttraumatic Deformities.* New York, NY: Stuttgart, Thieme; 2008.

Paley D. *Principles of Deformity Correction.* Berlin, Germany: Springer-Verlag; 2002.

CHAPTER 4

Biomechanics and Biomaterials

Frank A.B. Gottschalk

BIOMECHANICS

I. Introduction—Biomechanics of the musculoskeletal system is the study of the effect of forces on the musculoskeletal system. Forces may be generated by muscle contractions or from externally applied sources. When a force is applied by an outside source, acceleration occurs and thus movement of an extremity. External forces can be explained using Newton's laws of motion. The application of external loads on materials and their effect is determined by the stress and strain of the material.

A. Definitions
   1. Biomechanics—Biomechanics is the study of the effects of forces on the musculoskeletal system.
   2. Statics—Statics is the branch of physics concerned with the analysis of loads (Force = Torque/Moment) on physical systems in static equilibrium.
   3. Kinematics—Kinematics is a branch of dynamics that describes the motion of objects without consideration of the circumstances leading to the motion. Motions may be within the body (joint kinematics) or may be during gait.
   4. Scalars—Scalars have magnitude but no direction. These include mass, age, time and height.
   5. Vectors—Vectors have magnitude and direction. These include force, velocity, acceleration, torque, stress, and strain. Vectors may be resolved into components that are perpendicular to each other, so that one is normal (perpendicular) and the other is parallel to a plane.

B. Newton's Laws—Newton's laws form the basis of biomechanical principles; they are:
   1. A physical body will remain at rest, or continue to move at a constant velocity along a straight path, unless an external net force acts upon it.
   2. The rate of change of momentum is proportional to the resultant force producing it and takes place in the direction of that force (Force = Mass × Acceleration).
   3. Every action has an equal and opposite reaction.

C. Forces
   1. A *force* is the quantity that changes velocity and/or the direction of an object (i.e., the vectors having magnitude and direction). The magnitude of a force is equal to the mass of the object multiplied by the acceleration of the object. The unit of force is $kg\ m/s^2$, which is a newton (N).
   2. Forces, stresses, and strains can be resolved into normal and shear components with respect to any arbitrary plane at any point of application on the structure.
   3. Normal stress—Normal means perpendicular to a particular plane. Normal stress may be compressive or tensile.
   4. Shear stress—Shear means parallel to a particular plane.

D. Moment
   1. A moment is the quantity that changes the angular velocity. It is the action of a force that tends to rotate an object about an axis.
   2. Moments are vectors. The magnitude of a moment = force × perpendicular distance to the axis of rotation; that is, it is equal to the mass moment of inertia of the object and its angular acceleration. The unit of the moment is the newton-meter (N·m). The direction of the moment is given by the right-hand rule.

E. Equilibrium
   1. The concept of static equilibrium is used for solving problems related to orthopaedic biomechanics.
   2. Static equilibrium is the situation in which no acceleration occurs in the system. (The system is at rest or moving at a constant velocity.)

3. Carrying objects—A weight held by the arm creates a moment about the elbow, the magnitude of which is calculated as the product of the force acting on the hand and the perpendicular distance between the line of action of the force and the center of rotation of the joint (Fig. 4-1).

4. Stance—The forces acting about the hip joint during single leg stance include the body weight, abductor muscle force to counteract the body weight, and the vector sum of these forces acting through the hip joint (joint reaction force). The abductor muscle force acts through a shorter moment arm than the body weight force; thus, the abductor muscle forces are approximately twice the body weight force. The result is the joint reaction force and is 3 to 4 times body weight. ***Using a cane in the opposite hand reduces the abductor muscle force and thus the joint reaction force by providing a moment that counters the body weight moment.***

5. Stair climbing—Stair climbing with the knee less flexed reduces the moment arm of the body weight force.

F. Linear Elasticity
   1. Linear elasticity is the model for material behavior and has three basic assumptions: stress and strain are proportional to each other; this proportionality constant is the modulus of elasticity, E (Young's modulus); and strain is reversible

when the stress is removed. The rate of application of the load does not have an effect. If stress is plotted against strain, the relationship between the calculated stress and the measured strain is linear, so the ratio of stress to strain is constant. The ratio of stress to strain depends on the material being tested and not the shape of structure being tested.

   2. Stress = elastic modulus × strain. Stress is the internal reaction to an externally applied force (or torque) distributed over the cross section of the material ($\sigma = E\varepsilon$). Testing of a material is usually done as an axial tensile load. The load is resisted internally over the surface of the material's cross section. Stress on a small piece of cross section is defined as internal force divided by surface area over which it acts; that is, stress = force / area. Unit of stress is N/m^2; $1 N/m^2$ is a Pascal (Pa). A force perpendicular to the cross section is called normal stress. Cross sections that are not perpendicular to the applied load have the force acting parallel to the surface of the cross section and this produces shear stress.

   3. Strain—Strain is internal deformation of a material in response to an applied stress; strain = the change in a dimension / the original dimension (Fig. 4-2). This may also be written as the following: normal strain = change in length / unit length. If positive, it is tensile and if negative, it is compressive. Strain is a ratio without units and is presented as a percentage or micro strain. Shear strain occurs when there is a change in the angle between two adjacent surfaces that were perpendicular to each other. Shear strain is expressed in units of radians.

G. Geometric Properties
   1. Cross-sectional area is important in resisting axial loading (tension or compression).
      • Axial load is the simplest loading that a structure can experience. As an example, ligaments support loads in tension and this

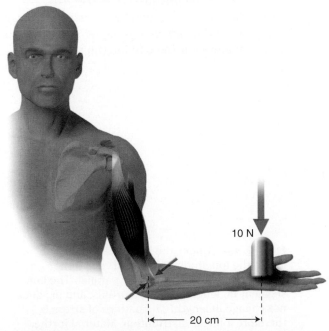

10 N

|← 20 cm →|

FIGURE 4-1 A 10-N weight in the hand creates a 2-N m moment about the elbow.

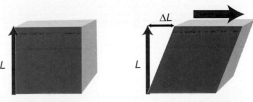

ΔL

L

L

FIGURE 4-2 When load is applied parallel to the face of a cube of material, the cube distorts, so that the edges of the cube are no longer right angles. The distortion (approximately equal to $\triangle L$, divided by L in radians) is the shear strain, where L is the length.

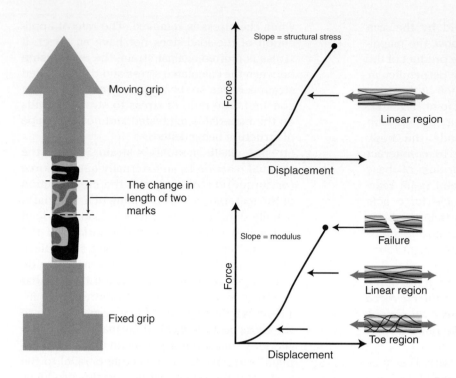

FIGURE 4-3 A patellar ligament is subjected to a uniaxial tensile test. The stiffness is the slope of the linear portion of the resulting force–displacement graph. If load is converted to stress and displacement to strain, the slope of the stress–strain graph is the elastic modulus of the ligament tissue. The strength is the maximum stress that the ligament can withstand before rupture.

is called tensile axial loading. The ligament elongates because the fibers elastically deform (Fig. 4-3).

(a) Structural stiffness is the ability of the structure to maintain its shape while under load. Structural stiffness can be altered by changes in geometry or by elastic modulus.

(b) The strength of a structure is defined as the maximum load that the structure can withstand without material failure.

• Centroid is the geometric center of the area or of the volume.

• Bending loads produce stresses in a material (e.g., bone, and therefore distribution of the loads through the structure).

(a) Application of a bending load to a rectangular structure results in the slight deformation of the material such that there is tension on the convex side and compression on the concave side. The mid portion of the structure (the neutral axis) experiences no tensile or compressive stress (Fig. 4-4).

(b) Material in the rectangular structure away from the midline has higher stresses than material at the midline (no stress).

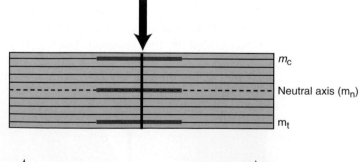

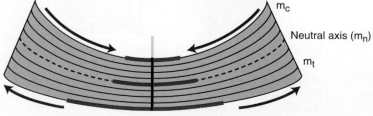

FIGURE 4-4 Under the influence of bending loads, the longitudinal lines curve and the transverse lines are no longer parallel. The line segment m_t lengthens, m_c shortens, and m_n does not change in length. The pattern of stress is therefore a linear distribution. Material further away from the midline has higher stress than the neutral axis, which experiences no stress.

(c) The distribution of mass about the midline is described by the area of moment of inertia (I). This is calculated by adding each increment of cross-sectional area in the structure multiplied by the square of the distance from the increment of cross section to the neutral axis. $I = (1/12) wd^3$ where w is width and d is thickness. Doubling the thickness of the rectangular structure increases resistance to bending by a factor of 8.

(d) The strength of a beam is the largest bending moment a beam can carry without causing stress in the material to exceed a critical limit. In biologic structures and implants that undergo cyclic bending loads, the critical limit is the fatigue strength of the material.

(e) Bending loads applied to long bones usually result in the intensities of the induced compressive and tensile stresses to be almost equal because of the relative symmetry of the bones. ***Bone is weaker under tension (tensile loading) than under compression (compressive loading), and failure starts in the region of highest tensile stress.***

- Torsional load is another mode of loading. Torsional loads produce moments that tend to twist the structure.

(a) A common occurrence is torsional loading of the tibia that occurs while skiing. A load applied perpendicular to the ski tip produces a torsional moment, resulting in external rotation of the tibia. Using static equilibrium, there is a moment applied to the internal cross section of the tibia proximally that is equal to the external applied moment but in the opposite direction. The internal torque is constant along the length of the tibia. This is different from bending moments, which vary along the length of the bone.

(b) Torsional load applied to a beam or cylinder leads to one end rotating relative to the other. A straight longitudinal line on the surface will twist into a helix providing a helix angle α. The total deformation (θ) is proportional to the applied torque and the length of the structure (L). The proportional constant between the torque and the angle of deformation (torsional stiffness) depends on the material property and geometric property of the structure. The material property is

the shear modulus, which, in metallic alloys, is related to the elastic modulus. An example is that stainless steel 316L has twice the elastic modulus as titanium; therefore, stainless steel shear modulus is twice as great as titanium.

(c) Torsional strength also depends on the material property and the cross-sectional property. The material property is the ultimate shear stress and the cross-sectional property is the ratio of the polar moment of inertia to the radius of the cylinder (Fig. 4-5).

- Polar moment of inertia (J) measures the average of the square of the perpendicular distance of each minute section of material from the axis of torsion. It is always positive. Its importance is in describing resistance to torsion.

(a) For a solid cylinder, $J = \frac{1}{2} \pi r^4$ where r = radius of the cylinder. Doubling the radius of a cylinder increases the resistance to torsion by a factor of 16.

- Centroid is the geometric center of the area or volume. Because the strength of the cross section depends on the radius, torsional

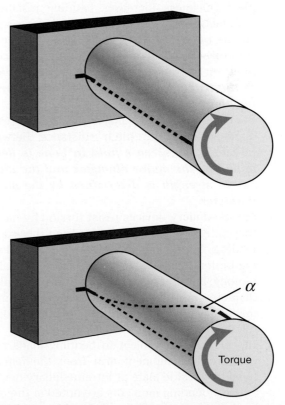

FIGURE 4-5   A cylinder is fixed at one end and has a torque applied to the other end. The torque causes an angular twist to the rod.

fractures start at the surface of the cross section that is closest to the centroid (the part with the smallest radius).

H. Application to Bone—Fractures resulting from torsional loading occur most often in the distal third of the tibia. This can be explained by the axis of the tibia and that the bone in the middle and proximal parts of the tibia are farther away from the axis of the tibia and are better able to resist torsional loading. Another example would be a pin or screw hole in the distal third of the tibia, which weakens the bone more than if the location was in the proximal third where the bone has a larger radius. A bending load applied at the mid-tibia produces strains that are greater than those when a bending load applied at the proximal tibia, thus increasing the fracture potential. If a hole is located at the bending loading site, the weakening effect is more profound.

I. Orthopaedic Implants—All orthopaedic implants will have bone contact at certain points, so as to be able to transmit or receive loads. Loads may be transmitted over large areas or at localized points. **Load transmission may be load sharing or load transfer.**

   1. Bone plates resistance to bending is proportional to the thickness cubed; thus doubling the plate thickness increases bending resistance by a factor of 8. Plates resist tensile forces and should be placed where possible on the tensile side of bone. They may also be used for compression or graft support. **Screws placed close to the fracture site reduce the unsupported length of the plate.**

   2. Bone screws have a major and minor (root) diameter and the pitch (distance between threads). **The screw's hold in bone is determined by the major diameter and the pitch. Screw strength is determined by the minor diameter.**

   3. Intramedullary devices resist torsion by having the material distributed away from the axis of loading; larger implants resist torsional loading better. Reaming affects the fracture healing biology; and fracture comminution and implant diameter impact fracture stability. Solid intramedullary devices are stiffer compared to open (slotted) designs.

   4. Hip screws are subject to bending loads as a result of the moment arm from the femoral head to the side plate or intramedullary device. Smaller bending moments are noted in the intamedullary device. Compression hip screws, depending on the angle of the side plate, allow for some impaction of the fracture fragments. Blade plates resist torsion but do not provide fracture impaction. They are best used for reverse obliquity intertrochanteric fractures.

   5. External fixators provide best stability by allowing fracture ends to be in contact with each other. Other factors that improve stability are increased pin diameter (second most important factor), bending is proportional to the fourth power of diameter; additional pins; decreased bone-rod distance (pin stiffness is proportional to the third power of bone-rod distance); pins in different planes; stacked rods; increased distance between pins.

   6. Circular external fixators use thin 1.8-mm wires fixed under tension. The optimum orientation of implants on the ring is at 90° to one another where possible. Half pins provide better purchase in diaphyseal bone. The bending stiffness of the frame is independent of the loading direction because the frame is circular. Tensioned wires should be positioned opposite to each other and not on the same side of the ring. Enhanced stability of circular external fixators includes the use of larger diameter wires and half pins, smaller ring diameter, olive wires, wires that cross at 90°, increased wire tension up to 130 kg, placement of the two central rings close to the fracture site, decreased spacing between adjacent rings and the use of more rings.

BIOMATERIALS

The term "biomaterials" refers to synthetic materials used to augment or replace tissues and their functions.

A. Mechanical Properties of Material

   1. Generalized Hooke's law—It states that in a particular direction, stress is proportional to strain. The proportionality constant is the material's elastic modulus in that direction.

   2. Measurements of properties of materials are done using standardized specimens that are subjected to tension, compression, and shear (torque) by a mechanical testing machine.

   • Stress–strain curves describe material behavior, and force–displacement curves describe structural behavior.

   • In experimental conditions, converting a force–displacement curve to a stress–strain curve is not always possible.

B. Material Properties

The stress–strain relationships for an isotropic material are characterized by the elastic modulus and Poisson's ratio. In the study of mechanical properties of materials, "isotropic" means having identical values of a property in all crystallographic directions (from Greek: *Iso* means equal and *tropos* means direction). Poisson's ration is the ratio of the relative contraction strain, or transverse strain (normal to the applied load), divided by the relative extension strain, or axial strain (in the direction of the applied load).

1. Elastic, or Young's, modulus (E) is the slope of the initial linear portion of the curve on a stress–strain graph. It is the proportionality between stress and strain for that particular material (Fig. 4-6). Elastic modulus is characteristic of the material and cannot be changed without changing the material itself.

2. Poisson's ration (v) for a specimen in tension is the ratio of the transverse strain to the axial strain (see above).
   • v = (change in diameter / original diameter) / (change in length/original length) If v = 0, the

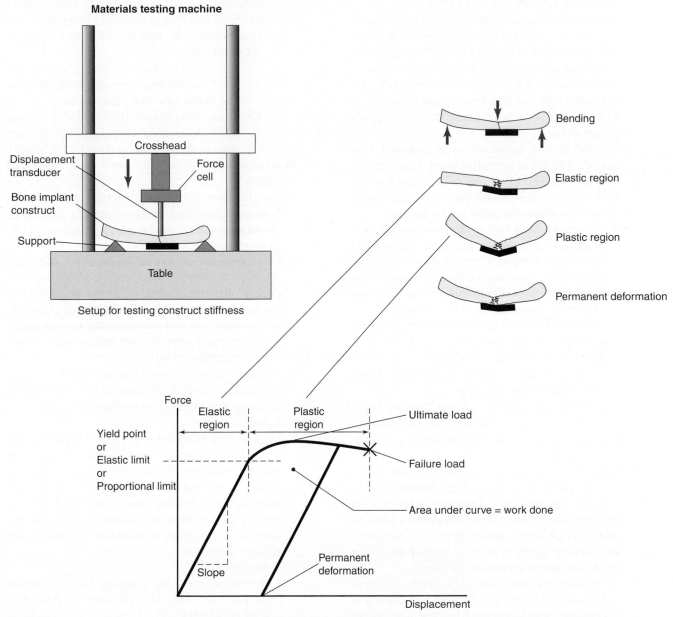

FIGURE 4-6 *Top left:* A fixation construct (bone–fixation–bone) set up in a mechanical testing machine. In this example, a long bone is fixed with a plate and subjected to bending. *Top right:* The construct during loading in the elastic region, plastic region, and with permanent deformation. *Bottom:* The resulting measurements from the testing machine, which measures foced applied and displacement at the point of the applied load. The graph demonstrates the elastic region, in which the construct acts like a spring, returning to its original shape after the load is released; the plastic region, in which the plate may have permanently bent; and the failure load, in which the fixation fails. (Adapted from Tencer AF. Biomechanics of fractures and fracture fixation. In: Bucholz RW, Court-Brown CM, Heckman JD, et al., eds. *Rockwood and Green's Fractures in Adults.* 7th ed. Philadelphia, PA: Lippincott Williams & Wilkins; 2010, with permission.)

material is highly compressible and if ν = 1, the material incompressible.

3. Yield point (or region) is the point at which the material behavior deviates from elastic to plastic deformation (Fig. 4-6). Strains applied beyond the yield point are not completely reversible since plastic deformation has occurred.

4. Failure point is the point at which the material fails (Fig. 4-6).

5. Ductility is a measure of a material's ability to deform plastically before failure.

6. Resilience is the amount of energy returned on release of a strain while the material is elastically deformed. In Figure 4-6, it is the area under the linear portion of the stress–strain curve.

7. Toughness is the amount of energy per unit volume a material can absorb before failure. In Figure 4-6, it is the area under the entire stress strain curve.

8. Fatigue is the property of a material that causes it to fail at a relatively low load applied many times and is usually a load much lower than that which causes failure in a single cycle. Several biologic materials fail by fatigue.
   • Endurance limit is the theoretic upper limit of stress for which a material will not fail by fatigue. Fatigue is a cumulative phenomenon and is accelerated by corrosion. Bone remodeling prevents failure in bone material that is damaged as a result of fatigue.

9. Isotropic properties denote that the material properties do not vary with the direction of loading. Stress–strain relationships are characterized by two material properties: elastic modulus and Poisson's ratio.

10. Anisotropic properties indicate that the material properties do vary with the direction of loading. Stress–strain relationships are difficult to characterize.

11. Orthotropic properties mean that the material properties do not change appreciably in a particular direction. ***Cortical bone is considered orthotropic with properties that do not change in the axial direction, across a transverse section, or in a radial direction within a specific sample of bone.***

12. Viscoelasticity indicates that a material's properties vary with the rate of loading. Loading and unloading curves are not identical and not all energy applied to the material during loading is recovered on unloading. The loss of strain energy (in the form of heat) is called hysteresis.

13. Creep (cold flow) is the phenomenon of a material exhibiting increasing strain (deformation) under a constant applied load. Relaxation from stress occurs after the application of a displacement load, and after some time with the same displacement, the stress decreases. Creep and stress relaxation describe similar behavior. Examples of materials which are subject to creep include vertebral discs, polyethylene, bone, skin, and glass.

14. Viscosity (η) is a fluid's resistance to flow and is analogous to the modulus of elasticity. Viscosity (η) = shear strain / shear rate.
   • Newtonian fluids—Viscosity is independent of shear rate (e.g., water and plasma).
   • Non-Newtonian fluids—Viscosity depends on shear rate.
     (a) Shear-thickening or dilatant fluids exhibit increasing viscosity with increasing shear rate (e.g., emulsions).
     (b) Shear-thinning or thixotropic fluids exhibit decreasing viscosity with increasing shear rate (e.g., synovial fluid, blood).

C. Molecular Structure Influence on Material Properties

1. Metals have a crystal structure and metallic bonding. They may be commercially pure (e.g., titanium) or they may be alloys (mixtures of two or more metals, e.g., Ti-6Al-4V).

2. Polymers are chains of molecules covalently bonded together. Secondary bonding may occur by hydrogen chains or van der Waals forces.

3. Ceramics are materials created by ionic bonding of a metallic ion and a nonmetallic ion (oxygen). They are hard, strong, and brittle (e.g., aluminum oxide, zirconium).

4. Composites involve mechanical bonding between materials. Chemical, physical, or true mechanical bonding may occur (e.g., laminates, bone).

D. Tribology

1. Friction is a coefficient of force / applied load. μ = frictional force / applied load. Static coefficient describes the condition in which the object is at rest and the dynamic coefficient describes the friction when the object has begun to move. Wear properties depend on the particular materials in contact, lubricant, and relative velocity.

2. Lubrication
   • Hydrodynamic—Surfaces are fully separated by the lubricant. The viscosity of the lubricant is primary.
   • Hydrostatic—Lubricant is pressurized to maintain separation of surfaces.
   • Boundary layer—A thin, slippery surface adherent layer that minimizes contact. Higher wear can occur than in situations where the surfaces are completely separated.

- Elastohydrodynamic—Elasticity of the bearing surfaces allows adaptation of surface irregularities without plastic deformation. This allows for a thicker film of lubricant. Low wear rates occur but subsurface fatigue may occur with breakdown of the material (e.g., knee polyethylene).
- Weeping—One surface is porous and fluid is forced out of the surface (e.g., normal joints).

3. Wear mechanisms
   - Adhesive—Particles of each bearing surface can adhere to the other surface.
   - Abrasive—The harder material abrades the softer material's surface.
   - Transfer is similar to adhesive wear but with a film of material transferred from one to the other.
   - Fatigue of the softer material is usually due to subsurface stresses. It occurs with polyethylene delamination.
   - Third body wear occurs when particles from a different source are interspersed between two bearing surfaces (e.g., cement in a total hip or knee).
   - Corrosive wear is seen when electrochemical reactions occur around a bearing surface.
   - Fretting wear is seen with cyclic loading with very small oscillations (e.g., screw head in contact with plate).

E. Corrosion
   Corrosion is the gradual breaking down of a material due to chemical reactions with its surroundings. This means the loss of electrons of metals reacting with water and oxygen. Corrosion can be concentrated locally to form a pit or crack, or it can extend across a wide area to produce general deterioration.
   1. Metals are degradable by corrosion.
   2. Polymers undergo chemical degradation usually observed by discoloration.
   3. Ceramics may also undergo corrosion but this is usually a longer and very slow process.
   4. Passivation is a thin film of corrosion products that form on a metal's surface spontaneously, acting as a barrier to further oxidation. This layer stops growing at less than a micrometer thick and can be used under conditions to minimize surface wear. Commercially pure titanium and some stainless steels form passivation layers spontaneously. Implants are manufactured with a passivation layer by treatment in a weak acid solution.
   5. Types of corrosion
      - Uniform corrosion is the continuous degradation of a material throughout its surface.

These materials are not used for implantation (e.g., iron).
   - Galvanic corrosion occurs when two different metals in direct contact are immersed in an electrolyte. In order for galvanic corrosion to occur, an electrically conductive path and an ionically conductive path are necessary. Of the two metals, one is the anode giving up electrons and is reduced by oxidation. The other metal is the cathode and is protected. Combinations of other metals with stainless steel are bad.
   - Crevice corrosion is a localized form of corrosion occurring in spaces in which the access of the working fluid from the environment is limited, and, as a result, concentration of metallic ions (positive) and chloride or hydrogen ions (negative) results.
   - Pitting is a localized occurrence of corrosion, similar to crevice corrosion. It is usually seen with breakdown of the passivation process.
   - Intergranular corrosion is corrosion within a metal, at the boundaries between the metal grains, as a result of a localized galvanic cell. The presence of debris in the metal is a contributing factor. Low-carbon steel used in surgical application reduces the precipitation of chromium carbides and minimizes intergranular corrosion.
   - Stress corrosion cracking is the cracking of a material in a corrosive environment. Stress-induced cracks may accelerate the corrosion process, and cyclic loading may interfere with the material's ability to re-form a passive layer.

F. Mechanical Properties of Orthopaedic Materials
   1. Modulus of elasticity (Fig. 4-7)—The values are ranked from lowest to highest. Cancellous bone has the lowest modulus of elasticity, followed by polyethylene and polymethylmethacrylate up to aluminum oxide.
   2. Ultimate strength of a material is shown in Figure 4-8. The values are ranked from minimum to maximum, from cancellous bone to cobalt chrome.
   3. Values of elastic modulus and ultimate strength are shown in Table 4-1. The values are approximate because testing conditions may vary.
   4. Bone as a material.
      - Composite material—Bone is formed predominantly of type I collagen and has a mineralized matrix of hydroxyapatite.
      - Anisotropic properties—Bone is modeled as transverse isotropic and has continuous remodeling of its mineral content by resorption and deposition. Fatigue damage is minimized by the remodeling process.

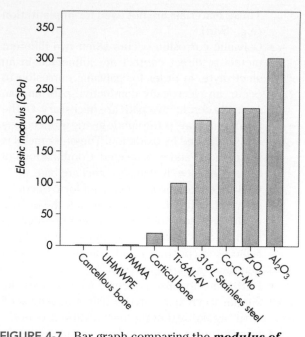

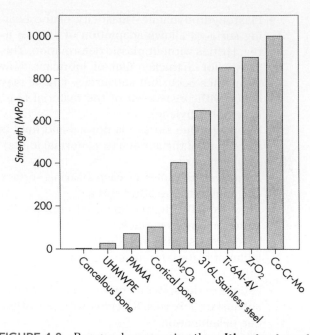

FIGURE 4-7 Bar graph comparing the ***modulus of elasticity*** for various biomaterials. The values shown are not exact. See Table 4-1 for approximate values. *Co–Cr–Mo*, Cobalt–chromium–molybdenum; *UHMWPE*, ultrahigh-molecular-weight polyethylene.

FIGURE 4-8 Bar graph comparing the ***ultimate strength*** for various biomaterials. The value shown for PMMA bone cement is compressive strength; the values shown for ZrO_2 and Al_2O_3 are for bending strength. The values shown are not exact. See Table 4-1 for approximate values. *Co–Cr–Mo*, Cobalt–chromium–molybdenum; *UHMWPE*, ultrahigh-molecular-weight polyethylene.

TABLE 4-1

Material Properties for Various Biomaterials

Modulus of Elasticity (GPa)[a]	
Cancellous bone	0.5–1
Polyethylene (ultrahigh molecular weight)	1
PMMA bone cement	2
Cortical bone	15–20
Ti-6Al-4V	100
316L stainless steel	200
Cobalt–chromium–molybdenum alloy	220
ZrO_2	220
Al_2O_3	300
Ultimate Strength (MPa)[a]	
Cancellous bone	2
Polyethylene (ultrahigh molecular weight)	25
PMMA bone cement	70 (compressive strength)
Cortical bone	100
Al_2O_3	400 (bending strength)
316L Stainless steel	500–800
Ti-6Al-4V	850
ZrO_2	900 (bending strength)
Cobalt–chromium–molybdenum alloy	650–1,100

Note: Values are representative and are not intended to be exact.
[a]The SI unit for stress is the pascal (Pa). 1 GPa (gigapascal) = 10^9 Pa; 1 MPa (megapascal) = 10^6 Pa; 1 MPa = 145 psi (pounds per square inch).

- Mineral component—This varies throughout the bone and continuously over time.
- Structural adaptation attempts to compensate for weakening of bone. The diameter of the inner and outer femoral cortex increases with age. Mechanically, the structural resistance to bending is increased, as is the torsion resistance while the bone becomes weaker due to the loss of mineral content.
- Strength and modulus are approximately proportional to the square of the density. This is used in quantitative computed tomography and dual-energy X-ray absorptiometry bone mineral measurements.
- Fractures occur along haversian canals, cement lines, and lacunae. When the strain rate is very high, fracture patterns become random. Failure increases 10% for every tenfold increase in strain rate. Comminution results from the release of energy stored in bone before fracture.
- Fracture patterns may indicate the mechanism of loading resulting in fracture.
  - (a) Transverse fracture pattern indicates tensile loading.
  - (b) Spiral fracture pattern indicates torsional loading.
  - (c) Transverse fracture pattern with butterfly fragments indicates bending load as seen with the case of a pedestrian hit by a car bumper resulting in tibial fracture.
  - (d) Oblique fracture pattern indicates compressive loading.

SUGGESTED READINGS

Recent Articles

Brinker MR, O'Connor DP. Biomaterials and biomechanics. In: Miller MD, ed. *Review of Orthopaedics*. Philadelphia, PA: Saunders Elsevier; 2008.

Mow VC, Flatow EL, Ateshian GA. Biomechanics. In: Buckwalter JA, Einhorn TA, Simon SR, eds. *Orthopaedic Basic Science*. Rosemont, IL: American Academy of Orthopaedic Surgeons; 2000.

Wright TM, Li SL. Biomaterials. In: Buckwalter JA, Einhorn TA, Simon SR, eds. *Orthopaedic Basic Science*. Rosemont, IL: American Academy of Orthopaedic Surgeons; 2000.

Wright TM, Maher SA. Musculoskeletal biomechanics. In: *Orthopaedic Knowledge Update 9*. Rosemont, IL: American Academy of Orthopaedic Surgeons; 2008.

Textbooks

Black J. *Orthopaedic Biomaterials in Research and Practice*. New York, NY: Churchill Livingstone; 1988.

Brinker MR. Basic sciences. In: Miller MD, Brinker MR, eds. *Review of Orthopaedics*. 3rd ed. Philadelphia, PA: WB Saunders.

Chao EYS, Aro HT. Biomechanics of fracture fixation. In: Mow VC, Hayes WC, eds. *Basic Orthopaedic Biomechanics*. New York, NY: Raven; 1991.

Cochran GVB. *A Primer of Orhtopaedic Biomechanics*. New York, NY: Churchill Livingstone; 1982.

Kaplan FS, Hayes WC, Keaveny TM, et al. Form and function of bone. In: Simon SR, ed. *Orthopaedic Basic Science*. Rosemont, IL: American Academy of Orthopaedic Surgeons.

Litsky AS, Spector M. Biomaterials. In: Simon SR, ed. *Orthopaedic Basic Science*. Rosemont, IL: American Academy of Orthopaedic Surgeons; 1994.

Mow VC, Flatow EL, Foster RJ. Biomechanics. In: Simon SR, ed. *Orthopaedic Basic Science*. Rosemont, IL: American Academy of Orthopaedic Surgeons; 1994.

SECTION II

Adult Trauma

CHAPTER 5

Fractures of the Femoral Neck and Intertrochanteric Region

Robert Victor Cantu and Kenneth J. Koval

I. Introduction—Osteoporosis and resulting hip fractures have a substantial economic and social impact. It is estimated that worldwide, 323 million people suffer from osteoporosis and that number is projected to be 1.55 billion by the year 2050. It has been predicted that the number of hip fractures in the year 2050 will be 6.3 million. Despite improvements in patient care and operative technique, hip fractures account for a significant amount of health care expenditure.

II. Femoral Neck Fractures

A. Overview—Femoral neck fractures are intracapsular fractures that occur in the region from just above the intertrochanteric region to just below the articular surface of the femoral head. There is a bimodal distribution of femoral neck fractures, with the majority occurring in the geriatric population from low energy falls, and a smaller number occurring in younger individuals from high-energy mechanisms. The approach to treatment is different in these two groups, in that an attempt is made to reduce and fix almost all femoral neck fractures in young adults, while most displaced fractures in elderly patients are treated with arthroplasty.

B. Evaluation

1. Physical examination—If a patient is suspected of having a femoral neck fracture, range of motion of the hip should be avoided until radiographs of the proximal femur have been obtained, to avoid displacement of the fracture. Patients who have a displaced femoral neck fracture will present with the affected leg in a

shortened and externally rotated position. With nondisplaced fractures, the injured extremity lacks these obvious deformities.

- Elderly population—In elderly patients who have sustained a fall and resulting hip fracture, the cause of the fall should be elucidated. Nonmechanical reasons for falling such as syncope, presyncope, myocardial infarction, and stroke are all possible etiologies. The patient should be evaluated for other injuries. The distal radius and proximal humerus are regions commonly affected by osteoporosis, and should be evaluated for possible fracture.
- Younger population—Hip fractures in younger patients typically result from high-energy mechanisms. These patients require a complete primary and secondary survey with special attention paid to the ipsilateral femoral shaft. *Approximately 2.5% of femoral shaft fractures are associated with an ipsilateral femoral neck fracture*.

2. Radiographic evaluation—The standard radiographic evaluation for patients suspected to have a hip fracture includes an anteroposterior (AP) view of the pelvis and hip and a cross-table lateral view of the hip. The AP pelvis view allows for comparison with the contralateral hip; this comparison may reveal subtle impaction or fracture displacement. The cross-table lateral is preferred to the frog lateral, since the latter can result in increased pain and fracture

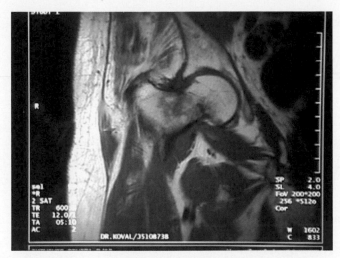

FIGURE 5-1 T1-weighted MRI showing a nondisplaced femoral neck fracture.

displacement. Ideally, the AP hip view should be obtained with the hip in 15° of internal rotation to compensate for the anatomic anteversion of the femoral neck and provide an en face view

of the proximal femur. This view can help diagnose nondisplaced fractures. If all radiographs appear normal but the clinical suspicion for hip fracture is high, a technetium bone scan or magnetic resonance image (MRI) should be obtained (Fig. 5-1). The MRI is sensitive for occult hip fracture within 24 hours, whereas the bone scan may take 48 to 72 hours to demonstrate the fracture.

C. Injury Classification—The Garden classification is commonly used and consists of four grades: Grade 1 is an incomplete or valgus impacted fracture, Grade 2 is a complete and nondisplaced fracture, Grade 3 is a partially displaced fracture, and a Grade 4 is completely displaced (Fig. 5-2). The risk of nonunion and osteonecrosis is substantially higher for Grades 3 and 4. The Pauwel classification is based on the angle formed by the fracture line and a horizontal line with simulated standing. Pauwel's classification consists of three types: Type 1 has an angle less than 30°, Type 2 has an angle between 30° and 50°, and Type 3 has and angle greater than 50° (Fig. 5-3). ***The more vertical the fracture line***

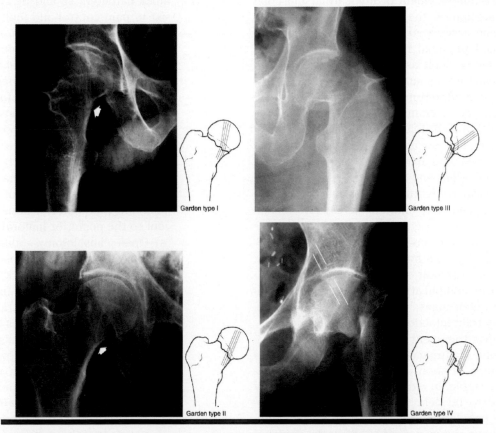

Garden type I

Garden type III

Garden type II

Garden type IV

FIGURE 5-2 Garden's classification of femoral neck fractures. (From Keating J. Femoral neck fractures. In: Bucholz RW, Heckman JD, Court-Brown C, et al., eds. *Rockwood and Green's Fractures in Adults*. 7th ed. Philadelphia, PA: Lippincott Williams & Wilkins; 2010, with permission.)

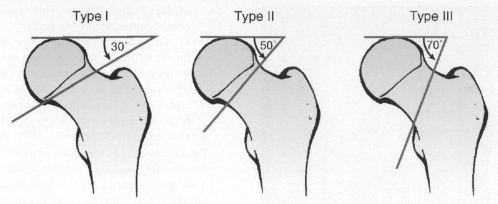

Type I Type II Type III

FIGURE 5-3 The Pauwel classification of femoral neck fractures is based on the angle the fracture forms with the horizontal plane. As fracture type progresses from Type 1 to Type 3, the obliquity of the fracture line increases and, theoretically, the shear forces at the fracture site also increase. (From Keating J. Femoral neck fractures. In: Bucholz, RW, Heckman JD, Court-Brown C, et al., eds. *Rockwood and Green's Fractures in Adults.* 7th ed. Philadelphia, PA: Lippincott Williams & Wilkins; 2010, with permission.)

is, the higher the Pauwel's angle, and the higher the shear forces across the fracture.

D. Associated Injuries

1. Elderly population—In elderly patients a cerebral vascular accident or myocardial infarction may precipitate the fall resulting in fracture. Common associated injuries include distal radius and proximal humerus fractures. Closed head injury such as subdural hematoma can also result from a fall.

2. Younger population—In young patients the high-energy mechanisms can result in associated orthopaedic injuries of the ipsilateral tibia, femur, and pelvis/acetabulum. Injuries to the head, chest, and abdomen are also common.

E. Treatment Options and Rationale

1. Nonoperative treatment—Nonoperative treatment is generally limited to elderly nonambulators who are considered too high risk for surgery or who have minimal pain with mobilization. The goal for these patients should be early bed to chair mobilization in attempt to limit the complications of prolonged recumbence: atelectasis, thromboembolic disease, urinary tract infection, and decubitus ulcers.

2. Operative treatment

• Timing of surgery—Patients should undergo surgery as soon as they are deemed medically stable. In elderly patients, surgery may need to be delayed until fluid and electrolyte imbalances are corrected. Recent studies have shown some benefit to the model of orthopaedic and geriatric medicine cocare in reducing complications such as delirium and improving survival. *In young patients, displaced femoral neck fractures are treated*

emergently with ORIF to help reduce the risk of osteonecrosis.

• Anesthetic considerations—For patients unable to undergo early surgery, femoral nerve block catheters should be considered to assist in pain control and limit narcotic use in the elderly. Studies have not shown a consistent difference in perioperative mortality with general versus regional anesthesia.

• Nondisplaced femoral neck fractures—Recommended treatment for nondisplaced femoral neck fractures consists of internal fixation with multiple lag screws placed in a parallel fashion. Either three or four screws should be used. If three screws are used, an inverted triangle pattern can be used with the inferior screw adjacent to the inferior neck and the posterior superior screw adjacent to the posterior femoral neck.

(a) Open capsulotomy—Some authors have recommended open capsulotomy for nondisplaced femoral neck fractures, with the theory that capsulotomy relieves pressure from the intracapsular hematoma and in turn reduces the risk of osteonecrosis. Controversy exists as to whether capsulotomy actually lowers the rate of osteonecrosis; however, it does have its advocates, especially for young patients. *Prior to surgery, allowing the leg to assume a flexed, abducted, and externally rotated position has also been shown to decrease intracapsular pressure.*

• Displaced femoral neck fractures—Treatment of displaced femoral neck fractures largely depends on the patient's age and activity

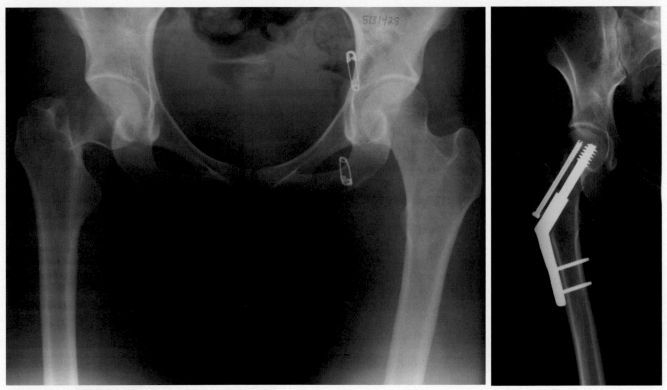

FIGURE 5-4   Preop and 3-month postop X-rays of a displaced femoral neck fracture in a 26-year-old man treated with open reduction and internal fixation.

level. In younger patients, closed or open reduction is performed followed by internal fixation (Fig. 5-4). The goal is anatomic reduction and it may be necessary to perform either a Smith-Petersen or a Watson-Jones approach to ensure proper reduction. In older, less active patients, most authors recommend prosthetic replacement of the femoral head. ***Trials comparing ORIF to hemiarthroplasty for displaced femoral neck fractures in the elderly have consistently shown improved outcomes and lower reoperation rates for the arthroplasty group***.

(a) Internal fixation—When internal fixation is chosen, anatomic reduction is essential to try to minimize complications such as nonunion and osteonecrosis. If attempts at closed reduction do not clearly result in anatomic reduction, then open reduction should be performed and fixation achieved typically with multiple parallel screws. For basi-cervical fractures, fixation with a sliding hip screw is another alternative.

(b) Prosthetic replacement of the femoral head—Prosthetic replacement can take the form of either hemiarthroplasty with a monopolar or a bipolar prosthesis, or total hip arthroplasty. The bipolar prosthesis has a theoretic advantage over the unipolar, as the second articulation in the bipolar has been suggested to decrease acetabular wear. In practice, however, it has been shown that the second articulation in a bipolar often ceases to function and it essentially becomes a unipolar construct. Additionally, unlike the monopolar, the bipolar typically has a metal-polyethylene articulation, which, if it does function as designed, can lead to polyethylene wear and osteolysis. For most low-demand elderly patients, the unipolar replacement is the recommended prosthesis (Fig. 5-5).

(c) Total hip replacement—Patients with pre-existing degenerative disease of the hip (i.e., rheumatoid arthritis, Paget's disease, osteoarthritis) and a femoral neck fracture should be considered for total hip arthroplasty. Some studies have suggested improved outcomes regarding pain and function for total hip arthroplasty compared with hemiarthroplasty even for elderly patients without arthritis. On the other hand, total hip replacement does have a higher dislocation rate and generally should be avoided in patients with dementia who are unable to comply

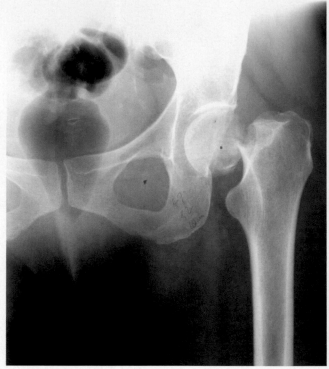

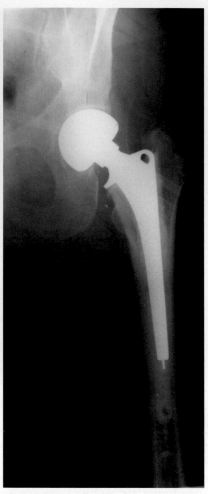

FIGURE 5-5 Preop and postop hip radiographs of an elderly patient with a displaced femoral neck fracture treated with hemiarthroplasty.

with hip precautions. Patients with neurologic conditions such as Parkinson's or paralysis from a prior cerebrovascular accident are also at increased risk of dislocation and generally should be treated with a hemiarthroplasty.

- Postoperative management—Recommendations regarding weight-bearing status after femoral neck fixation have ranged from complete nonweight bearing to weight bearing as tolerated. Biomechanical studies have shown that even when a person attempts to be nonweight bearing, there are substantial joint reactive forces across the hip and knee due to muscular contractions. Many elderly patients cannot comply with restricted weight bearing. For these reasons, it is recommended that elderly patients be allowed to weight bear as tolerated to assist with mobilization and avoid the complications of prolonged recumbence. For younger patients restriction of weight bearing may be considered if fracture fixation is in question.

F. Complications of the Injury
  1. Nonunion—The nonunion rate for femoral neck fractures is determined largely by fracture displacement. Nondisplaced or impacted femoral neck fractures have a nonunion rate of approximately 5% or less after fixation. Displaced fractures have a nonunion rate closer to 30% after ORIF. *For young patients who have undergone ORIF, nonunion is the most common complication.* Additional risk factors for nonunion include nonanatomic reduction and metabolic conditions such as dialysis dependent renal failure. Nonunion typically presents with groin or thigh pain. Most femoral neck nonunions require further surgery. *For young patients attempt is usually made to preserve the femoral head with a valgus intertrochanteric osteotomy with plate fixation. In older patients nonunion is treated with hemiarthroplasty of the hip.*
  2. Osteonecrosis—Due largely to its retrograde blood supply, the femoral head is prone to osteonecrosis after femoral neck fracture. Similar to nonunion, osteonecrosis rates are strongly

correlated with the degree of fracture displacement. Nondisplaced or impacted fractures have an osteonecrosis rate of 8% or less, while Garden's Grade 4 fractures have a rate of 30% or more. Magnetic resonance imaging is more sensitive than plain radiographs at demonstrating early signs of osteonecrosis. Late changes can be seen on X-rays which include subchondral collapse and femoral head deformity. Symptoms include groin or thigh pain and about 33% of patients require further surgical procedures. In younger patients, attempts to revascularize the femoral head such as drilling and bone grafting can be considered. In older patients with advanced osteonecrosis, the treatment is typically prosthetic replacement.

3. Mortality—For elderly patients, in hospital mortality from hip fracture is approximately 3% to 5% in most studies. The 1-year mortality after hip fracture is substantially higher than age matched controls and ranges between 20% and 40%. Risk factors for increased mortality include pre-existing cardiac or pulmonary disease, cognitive impairment, pneumonia, and male gender.

4. Thromboembolic disease—Even with prophylaxis, the rate of thromboembolic disease after hip fracture is substantial, with some reports as high as 23%. Multiple agents have been used to prevent deep venous thrombosis (DVT) and pulmonary embolism (PE), including low-molecular weight heparin, warfarin (Coumadin), aspirin as well as pneumatic compression boots. For patients suspected of having a DVT, ultrasonography is the least invasive means of diagnosis. For diagnosis of PE, spiral CT has largely replaced ventilation/perfusion scan as the modality of choice.

G. Complications of Treatment
1. Fixation failure—Risk factors for implant failure include osteopenia, fracture comminution, and nonanatomic reduction. Patients typically present with groin pain, buttock pain, or both. Treatment options consist of revision internal fixation, valgus osteotomy, hemiarthroplasty, or total hip arthroplasty. The revision/osteotomy options are generally performed on younger patients, while prosthetic replacement is generally the preferred options for elderly patients.

2. Subtrochanteric femur fracture—*Subtrochanteric femur fracture can result from multiple unfilled drill holes in the lateral femur, or starting holes for fracture fixation that are distal to the lesser trochanter.* Treatment options for the fracture include revision to a sliding hip screw with a long side plate, or conversion to an intramedullary hip screw. Either option requires care to maintain anatomic reduction of the femoral neck.

3. Failed arthroplasty—Prosthetic replacement can fail due to aseptic loosening, infection, or acetabular wear. Superficial infections can be treated with wound debridement and IV antibiotics, while deep infections may require staged revision or resection arthroplasty. Acetabular wear can occur with either a unipolar or a bipolar hemiarthroplasty. Studies have shown many bipolar implants function essentially as a unipolar within the first year. Advanced acetabular wear after a hemiarthroplasty typically results in groin pain and treatment generally consists of conversion to a total hip replacement. Femoral stem loosening can often be seen radiographically before symptoms such as thigh pain develop.

H. Special Considerations
1. Femoral neck stress fractures—In patients with osteopenic bone, femoral neck stress fractures can occur with repetitive loading from normal daily activities. In younger patients with healthy bone, stress fractures can result from unusually heavy and repetitive load such as seen in military recruits or long distance runners. Stress fractures result in new onset groin pain. Plain radiographs may not demonstrate the fracture acutely and either MRI or bone scan should be obtained if the diagnosis is in question.

2. Ipsilateral femoral neck and femoral shaft fractures—*Ipsilateral femoral neck fractures occur in about 2.5% of femoral shaft fractures.* Assuming the femoral neck fracture is nondisplaced, secure internal fixation of the femoral neck should be obtained before insertion of intramedullary nails to prevent displacement. *A sliding hip screw can be used to obtain fixation of the femoral neck fracture, followed by reamed retrograde nailing of the femoral shaft fracture.* Displaced femoral neck fractures in younger patients often require open reduction through either a Smith-Petersen or a Watson-Jones approach to ensure anatomic reduction.

3. Neurologic impairment—In patients with severe neurologic impairment such as advanced Parkinson's disease, paralysis from previous stroke, or severe dementia an anterior approach to the hip should be considered when performing hemiarthroplasty. This helps prevent both wound contamination as well as hip dislocation from noncompliance. Some patients have a significant adductor contracture and should undergo adductor release at the time of arthroplasty.

4. Chronic renal disease—Patients with advanced renal failure often have poor bone quality making them poor candidates for internal fixation. In these patients, even nondisplaced fractures may best be treated with femoral head replacement.

5. Paget's disease—Patients with Paget's disease are prone to proximal femoral deformity and excessive bleeding at surgery. If the acetabulum is involved, treatment should consist of total hip arthroplasty.

6. Pathologic fracture—A pathologic fracture is a contraindication to internal fixation. Patients should be evaluated for metastases before surgery, including full pelvis and femur films. Before surgery, it should be clear as to whether the fracture is from a primary tumor or a metastasis, as the treatment may be quite different.

III. Intertrochanteric Femur Fractures
   A. Overview—The majority of intertrochanteric fractures occur in elderly patients from low energy falls. The intertrochanteric region consists of the extracapsular bone running between the greater and lesser trochanters. The bone in this area is primarily cancellous and has an excellent blood supply, thereby making the risk of nonunion lower than with femoral neck fractures. The calcar femorale is the proximal continuation of the linea aspera found in the posteromedial femoral shaft and the posterior femoral neck. It receives substantial forces during weight bearing as stress is transferred from the hip region to the femoral shaft.
   B. Evaluation—The physical examination and radiographic evaluation for patients with intertrochanteric fractures is the same as for patients with femoral neck fractures. Patients with intertrochanteric fractures tend to have more tenderness over the greater trochanter.
   C. Injury Classification—The Evans classification of intertrochanteric fractures was developed in 1949; it stresses the importance of an intact posteromedial cortex for maintaining a stable reduction. The classification has not been shown to have good reproducibility and it may be better to simply classify fractures as stable or unstable. Unstable fractures include those with comminution of the posteromedial cortex, subtrochanteric extension, or reverse obliquity patterns.
   D. Associated Injuries—Common associated injuries in elderly patients include distal radius fracture, proximal humerus fracture, subdural hematoma, myocardial infarction, and cerebrovascular accident.

E. Treatment
   1. Nonoperative treatment—Nonoperative treatment should only be considered in nonambulators who are deemed too high-risk for operative intervention or who have minimal pain with mobilization. If nonoperative treatment is elected, it is an option to mobilize the patient with early bed to chair activity, with the goal of preventing the sequelae of prolonged bedrest (e.g., thromboembolic disease, atelectasis, pneumonia). If fracture deformity occurs, a reconstructive procedure may be indicated later on if the patient's medical condition improves. The other option is to maintain the patient in skeletal traction in an attempt to maintain fracture alignment during healing. The latter form of treatment makes nursing care very difficult and carries with it all the risks of prolonged recumbence.
   2. Operative treatment—Surgery is the treatment for virtually all patients who can tolerate an operation. Surgery should be performed as soon as all comorbid medical conditions, including cardiopulmonary, fluid, and electrolyte imbalances have been assessed and optimized.
      • History—Some of the earliest devices used to treat intertrochanteric hip fractures were fixed angle nail-plate implants such as the Jewett nail. These devices provided fracture fixation, but did not allow for fracture impaction. Failure tended to occur as a result of nail penetration into the hip joint, nail "cutout" from the femoral head, or hardware breakage. In an effort to combat the high failure rate for unstable fractures, reduction techniques were developed in an attempt to restore the posteromedial buttress. Examples included the Hughston–Dimon medial displacement osteotomy, the Sarmiento valgus osteomy, and the Wayne County lateral displacement reduction. The next generation of implants, such as the Massie nail, allowed for the nail fixation in the femoral head to telescope within the barrel of the side plate, similar to present day sliding hip screws. This design improved osseous contact but still risked nail cutout because of poor fixation in the femoral head and sharp edges on the nail. The modern sliding hip screw provides improved fixation in the femoral head with the large outside thread diameter of the lag screws (Fig. 5-6).
      • Sliding hip screw—Before inserting a sliding hip screw, fracture reduction should be

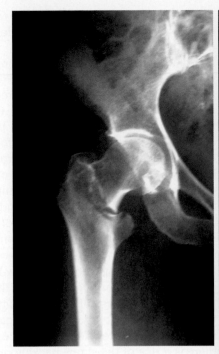
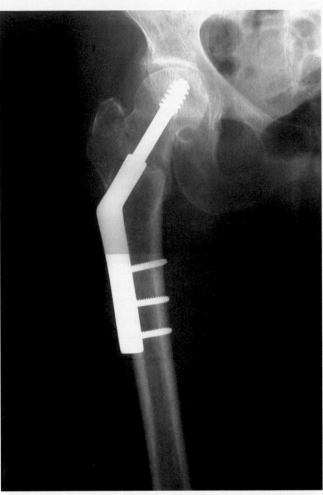

FIGURE 5-6 Preop and 3-month postop X-rays of a stable intertrochanteric fracture treated with a sliding hip screw.

obtained. This is typically done on the fracture table with the affected leg in traction. The leg is internally rotated and reduction examined using fluoroscopy on AP and lateral views. Care should be taken to avoid malrotation, varus alignment, and posterior sag. Posterior sag can be corrected by placing a crutch under the hip or by using an elevator during surgery. After reduction, a lateral approach to the proximal femur is performed. Lag screw placement is performed next with care to *position the screw in the center of the femoral head on both the AP and lateral views. Screws should be placed within 1cm of the subchondral bone as a tip–apex distance of greater than 2.5 cm has been associated with increased risk of failure.* Plate angles between 130° and 150° are most commonly used. The advantages of higher angle plates are improved sliding characteristics between the screw and barrel and decreased varus moment acting on the implant. The

disadvantages include difficulty with screw placement in the center of the femoral head and an increased cortical stress riser because of the necessity for a distal starting hole for screw placement. The most common angle used is the 135° side plate which allows for proper lag screw placement and minimizes the cortical stress riser. Newer implants have the ability to adjust the barrel plate angle to match the patient's anatomy. Side plate application is performed next. *Although biomechanical studies have shown that a two-hole side plate may provide adequate fixation, this assumes both screws have good purchase in bone. If there is any question, a four-hole plate should be used.* If there is comminution or displacement of the greater trochanter, reduction and fixation can be achieved with a tension band technique. If the greater trochanter is not reduced, the abductor mechanism may be compromised with resulting Trendelenburg gait pattern.

- Intramedullary hip screw—The intramedullary hip screw consists of a sliding hip screw coupled to an intramedullary nail. Theoretic advantages include limited fracture exposure and a lower bending moment than with the sliding hip screw. Studies have shown no consistent difference between IM hip screws and sliding hip screws with respect to operating time, blood loss, infection rate, screw cutout, or screw sliding. Recent studies have shown, however, a dramatic increase in the use of IM hip screws for intertrochanteric fractures. Short IM hip screws do have an increased risk of femoral shaft fracture at the nail tip or at the distal locking screw insertion points.
- Prosthetic replacement—Prosthetic replacement has been used for comminuted, unstable intertrochanteric fractures. Prosthetic replacement is a more extensive surgical procedure with increased blood loss and does introduce the risk of hip dislocation. For some patients, particularly those with advanced osteoporosis as seen in renal disease, prosthetic replacement may provide a more predictable result than ORIF. Prosthetic replacement can also be used as a salvage for failed internal fixation.
- Postoperative management—Postoperatively patients are mobilized as soon as possible and generally are allowed to weight bear as tolerated. Thromboprophylaxis should be administered until patients are ambulatory.

F. Complications of the Injury—The risk of thromboembolic disease and mortality are essentially the same as for patients with femoral neck fractures. Due largely to the improved blood supply to the intertrochanteric region, the risk of osteonecrosis and nonunion is much less than for femoral neck fractures.

G. Complications of Treatment
   1. Varus displacement of the proximal fragment—Varus displacement of the proximal fragment is usually associated with unstable fractures with a lack of restoration of the posteromedial buttress. This may result in implant breakage, screw cutout, screw penetration into the joint, and dissociation of the side plate from the femur. Potential causes of this complication include anterosuperior femoral screw placement, improper reaming creating a second lag screw channel, lack of stable reduction, excessive fracture collapse (exceeding the sliding capacity of the device), and severe osteopenia leading to poor screw fixation. Management options

include revision ORIF, conversion to joint arthroplasty, or acceptance of the deformity in nonambulatory, pain-free patients.
   2. Malrotation deformities—Malrotation can occur with either excessive internal or external rotation of the distal fragment. During reduction of unstable fracture patterns, excessive internal rotation of the distal fragment should be avoided and fixation should generally be performed with the leg in neutral or slight external rotation.
   3. Nonunion—The risk of nonunion of intertrochanteric fractures using a sliding hip screw is approximately 2%. Symptoms include buttock or groin pain. Treatment consists of either revision internal fixation or conversion to a joint arthroplasty.
   4. Screw-barrel disengagement—Screw-barrel disengagement is a rare complication that can be prevented by the use of a compression screw if there is insufficient screw-barrel engagement. If a compression screw is left in place, however, there is a risk of the screw backing out, becoming symptomatic, and requiring a second operation for removal.
   5. Bleeding—With the lateral approach to the proximal femur for fixation of an intertrochanteric fracture, bleeding encountered as the vastus lateralis muscle is elevated is most likely from a branch of the profunda femoris artery.

H. Special Considerations
   1. Basilar neck fractures—Basilar femoral neck fractures are extracapsular, and behave more like intertrochanteric fractures. Fixation can be achieved with either cannulated screws or a sliding hip screw. If a sliding hip screw is used, there is a tendency for the femoral head to rotate, especially in patients with good bone quality. To prevent the rotation, an antirotation screw is placed superior to the lag screw guide wire before insertion of the lag screw.
   2. Reverse obliquity fractures—In reverse obliquity fractures, the fracture line runs from superomedial to inferolateral (Fig. 5-7). The sliding axis of the hip screw is parallel to the fracture line in reverse obliquity fractures, as opposed to perpendicular with standard intertrochanteric fractures. The impaction benefits of the sliding hip screw are lost and the result is suboptimal fixation with the potential for medialization of the femoral shaft relative to the proximal fragment. ***This fracture pattern is better treated with either an intramedullary hip screw or a fixed angle device such as a 95° dynamic condylar screw or a blade plate.***

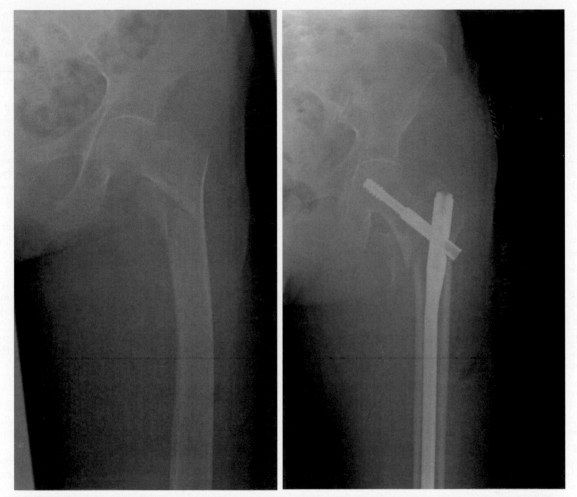

FIGURE 5-7 Preop and postop X-rays of an intertrochanteric hip fracture with reverse obliquity subtrochanteric extension treated with a cephalomedullary IM nail.

3. Severe osteopenia—With severe osteopenia, fixation in the femoral head and the femoral shaft may be compromised. Methylmethacrylate has been used to improve implant fixation. Locked plates designed for the proximal femur can be used. Alternatively, joint arthroplasty can be performed.

4. Isolated greater trochanteric fractures—Isolated greater trochanteric fractures are rare and typically occur in elderly patients who have sustained a direct blow to the greater trochanter. Patients present with lateral hip or buttock pain with weight bearing or hip range of motion. The fracture can usually be treated nonoperatively with weight bearing as tolerated using assistive devices. Operative treatment is generally reserved for physiologically young patients with widely displaced fractures.

5. Isolated lesser trochanteric fractures—Isolated lesser trochanteric fractures can occur in adolescents from a forceful iliopsoas contraction resulting in avulsion of the lesser trochanteric apophysis. Treatment is usually symptomatic. *In elderly patients, isolated lesser trochanteric fractures should be considered pathognomonic for a pathologic lesion of the proximal femur.* Treatment is based on the nature and extent of the pathologic process. If it turns out there is no pathologic involvement, treatment is symptomatic.

SUGGESTED READINGS

Classic Articles

Arnold WD. The effect of early weight-bearing on the stability of femoral neck fractures treated with Knowles pins. *J Bone Joint Surg.* 1984;66A:847–852.

Barnes R, Brown JT, Garden RS, et al. Subcapital fractures of the femur. *J Bone Joint Surg.* 1976;58B:2–24.

Boyd HB, Griffin LL. Classification and treatment of trochanteric fractures. *Arch Surg.* 1949;58:853–866.

Dahl E. Mortality and life expectancy after hip fractures. *Acta Orthop Scand.* 1980;51:163–170.

Evans EM. The treatment of trochanteric fractures of the femur. *J Bone Joint Surg.* 1951;33B:190–203.

Garden RS. Low angle fixation in fractures of the femoral neck. *J Bone Joint Surg.* 1961;43B:647–663.

Garden RS. Malreduction and avascular necrosis in subcapital fractures of the femur. *J Bone Joint Surg.* 1971;53B:183–197.

Kyle RF, Gustilo RB, Premer RF. Analysis of 622 intertrochanteric hip fractures: a retrospective study. *J Bone Joint Surg.* 1979;61A:216–221.

Kyle RF, Wright TM, Burstein AH. Biomechanical analysis of the sliding characteristics of compression hip screws. *J Bone Joint Surg.* 1980;62A:1308–1314.

Stromquist B, Hansson L, Nilsson L, et al. Hook pin fixation in femoral neck fractures: a two year follow-up study of 300 cases. *Clin Orthop.* 1987;318:58–62.

Swiotkowski MF, Winquist RA, Hansen ST. Femoral neck fractures in patients aged 12–49. *J Bone Joint Surg.* 1984;66A:837–846.

Swiontkowski MF, Harrington RM, Keller TS, et al. Torsion and bending analysis of internal fixation techniques for femoral neck fractures: the role of implant design and bone density. *J Orthop Res.* 1987;5:433–444.

Recent Articles

Al-Ani AN, Samuelsson B, Tidermark J, et al. Early operation on patients with a hip fracture improved the ability to return to independent living. A prospective study of 850 patients. *J Bone Joint Surg Am.* 2008;90(7):1436–1442.

Aros B, Tosteson AN, Gottlieb DJ, et al. Is a sliding hip screw or im nail the preferred implant for intertrochanteric fracture fixation? *Clin Orthop Relat Res.* 2008;466(11):2827–2832.

Anglen JO, Weinstein JN. American Board of Orthopaedic Surgery Research Committee. Nail or plate fixation of intertrochanteric hip fractures: changing pattern of practice. A review of the American Board of Orthopaedic Surgery Database. *J Bone Joint Surg Am.* 2008;90(4):700–707.

Blomfeldt R, Tornkvist H, Ponzer S, et al. Comparison of internal fixation with total hip replacement for displaced femoral neck fractures. Randomized, controlled trial performed at four years. *J Bone Joint Surg Am.* 2005;87(8):1680–1688.

Gotfried Y. Integrity of the lateral femoral wall in intertrochanteric hip fractures: an important predictor of reoperation. *J Bone Joint Surg Am.* 2007;89(11):2552–2553.

Heetveld MJ, Raaymakers EL, Luitse JS, et al. Rating of internal fixation and clinical outcome in displaced femoral neck fractures: a prospective multicenter study. *Clin Orthop Relat Res.* 2007;454:207–213.

Keating JF, Grant A, Masson M, et al. Randomized comparison of reduction and fixation, bipolar hemiarthroplasty, and total hip arthroplasty. Treatment of displaced intracapsular hip fractures in healthy older patients. *J Bone Joint Surg Am.* 2006;88(2):249–260.

Zlowodzki M, Jonsson A, Paulke R, et al. Shortening after femoral neck fracture fixation: is there a solution? *Clin Orthop Relat Res.* 2007;461:213–218.

Review Articles

Koval KJ, Zuckerman JD, Hip fractures I. Overview and evaluation and treatment of femoral-neck fractures. *J Am Acad Orthop Surg.* 1994;2(3):141–149.

Koval KJ, Zuckerman JD. Hip fractures. II. Evaluation and treatment of intertrochanteric fractures. *J Am Acad Orthop Surg.* 1994;2(3):150–156.

Textbooks

Koval KJ, Cantu RV. Intertrochanteric fractures. In: Bucholz RW, Heckman JD, Court-Brown C, et al., eds. *Rockwood and Green's Fractures in Adults.* 6th ed. Philadelphia, PA: Lippincott Williams & Wilkins; 2006.

Swiontkowski MF. Intracapsular hip fractures. In: Browner BD, Jupiter JB, Levine AM, et al., eds. *Skeletal Trauma.* Vol 2. 2nd ed. Philadelphia, PA: WB Saunders; 1998.

CHAPTER 6

Fractures of the Femoral Shaft and Subtrochanteric Region

Sean E. Nork

I. Overview
   A. Divisions of the Femur—The femur may be divided into five general anatomic regions: head and neck, intertochanteric, subtrochanteric, shaft, and supracondylar/intercondylar.
      1. Subtrochanteric region—The subtrochanteric zone of the femur is typically defined as the area extending from the lesser trochanter to a point 5 cm distally. Fractures with a component occurring within this region are usually reported as subtrochanteric fractures, even if fracture extensions proximally and distally are observed.
      2. Femoral shaft—The shaft of the femur begins at the top of the femoral isthmus and extends to the distal metadiaphyseal junction, an indistinct transitional zone contiguous with the supracondylar region.
   B. Incidence and Mechanisms of Injury
      1. Subtrochanteric fractures—Subtrochanteric fractures may occur across all age groups. There is an asymmetric age- and gender-related bimodal distribution of fractures. High-energy injuries are typically seen in young males and low-energy injuries are frequently observed in elderly females. Subtrochanteric fracture extensions occur commonly in elderly patients who sustain a hip fracture due to a fall. Typical high-energy mechanisms that predominate in younger patients result from motor vehicle crashes, falls from heights, and penetrating trauma. Although uncommon, fractures can occur in the subtrochanteric region as a complication of screw fixation for a femoral neck fracture, especially if screws are placed below the level of the lesser trochanter, or if an apex proximal triangle configuration of three screws was used.
      2. Femoral shaft fractures—Similar to subtrochanteric fractures, femoral shaft fractures are observed in all age groups. However, younger patients with high-energy blunt mechanisms are most common. The majority (70%) occurs in male patients with an average age below 30 years. Transverse and oblique patterns are the most common configurations in young patients. Older patients, especially females, may sustain a femoral shaft fracture due to a lower energy mechanism such as a fall from standing. Spiral patterns are commonly seen in older patients.
   C. Anatomy—Subtrochanteric and shaft regions of the femur are encased in a thick muscular envelope. The muscular attachments typically determine the primary displacements following fracture. Subtrochanteric fractures occurring entirely below the lesser trochanter have the typical deformities of flexion, abduction, and external rotation of the proximal segment. Shortening is common in both shaft and subtrochanteric patterns. The osseous anatomy of the proximal femur has considerable variation. The femoral neck is anteverted an average of $13° \pm 7°$ and is translated 1.0 to 1.5 cm anterior to the axis of the femoral shaft. The neck–shaft angle averages $133° \pm 7°$ in women and $129° \pm 7°$ in men. The adult femur has an asymmetrical anterior bow with an average radius of curvature between 109 and 120 cm. The linea aspera is the posterior cortical thickening of the femoral diaphysis, is a muscular attachment site, and buttresses the concavity of the femoral shaft.

II. Evaluation
   A. Initial Management—Due to the high-energy mechanisms observed in young patients, associated injuries are common. The initial management includes adequate resuscitation using advanced trauma life support guidelines and should include fluid replacement for blood loss (up to three units

of blood loss can be expected per femur fracture). For older patients with low-energy mechanisms of injury, pathologic (including metabolic) etiologies should be investigated.

B. Physical Findings—Typical findings on physical examination include pain, swelling, and deformity. Associated injuries can be distracting. A visual inspection should include a circumferential evaluation of the limb as well as palpation of all extremities, the pelvis, and the spine. The ipsilateral knee and hip should be examined to determine if there are associated noncontiguous fractures or ligamentous injuries. Subtrochanteric fractures tend to shorten and present with fracture extension (the iliopsoas causes flexion of the proximal fragment) and varus (the hip muscles cause abduction and external rotation of the proximal fragment). Shaft fractures present with limb shortening and variable rotation and translation.

C. Emergency Treatment—Emergency treatment should include realignment of the injured extremity using skeletal traction (preferable at the distal femur using a small diameter tensioned wire) to prevent additional soft-tissue injury, to decrease muscle spasm, to limit ongoing blood loss, and to decrease pain. Open wounds should be irrigated and a sterile dressing should be applied. Pulses should be symmetrical, and the ankle–arm index (AAI) should be equal in both extremities. An AAI of less than 0.9 is an indication for vascular consultation and arterial imaging.

D. Radiographic Imaging—Imaging should allow visualization of the entire femoral shaft, the ipsilateral hip, and the ipsilateral knee joint in both the anteroposterior and lateral planes. The femoral neck should be scrutinized for fracture in both subtrochanteric and femoral shaft fractures. This can be accomplished with dedicated hip radiographs, after review of a pelvic CT or both if applicable. The fracture configuration and location, as well as the femoral anatomy can be determined primarily from biplanar radiographs. Bone loss, bone quality, and the femoral canal diameter can be determined. Contralateral femur radiographs can be useful in segmental or highly comminuted patterns, in anticipation of difficulty with length and rotational determination at the time of treatment.

III. Injury Classifications
  A. Subtrochanteric Fractures—There are numerous classifications for fractures of the subtrochanteric region.

1. Russell-Taylor classification—The Russell-Taylor classification (Fig. 6-1) has gained acceptance because it is a useful guide in selecting the best type of internal fixation from both a biomechanical and a biological perspective.

2. Orthopaedic Trauma Association (OTA) classification based on the AO/ASIF
   • Types 32-A1.1, 32-A2.1, and 32-A3.1 are elementary patterns without comminution (spiral, oblique, and transverse).
   • Types 32-B1.1, 32-B2.1, and 32-B3.1 have butterfly comminution (spiral wedge, bending wedge, fragmented wedge).
   • Types 32-C1.1, 32-C2.1, and 32-C3.1 are comminuted versions of the elementary patterns.

3. Fielding and Magliato classification
   • Type I fractures occur at the level of the lesser trochanter.
   • Type II fractures occur within 1 inch below the lesser trochanter.
   • Type III fractures occur 1 to 2 inches below the lesser trochanter.

4. Older classifications—Older classifications include those of Seinsheimer, Waddell, and Boyd and Griffin.

B. Femoral Shaft Fractures—Femoral shaft fractures are initially described according to location, pattern (e.g., transverse, oblique, spiral), and any associated soft-tissue injury. The location is typically described as proximal third, middle third, or distal third; or at the junctions of these approximate locations. Additionally, the location of the fracture relative to the isthmus is important for communication.

1. OTA classification—The OTA (AO/ASIF) classification (Fig. 6-2) describes fractures based on morphology and suggests the mechanism of the applied force. Type A fractures are simple in configuration and are divided into spiral, oblique, and transverse patterns. Type B fractures have components of comminution and include spiral and bending wedge patterns; as well as fragmented wedge patterns. Type C fractures have segmental comminution.

2. Winquist-Hansen classification—The Winquist-Hansen classification was devised to describe comminution as related to the need for interlocking screw fixation in early nail designs (Fig. 6-3). Grade 0 and I fractures were considered axially stable and interlocking was therefore not necessarily needed. Grade III, IV, and V fractures were considered axially unstable and therefore required interlocking to prevent

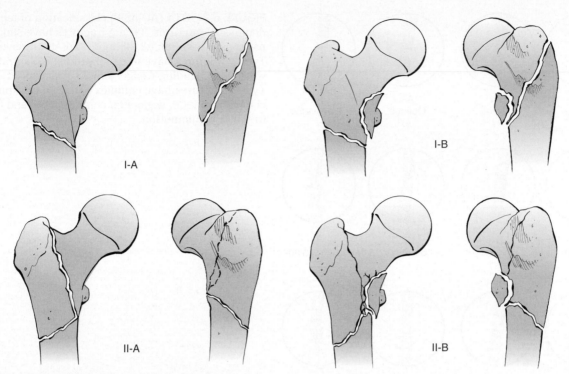

FIGURE 6-1 Russell-Taylor classification of subtrochanteric fractures. **Type 1A,** Fracture extension with any degree of comminution from below the level of the lesser treochanter to the isthmus with no extension into the piriformis fossa. **Type 1B,** Fracture extension involving the lesser trochanter to the isthmus with no extension into the piriformis fossa. **Type IIA,** Fracture extension into the piriformis fossa without lesser trochanter involvement (with medial cortex stability). **Type IIB,** Fracture extension into the piriformis fossa and involving the lesser trochanter (without medial cortex stability). (Reprinted with permission from Haidukewych G, Langford J. Subtrochanteric fractures. In: Bucholz RW, Heckman JD, Court-Brown C, et al, eds. *Rockwood and Green's Fractures in Adults.* 7th ed. Philadelphia, PA: Lippincott Williams & Wilkins; 2006.)

shortening and rotational malunion. However, because of the possibility of unrecognized comminution and the currently predictable performance of statically locked nails, this classification system is now largely used for the purpose of describing communication.

C. Open Fractures—The soft-tissue injuries associated with open fractures are extrapolated from the original system of Gustilo and colleagues. Although not a perfect translation to the femur, it is still used.

1. Type I is an open fracture with a clean wound shorter than 1 cm.

2. Type II is an open fracture with a wound longer than 1 cm and without extensive soft-tissue damage, flaps, or avulsions.

3. Type IIIA open fractures have adequate soft-tissue coverage of the bone despite extensive soft-tissue laceration or flaps; these include open fractures with segmental comminution and fractures caused by a gunshot.

4. Type IIIB signifies periosteal stripping with inadequate soft-tissue coverage of the fractured bone.

5. Type IIIC is an open fracture associated with an arterial injury requiring repair.

IV. Associated Injuries

A. Open Fractures—Open fractures may occur from indirect trauma (e.g., motor vehicle crashes) or from penetrating trauma (e.g., gunshot injuries). These injuries are typically the result of high-energy mechanisms and associated vascular injuries are commonly observed. Intramedullary stabilization remains the treatment of choice for most open fractures. Exceptions include gross contamination that cannot be adequately debrided and substantial surgical delay to treatment. In these cases, a period of skeletal traction with repeated debridements until soft-tissue contamination is reduced is recommended prior to definitive intramedullary stabilization.

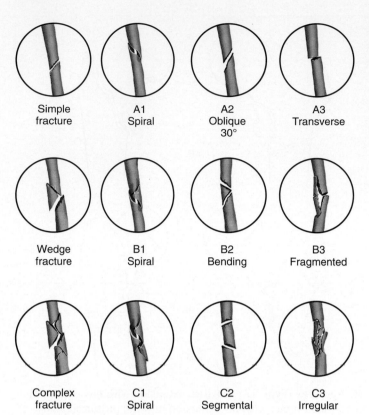

FIGURE 6-2 OTA (AO-ASIF) classification of femoral diaphyseal fractures. Type A fractures have simple patterns: A1, spiral; A2, oblique; and A3, transverse. Type B fractures have wedge patterns: B1, spiral wedge; B2, bending wedge; and B3, fragmented wedge. Type C fractures have complex patterns: C1, spiral comminution; C2, segmental comminution; and C3, irregular comminution.

Low-velocity gunshot injuries do not require an open debridement before intramedullary nailing assuming that no foreign material has been brought into the wound with the projectile. Brumback had no infections in 62 Gustilo Type I, II, and IIIA open fractures and only three infections in 27 Type IIIB injuries (two had delayed treatment). Grosse reported three infections in 115 open femoral shaft fractures, all of which were treated with early IM nailing.

B. Ipsilateral Femoral Shaft and Neck Injuries—*Concomitant femoral neck fractures occur in 3% to 10% of patients with femoral shaft fractures. The femoral neck fracture is often nondisplaced and is missed in 30% to 50% of cases.* Most commonly, the femoral neck fracture is basicervical in location (55%), although vertically oriented intracapsular patterns are seen in approximately 35% of patients. Because of the high incidence of missed femoral neck fractures, all patients should undergo a careful review of all available radiographic studies and dedicated hip radiographs. Treatment should be prioritized based on the patient's overall condition. An accurate reduction and treatment of the femoral neck should take precedence.

C. Floating Knee Injuries—Floating knee injuries (ipsilateral femoral and tibial fractures) are best treated with early stabilization of both injuries, ideally with intramedullary nailing. *The femur should be stabilized first.* In the event that the patient becomes medically unstable during surgery and both surgeries cannot be completed, femoral fixation allows the patient to sit upright (decreasing the risk of pulmonary complications) and controls pain. The presence of a tibia fracture should not affect the method or direction (antegrade versus retrograde) of medullary stabilization.

D. Fat Embolism—Fat embolism occurs in many trauma patients with long bone fractures, but is usually subclinical. In young patients, a delay in medullary stabilization is associated with an increased incidence of clinically significant fat embolism syndrome.

E. Knee Ligamentous and Meniscal Injuries—Ipsilateral knee ligamentous and meniscal injuries occur commonly in association with femoral shaft fractures. Ligamentous laxity on physical examination is seen in approximately 50% of patients and meniscal tears occur in approximately 30% of patients. Ligamentous stability is best assessed under anesthesia immediately after fracture stabilization.

F. Nerve Injuries—Nerve injuries occur rarely and are more likely following penetrating trauma.

G. Vascular Injuries—Associated vascular injuries are rare, but they represent a surgical emergency.

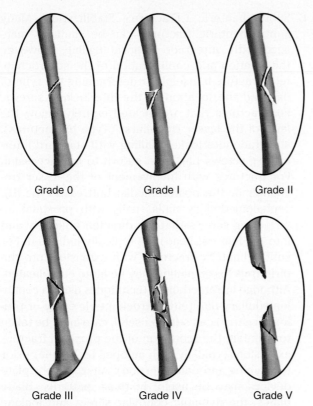

Grade 0   Grade I   Grade II

Grade III   Grade IV   Grade V

FIGURE 6-3 Winquist and Hansen's classification of femoral shaft fracture comminution. Grade 0 has no comminution. Grade I has a small butterfly fragment. Grade II has a large butterfly fragment of less than 50% of the width of the bone (leaving 50% or more of the cortex of the proximal fragment in contact with the cortex of the distal fragment). Grade III has a large butterfly fragment of more than 50% of the width of the bone (leaving less than 50% of the cortex of the proximal fragment in contact with the cortex of the distal fragment). Grade IV has segmental comminution. Grade V has a segmental bone defect.

Vascular flow to the extremity should be reestablished within 6 hours if possible to maximize limb salvage rates. Temporary shunting followed by orthopaedic stabilization and definitive vascular repair may be necessary if a time delay exists. In most instances, definitive femoral stabilization can be performed during the same surgical procedure as the vascular repair.

H. Bilateral Injuries—Patients with bilateral femur fractures have a worse overall prognosis and higher mortality than patients with unilateral fractures. This is likely due to increased blood loss, a higher risk of respiratory distress syndrome, and a higher prevalence of associated injuries. Treatment with reamed nails can be safely performed even in patients with bilateral fractures.

I. Associated Head Injury—Timing for femoral stabilization in patients with an associated head injury remains controversial. The primary concern is the impact of any associated intraoperative hypotension (and hypoxia) on the neurological outcome in these patients. While intraoperative hypotension and decreased cerebral perfusion pressure is common during femoral nailing procedures, the association with neurological injury has yet to be demonstrated. There is an increased rate of pulmonary complications when femoral stabilization is delayed due to an associated head injury.

J. Skeletal Immaturity and Open Physes—Skeletal immaturity and open physes alter the treatment decision. An open capital femoral epiphysis is usually a contraindication to treatment with a piriformis entry reamed nail. Younger patients (depending on the patient's weight and the fracture location) may be treated with flexible (elastic) intramedullary nails. External fixation and plates also have a role depending on the patient's associated injuries and the fracture pattern.

V. Treatment and Treatment Rationale

A. Overview—Fractures of the femoral shaft and subtrochanteric region will heal with immobilization. However, traction and casting are associated with numerous problems including knee stiffness, malunion (shortening, angulation, rotational malalignment), prolonged recumbency, and pulmonary demise. Operative treatment is standard for virtually all femoral shaft and subtrochanteric fractures.

B. Multiple Injuries—The timing and type of treatment of the polytraumatized patient with a femoral shaft fracture remains controversial. Early stabilization of the femoral shaft is necessary. However, the method of stabilization is dependent on multiple factors including any associated chest, head, or other injuries. In most patients, early and definitive stabilization with a reamed intramedullary nail can be performed. In a prospective and randomized study by Bone et al. in 1989, early (<24 hours) and late stabilization (>48 hours) were compared. Early stabilization was associated with a lower incidence of acute respiratory distress syndrome (ARDS), fat embolism, and pulmonary dysfunction in patients with an injury severity score (ISS) higher than 18. Length of care in both the intensive care unit and the hospital, as well as hospital costs, were reduced in the early stabilization group. However, there may exist a subgroup of patients, typically termed "borderline" patients or patients in extremis, who may benefit from early stabilization with external fixation followed by delayed (typically 5 to 7 days later) conversion to internal fixation. This has been shown to be a safe approach and may be indicated in some patients with an associated pulmonary injury or in patients who will not tolerate a lengthy operative procedure.

C. IM Nailing for Femoral Shaft Fractures—Most femoral shaft fractures can be treated with intramedullary nailing. This is the treatment of choice for femoral shaft fractures as it can typically be performed in a closed fashion, thereby maintaining the fracture hematoma and the associated soft-tissue envelope. Results of reamed, antegrade, statically locked intramedullary nailing for femoral shaft fractures has shown union rates that range from 94% to 100%. In Winquist and Hansen's series of 520 femoral shaft fractures, the rate of union was 99% with an infection rate of less than 1%. More recently, in a series of 551 fractures reported by Wolinksy et al., fracture healing after the index intramedullary procedure was 94%. Including minor secondary procedures and exchange nailings, union was ultimately achieved in 99% of patients.

D. Alternative Treatments for Femoral Shaft Fractures—Although intramedullary nailing is considered the optimal treatment for most femoral shaft fractures, an alternative treatment approach may be necessary in some patients. This decision may be influenced by the availability of implants and fluoroscopy, the size of the medullary canal, and other factors.

1. Skeletal traction and bracing—The use of a period of traction, roller traction, cast braces and other methods are usually reserved for the rare situation where the patient cannot tolerate a surgical procedure. Young children may be treated with a period of traction followed by casting.

2. External fixation—In an adult patient, it is rare to use external fixation as a definitive treatment method. However, external fixation may be useful as a temporary form of stabilization in the severely injured patient or in cases where severe contamination necessitates a deep secondary debridement. Conversion to a medullary implant at the appropriate time (preferably within 2 weeks) is optimal.

3. Plate stabilization—The relative indications for plate stabilization of a femoral shaft fracture include: associated ipsilateral femoral neck fracture, a narrow medullary canal that cannot be treated with a nail, previous malunion, and skeletal immaturity.

4. Flexible IM nails—Flexible IM nails are generally reserved for fractures in the skeletally immature patient. These may be inserted either retrograde or antegrade, avoiding the femoral growth plates.

E. Subtrochanteric Fracture Stabilization—Many subtrochanteric fractures can be similarly managed with antegrade femoral nailing. However, the location and configuration of the subtrochanteric fracture is useful for determining the type of nail and the location of the interlocking screws. For fractures that are located entirely below the level of the lesser trochanter (Type IA fractures), antegrade interlocked nailing with standard interlocking screws has been shown to be successful. For fractures with involvement of the lesser trochanter or the posteromedial buttress (Type IB), cephalomedullary nails (nails with proximal interlocking screws that are directed obliquely and into the femoral head) are typically indicated. For subtrochanteric fractures with extension into the piriformis fossa, nailing may be more complicated. Although intramedullary techniques using a cephalomedullary nail (either trochanteric entry or piriformis entry) can still be useful, care must be taken to maintain the reduction of the proximal fracture extension (typically with an open technique) prior to reaming and nail insertion). Alternatively, plate devices may be useful in these patterns. Blade plates, the dynamic condylar screw, and locking plate devices may all be useful for complex and simple patterns. Submuscular plate application, indirect reduction techniques, and avoidance of any additional medial dissection all contribute to a higher success rate with lateral plate devices. Acute bone grafting is not necessary with plate fixation in these fractures. The results of treatment of subtrochanteric femur fractures with a 95° angled blade in experienced hands can be favorable. In a longitudinal cohort study by Kinast et al., indirect reduction techniques and avoidance of acute bone grafting was associated with a decrease in nonunion rates (from 16.6% to 0%) by avoiding an extensive surgical dissection for placement of the implant. Whether a plate or nail is chosen, the surgical goals are identical and include restoration of length, alignment and rotation of the femur with re-establishment of the normal neck-shaft angle of the proximal femur.

VI. Anatomic and Biomechanical Considerations and Surgical Techniques

A. Anatomic Considerations—In subtrochanteric fractures, the deforming forces on the proximal fragment make the reduction using longitudinal traction difficult. The proximal fragment is usually flexed, abducted, and externally rotated, while the distal segment is typically shortened and medially displaced. This makes identification and delivery of the starting point for an intramedullary nail difficult. The displacement patterns for femoral shaft fractures are more variable and are dependent on the level of the fracture relative to the muscular origins and insertions.

B. Biomechanical Considerations—Important biomechanical considerations include the nail radius of curvature (relative to the femoral bow), the nail entry site (see the section on surgical techniques), and the nail stiffness and strength.

1. IM nail curvature—The normal femur has an anterior bow with a radius of curvature of approximately 120 cm. Most nail designs have a larger radius of curvature (i.e., a less bowed design) with a range from 150 to 300 cm. As a result, care must be taken, especially in proximal shaft or subtrochanteric fractures, to avoid penetration of the anterior cortex distally. This is especially relevant in elderly patients and in cases where there is a significant mismatch between the nail and the femoral anatomy.

2. IM nail stiffness—The bending stiffness of an IM nail increases with the nail diameter, increasing wall thickness, and interlocking capabilities. Torsional stiffness is increased in closed section nails compared with open section nails. Stiffness is also a function of nail composition: steel is stiffer than titanium.

3. Small diameter nails—The use of small diameter nails typically requires placement of smaller interlocking screws. These screws are at a higher risk for fatigue failure.

4. IM nail breakage—Larger diameter nails with larger locking screws are associated with a decreased incidence of nail breakage. However, with the improved designs from most implant manufactures, early fatigue failure is rare when the implant is appropriately matched to the femoral canal. Extensive reaming to allow placement of an extremely large nail is now rarely required. Fatigue failure of nails is usually an indication of nonunion. Ideally, 5 cm should separate the nearest extension of the fracture from the interlocking screws; but this is not absolutely imperative depending on the reduction and the patient's size.

5. Plates—Because of the eccentric location of the plate relative to the mechanical and anatomical axes of the femur, greater mechanical demands are placed on a plate than on an IM nail. As a result, plates usually require weight bearing restrictions that are unnecessary in most patients treated with an intramedullary nail.

C. Surgical Techniques

1. IM nailing—The patient may be positioned either supine or lateral for antegrade IM nailing. Supine positioning is used for retrograde nailing. A fracture table can be used for IM nailing with the patient positioned either supine or lateral. Alternatively, the injured leg can be prepped free and intramedullary nailing can be performed on a radiolucent table. The supine position may be advantageous in patients with multiple injuries or where access to the abdomen and chest is desirable. Placement of an IM femoral nail with the patient in the lateral position is associated with *valgus* deformity, especially in fractures distal to the femoral isthmus.

• Antegrade piriformis starting point—The piriformis fossa was identified by Johnson and Tencer as the ideal starting point because it coincides with the neutral axis of the medullary canal. Anterior displacement of the starting point by more than 6 mm is associated with high-hoop stresses, potentially resulting in bursting of the femoral cortex with nail insertion. This is especially important in stiff or large diameter intramedullary nails. Lateral and medial starting point displacements are associated with varus and valgus deformities, especially in proximal or subtrochanteric fractures. One difficulty associated with the use of a cephalomedullary nail that does not have a lateral bend is the alignment of the nail with the medullary canal while simultaneously aligning the proximal interlocking screws with the neck of the femur. The femoral neck is typically offset anteriorly relative to the femoral shaft. For subtrochanteric fractures, especially those with proximal extension, the starting point may be biased anteriorly (by up to 5 mm), since hoop stresses are dissipated by the proximal fracture.

• Antegrade trochanteric starting point—Trochanteric entry nails were designed because of perceived difficulties identifying the piriformis fossa. Each nail manufacturer has a specific lateral bend which ranges from 4° to 10°. *If the starting point is placed too laterally, a varus malreduction is likely in proximal fracture patterns.*

• Retrograde starting point—The location of the proper starting point is anterior to the posterior cruciate ligament and at the intercondylar sulcus in line with the canal of the femur. Radiographically, this is at the anterior extension of Blumensaat's line on the lateral view. The entrance should be collinear with the longitudinal axis of the femoral canal on the anteroposterior radiographic projection and not perpendicular to the knee joint femoral articulation (which is in valgus). Knee flexion of 35° to 50° is necessary to allow identification of the starting point. Proximally the nail should be placed so that the most proximal portion of the nail extends above the level of the lesser trochanter.

- Reaming—Sharp, flexible reamers with deep flutes and a thin flexible shaft should be used to decrease the risk of thermal injury and elevated intramedullary pressures. The canal is usually reamed 1.0 to 1.5 mm larger than the chosen nail diameter. There is no need for excessive reaming with current interlocking nail designs.
- Interlocking—All femoral fractures should be statically locked. There is no evidence that dynamic interlocking offers any advantage with regards to healing. Additionally, in patients with unrecognized fracture comminution, shortening is a concern.

2. Plating—For plating of subtrochanteric and femoral shaft fractures, open extensile and minimally invasive techniques are both useful. No matter the technique, the deep dissection should be limited as much as possible. For an open approach to the femur, a lateral subvastus approach is used, reflecting the vastus lateralis from the lateral intermuscular septum. Perforating branches of the profunda femoris artery should be identified and ligated. For comminuted fracture patterns, bridge plating using biological principles should be used with indirect reduction of any intercalary fragments. A broad, large fragment compression plate is typically required. There are very few disadvantages to using a longer plate; the number of cortices on each side of the fracture is less important than the plate length.

3. External fixation—External fixation of the femur can be performed with a unilateral configuration using 5- or 6-mm pins. The pins are usually placed from lateral to medial with two pins on either side of the fracture. Anterolateral and anterior entry sites can be used as well. Since external fixation is usually a temporizing measure until a definitive procedure can be performed, maximization of the biomechanical strength is not necessary.

If temporary spanning external fixation of a high-subtrochanteric fracture is necessary and proximal femoral fixation cannot be obtained, the external fixation can be extended to the pelvis to span the hip joint.

VII. Acute Injury Complications
   A. Pulmonary Complications—Fat emboli syndrome (FES), ARDS, and pulmonary dysfunction are complications associated with femoral shaft fractures. Patients with multiple injuries, especially concomitant thoracic or pulmonary trauma, are at particular risk. Early fracture stabilization is associated with a decreased risk of FES.
   B. Thigh Compartmental Syndrome—Thigh compartmental syndrome is rare. However, because of the potential consequences of missing this entity, early diagnosis is critical. Clinical signs and symptoms include severe and tense swelling, pain with passive knee motion, and pain out of proportion to the injury. However, all of these indicators are present with any femur fracture, making diagnosis difficult. Pressure measurements can helpful if the diagnosis is questionable or in an unconscious patient. Thigh compartmental syndrome is treated by immediate fasciotomies.

VIII. Complications of Treatment and Long-Term Sequelae
   A. Pulmonary Dysfunction or FES—The process of instrumenting the femoral canal, either with a medullary implant, a reamer, or a starting awl; is associated with embolization of marrow or fat into the venous circulation. Although controversial, this has been hypothesized to contribute to pulmonary dysfunction, especially in patients with thoracic or pulmonary injuries. However, a retrospective study by Bosse et al. demonstrated no difference in pulmonary complications when femoral plating versus reamed nailing was retrospectively compared at two institutions.
   B. Nerve Injury—Iatrogenic nerve injury is infrequent following femoral nailing. The primary nerves at risk are the femoral, sciatic, peroneal, and pudendal. Patient positioning on a traction table can injure the pudendal nerve due to direct pressure from the perineal post. Prolonged and sustained traction should be avoided. Over distraction or vigorous reduction maneuvers can put the sciatic nerve at risk.
   C. Muscle Weakness—In antegrade femoral nailing, injury to the hip abductors and external rotators may occur and is related to the site of

nail insertion. Trochanteric entry nails injure the abductor insertion, although studies have not shown an increased risk of abductor dysfunction following trochanteric nailing. Quadriceps impairment is common following femoral fracture, although this is likely due to the injury and not the method of treatment.

D. Knee Stiffness, Knee Pain, Hip Pain—Temporary knee stiffness is common following treatment of a femoral shaft fracture. Treatment with plate fixation has been assumed to contribute to knee stiffness, although several larger studies have failed to identify this relationship. Retrograde nailing may be associated with knee stiffness, although several prospective and randomized studies have failed to demonstrate this. Knee pain is associated with retrograde nailing; and hip pain is associated with antegrade nailing. The incidence of hip pain following antegrade nailing ranges from 10% to 40%. The incidence of knee pain following retrograde nailing ranges from 30% to 40%.

E. Heterotopic Ossification (HO)—The formation of heterotopic bone at the nail entry site following antegrade nailing ranges from 9% to 60%; however, clinically significant bone formation is uncommon and is reported in 5% to 10% of patients. Heterotopic bone formation is loosely associated with male gender, a delay to surgery, prolonged intubation, and an associated head injury. There is a higher incidence of HO following reamed nails than with unreamed nails.

F. Refracture—Refracture following plating is uncommon and is usually an indication of nonunion. Fracture can occur at the end of a plate, although this usually requires a substantial injury.

G. Implant Complications—Broken nails, screws: With advances in nail design, fatigue failure prior to healing occurs infrequently. Broken nails are indicative of nonunion. Broken screws and nails can be challenging to remove and numerous techniques have been described to allow for successful extraction.

H. Angular Malalignment—An angular deformity is usually defined as 5° in either the coronal or sagittal plane. This is more common in proximal or distal fractures where the intimate fit between the medullary implant and the femoral isthmus is not present. For proximal fractures, the starting point of the nail is critical for ensuring proper alignment. In subtrochanteric fractures treated with intramedullary nails, the alignment should be corrected and maintained throughout the procedure (from the identification of the starting point through the placement of interlocking screws) to ensure proper alignment.

I. Rotational Malalignment—The amount of femoral rotation that is well tolerated is largely unknown, but there appears to be increased symptoms with over 15° of rotational malalignment. Femoral rotation can be determined intraoperatively using several methods of clinical and radiological evaluation. Symmetry of the cortical thicknesses is useful but not reliable. The shape and appearance of the lesser trochanter in known rotation (compared with the uninjured femur) is a reliable method of determining rotation of the femur. A CT scan following stabilization can be used if there is a question regarding rotational alignment. This CT is performed by binding bilateral lower extremities together with straps so that the legs can not move and scanning both proximal and distal femurs to compare their relative rotations (proximal versus distal on the injured and uninjured side).

J. Femoral Nail Removal—The need and timing of femoral nail removal following fracture healing remains unknown. Complete radiographic and clinical healing should be assured prior to removal. Nail removal should likely be restricted to symptomatic patients only as the procedure is associated with complications and the improvement in discomfort is inconsistent. In a study on over 100 patients followed for 2 years after femoral nail removal, over 20% of patients were no better or worse.

IX. Nonunion

Nonunion is uncommon following intramedullary nailing of femoral shaft and subtrochanteric fractures. However, the incidence is likely more frequent than some studies indicate. Several larger series indicate delayed or nonunion in 6% to 12% of patients. Treatment options include femoral exchange nailing, conversion to a plate with or without bone grafting, and plating around the nail. Dynamization has not been shown to be consistently effective for the treatment of femoral nonunions. Femoral exchange nailing involves nail removal, reaming, and insertion of a larger diameter implant, typically 1 to 3 mm larger than the original nail. Success varies and ranges from 53% to 96%. Conversion from a nail to plate, with or without bone grafting depending on the type of nonunion, has been successful in over 90% of patients as reported by Bellabarba et al. Finally, augmentative plating around a nail has been associated with a high success rate. This is thought to be primarily due to the increased torsional stability in fractures/nonunions that had some persistent rotational instability following intramedullary nailing.

X. Malunion

Angular femoral malunion is more commonly associated with closed fracture treatment than with operative fixation. However, subtrochanteric fractures are more difficult to accurately reduce and control than shaft fractures, thus resulting in a larger incidence of angular malunion. Limb length inequality may be associated with an angular malunion or may occur in isolation. Angular corrections typically require treatment with a femoral osteotomy. Limb length inequality may be treated with a lengthening procedure on the affected side or a closed shortening of the contralateral side. Torsional malunions can occur with fractures in any location. Correction of torsional deformities should be considered if the rotational malalignment is greater than 15° as compared to the normal side.

XI. Other Issues and Special Coniderations

A. Pathologic Fractures—The femur may be weakened by pathologic (e.g., metabolic, neoplastic) processes, resulting in a fracture or impending fracture. Cephalomedullary nails are particularly useful for pathologic fractures of the femur, as these implants simultaneously stabilize the femoral shaft and femoral neck.

B. Periprosthetic Fractures—There are several classification systems for periprosthetic fractures; the most often used is the Vancouver system which takes into account the fracture location, the integrity of the prosthesis, and any associated bone deficiencies that need to be addressed. In general, fractures proximal to the tip of a hip arthroplasty are treated with revision while fractures distal to the tip of a well-fixed femoral prosthesis can be treated with standard fracture reduction techniques. Multiple techniques are described for obtaining fixation around the prosthesis.

SUGGESTED READINGS

Classic Articles

Benirschke SK, Melder I, Henley MB, et al. Closed interlocking nailing of femoral shaft fractures: assessment of technical complications and functional outcomes by comparison of a prospective database with retrospective review. *J Orthop Trauma.* 1993;7(2):118–122.

Bone LB, Johnson KD, Weigelt J, et al. Early versus delayed stabilization of femoral fractures. A prospective randomized study. *J Bone Joint Surg Am.* 1989;71(3):336–340.

Brumback RJ, Uwagie-Ero S, Lakatos RP, et al. Intramedullary nailing of femoral shaft fractures. Part II: Fracture-healing with static interlocking fixation. *J Bone Joint Surg Am.* 1988;70(10):1453–1462.

Johansen K, Lynch K, Paun M,et al. Non-invasive vascular tests reliably exclude occult arterial trauma in injured extremities. *J Trauma.* 1991;31(4):515–519; discussion 519–522.

Kinast C, Bolhofner BR, Mast JW, et al. Subtrochanteric fractures of the femur. Results of treatment with the 95 degrees condylar blade-plate. *Clin Orthop.* 1989;(238):122–130.

Michelson JD, Myers A, Jinnah R, et al. Epidemiology of hip fractures among the elderly. Risk factors for fracture type. *Clin Orthop Relat Res.* 1995;(311):129–135.

O'Brien PJ, Meek RN, Powell JN, et al. Primary intramedullary nailing of open femoral shaft fractures. *J Trauma.* 1991;31(1):113–116.

Riemer BL, Butterfield SL, Burke CJ 3rd, et al. Immediate plate fixation of highly comminuted femoral diaphyseal fractures in blunt polytrauma patients. *Orthopedics.* 1992;15(8):907–916.

Riemer BL, Butterfield SL, Ray RL, et al. Clandestine femoral neck fractures with ipsilateral diaphyseal fractures. *J Orthop Trauma.* 1993;7(5):443–449.

Tencer AF, Sherman MC, Johnson KD. Biomechanical factors affecting fracture stability and femoral bursting in closed intramedullary rod fixation of femur fractures. *J Biomech Eng.* 1985;107(2):104–111.

Winquist RA, Hansen ST Jr, Clawson DK. Closed intramedullary nailing of femoral fractures. A report of five hundred and twenty cases. *J Bone Joint Surg Am.* 1984;66(4):529–539.

Wiss DA, Brien WW. Subtrochanteric fractures of the femur. Results of treatment by interlocking nailing. *Clin Orthop.* 1992;(283):231–236.

Wiss DA, Brien WW, Stetson WB. Interlocked nailing for treatment of segmental fractures of the femur. *J Bone Joint Surg Am.* 1990;72(5):724–728.

Wolinsky PR, Sciadini MF, Parker RE, et al. Effects on pulmonary physiology of reamed femoral intramedullary nailing in an open-chest sheep model. *J Orthop Trauma.* 1996;10(2):75–80.

Recent Articles

Bellabarba C, Ricci WM, Bolhofner BR. Results of indirect reduction and plating of femoral shaft nonunions after intramedullary nailing. *J Orthop Trauma.* 2001;15(4):254–263.

Bhandari M, Guyatt GH, Tong D, et al. Reamed versus non-reamed intramedullary nailing of lower extremity long bone fractures: a systematic overview and meta-analysis. *J Orthop Trauma.* 2000;14(1):2–9.

Bosse MJ, MacKenzie EJ, Riemer BL, et al. Adult respiratory distress syndrome, pneumonia, and mortality following thoracic injury and a femoral fracture treated either with intramedullary nailing with reaming or with a plate. A comparative study. *J Bone Joint Surg Am.* 1997;79(6):799–809.

Brinker MR, O'Connor DP. Exchange nailing of ununited fractures. *J Bone Joint Surg Am.* 2007;89-A:177–188.

Brumback RJ, Toal TR Jr, Murphy-Zane MS, et al. Immediate weight-bearing after treatment of a comminuted fracture of the femoral shaft with a statically locked intramedullary nail. *J Bone Joint Surg Am.* 1999;81(11):1538–1544.

Buttaro M, Mocetti E, Alfie V, et al. Fat embolism and related effects during reamed and unreamed intramedullary nailing in a pig model. *J Orthop Trauma.* 2002;16(4):239–244.

Canadian Study Group. Nonunion following intramedullary nailing of the femur with and without reaming. Results of a multicenter randomized clinical trial. *J Bone Joint Surg Am.* 2003;85-A(11):2093–2096.

Dora C, Leunig M, Beck M, et al. Entry point soft tissue damage in antegrade femoral nailing: a cadaver study. *J Orthop Trauma.* 2001;15(7):488–493.

Egol KA, Chang EY, Cvitkovic J, et al. Mismatch of current intramedullary nails with the anterior bow of the femur. *J Orthop Trauma.* 2004;18(7):410–415.

French BG, Tornetta P 3rd. Use of an interlocked cephalomedullary nail for subtrochanteric fracture stabilization. *Clin Orthop.* 1998;(348):95–100.

Giannoudis PV, MacDonald DA, Matthews SJ, et al. Nonunion of the femoral diaphysis. The influence of reaming and non-steroidal anti-inflammatory drugs. *J Bone Joint Surg Br.* 2000;82(5):655–658.

Kloen P, Rubel IF, Lyden JP, et al. Subtrochanteric fracture after cannulated screw fixation of femoral neck fractures: a report of four cases. *J Orthop Trauma.* 2003;17(3):225–229.

Lundy DW, Acevedo JI, Ganey TM, et al. Mechanical comparison of plates used in the treatment of unstable subtrochanteric femur fractures. *J Orthop Trauma.* 1999;13(8):534–538.

Meyer RS, White KK, Smith JM, et al. Intramuscular and blood pressures in legs positioned in the hemilithotomy position: clarification of risk factors for well-leg acute compartment syndrome. *J Bone Joint Surg Am.* 2002;84-A(10):1829–1835.

Nowotarski PJ, Turen CH, Brumback RJ, et al. Conversion of external fixation to intramedullary nailing for fractures of the shaft of the femur in multiply injured patients. *J Bone Joint Surg Am.* 2000;82(6):781–788.

Oakey JW, Stover MD, Summers HD, et al. Does screw configuration affect subtrochanteric fracture after femoral neck fixation? *Clin Orthop Relat Res.* 2006;443:302–306.

Ostrum RF, Agarwal A, Lakatos R, et al. Prospective comparison of retrograde and antegrade femoral intramedullary nailing. *J Orthop Trauma.* 2000;14(7):496–501.

Ostrum RF, Marcantonio A, Marburger R. A critical analysis of the eccentric starting point for trochanteric intramedullary femoral nailing. *J Orthop Trauma.* 2005;19(10):681–686.

Pape HC, Grimme K, Van Griensven M, et al. Impact of intramedullary instrumentation versus damage control for femoral fractures on immunoinflammatory parameters: prospective randomized analysis by the EPOFF Study Group. *J Trauma.* 2003;55(1):7–13.

Pape HC, Hildebrand F, Pertschy S, et al. Changes in the management of femoral shaft fractures in polytrauma patients: from early total care to damage control orthopedic surgery. *J Trauma.* 2002;53(3):452–461.

Ricci WM, Bellabarba C, Evanoff B, et al. Retrograde versus antegrade nailing of femoral shaft fractures. *J Orthop Trauma.* 2001;15(3):161–169.

Ricci WM, Bellabarba C, Lewis R, et al. Angular malalignment after intramedullary nailing of femoral shaft fractures. *J Orthop Trauma.* 2001;15(2):90–95.

Ricci WM, Schwappach J, Tucker M, et al. Trochanteric versus piriformis entry portal for the treatment of femoral shaft fractures. *J Orthop Trauma.* 2006;20(10):663–667.

Roberts CS, Nawab A, Wang M, et al. Second generation intramedullary nailing of subtrochanteric femur fractures: a biomechanical study of fracture site motion. *J Orthop Trauma.* 2002;16(4):231–238.

Salminen ST, Pihlajamaki HK, Avikainen VJ, et al. Population based epidemiologic and morphologic study of femoral shaft fractures. *Clin Orthop.* 2000;(372):241–249.

Scalea TM, Boswell SA, Scott JD, et al. External fixation as a bridge to intramedullary nailing for patients with multiple injuries and with femur fractures: damage control orthopedics. *J Trauma.* 2000;48(4):613–621.

Starr AJ, Hay MT, Reinert CM, et al. Cephalomedullary nails in the treatment of high-energy proximal femur fractures in young patients: a prospective, randomized comparison of trochanteric versus piriformis fossa entry portal. *J Orthop Trauma.* 2006;20(4):240–246.

Starr AJ, Hunt JL, Chason DP, et al. Treatment of femur fracture with associated head injury. *J Orthop Trauma.* 1998;12(1):38–45.

Stephen DJ, Kreder HJ, Schemitsch EH, et al. Femoral intramedullary nailing: comparison of fracture-table and manual traction. A prospective, randomized study. *J Bone Joint Surg Am.* 2002;84-A(9):1514–1521.

Tornetta P 3rd, Tiburzi D. Reamed versus nonreamed anterograde femoral nailing. *J Orthop Trauma.* 2000;14(1):15–19.

Watson JT, Moed BR. Ipsilateral femoral neck and shaft fractures: complications and their treatment. *Clin Orthop.* 2002;(399):78–86.

Weresh MJ, Hakanson R, Stover MD, et al. Failure of exchange reamed intramedullary nails for ununited femoral shaft fractures. *J Orthop Trauma.* 2000;14(5):335–338.

Wolinsky PR, McCarty E, Shyr Y, et al. Reamed intramedullary nailing of the femur: 551 cases. *J Trauma.* 1999;46(3):392–399.

Textbooks

Court-Brown CM. Femoral diaphyseal fractures. In: Browner BD, Jupiter JB, Levine AM, eds. *Skeletal Trauma: Basic Science, Management and Reconstruction.* 3rd ed. Philadelphia, PA: Saunders; 2003:1879–1883.

Fischgrund JS. *Orthopaedic Knowledge Update 9.* 1st ed. Rosemont, IL: American Academy of Orthopaedic Surgeons; 2008.

Leung K. Subtrochanteric fractures. In: Bucholz RW, Heckman JD, Court-Brown C, eds. *Rockwood and Green's Fractures in Adults.* 6th ed. Philadelphia, PA: Lippincott Williams & Wilkins; 2005:1827–1844.

Nork SE. Fractures of the shaft of the femur. In: Bucholz RW, Heckman JD, Court-Brown C, et al, eds. *Rockwood and Green's Fractures in Adults.* 6th ed. Philadelphia, PA: Lippincott Williams & Wilkins; 2005:1845–1914.

Russell TA. Subtrochanteric fractures of the femur. In: Browner BD, Jupiter JB, Levine AM, eds. *Skeletal Trauma: Basic Science, Management and Reconstruction.* 3rd ed. Philadelphia, PA: Saunders; 2003:1832–1878.

CHAPTER 7

Fractures of the Supracondylar Femoral Region

Milan K.Sen

I. Evaluation
  A. History—As with all extremity injuries, preliminary evaluation of fractures of the supracondylar femoral region must include an account of the mechanism of injury, assessment of comorbidities, history of prior surgery in the affected area, preinjury symptoms, and preinjury level of function. Often these patients fall into two categories:
    1. The elderly or osteopenic patient with a fracture after a low-energy injury due to a fall from standing or a twisting injury.
    2. The younger, healthier patient who sustains a high-energy injury due to a motor vehicle accident or a fall from a significant height.
    In either case, the force is usually transmitted through a flexed knee. Additional clues as to the energy of the injury can be obtained from the physical findings and X-ray pattern. Together, this information allows the surgeon to make appropriate management decisions, look for associated injuries, and prevent complications.
  B. Physical Examination—In the setting of polytrauma, initial examination includes ATLS protocol, prioritizing the ABCs (airway, breathing, and circulation). Once this assessment is complete, evaluation of the extremities is performed. Deformity in and around the knee, bruising, swelling, and open wounds should be noted. In addition, a proper neurovascular exam is critical.
    1. Neurologic—Evaluation of motor and sensory function of the tibial nerve, superficial peroneal, and deep peroneal nerves should be performed, and the results documented. Often, the exam is limited by pain, level of consciousness, sedation, or neurologic injury, and this should also be documented in the patient record.
    2. Vascular—Palpable pulses are a good indicator of limb perfusion. If the pulses are not palpable, then a Doppler examination should be performed. Realignment of the limb using traction and splinting can help with restoration of pulses and limb perfusion. If pulses are unequal, or not detectable on Doppler examination, an ankle–brachial index (ABI) or arteriogram should be performed. An ABI of less than 0.9 warrants further workup. If pulses are initially absent but return after manipulation of the limb, an arteriogram should strongly be considered to rule out an intimal tear that could lead to thrombosis.
    3. Soft tissues—Initial evaluation should include documentation of open wounds. Attention should be paid to the posterior aspect of the limb to make certain that wounds on the back of the leg are not missed. Patients with open fractures should receive antibiotic coverage for gram-positive organisms. Grossly contaminated wounds should also receive gram-negative coverage. Wounds contaminated with dirt should receive anaerobic coverage as well.
    4. Compartment syndrome—Compartment Syndrome should be ruled out in all patients with extremity injuries. Special attention should be paid to the polytrauma patient who may have distracting injuries or is sedated. If the clinical exam is suggestive of compartment syndrome, fasciotomies should be performed. If the patient is not examinable, compartment pressure measurements should be performed. If the patient undergoes a revascularization procedure, prophylactic fasciotomies should be performed to account for edema associated with reperfusion injury.

5. Associated injuries—Particularly in the setting of polytrauma, associated injuries should be ruled out. Often, these are not obvious on the secondary survey and must be evaluated on tertiary survey or on exam under anesthesia in the operating room. Musculoskeletal injuries commonly seen in the ipsilateral limb include tibial shaft fractures (floating knee), femoral neck fractures or hip dislocations, patella fractures, and ligamentous knee injuries or dislocations. Falls from significant height may also result in calcaneus or pilon fractures, or fractures of the pelvis, acetabulum, or spine.

C. Radiographs

1. AP and lateral X-ray images of the hip, femur, and knee should be obtained. X-rays should be scrutinized for intra-articular fractures, and **Hoffa fragments** (Fig. 7-1).

2. More comminuted fractures and those with extension into the diaphysis are often the result of higher-energy mechanisms of injury and should prompt the surgeon to look for other associated injuries.

3. Intrarticular fractures should be imaged with CT scan. This is more valuable if provisional realignment has been performed with traction and splinting, or external fixation.

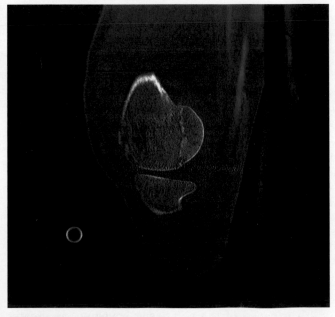

FIGURE 7-1   Sagittal cut from a CT scan of the distal femur demonstrates the fracture of the posterior condyle of the femur (Hoffa fragment). This fracture line is easily missed on plain X-rays.

4. If a ligamentous knee injury or dislocation is suspected, an MRI should be considered prior to instrumentation and after consultation with a specialist.

5. If a vascular injury is suspected—Often in association with a knee dislocation—A CT angiogram should be performed.

D. Classification—Orthopaedic Trauma Association Classification (Fig. 7-2)

II. Initial Management

A. Reduction using traction and splinting is usually sufficient for temporary stabilization of isolated supracondylar femur fractures. Skeletal traction is usually not necessary.

B. External fixation spanning the knee is indicated when definitive fixation is delayed due to soft tissue injury or wound contamination, and in the setting of a vascular repair. Ideally, external fixation should be converted to definitive internal fixation within 2 weeks to decrease the infection risk secondary to pin track colonization.

III. Definitive Treatment

A. Principles of ORIF

The goal of open reduction and internal fixation is to restore anatomic alignment of the limb while providing a stable environment for healing and sufficient stability to allow for early range of motion. This is accomplished by following these steps:

1. Anatomic reduction of the articular surface—In fractures with intra-articular extension, the first goal should be to restore articular congruity. This is best achieved using interfragmentary screws. Cancellous, and sometimes cortical screws, ranging from 3.5 to 6.5 mm are commonly used. Smaller screws (2.0 to 3.0 mm) should also be available for fixation of smaller fragments in the setting of fracture comminution. Care must be taken to keep the starting point and trajectory of these screws from interfering with a subsequent intramedullary nail, or plate and screw positioning. One must consider the three-dimensional structure of the distal femur to avoid violation of the notch anteriorly and also the fossa posteriorly. Prominent screw penetration medially may also lead to irritation of the soft tissues along the medial condyle.

2. Restoration of mechanical axis—Realignment of the axis of the femur can be achieved with the use of plates and screws, or an intramedullary implant such as a supracondylar nail. In the setting of intra-articular fractures, a plate-and-screw construct is often preferred

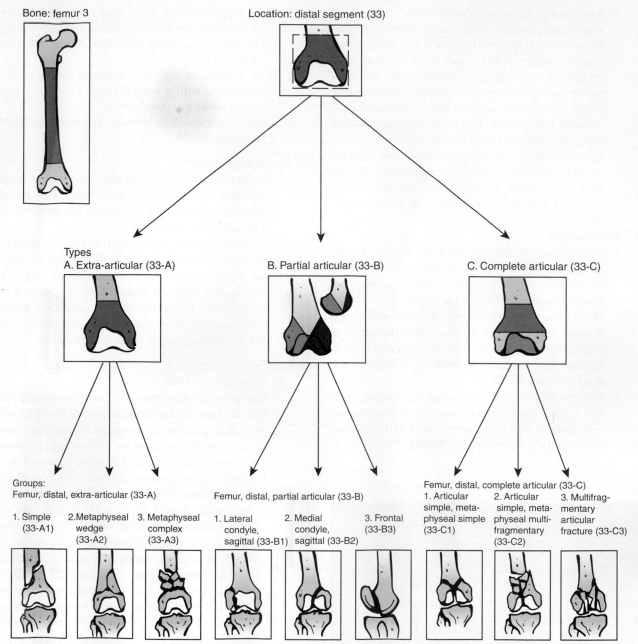

FIGURE 7-2 The Orthopaedic Trauma Association classification of distal femur fractures. The alphanumeric code used to classify these fractures is made up of a number for the bone *segment*—in this case 33 (for femur, distal)—followed by a letter to describe the general *type* of fracture. Fractures classified as 33-A are extra-articular fractures in the metadiaphyseal region. 33-B refers to partial articular fractures, where at least one portion of the articular surface is in continuity with the diaphysis. 33-C fractures are complete articular fractures, where no part of the articular surface remains in continuity with the diaphysis. More extensive classification is possible, with subdivision into *groups*. (From Collinge CA, Wiss DA. Distal femur fractures. In: Bucholz RW, Court-Brown CM, Heckman, JD, et al, eds. *Rockwood and Green's Fractures in Adults.* 7th ed. Philadelphia, PA: Lippincott Williams & Wilkins, 2010, with permission.)

to avoid displacing the articular reduction or fixation. Ultimately, implant selection depends on surgeon experience and preference.

    B. ORIF with Plate Fixation

        Fixed angle plates provide excellent fixation for maintaining reduction, but this comes at the

expense of the soft-tissue envelope, as greater dissection is required for insertion.

    1. Plate fixation is usually achieved from the lateral side. In simple fracture patterns, this is sufficient, as stability of the medial column of the femur is provided by restoration of bony

alignment and contact. In comminuted fractures, no stability is provided by restoration of bony alignment alone.

2. Locking plates now play an important role in the management of these types of fractures. Their fixed angle construct has allowed for stable fixation of fractures in the setting of comminution, avoiding the need for additional medial plates, and with easier insertion than older fixed-angle devices (Fig. 7-3).

3. The development of minimally invasive plate osteosynthesis (MIPO) techniques have also been helped by the design of these plates, which are very amenable to MIPO insertion.

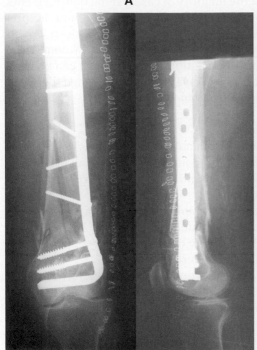

A

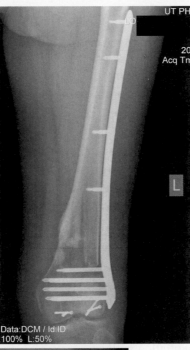

B

FIGURE 7-3 **A.** AP and lateral X-ray of a supracondylar fracture stabilized with a 95° blade plate. **B.** AP X-ray of an intercondylar femur fracture stabilized with a Less Invasive Stabilization System (LISS) plate. **C.** AP X-ray of a periprosthetic distal femur nonunion stabilized with a locking condylar plate. (Part A from Collinge CA, Wiss DA. Distal femur fractures. In: Bucholz RW, Court-Brown CM, Heckman, JD, et al, eds. *Rockwood and Green's Fractures in Adults.* 7th ed. Philadelphia, PA: Lippincott Williams & Wilkins, 2010, with permission.)

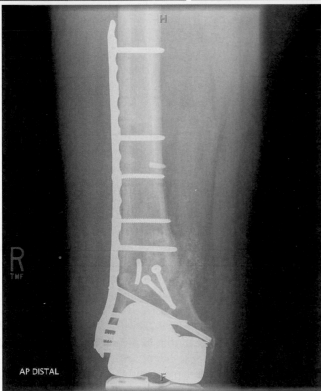

C

C. ORIF with Intramedullary Implant—Intramedullary nails can also be used for realignment of the femur but have several limitations.
   1. Theoretically, their insertion causes additional injury to the articular surface.
   2. Intramedullary nails are not canal filling at the level of the distal femur. Fixation is minimal, and the nail is not as capable of controlling motion in the varus–valgus plane, which can lead to a "windshield wiper" effect.
   3. Special "supracondylar nails" are available and offer more points of fixation for these types of fractures. Blocking screws can also be used to control alignment and increase the stability of the construct (Fig. 7-4).
D. Special Considerations
   1. Periprosthetic fractures
      The first thing that needs to be determined in the setting of a periprosthetic fracture of the distal femur is whether the implant is loose. If it is loose, infection must be ruled out. If a cruciate sparing total knee prothesis was used, either a plate and screw construct or a supracondylar nail may be used (Fig. 7-5). If a cruciate sacrificing prosthesis was used, the CAM will not allow for placement of a supracondylar nail. Similarly, the CAM will block the trajectory of some of the locking screws, and this needs to be taken into consideration in the selection and positioning of a fixed-angle implant. If the prosthesis is loose, consultation with an arthroplasty specialist is recommended.
   2. Pre-existing knee arthritis
      Primary TKA in a patient with pre-existing knee arthritis is an option. One must consider the severity and duration of the symptoms preoperatively, the patient's pre-existing level of function, and whether the fracture pattern is amenable to this form of treatment. Often these are more challenging cases than a typical primary TKA, as the prosthesis will require augments and/or stems for stability of the implant. Comminuted intra-articular fractures in osteopenic bone are a better indication for primary TKA than extra-articular fractures are. In the majority of cases, it is preferable to obtain anatomic realignment of the femur to allow for healing with enough bone stock for a primary TKA in the future, if needed.
   3. Open fractures
      • Antibiotics need to be started on presentation in the emergency room.
      • Tetanus status must be verified.
      • A thorough surgical debridement is paramount, removing all contaminated and

devitalized tissue (including bone), and foreign material. Wounds must be extended to allow for removal of all debris, and exposure of the bone for proper debridement. No amount of irrigation or antibiotics will compensate for an inadequate debridement.
      • In clean wounds with good soft-tissue coverage, immediate ORIF may be considered.
      • In the majority of cases, serial debridements being performed every 48 hours is preferred. ORIF is delayed until a clean wound is obtained. Negative pressure wound therapy or an antibiotic bead pouch can be used for provisional wound coverage between debridements.

IV. Perioperative Plan
   A. Instrumentation and Equipment
      It is important to make certain that all of the necessary instrumentation is pulled for your case. This includes:
      1. The desired implant—Typically a locking plate or an intramedullary nail.
      2. Multiple screw options in the case of an intra-articular fracture.
      3. Various reduction clamps, including large periarticular reduction tenaculums.
      4. Kirschner wires.
      5. A radiolucent operating table.
      6. C-arm fluoroscopy.
      7. Equipment for adjustment or removal of an external fixator, if present.
      8. A femoral distractor should be available to assist with reduction of the femur. When spanning the knee, the distractor can greatly improve the visualization of the articular surface.
   B. Positioning
      1. The patient is positioned supine.
      2. A bump is placed under the distal femur at the level of the apex of the fracture. This helps reduce the apex posterior deformity by allowing the knee to flex and reduces the tension on the gastroc's origin, which pulls the distal fragment into extension. It also elevates the femur for fluoroscopic visualization of the fracture site on a lateral projection.
      3. Alternatively, blankets layered underneath the tibia, elevating and supporting it in a plane horizontal to the ground may be used (Fig. 7-6). Prefabricated "triangles" are also available in a variety of material and serve the same purpose.
      4. Prepping out the uninjured leg allows for intraoperative assessment of bilateral limb

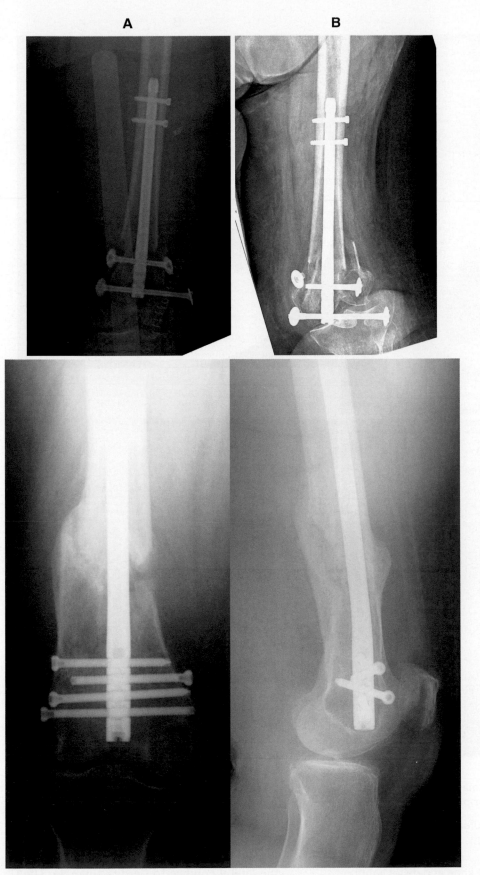

A

B

C

FIGURE 7-4   When a femoral nail is used for fixation of distal femur fractures, it is important that the construct is stable enough to maintain reduction. **A.** AP image of a supracondylar nail with minimal fixation. Not enough stability is obtained, and the nail is akin to a "pencil in a trashcan." **B.** This goes on to catastrophic failure. A properly used intramedullary nail with multiple points of fixation can provide good stability. **C.** Radiographs show stable fixation of the condyles using a modern nailing system that allows for maintenance of alignment. (Part C from Collinge CA, Wiss DA. Distal femur fractures. In: Bucholz RW, Court-Brown CM, Heckman, JD, et al, eds. *Rockwood and Green's Fractures in Adults.* 7th ed. Philadelphia, PA: Lippincott Williams & Wilkins, 2010, with permission.)

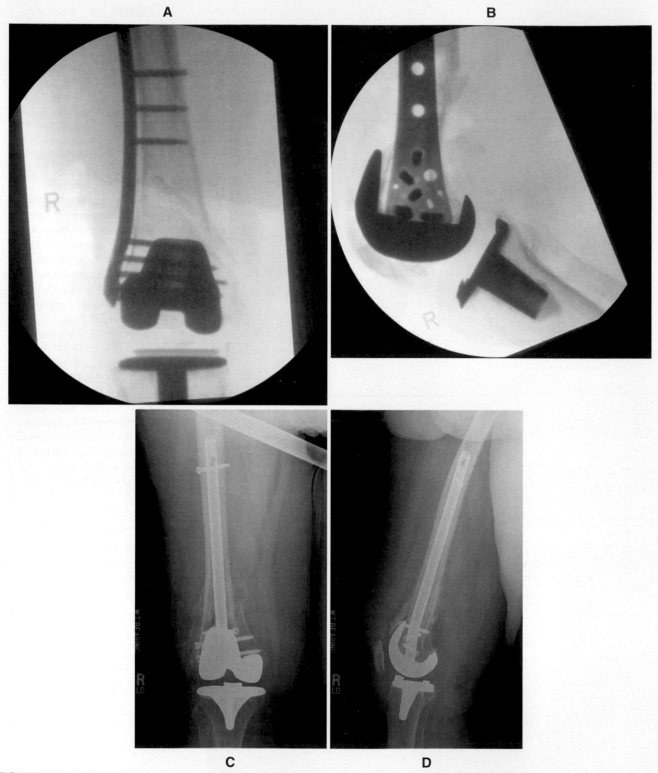

A

B

C

D

FIGURE 7-5 **A.** AP and **B.** Lateral images of a periprothetic supracondylar femur fracture stabilized with a locking plate. **C.** AP and **D.** Lateral images of a periprothetic supracondylar femur fracture stabilized with an intramedullary nail.

alignment; this is particularly useful for evaluating rotational alignment.

C. Exposure
1. A lateral approach to the knee and distal femur is the workhorse for this fracture when using

a plate and screw construct, or when intra-articular visualization is necessary. An incision is made extending in a curvilinear fashion from the lateral condyle to Gerdy's tubercle. The IT band is incised longitudinally along with the

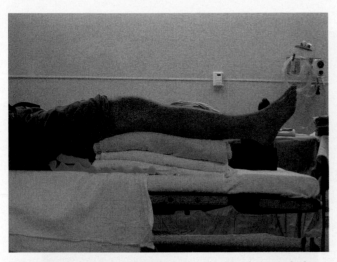

FIGURE 7-6 Blankets positioned under the leg can help reduce the deformity in the saggital plane while also elevating the leg for easier intraoperative imaging.

joint capsule. The capsule can be elevated anteriorly to allow for retraction of the patella and exposure of the articular surface of the distal femur underneath the extensor mechanism.

2. If a closed reduction is obtainable, the fracture may be amenable to intramedullary nail fixation. Again, the knee is positioned in slight flexion to improve alignment. This also allows access to the starting point for nail insertion. If the knee is flexed too little, the starting point is not accessible. If the knee is flexed too much, the inferior pole of the patella may limit access. An incision through the medial retinaculum of the patella is made. Alternatively, the patellar tendon may be split. The incision needs be large enough for nail insertion. Some surgeons prefer larger incisions to allow for adequate removal of reaming debris from the joint. ***The ideal starting point is centered in the notch on the AP view, and 1 to 2 mm anterior to the tip of Blumenstat's line on the lateral to avoid inadvertent injury to the PCL origin.***

D. MIPO

MIPO techniques and principles are often employed when performing ORIF with plate and screws for the fractures.

1. A lateral exposure is used. The exposure needs to be sufficient for the use of direct and indirect reduction techniques to obtain anatomic reduction of the articular surface, and for realignment of the femur. The fracture line and comminution in the metaphyseal region is often not exposed.

2. A locking plate is then slid submuscularly underneath the vastus lateralis in retrograde

fashion and positioned under fluoroscopy. Distal fixation is obtained through the surgical wound, and proximal fixation is obtained with the use of a jig or guide connected to the plate. This allows for accurate targeting of the proximal screws and insertion through small stab incisions (Fig. 7-7). Special attention must be paid to the fluoroscopic images when using this technique.

3. Positioning of the plate on the anterior half of the lateral femoral condyle is necessary to avoid medialization of the distal fragment. The plate must be positioned so as not to pull the femur into varus or valgus malalignment.

4. At the proximal end, care must be taken to make sure that the plate is positioned against the lateral cortex of the femur and well centered on the lateral X-ray (Fig. 7-8). There is a tendency for the plate to drift anteriorly along the proximal diaphysis, leading to prominence of the plate and poor screw purchase, which may lead to instability and failure of fixation.

E. Postoperative Protocol

1. Patients should begin immediate ROM exercises for the hip, knee, and ankle. This is especially important for nutrition of the articular cartilage; it also helps regain motion in the injured joint.

2. An extension splint should be worn between exercises and at night to maintain knee extension and prevent contracture.

3. Hinged knee braces are sometimes useful to protect against varus/valgus forces.

4. The use of sequential compression devices and routine thromboprophylaxis is recommended.

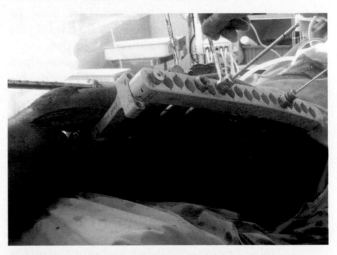

FIGURE 7-7 MIPO technique for distal femoral fracture fixation. The external targeting device allows for the placement of proximal locking screws through small stab incisions.

A   **B**

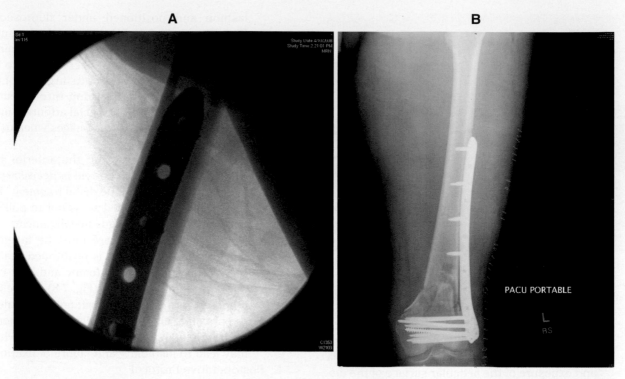

<u>FIGURE 7-8</u>   **A.** Intraoperative lateral fluoroscopic image demonstrates proper central positioning of the proximal portion of the plate on the lateral aspect of the femur. **B.** AP X-ray of a different patient with a supracondylar femur fracture properly stabilized with a locking plate.

V. Preventing Complications of Treatment
   A. Infection
      1. Respecting the soft tissues
         • No surgical incision should be made through a compromised soft-tissue envelope. In the setting of contusion, edema, or fracture blisters, surgery should be delayed until these conditions improve.
         • Dissection should minimize additional trauma to the soft tissues. Care must be taken not to devitalize bone fragments that can then become a nidus for infection.
         • Proper debridement of open fractures—Open fractures must be extensively debrided. This includes exposure and debridement of the fracture site. ORIF should be deferred until the wound is clean and free of necrotic tissue and debris.
      2. Early detection and treatment—Early postoperative wound infection often presents between 7 and 14 days postoperatively. Superficial wound infections, when treated early, are often successfully managed with oral antibiotics.
   B. Loss of Motion
      1. Stable fixation—Whatever fixation construct is chosen, one of the main goals is to obtain enough stability to allow for early range of motion.
      2. Early range of motion

         • Joints do not tolerate immobilization well, and so initiation of active, active–assisted, and gentle passive exercises is important for regaining range of motion of the knee.
         • Movement of the knee joint also helps with nutrition of articular cartilage.
      3. Extension splinting—The use of static extension splints, often at nighttime, can help prevent flexion contractures of the knee.
   C. Nonunion
      1. Prevent infection (see above).
      2. Maintain soft-tissue attachments—The use of indirect reduction techniques and meticulous handling of the soft tissues prevent devitalization of bone, which can lead to nonunion.
      3. Stable fixation—Too much motion at the fracture site can contribute to nonunion, especially in simple fracture patterns.
   D. Malunion
      1. Careful preoperative planning is essential.
         • Scrutinize X-rays and identify all fracture lines and fragments.
         • Contralateral X-rays can be useful as a template for reconstruction and alignment.
         • CT scan should be obtained for intra-articular fractures.
         • Preoperative drawings are a very useful way to walk through the steps of the surgery and

to plan for reduction techniques and implant selection and insertion.

2. Intraoperative assessment of alignment
   - Comparison to the uninjured leg is a valuable way to assess alignment, particularly rotation. This can be accomplished by prepping out both legs.
   - Intraoperative fluoroscopy is prone to distortion of alignment at the periphery of the beam. Formal radiographs should be performed intraoperatively to verify alignment.
3. Familiarity with the implants—Modern implants have particular methods of insertion and techniques to assess orientation of the implants. Familiarizing yourself with these implants, the insertion tools, and the particulars of the implant's design will make proper insertion and positioning of these implants easier. This leads to fewer problems with malalignment and/or loss of fixation.

SUGGESTED READINGS

Classic Articles

Daoud H, O'Farrell T, Cruess RL. The Judet technique and results of six cases. *J Bone Joint Surg Br.* 1982;64(2):194–197.

Thompson TC. Quadricepsplasty to improve knee function. *J Bone Joint Surg.* 1944;26A:366–379.

Recent Articles

Rolston LR, Christ DJ, Halpern A, et al. Treatment of supracondylar fractures of the femur proximal to a total knee arthroplasty. A report of four cases. *J Bone Joint Surgery Am.* 1995;77:924–931.

Sanders R, Regazzoni P, Ruedi T. Treatment of supracondylar-inlraarticular fractures of the femur using the dynamic condylar screw. *J Orthop Trauma.* 1991;3:214–346.

Sanders R, Swiontkowski M, Rosen H, et al. Double-plating of comminuted unstable fractures of the distal part of the femur. *J Bone Joint Surg.* 1991;73A:341–346.

Simon RG, Brinker MR. Use of Ilizarov external fixation for a periprosthetic supracondylar femur fracture. *J Arthroplasty.* 1999;14:118–121.

Review Articles

Warner JJ. The Judet Quadricepsplasty for management of severe post-traumatic extension contracture of the knee: a report of a bilateral case and review of the literature. *Clin Orthop.* 1990;256:169–173.

Textbooks

Clemente CD, ed. *Gray's Anatomy.* 30th ed. Philadelphia, PA: Lea & Febiger; 1985.

Femur: Trauma. In: Poss R, Buchholz RW, Frymoyer JW, et al, eds. *Orthopaesdic Knowledge Update 4: Home Study Syllabus.* Rosemount, IL: American Academy of Orthopaedic Surgeons; 1993.

Helfet DL. Fractures of the distal femur. In: Browner BD, Jupiter JB, Levine AM, et al, eds. *Skeletal Trauma: Fractures, Dislocations, Ligamentous Injuries.* Vol 2. 2nd ed. Philadelphia, PA: WB Saunders; 1992.

Johnson KD. Femoral shaft fractures. In: Browner BD, Jupiter JB, Levine AM, et al, eds. *Skeletal Trauma: Fractures, Dislocations, Ligamentous Injuries.* Vol 2. 2nd ed. Philadelphia, PA: WB Saunders; 1992.

Taylor JC Delayed union and nonunion of fractures. In Crenshaw, A.M., ed. *Campbell's Operative Orthopaedics.* Vol 2. St. Louis, MO: Mosby; 1992:1287–1345.

CHAPTER 8

Knee Dislocations, Fracture-Dislocations, and Traumatic Ligamentous Injuries of the Knee

Bryon Hobby, Kris Moore, Krishna Tripuraneni, Dustin Richter, and Robert C. Schenck Jr.

I. Introduction—Knee trauma involves a continuum of velocity and energy that changes a knee injury from what is classically considered sports injury (low velocity, low energy) to motor-vehicle injury (high velocity, high energy). Frequently, there is blurring of this distinction based on either energy or velocity, since overlap of injury type exists in both groups. Associated injuries, such as soft-tissue injuries (open vs. closed), fractures, and neural or vascular injuries, are more frequent in motor vehicle trauma, but can be present in sporting injuries as well. The terms *dislocation* and *fracture-dislocation* can be confusing, but are important to distinguish. Fracture-dislocation can be considered part of a continuum of fracture and ligamentous injuries, from the classic tibial plateau fracture (in which the ligaments are not torn), to fracture-dislocation (usually a tibial or femoral condyle fracture with a ligament injury), to pure ligamentous injuries (knee dislocations [KDs]). These distinctions are important clinically, especially in recognition of an associated vascular injury in regards to the surgical treatment. Lastly, approximately 20% of KDs frequently reduce spontaneously after the initial injury, and may not be recognized on cursory plain radiograph inspection. The concepts of examination under anesthesia (EUA) and acute versus chronic management of knee ligament injuries (e.g., repair or reattachment vs. reconstruction) are important in the management of knee trauma.

II. Knee Dislocations
   A. Introduction—Knee dislocations (KDs) classically involve pure ligamentous injuries (but also include avulsions of ligaments) of the knee wherein the tibiofemoral joint is completely displaced at the time of injury. *Initially, KDs were felt to occur only with tearing of both cruciate ligaments, but dislocations have since been shown to occur with an intact anterior cruciate ligament (ACL) or poster cruciate ligament (PCL)* (Figs. 8-1 and 8-2).
   B. Classifications—In the literature, three systems are used regularly to classify KDs and involve one of three types: (a) joint position after dislocation, (b) velocity or energy of the injury, and most recently, (c) anatomic structures torn. All three systems are useful but serve different purposes in diagnosis and treatment.
      1. Joint position after dislocation—Initially described by Kennedy, joint position after dislocation places dislocations in one of five groups: (a) anterior, 40%, (b) posterior, 33%, (c) medial, 4%, (d) lateral 18%, and (e) rotatory, 5%. Position is based on standard orthopaedic nomenclature and is named by the position of the distal articulating structure (tibia) as related to the proximal one (femur). Joint position is useful in classifying KDs, especially as related to reduction maneuvers. Rotatory dislocation most commonly involves a posterolateral dislocation (torn ACL, PCL, or medial collateral ligament [MCL]), is a complex dislocation (that requiring open reduction due to interposed soft tissue preventing closed reduction as seen in a posterolateral KD with an invaginated MCL and medial knee skin furrowing), is associated with peroneal nerve palsy, and is at high risk for soft tissue necrosis. Over 20% of KDs spontaneously reduce after injury, and hence cannot be classified by position. Furthermore, position does not determine what ligaments are torn (i.e., anterior dislocations

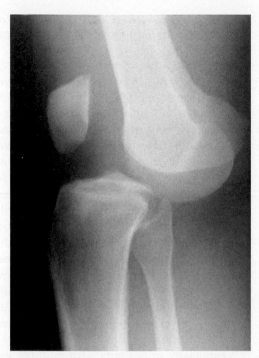

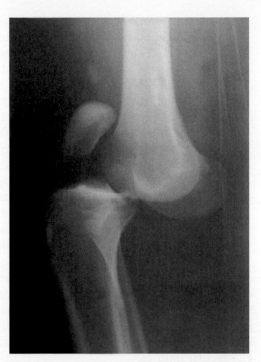

FIGURE 8-1 Lateral radiograph revealing an anterior KD that reduced with axial traction. The widened distance between the patella and the femur is characteristic of a KD with both an ACL and a PCL injury. There is greater anterior translation of the tibia on the femur. (Reprinted with permission from Stannard JP, Schenck RC Jr, Fanelli GC. Knee dislocations and fracture-dislocations. In: Bucholz RW, Heckman JD, Court-Brown C, et al., eds., *Rockwood and Green's Fractures in Adults.* 7th ed. Philadelphia, PA: Lippincott Williams & Wilkins; 2006.)

FIGURE 8-2 Lateral radiograph of a PCL-intact KD. Note the proximity of the patella to the femur as compared to that in Figure 8-1. (Reprinted with permission from Stannard JP, Schenck RC Jr, Fanelli GC. Knee dislocations and fracture-dislocations. In: Bucholz RW, Heckman JD, Court-Brown C, et al., eds., *Rockwood and Green's Fractures in Adults.* 7th ed. Philadelphia, PA: Lippincott Williams & Wilkins; 2006.)

can occur with or without tearing of the PCL), and treatment depends on the ligaments and tendons injured. Thus the position classification is useful, but has limitations, especially in directing definitive ligamentous treatment.

2. Velocity or energy of the injury—High-energy, high-velocity motor vehicle injuries account for over 50% of all KDs, and low-energy, low-velocity sporting injuries account for approximately one-third (33%). Although velocity and energy are not interchangeable, sports KDs are considered low velocity or low energy and are considered to have a lower incidence of associated vascular injury as compared with motor vehicle injuries. Regardless of the energy of injury (high or low), the risk of popliteal arterial injury still exists and must be ruled out with the initial clinical evaluation.

3. Anatomic structures torn—The anatomic classification was developed by Schenck to classify KDs by the ligaments torn and thus help direct treatment, compare injuries, and use

with all dislocations, even those with spontaneous reduction (those unclassifiable by the joint position system). *The anatomic classification requires a standard ligamentous examination to determine which ligaments are torn* (Table 8-1). The numeric system uses the two cruciates and two corners (medial or lateral) in combination to describe what can potentially be torn. Increasing numbers in the anatomic system usually implies increasing severity/energy of injury. The anatomic classification uses four classes with five basic injury patterns: *KD-I, a single cruciate ligament-intact KD,* such as a PCL-intact KD in which the ACL and posterolateral corner are torn, or the ACL-intact KD (tibia is dislocated posteriorly, PCL is torn), which has also been described but is rare; *KD-II, ACL and PCL torn* and the collaterals are structurally/clinically intact (rare); *KD-IIIM (medial) ACL, PCL, and MCL and posteromedial corner torn and the lateral side is clinically intact (most common); KD-IIIL (lateral), ACL, PCL, and posterolateral corner torn, and the medial side is intact; KD-IV, all four ligaments torn (highest energy of injury)*. The distinction of a clinically intact corner, such as the posterolateral corner in the KD-IIIM, is based on EUA. For example, the KD-IIIM on MRI may have subtle injury changes to the posterolateral corner, but on EUA, the lateral ligaments are structurally competent, thus its distinction from a KD-IV Injury. The increasing number implies increasing severity and energy of injury. The modifiers *C* and *N* are used for arterial or neural injuries, respectively (C as in Gustilo type IIIC injury and N as in nerve injury). Although surgical techniques change over time, basing the classification on what is torn directs treatment and the appropriate surgical exposure (Fig. 8-3).

C. Associated Injuries—KDs have a wide variation of associated injuries and include vascular injuries, neurologic injuries, fractures, soft-tissue injuries, tendinous injuries, meniscal and hyaline injuries, and of course ligamentous injuries.

1. Vascular injuries
   - Popliteal artery—Anatomically, the popliteal artery is rigidly fixed at the adductor hiatus proximally and at the soleus arch distally; tibiofemoral displacement can injure the vessel by traction or direct transection. Collateralization is rich about the knee but insufficient to perfuse the extremity. *Limb loss is imminent if revascularization is not performed within 6 to 8 hours from the time of popliteal artery injury. The overall incidence of arterial injury is 20% and varies dependent on population studied.* Low-velocity KDs have a lower incidence of arterial injury (approximately 8%).
   - Clinical examination—An initial clinical vascular examination of the knee is absolutely necessary (Fig. 8-4). *The presence of pulses does not rule out an arterial injury,* especially if there is an intimal injury or collateral rupture. However, the absence of pulses (or equivocal findings of vascularity) implies an arterial injury and cannot be considered a temporary finding of spasm that will resolve with time. *After adequate joint reduction has been emergently performed, the presence of continued vascular insufficiency requires emergent revascularization, which should not be delayed for arteriography. Recent studies have documented the usefulness and safety of sequential clinical examinations (pulses) to rule out arterial injury. However, any evidence of vascular insufficiency must be further evaluated with vascular consultation, ultrasonography (if available) or arteriography.*
   - Arteriography—The indications for use of arteriography have become controversial, but arteriography still remains the gold standard for ruling out an arterial injury. *Decision making in the presence of vascular insufficiency usually involves a one-shot intraoperative arteriogram before vascular exploration and revascularization.* In the past, decision making in the presence of normal pulses has always required arteriography. More recently, clinical observation of normal palpable pulses and the use of noninvasive arterial Doppler studies with ankle–brachial indices have been shown as reliable in the presence of a normal vascular examination. Ankle–brachial indices of less than 0.90 are strongly predictive for vascular injury. Arteriography is still frequently used, especially in patients with multiple injuries or in the patient with closed head trauma. *The onus is on the clinician to rule out an arterial injury*.
   - Compartment syndrome—Severe leg pain in the presence of a KD or stocking-glove paresthesias of the leg (indicating a late compartment syndrome) implies a compartment syndrome. Vascular examination should involve consideration of compartment syndrome and if indicated requires compartment pressure measurement and a fasciotomy if pressures are above 35 mm Hg. (The indications for fasciotomy change if the systemic blood pressure is low or if revascularization is performed.)

2. Neurologic injuries—Injury to nerves from simple mechanical displacement produces neurologic injury, most commonly axonotmesis. Complete disruption of the nerve (neurotmesis) can occur but is much less common. *The peroneal nerve is most commonly involved (20% of all KDs)* and is most commonly associated with lateral-sided injuries (KD-IIIL) or a posterolateral KD. Tibial nerve involvement is rare, but can be seen with vascular injury. Loss of protective sensation of the foot (the sole of the foot) with a complete tibial nerve injury associated with a vascular injury may result in amputation. In contrast, peroneal nerve involvement is a functional problem from the motor abnormalities and is frequently a significant factor in the patient's disability.

TABLE 8-1

Physical Examination of the Knee

Examination	Method	Significance
McMurray	External/internal rotation and varus/valgus stress-extension	Meniscal pathology or chondromalacia of the articular surface
Varus/valgus stress	30°	MCL/LCL laxity (Grades I–IV)
Varus/valgus stress	0°	MCL/LCL and PCL/posterior capsule laxity
Apley's	Prone-flexion compression	DJD, meniscal pathology
Lachman	Tibia forward at 30° of flexion	ACL (most flexible)
Stabilized Lachman	Examiner's thigh under the patient's knee	ACL (use the posterior Lachman test to guage the PCL)
Finacetto	Same as Lachman test, with the tibia subluxing beyond the posterior horns of the menisci	ACL (severe)
Anterior drawer	Tibia forward at 90° of flexion	ACL
Internal rotation driver	Foot internally rotated with drawer	Tighter, normal, looser, ALRI
External rotation driver	Foot externally rotated with drawer	Loose, normal, looser, AMRI
Pivot shift	Flexion with the internal rotation and valgus	ALRI
Flexion-rotation drawer	Shift with axial load, less valgus	ALRI
Slocum	Supine-side flexion and pivot	ALRI
Pivot jerk	Extension with internal rotation and valgus	ALRI
Posterior drawer	Tibia backward at 90° of flexion	PCL
Tibial sag	Flexion at 90°, observation	PCL
90° quadriceps active	Extension of flexed knee	PCL
External rotation recurvatum	Picking up of great toes	PLRI
Reverse pivot shift	Extension with external rotation and valgus	PLRI
External rotation at 30 and 90	Increased external rotation associated with PLRI	PLRI
Posterolateral drawer	Posterior drawer, lateral > medial	PLRI

MCI, Medial collateral ligament; LCL, lateral collateral ligament; PCL, posterior cruciate ligament; DJD, degenerative joint disease; ACL, anterior cruciate ligament; ALRI, anterolateral rotatory instability; AMRI, anteromedial rotatory instability; PLRI, posterolateral rotatory instability.
Source: Modified from Miller M. *Review of Orthopaedics*. 3rd ed. Philadelphia, PA: W B Saunders; 2000, with permission.

3. Fractures—Joint-surface fractures of the tibia or femur create an injury best described and classified as a fracture-dislocation. Ligamentous avulsions are common in KDs and change the character of the injury and can often simplify treatment.

- Multitrauma KDs are commonly seen in multitrauma (multiple fractures severe trauma) and can be missed when there are multiple complex injuries. As noted previously, spontaneous reduction of KDs can make a multiligamentous knee injury less obvious, and careful attention during the skeletal survey is important to evaluate for a severe knee injury. Gross knee swelling in the presence of multiple trauma necessitates consideration of a dislocation, despite the presence of a reduced knee joint on radiographic evaluation. In the presence of multiple trauma, a lower threshold for arteriography may be necessary, as the treatment (i.e., immediate femoral nail fixation) in such situation does not readily allow for the observation of noninvasive studies. Furthermore, a noncooperative patient in light of a closed head injury often pushes the clinician to consider arteriography in evaluation of the vascular tree in the dislocated knee. The treatment of musculoskeletal injuries in multiple trauma is frequently prioritized, and the ligamentous management of dislocations is frequently delayed for days to weeks and follows stabilization of long-bone fractures. KDs in multiple trauma are also acceptably stabilized with external fixation, which will facilitate patient transfer and allows for visualization of the knee and extremity.

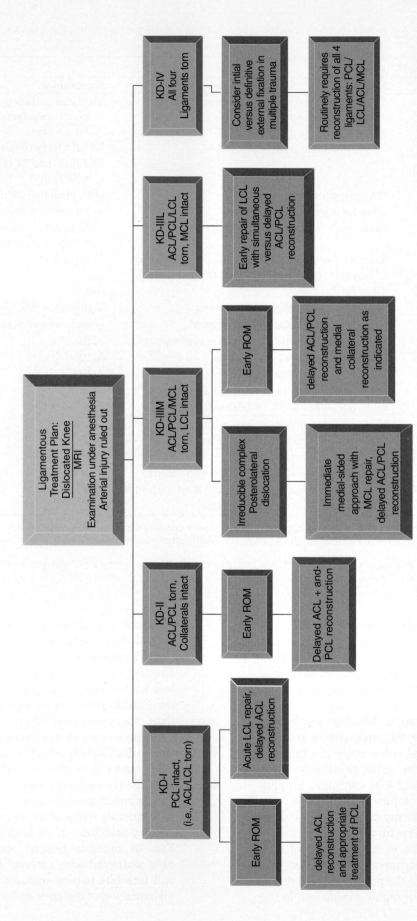

FIGURE 8-3 Suggested ligamentous management plan for KDs based on the anatomic classification system. Delayed surgical treatment is usually 6 to 8 weeks following injury or until full ROM is attained. When combining ACL/PCL reconstruction, one should tension the PCL repair before the ACL; tensioning the ACL first will result in posterior tibiofemoral knee subluxation. *LCL*, Lateral collateral ligament but includes structures of the posterolateral corners; *MRI*, magnetic resonance imaging; *ROM*, range of motion.

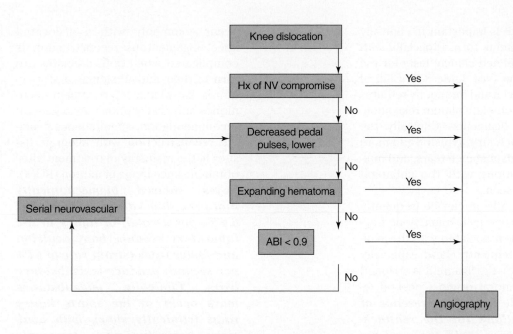

FIGURE 8-4 Suggested vascular evaluation algorithm for managing KDs.

- Microfractures—Bone bruises occur, but, in the past, have been underreported because of the need for magnetic resonance imaging (MRI) to document the injury. Chondral injuries are classified according to standard grading systems but are usually observed unless a reparable surface fracture exists.
4. Soft-tissue injuries—Soft-tissue injuries include the soft tissue envelope and the menisci.
   - Soft-tissue envelope—With any high-energy or motor-vehicle trauma, the status of the soft tissues is extremely important. Even with a closed KD, the magnitude of the displacement frequently separates the knee joint proper from its attachments to the subcutaneous tissues. Gross and widespread ecchymosis, as well as subcutaneous crepitus from the soft tissue separation, is a common finding. As an aside, exploration for open ligamentous repair is frequently simplified by the underlying displacement and soft tissue injury. Open joint injuries occur, especially with high-energy trauma, and can compound the eventual ligamentous management with the need for external fixation and eventual soft tissue coverage. Open knee joint injuries from a dislocation require careful evaluation for vascular and neural injuries as a result of the degree of displacement required to cause an open injury. Treatment of an open KD requires the standard approach of debridement, pulsatile lavage, and bony joint stabilization, which frequently requires external fixation, with delayed ligamentous reconstruction.

- Meniscus—With the multiple ligamentous involvement in producing a KD, meniscal tears are variable in presentation and include displaced bucket-handle tears, peripheral tears, crush injuries with nonreconstructable meniscal damage, and coronary ligament avulsions with gross meniscal instability. Intraoperative evaluation requires inspection of both menisci and repair if possible. The inspection of medial and lateral meniscal injuries and the meniscofemoral ligaments is important.
5. Tendinous injuries—Ruptures of supporting tendinous structures about the knee are frequent and should be suspected. Avulsions or ruptures of the patellar, biceps femoris, iliotibial band, and popliteus tendons are common; the last three are usually associated with lateral sided injury. Patellar tendon injuries are problematic if missed and should be evaluated clinically with a straight leg lift, radiographs (patella alta), MRI, or a combination thereof. Quadriceps tendon ruptures can occur and are usually associated with an open injury.
6. Ligamentous injuries—Ligamentous injuries are not truly associated injuries but are the primary reason for the other injuries. As noted in the section on avulsions, ligamentous involvement in KD is usually more complex, extensive, and severe than subluxation injuries involving the isolated collaterals or cruciates.
   - Specific injuries—As noted previously, KDs present with varying combinations of ligament involvement. KD (complete tibiofemoral displacement) can occur with an intact

PCL or ACL. Thus it is important to clinically diagnose the ligaments torn, especially with the current well-defined clinical tests for the ligament evaluation (see Table 8-1). Clinical examination is crucial and frequently requires an anesthetic for complete patient relaxation.

(a) The cruciate ligaments—Clinically the two patterns of injury, avulsion and more commonly midsubstance tears, and multiple combinations with the collateral ligaments are seen.

- Avulsion—Avulsion can be frequently seen in high-energy trauma. Bone fragments can be associated with the avulsion, but, frequently (and especially with the PCL), the ligament is stripped from the femoral origin ("peel-off lesion") (Table 8-2). *The presence of avulsion allows for the reattachment and may avoid the need for reconstruction of the involved cruciates. The "peel-off lesion" of the PCL can be reattached with heavy, nonabsorbable, braided sutures using the Krackow locking suture technique if recognized early* (Fig. 8-5). Repair techniques can be performed arthroscopically, but are most easily performed open using drill tunnels and suture anchors. MRI is useful in identifying avulsions/midsubstance tears, and is especially useful for preoperative planning used in conjunction with careful EUA. EUA allows for determination of ligament function and when combined with MRI can allow for thorough preoperative planning.
- Midsubstance—Commonly seen in the isolated rupture of the ACL, midsubstance tears of the cruciates also

occur commonly with a dislocated knee. Ligamentous reconstruction is complicated when both cruciates are torn in their midsubstance, and it requires knowledge of treatment techniques and graft options. As a general recommendation, simultaneous cruciate reconstruction with allograft tissues is the mainstay of treatment after obtaining knee range of motion (ROM). *Noyes showed biomechanically that very slow rates (strain rate of 0.67% per second) of injury in the laboratory produce bony avulsion and faster rates (strain rate of 67% per second) produce midsubstance tears. Clinically, midsubstance tears occur at the sports injury rates (clinically slow), with avulsions occurring more commonly in high-velocity (clinically fast) injuries.* Clinically fast rates are much higher that what can be produced in the laboratory, and avulsions occur from the higher, clinically applicable injury strain rate.

(b) Collateral ligaments and capsule—Unlike combined injuries of the ACL and MCL, the collateral and capsular injuries in KDs are frequently complete, extensive, and require operative attention. Clinical examination is important to determine partial versus complete tears of the corners, especially when evaluating varus and valgus stability in extension and 30° of flexion. MRI can reinforce these findings of collateral injury, especially with retraction of the MCL, LCL, and popliteus tendon. *Although injury to a collateral ligament can be seen on MRI, the clinical EUA is paramount in determining treatment.* Surgical exploration and reconstruction or repair of capsular, collateral, and tendinous (popliteus) structures is necessary and can be performed only with open surgery (Fig. 8-6). Most treatment algorithms recommend early lateral corner repair (KD-IIIL) and allow for early range of motion of the KDIIIM with the treatment of medial sided structures as indicated at the time of bicruciate reconstruction.

- Examination—Careful examination is mandatory and includes a vascular and neurologic

TABLE 8-2

ACL and PCL Avulsions in KDs

Author (Year)	No. of Knees	No. (%) of Cases with Avulsed Ligament	
		ACL	PCL
Sisto and Warren (1985)	16	10 (63%)	14 (88%)
Frassica et al. (1991)	13	6 (46%)	10 (77%)
Total	29	16 (55%)	24 (83%)

From Schenck RC Jr, Burke RL. *Perspect Orthop Surg.* 1991;2:119–134, with permission.

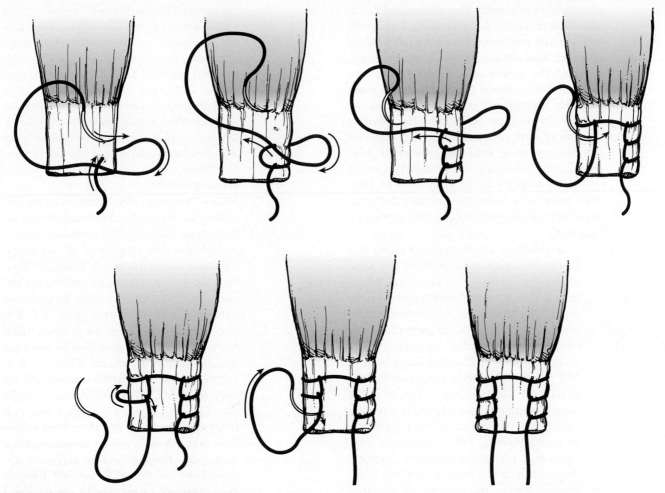

FIGURE 8-5 Sequential steps of placing Krakow locking loop ligament sutures for tendon or ligament repair.

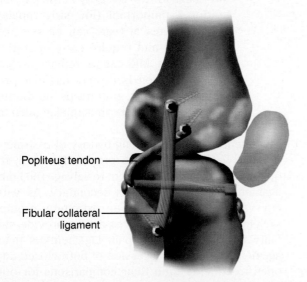

Popliteus tendon

Fibular collateral ligament

FIGURE 8-6 Anatomic posterolateral corner reconstruction (popliteus, popliteofibular ligament, lateral collateral ligament) using Achilles allograft.

examination, evaluation of the soft tissue envelope, extensor mechanism, and ligaments. Gross swelling is frequent, and such a finding on secondary survey (i.e., gross knee swelling, normal radiographs) should alert one to a KD with spontaneous reduction. Initial examination usually requires examination of the knee in extension and at 30° of flexion. The posterior drawer test is very specific for injury to the PCL, but is frequently too painful to perform without anesthesia at the time of injury. In contrast, varus and valgus stability in full extension and partial flexion (30°) in comparison to the normal knee is usually tolerated well by the patient. The Lachman test, and more commonly a stabilized Lachman test (examiner's left thigh supporting the patient's right knee and vice versa), allows evaluation of the anterior and posterior cruciate ligament translation endpoints. *The stabilized Lachman test is useful in examining ligaments in an acute presentation in which patient comfort and relaxation can be difficult. Placing the examiner's thigh under the injured knee allows for a relatively comfortable examination. Gross medial or lateral opening in full extension implies tearing of both cruciates, the affected collateral ligament, and the posterior capsule.* Subtle changes (improvement) in varus or valgus stability while extending to knee from a partially flexed to an extended position can imply integrity of one of the cruciate ligaments.

(a) EUA—EUA is an extremely important facet of surgical treatment of the knee as the integrity of a ligament determines the need for reconstruction or repair. Furthermore, determining the integrity of the PCL is necessary for evaluating the order of ligamentous reconstruction (PCL tensioning is first, ACL is second), and in the situation of a PCL-intact KD, integrity of the PCL can direct treatment to early ROM followed by an ACL reconstruction once motion is reestablished. With combined cruciate and collateral ligament injuries, the results of the drawer test are more dramatic than those with an isolated cruciate injury. Establishing a neutral point of tibiofemoral position based on condyle anatomy as well as comparison to the normal knee is important for clarifying the drawer position (whether it is anterior or posterior). Translation of 20 mm is common in a complete bicruciate KD when the anterior and posterior limits of the drawer are tested. Pivot-shift phenomenon is frequently not as instrumental in the clinical examinations of KDs, since the diagnosis is usually based on Lachman, drawer, and varus and valgus stress testing. Furthermore, pivot shift testing may redislocate the knee.

(b) Radiographs—Radiographic study is important for verifying reduction, ruling out joint surface fractures, and identifying avulsion injuries such as Segond's fracture (avulsion of the mid-third lateral capsule implying a complete tear of at least one cruciate) or the Gerdy tubercle (iliotibial band avulsion). In spontaneously reduced KDs, tibiofemoral widening on anteroposterior knee films may be one subtle sign of a spontaneously reduced KD. Although more useful for ruling out joint-surface fractures and avulsions, radiographs are helpful in evaluating subtle degrees of subluxation. Lastly, intraoperative radiographs are extremely important for documenting tibiofemoral reduction after surgical reconstruction.

(c) MRI—The use of MRI before surgery can determine ligament involvement and injury type (avulsion vs. midsubstance), meniscal tears, location of collateral ligament injury (femoral, tibial, or fibular), tendon involvement (especially patellar and popliteus), bone bruises, or extensive microfractures (Figs. 8-7, 8-8, and 8-9). *MR findings in a dislocated knee are wide ranging and depend on the ligaments involved. Classic findings in a KD-IIIM involve a peel-off injury of the PCL from its femoral origin* (see Fig. 8-8), *avulsion of the tibial collateral ligament from the tibial insertion* (see Fig. 8-7), *and a midsubstance ACL tear. The peel-off or stripped appearance of the PCL on MR images corresponds clinically to an avulsed PCL with minimal bone fragments with extension of Sharpies fibers onto the articular surface.* Inspection of the MR image for the integrity of the patellar tendon is important (for early repair). Locked meniscal tears can be seen on MR images and require early operative intervention. MRI cannot replace a clinical examination, but can be useful in predicting avulsions, graft needs, tendinous injuries, and long-term sequelae such as bone bruises.

D. Treatment—KDs have a long history of treatment options. Vascular injury, as previously noted, requires immediate management to salvage the limb, ligamentous management is secondary. As with any vascular injury about an extremity, prompt skeletal stabilization is necessary to provide stability for the vascular repair. Ligamentous management requires a discussion of both closed and open treatments (and their comparisons for outcome), complications, and prognosis. Many options exist for the treatment of bicruciate injuries

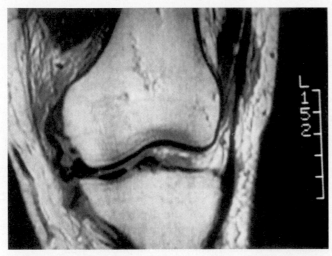

FIGURE 8-7   MRI image revealing a tibial avulsion of the MCL in a KD. (With permission from Schenck RC Jr. *Orthopaedic Special Edition.* 1998;4(3):1–4.)

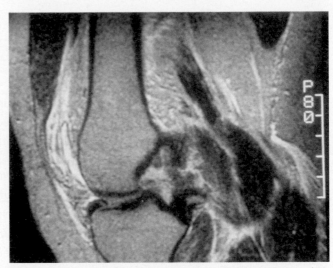

FIGURE 8-9   MRI image of the notch of a low-velocity KD (KD IIIM) revealing midsubstance tears of both the ACL and PCL. (With permission from Schenck RC Jr. *Orthopaedic Special Edition.* 1998;4(3):1–4.)

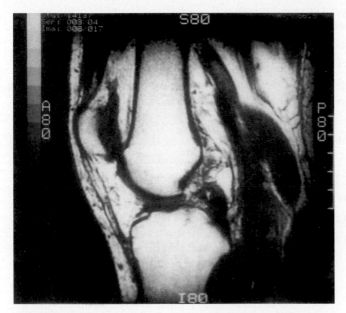

FIGURE 8-8   MRI image of a reduced KD, revealing a femoral avulsion of the PCL. The ligamentous injury is that of a stripping or peel-off from the medial condylar notch without a bony fragment. Frequently a portion of the hyaline cartilage surface is stripped in continuity with the ligament. (With permission from Schenck RC Jr. *Orthopaedic Special Edition.* 1998;4(3):1–4.)

and frequently depend on surgeon experience and patient presentation (Table 8-3).

1. Closed treatment—Although closed treatment has been maligned in the orthopaedic literature, there have been no prospective randomized trials comparing closed vs. open treatment of KDs. In a 1972 retrospective, non-randomized study evaluating closed and open treatment of KDs, *closed treatment gave satisfactory results when the knee was immobilized for 4 to 6 weeks*. Open treatment was performed only for open concomitant vascular injuries, and as expected, open treatment fared poorly as compared with the less complicated injuries that were treated closed. Current arthroscopic techniques, the knowledge of ligament anatomy, and reconstructive and rehabilitative options create a different environment for operative management from that in the 1970s. Furthermore, the complications of prolonged knee immobilization must be recognized with osteopenia, muscle atrophy, and arthrofibrosis. Nonetheless, in the patient who has multiple injuries and a KD or a KD complicated by an arterial repair, immobilization as outlined by Taylor et al. (1972) can be a useful guideline. *More recently, Wong et al. showed no statistical difference in ROM in a retrospective review comparing 11 KDs treated closed to 15 operatively treated KDs; however, operatively treated patients did have higher IKDC scores and a greater flexion contracture*. In general, closed treatment of uncomplicated KDs will have a significant degree of laxity and lower IKDC knee scores.

TABLE 8-3

The Dislocated Knee: Literature Review

Author (Year)	No. of Patients	Content
O'Donoghue (1955)	5	Advocated surgical ligament treatment
Quinlan and Sharrard (1958)	5	Discussed mechanism of injury with posterolateral dislocation
Hoover (1961)	14	Reported that eight of nine vascular injuries (89%) required amputation
Kennedy (1963)	22	Discussed classification system and cadaveric study and advocated surgical treatment
Shields et al. (1969)	24	Advocated surgical ligament repair
Reckling and Peltier (1969)	15	Discussed associated injuries
Meyers and Harvey (1971)	18	Advocated surgical ligament repair
Taylor et al. (1972)	41	Advocated nonsugical ligament treatment for uncomplicated KDs
Meyers et al. (1975)	53	Reemphasized surgical ligament repair
Green and Allen (1977)	41	Defined an average incidence of popliteal arterial injury in KDs
Jones et al. (1979)	22	Emphasized peripheral pulses as unreliable in verifying vascularity
Moore (1981)	132	Classified fracture-dislocation of the knee
Sisto and Warren (1985)	19	Advocated surgical ligament repair and emphasized the high incidence of ligament avusions
Frassica et al. (1991)	17	Advocated surgical repair
Kendall et al. (1993)	32	Discussed the clinical examination of KDs and the role of arteriography
Walker et al. (1994)	13	Advocated surgical repair based on the anatomic classification system
Fanelli et al. (1996)	20	Discussed delayed arthroscopic bicruciate ligament reconstruction
Wascher et al. (1997)	50	Bicruciate ligament injuries are equivalent to knee dislocation
Fanelli et al. (2002)	35	Advocated combined arthroscopic treatment of ACL/PCL injuries
Twaddle et al. (2003)	60	Described injury patterns and associated injuries
Mills et al. (2004)	38	Established ABI as important role in assessing for vascular injuries
Harner et al. (2004)	31	Advocated acute surgical ligament treatment
Tzubakis et al. (2006)	44	Advocated acute surgical ligament treatment

2. Open treatment—With the advent of ligament surgery about the knee, several authors have documented improved stability with early open surgery of a KD. ***Meyers and Harvey were the first to show (retrospectively) poorer results with nonoperative treatment and more predictable results with operative treatment***. Sisto and Warren also showed improved results with operative treatment, but with a small but significant chance for permanent stiffness. Current recommendations for KD ligament surgery involve early ligament repair (7 to 10 days after the injury) versus early ROM and simultaneous delayed cruciate reconstruction in the simple uncomplicated KD. Ligament surgery is always secondary to limb salvage, and a vascular injury must always be ruled out. In any traumatic injury to the extremity, associated injuries must be considered in designing a treatment plan. With a KD, the focus can be placed on ligamentous injuries, but must initially be focused on the vessels, nerves, and soft tissues. Once associated injuries are determined, the identification of the ligaments injured is crucial to treatment. The treatment of a PCL-intact KD (KD-I) is much different from that of an injury with involvement of the ACL, PCL, and posterolateral corner (KD-IIIL). Also, the type of ligament injury present, avulsion or midsubstance, determines the surgical option of reattachment versus reconstruction. With a functioning PCL, early ROM and delay

of arthroscopic ACL reconstruction until ROM is obtained is useful. The surgical options and timing depend on the ligaments involved specifically and not simply on the dislocation. Clinical examination (frequently required under anesthesia), plain radiographs, and MRI define the treatment algorithm (see Fig. 8-3). ***Because of the presence of a capsular injury and the risk of fluid extravasation with KDs, use of the arthroscope is avoided in early surgery (delayed until 7 to 10 days). Open surgery is recommended early, and arthroscopic reconstruction is delayed***. A complete injury to the posterolateral corner is best treated early and requires open surgery. Basic concepts for the order of ligament repair are as follows: first the PCL and the affected corner are reestablished, and second the ACL injury is addressed. ***The PCL forms the cornerstone of the knee, and in a KD with a complete PCL and ACL injury, the PCL must be treated first. Tightening of an ACL graft before reestablishing normal PCL mechanics will subluxate the tibia posteriorly on the femur***. Many dislocations are PCL-intact (including some partial PCL injuries) dislocations and can be treated with early ROM followed by a delayed ACL reconstruction.

- Open surgery—Early open surgery is recommended, especially when there is a complete injury to the posterolateral corner and a complete injury to the PCL and ACL. ***Some controversy currently exists regarding posterolateral corner repair versus reconstruction. Most studies have supported primary repair of a complete injury to the posterolateral corner***. In the patient with multiple injuries, a complete ACL/PCL/posterolateral corner injury may best be initially stabilized with an external fixator followed by eventual reconstruction. The success of KD ligamentous surgery depends on the associated injuries, and the surgery is best performed in the patient who has one or two isolated injuries.

- Delayed arthroscopic surgery—Arthroscopic surgery usually is performed on a delayed basis once range of motion is reestablished. Staged reconstructions where the PCL and posterolateral corner are reconstructed followed by delayed ACL reconstruction have been reported with successful results in the past. However, most surgeons follow the recommendations of Fanelli et al. and Wascher et al., who in separate reports discussed delayed, simultaneous ACL/PCL allograft reconstructions, after initial ROM exercises. The placement of simultaneous tibial tunnels for ACL and PCL grafts requires an appropriate bone bridge for a successful reconstruction. Nonetheless, early simultaneous ACL/PCL reconstructions can result in significant arthrofibrosis and are ideally performed once ROM has been reestablished and knee inflammation has resolved.

- Chronic dislocations—Very difficult problems can be treated with joint reduction and external fixation (hinged type also has been reported). A common scenario is a missed posterolateral dislocation (ACL, PCL, and MCL) with an invaginated MCL and a dislocated patellofemoral joint. This injury may have a concomitant peroneal nerve injury and requires open reduction to extract the MCL in what is defined as a complex dislocation. Results are often poor.

3. Closed versus open treatment—In the only study comparing closed versus operative treatment of KDs, Taylor et al. noted better results with closed treatment. The operative treatment was performed only in open, complex, or KDs with a vascular injury. (Similar injuries were not compared.) However, in most studies, operative treatment gives the most predictable results in the complete bicruciate KD injury. Either initial repair and delayed ACL reconstruction (staged cruciate reconstruction) or early ROM and simultaneous cruciate reconstruction after obtaining knee joint ROM is currently recommended. Initial ROM exercises followed by delayed ACL reconstruction gives a predictable result in PCL-intact KDs. In patients with multiple trauma with complicated KDs (vascular injuries, open KD-IV), external fixation with an anterior frame with the knee reduced is an effective initial management option. The external fixator (depending on injury and circumstance) is used for immobilization for 4 to 6 weeks, followed by fixator removal, manipulation of the knee under an epidural anesthesia, arthroscopic anterior release, and postoperative continuous passive motion (CPM) with an epidural for 48 to 72 hours. Late instability is reconstructed once motion is reestablished.

4. Complications—In the treatment of KDs, complications are frequent and are related to the initial severity of the injury. Late instability, arthritis, arthrofibrosis, and long-term peroneal nerve palsy are common.

- Stiffness—Clearly noted by Sisto and Warren, permanent stiffness of the knee can result with any operative treatment. Open surgery must be followed by immediate ROM exercises; otherwise the combination of the soft tissue injury from the dislocation and the immobilization can lead to permanent knee stiffness (despite attempts to correct this with arthroscopy, manipulation, and epidural-CPM). A fixed flexion contracture is a particularly difficult problem to manage and is functionally debilitating. Flexion loss was commonly noted after operative management. Stiffness is uncommon after closed treatment and usually results in an unstable knee with good range of motion. *One of the benefits of early ROM and delayed cruciate surgery is the prevention of knee stiffness after eventual operative reconstruction*. In most series of operative treatment of KDs, the need for post-reconstruction manipulation under anesthesia is approximately 20%.
- Vascular injury and limb loss—Vascular injury and limb loss is a disastrous complication that can be avoided with early recognition, vascular exploration and repair, and fasciotomy as needed. DeBakey and Simeone (from WWII data) noted an 80% amputation rate if repair of a popliteal arterial injury was not performed within 6 to 8 hours of injury. Vascular repair requires joint stabilization, and a simple anterior (external fixation) frame is useful for managing such injuries.
- Neurologic injury—Long-term disability from peroneal nerve palsy is common. Sisto and Warren noted improvement after neurolysis in two of eight patients with KDs. *Peroneal nerve injuries most commonly occur with lateral injuries* (KD-IIIL), and in such situations, repair of the posterolateral corner requires exploration of the peroneal nerve. Tibial nerve involvement is less common and frequently involves associated injuries (such as a vascular injury or open wounds) or gross joint displacement as would be seen with a KD-IV. There should be suspicion of a compartment syndrome if there is any sensory or motor nerve involvement.
- Arthritis—Arthrosis of the knee is common in KDs and is most likely the result of severe chondral contusions (bone bruises) associated with the injury. A difficult problem is that KDs frequently occur in a population

younger than 40 years of age, a group not well suited for knee-replacement surgery.
- Late instability—Late instability is usually not a difficulty with early surgery. Arthrofibrosis (stiffness) is usually the associated complication with early surgery. Late instability usually occurs with midsubstance cruciate repairs, early ROM, or no treatment with poor ligamentous healing. Combined PCL or posterolateral corner injuries are difficult to manage late and are best treated with early surgery. Abnormalities of gait (thrust, hyperextension) can be seen as a result of the instability pattern. Stiffness and late instability are opposing complications in the treatment of KDs.

5. Prognosis—The variety of KDs as well as the range of severity equates to a varied prognosis in ultimate function, ROM, arthritis, and stability. Comparing like injuries based on what is torn (anatomic system, KD-I to IV) allows one to prognosticate. Walker et al. (1994) noted that KD-IIIL injuries fared poorer than KD-IIIM injuries. Furthermore, in that study, KD-IV injuries had a higher incidence of neural and vascular involvement and resulted from higher-energy trauma.

III. Fracture Dislocations of the Knee
  A. Introduction—Fracture-dislocation, or fracture-subluxation, is an important concept in the diagnosis and management of injuries about the knee. Initially described by Tillman Moore, the concept of a knee fracture-dislocation is useful for recognizing fractures about the knee that involve ligamentous injuries. A review from Robertson et al. found the incidence of fractures of either the distal femur or proximal tibia with associated KD was 16%. *A fracture-dislocation implies that repair of both the fracture and ligament is often necessary for surgical management*.
  B. Tibial-Sided Fracture-Dislocations
    1. Classification (Fig. 8-10)—Moore et al. described a classification of tibial-sided fractures consisting of five types. Type 1 and 2 involve variations of medial tibial condyle fractures (similar to a Schatzker IV injury). *Type 1 has a coronal split of the medial condyle seen on a lateral radiograph. Type 2 involves the entire condyle* and although most commonly medial, can also be an isolated lateral condyle fracture. *Type 3, or "rim avulsion" (rim of the tibial plateau), is an enlarged lateral joint rim fracture, either an avulsion of the Gerdy's tubercle or an enlarged Segond's fracture*

(also known as the lateral capsular sign). Type 4, or "rim compression" with contralateral ligamentous injury, usually involves compression of the lateral tibial plateau edge with tearing of the MCL. Type 5 is described as a fracture involving four parts: both condyles, the tibial eminence, and the tibial shaft (the Schatzker V bicondylar fracture and/or the Schatzker VI metaphyseal diaphyseal dissociation). As with the Schatzker classification, the energy and severity of injury increase with the number (type), so the prognosis is poorer for higher classification numbers.

2. Vascular injury—A fracture-dislocation of the knee has a significant risk for vascular injury and should be suspected much like with KDs, especially with displacement of a large tibial condyle fracture. The risk of vascular injury depends on the type of fracture-dislocation: from Moore's study, type 1: 2%, type 2: 12%, type 3: 30%, type 4: 13% and type 5: 50%; *fracture-dislocation of the knee often requires arteriography to rule out a vascular injury.* Clinical examination is important, especially in considering compartment syndrome in addition to frank popliteal artery injury. Revascularization guidelines are similar to those for KD, and fracture fragment fixation and joint stabilization, with either internal or external fixation, should be performed at the time of revascularization.

3. Treatment—Operative management involves stable internal fixation of the tibial condyle and repair of the injured ligaments. *Ligamentous involvement depends on the type of fracture-dislocation present. Knee instability occurs in 60% of type 1 and type 2 injuries and 90% to 100% of type 3 to 5 injuries.* Ligament instability is best treated at the time of fracture fixation. Type 1 and 2 injuries can be treated with standard AO plate techniques and screws. (If the soft tissues are grossly swollen, cannulated screws and external fixation should be considered.) Displacement of the medial condyle and a varus deformity can occur when only cannulated screws are used. In high-energy medial condyle fractures, a medial buttress plate and screws are necessary considerations in fracture treatment. *A direct posterior or posteromedial approach may be used to fix type 1 fractures.* Type 3 injuries require reattachment of avulsions and repair of ligaments. Type 4 injuries (rim compression) can involve a large segment of the lateral plateau and may require open reduction with internal fixation of the compressed lateral plateau (with or without bone grafting) in addition to repair of the MCL. Type 5 injuries are high energy and are associated with

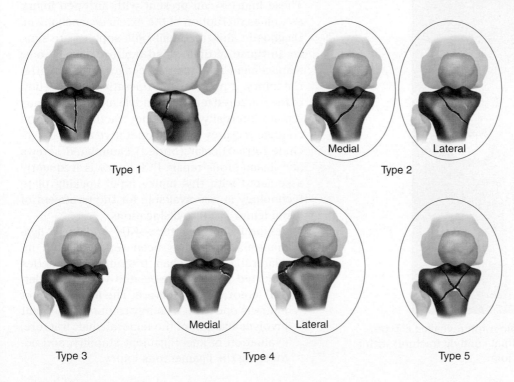

FIGURE 8-10 Classification of tibial-sided fractures of fracture-dislocations of the knee.

Type 1

Medial   Lateral

Type 2

Type 3

Medial   Lateral

Type 4

Type 5

vascular injury. Consideration of the soft tissue envelope is necessary in determining the surgical plan for type 5 injuries. Cannulated screw after joint-surface reduction is less invasive than standard plating and can be combined with external fixation to stabilize the condyles to the shaft. Injury of the cruciates in Type 5 injuries is related to the eminence fracture and may require late reconstruction. ***Locking plate technology has emerged as an excellent choice for internal fixation of proximal tibia fractures*** (Figs. 8-11 and 8-12).

4. Prognosis and complications—***Fracture-dislocation "involves some degree of long-term disability in almost all cases," as noted by Moore.*** Type 1 injuries have the best prognosis with rare neurovascular or ligamentous injuries. ***Type 5 injuries have the highest rate of vascular injury and have the worst prognosis.*** As noted by Moore, "patients with fracture-dislocations ultimately do better than those with classic dislocations, but not as well as those with plateau fractures."

C. Femoral-Sided Fractures—A rarer injury but seen in high-energy knee trauma and usually involving a direct blow to the knee, ***Femoral-sided***

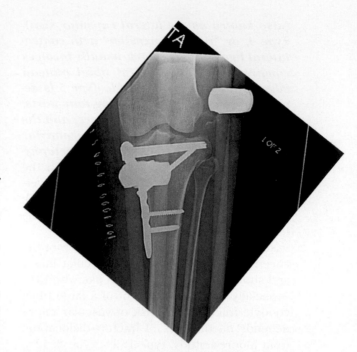

FIGURE 8-12 Postoperative radiograph after open reduction internal fixation (with a locking plate) of the medial tibial condyle fracture of the Type 2 fracture-dislocation shown in Figure 8-11. Additional spanning external fixation was required to adequately correct joint subluxation.

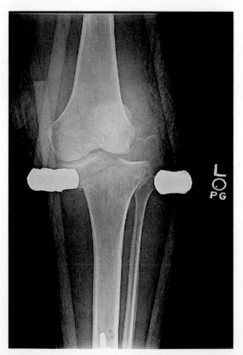

FIGURE 8-11 Preoperative radiograph revealing a Type 2 fracture-dislocation (medial tibial condyle fracture) with subluxation of the tibiofemoral joint.

fracture-dislocations involve a fracture of the femoral condyle at the level of Blumensaat's line with an associated ligamentous injury. These injuries can present with an open injury as well as disruption of the extensor mechanism. Diagnostic and treatment philosophies are similar to those of tibial-sided fracture-dislocations; management requires the recognition of an arterial injury, if present, and operative stabilization of the fractured femoral condyle and ligamentous repair. Internally fixing the fractured femoral condyle requires that the operative approach include intraarticular (buried) cannulated screws and ligamentous repair. PCL injury is frequently associated with this injury type. Locking plate technology is also available for the treatment of distal femur fracture-dislocations.

1. Femoral shaft fracture—KDs and knee ligamentous injury has been reported with ipsilateral femoral shaft fractures. One series reported five KDs associated with an ipsilateral femoral shaft fracture. The mechanism of injury is one of high-energy trauma. Treatment involves fixation of the femoral shaft fracture, evaluation of knee ligament stability, and addressing the ligamentous injury.

IV. Proximal Tibiofibular Dislocations

A. Introduction—Proximal tibiofibular dislocations are rare and frequently missed. Treatment is usually simple if recognized early. Dislocations can be acute or chronic in nature. Dislocation of the proximal tibiofibular joint has also been described as a Maisonneuve fracture equivalent.

B. Injury Pattern

1. Anatomy—The proximal tibiofibular joint is a synovial joint between the fibular head and the lateral tibial condyle. ***Ogden described two proximal tibiofibular joint types, oblique and horizontal, with 20° as the borderline between the two types.*** The horizontal joint type has more resistance to rotary forces. The tibiofibular joint capsule condenses anteriorly and posteriorly to create the proximal tibiofibular ligaments. Stability of the joint is rendered by the competence of the fibular collateral ligament (FCL). Other stabilizers of the joint include the biceps femoris tendon, popliteal tendon, arcuate ligament, fabellofibular ligament and popliteofibular ligament. Experimental models have shown dislocations to occur when the knee is flexed greater than 80°, relaxed FCL and when the FCL is sectioned.

2. Classification—Ogden described four types of dislocations. Type I is a subluxation which results in increased anteroposterior motion of the fibular head within the joint. This is most commonly seen in young children and adolescents and resolves with time. Type II is an anterolateral dislocation. This is the most common type (accounts for 85% of these dislocations) and is commonly seen in the sports population (Figs. 8-13 and 8-14). The mechanism of injury is knee flexion, external rotation of the leg, coupled with plantar flexion and internal rotation of the foot. Type III dislocations result from a direct blow to the fibular head with posteromedial dislocation. Type IV is a superior dislocation often the result of high-energy trauma.

3. Diagnosis—Diagnosis of proximal tibiofibular dislocations is a clinical and radiographic diagnosis. A high index of suspicion is necessary. AP and lateral radiographs of the knee are often sufficient, but comparison view of the contralateral knee may be needed. CT scan also may be necessary to make the diagnosis.

4. Treatment—Most dislocations can be treated with closed reduction. The knee is usually

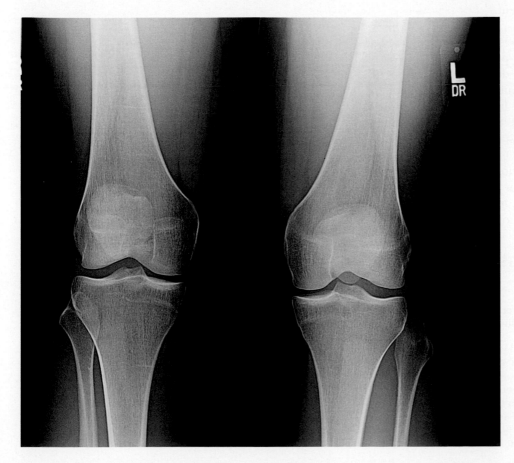

FIGURE 8-13 AP radiograph of a collegiate softball player with left knee Type II anterolateral proximal tibiofibular dislocation. Note the widening of the proximal tibiofibular joint on the left compared to the right.

A

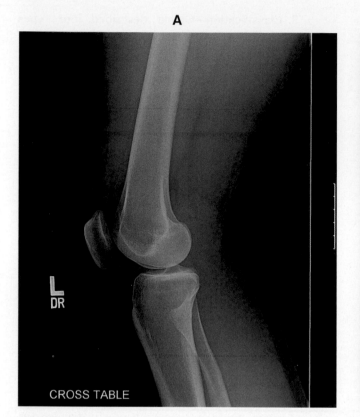

B

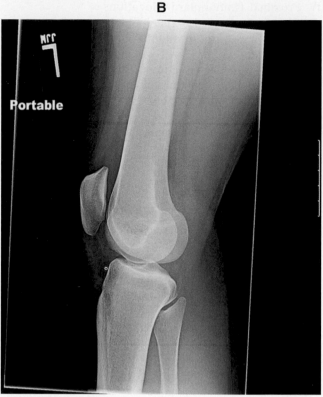

FIGURE 8-14 **A.** Prereduction lateral radiograph of the left knee from the athlete in Figure 8-13. Note the anterior displacement of the proximal tibiofibular joint. **B.** After closed reduction of the proximal tibiofibular joint with reestablished anatomic alignment.

placed in a flexed position, and direct reduction of the fibula is performed depending on the direction of the dislocation. Superior dislocations (rare) require manipulation of the fibula, pushing the fibular head in a distal direction to reduce the joint. The reduced tibiofibular joint is stable and rarely requires surgical treatment. Open reduction with temporary internal fixation is indicated for failed closed reduction. For chronic cases or those with peroneal nerve, irritation resection of the proximal fibula is recommended.

SUGGESTED READINGS

Classic Articles

Bunt TJ, Malone JM, Moody M, et al. Frequency of vascular injury with blunt trauma-induced extremity injury. *Am J Surg.* 1990; 160:226–228.

DeBackey M, Simeone F. Battle injuries of the arteries in World War II: An analysis of 2,471 cases. *Ann Surg.* 1946;123:534–579.

Dennis JW, Jagger C, Butcher JL, et al. Reassessing the role of arteriograms in the management of posterior knee dislocations. *J Trauma.* 1993;35(5):692–695.

Fanelli GC, Edson CJ. Arthroscopically assisted combined anterior and posterior cruciate ligament reconstruction in the multiple ligament injured knee: 2 to 10 year follow-up. *Arthoscopy.* 2002;18(7):703–714.

Frassica FS, Franklin HS, Staeheli JW, et al. Dislocation of the Knee. *Clin orthop.* 1992;263:200–205.

Green NE, Allen BL. Vascular injuries associated with dislocation of the knee. *J Bone Joint Surg Am.* 1977;59(2):236–239.

Harner CD, Waltrip RL, Bennett CH, et al. Surgical management of knee dislocations. *J Bone Joint Surg.* 2004; 86-A(3): 262–273

Hughston JC, Bowden JA, Andrews JR, et al. Acute tears of the posterior cruciate ligament. Results of operative treatment. *J Bone Joint Surg Am.* 1980;62(3):438–450.

Kennedy JC. Complete dislocation of the knee joint. *J Bone Joint Surg Am.* 1963;45:889–904.

Meyers MH, Harvey JP Jr. Traumatic dislocation of the knee joint. A study of eighteen cases. *J Bone Joint Surg Am.* 1971;53(1):16–29.

Mills WJ, Barei DP, McNair P. The value of the ankle-brachial index for diagnosing arterial injury after knee dislocation: A prospective study. *J Trauma.* 2004;56:1261–1265

Moore TM. Fracture-dislocation of the knee. *Clin Orthop Relat Res.* 1981;156:128–140.

Ogden JA. Subluxation and dislocation of the proximal tibiofibular joint. *J Bone Joint Surg Am.* 1974;56(1):145–154.

Sisto DJ, Warren RF. Complete knee dislocation. A follow-up study of operative treatment. *Clin Orthop Relat Res.* 1985;(198):94–101.

Taylor AR, Arden GP, Rainey HA. Traumatic dislocation of the knee. A report of forty-three cases with special reference to conservative treatment. *J Bone Joint Surg Br.* 1972;54(1):96–102.

Twaddle BC, Bidwell TA, Chapman JR. Knee dislocations: where are the lesions? A prospective evaluation of surgical findings in 63 cases. *J Orthop Trauma.* 2003;17(3):198–202.

Recent Articles

Burks RT, Schaffer JJ. A simplified approach to the tibial attachment of the posterior cruciate ligament. *Clin Orthop Relat Res.* 1990;(254):216–219.

Cooper DE, Speer KP, Wickiewicz TL, et al. Complete knee dislocation without posterior cruciate ligament disruption. A report of four cases and review of the literature. *Clin Orthop Relat Res.* 1992;(284):228–233.

Fanelli GC, Giannotti BF, Edson CJ. Arthroscopically assisted combined anterior and posterior cruciate ligament reconstruction. *Arthroscopy.* 1996;12(1):5–14.

Giannoudis PV. knee dislocation with ipsilateral femoral shaft fracture: a report of five cases. *J Orthop Trauma.* 2005;19(3): 205–210.

Horan J, Quin G. Proximal tibiofibular dislocation. *Emerg Med J.* 2006;23:e33.

Kendall RW, Taylor DC, Salvian AJ, et al. The role of arteriography in assessing vascular injuries associated with dislocations of the knee. *J Trauma.* 1993;35(6):875–878.

Krackow KA, Thomas SC, Jones LC. A new stitch for ligament-tendon fixation. Brief note. *J Bone Joint Surg Am.* 1986;68(5):764–746.

Laing AJ, Lenehan B, Ali A, et al. Isolated dislocation of the proximal tibiofibular joint in a long jumper. *Br J Sports Med.* 2003;37:366–367.

Laprade RF, Johansen S, Wentorf FA, et al. An Analysis of an anatomical posterolateral knee reconstruction: an in vitro biomechanical study and development of a surgical technique. *Am J Sports Med.* 2004;32:1405–1414.

Mandelbaum BR, Myerson MS, Forster R. Achilles tendon ruptures. A new method of repair, early range of motion, and functional rehabilitation. *Am J Sports Med.* 1995;23(4):392–395.

Muscat JO, Rogers W, Cruz AB, et al. Arterial injuries in orthopaedics: the posteromedial approach for vascular control about the knee. *J Orthop Trauma.* 1996;10(7):476–480.

Niall DM, Nutton RW, Keating JF. Palsy of the common peroneal nerve after traumatic dislocation of the knee. *JBJS (Br).* 2005;87-B(5):664–667.

Nonweiler DE, Schenck RC Jr, DeLee JC. The incomplete bicruciate knee injury. A report of two cases. *Orthop Rev.* 1993;22(11):1249–1252.

Patterson BM, Agel J, Swiontkowski MF, et al. Knee dislocations with vascular injury: Outcomes in the the Lower Extremity Assessment Project (LEAP) Study. *Am J Trauma.* 2007;63(4):855–858.

Reddy PK, Posteraro RH, Schenck RC Jr. The role of MRI in evaluation of the cruciate ligaments in knee dislocations. *Orthopedics.* 1996;19(2):166–170.

Robertson, A, Nutton RW, Keating JF. Dislocation of the knee. *J Bone and Joint Surg Br.* 2006;88-B:706–711.

Robinson Y, Reinke M, Heyde CE, et al. Traumatic proximal tibiofibular joint dislocation treated by open reduction and temporary fixation: a case report. *Knee Surg Sports Traumatol Arthosc.* 2007;15:199–201.

Schenck R, Burke R, Walker D. The dislocated knee: a new classification system. *South Med J.* 1992;85(9):3S–61S.

Schenck RC Jr, Kovach IS, Agarwal A, et al. Cruciate injury patterns in knee hyperextension: a cadaveric model. *Arthroscopy.* 1999;15(5):489–495.

Schenck RC Jr, McGanity PL, Heckman JD. Femoral-sided fracture-dislocation of the knee. *J Orthop Trauma.* 1997;11(6):416–421.

Schenck RC Jr, McGanity PL. Reattachment of avulsed cruciate ligaments: report of a technique. *Orthop Trans.* 1992;16:77.

Shelbourne KD, Porter DA, Clingman JA, et al. Low-velocity knee dislocation. *Orthop Rev.* 1991;20(11):995–1004.

Simonian PT, Wickiewicz TL, Hotchkiss RN, et al. Chronic knee dislocation: reduction, reconstruction, and application of a skeletally fixed knee hinge. A report of two cases. *Am J Sports Med.* 1998;26(4):591–596.

Stannard JP, Brown SL, Farris RC, et al. The posterolateral corner of the knee: repair versus reconstruction. *Am J Sports Med.* 2005;33(6): 881–888.

Tzurbakis M, Diamantopoulos A, Xenakis T, et al. Surgical treatment of multiple knee ligament injuries in 44 patients: 2–8 years follow-up results. *Knee Surg Sports Traumatol Arthrosc.* 2006;14:739–749.

Van Seymortier P, Ryckaert A, Verdonk P, et al. Traumatic proximal tibiofibular dislocation. *Am J Sports Med.* 2008;36(4): 793–798.

Walker D, Hardison R, Schenck R. A baker's dozen of knee dislocations. *Am J Knee Surg.* 1994;7(3):117–124.

Wascher DC, Becker JR, Dexter JG, et al. Reconstruction of the anterior and posterior cruciate ligaments after knee dislocation. Results using fresh-frozen nonirradiated allografts. *Am J Sports Med.* 1999;27(2):189–196.

Wascher DC, Dvirnak PC, DeCoster TA. Knee dislocation: initial assessment and implications for treatment. *J Orthop Trauma.* 1997;11(7):525–529.

Wong CH, Tan JL, Chang HC, et al. Knee dislocations-a retrospective study comparing operative versus closed immobilization treatment outcomes. *Knee Surg Sports Traumatol Arthrosc.* 2004;12(6):540–544.

Review Articles

Harner CD, Höher J. Evaluation and treatment of posterior cruciate ligament injuries. *Am J Sports Med.* 1998;26(3):471–482.

Schenck RC Jr. The dislocated knee. *Instr Course Lect.* 1994;43:127–136.

CHAPTER 9

Extensor Mechanism Injuries of the Knee

Luke S. Choi, Peter W. Ross, and Mark D. Miller

I. Patellar Fracture
  A. Anatomy—The patella is the largest sesamoid bone in the body. Its subcutaneous location leaves it susceptible to injury from direct blows (e.g., falls, dashboard injuries). Three-fourths of the patella's proximal posterior surface is covered with some of the thickest articular cartilage found in the human body. Its articular surface is divided by a longitudinal ridge separating it into medial and lateral facets. The bulk of the quadriceps tendon inserts directly into the proximal pole. Longitudinal extensions of the quadriceps tendon pass medial and lateral to the patella and insert directly on the anterior tibia. A thin layer of the fibers pass anterior to the patella and becomes confluent with the patellar tendon. Deep, transversely oriented fibers pass from the femoral epicondyles to the patella, making up the **patellofemoral ligaments**.
  B. Biomechanics—The extensor apparatus consists of the quadriceps muscle and tendon, the patella, and the patellar tendon. Secondary extensors of the knee include the iliotibial tract and the medial and lateral patellar retinacula. **The patella functions to improve the lever arm of the extensor mechanism**. Its contribution increases toward extension, increasing the force by nearly 30% at maximal extension. Through the patella, the quadriceps exerts an anteriorly directed translational force on the tibia that is exposed to complex loading consisting of tensile, bending, and compressive forces. The magnitudes of these forces vary with the degree of flexion, with **maximal tensile forces occurring at 45° to 60° of flexion**. Joint contact forces of 3.3-times body weight occur during stair climbing and up to 7.6-times body weight occurring during squatting. The size of the patellofemoral contact area is 2 to 4 cm^2, or 13% to 38% of the articular surface, and is oriented in a transverse band through most of the range of motion.

  C. Classification—Patellar fractures are most commonly classified based on the morphology of the fracture (Fig. 9-1). The most common mechanisms of injury consist of direct blows to the patella (e.g., dashboard injury), indirect trauma (e.g., sudden, rapid flexion of the knee against a maximally contracted quadriceps), or a combination thereof. **Direct trauma typically results in minimally displaced comminuted fractures, whereas indirect trauma usually results in displaced transverse fractures**. Osteochondral injuries that can occur with patellar dislocations usually involve the medial patellar facet. They are caused by impaction of the facet with the lateral ridge of the lateral femoral condyle, sometimes avulsing an osteochondral fragment from the lateral condylar ridge as well. A small, sometimes radiographically benign-appearing distal

Undisplaced   Transverse   Lower or upper pole   Multifragmented undisplaced

Multifragmented displaced   Vertical   Osteochondral

FIGURE 9-1 Classification of patellar fractures. (From Bedi A, Karunakar MA. Patella fractures and extensor mechanism injuries. In: Bucholz RW, Court-Brown CM, Heckman JD, et al, eds. *Rockwood and Green's Fractures in Adults*. 7th ed. Philadelphia, PA: Lippincott Williams & Wilkins, 2010, with permission.)

pole fragment, which can include a significant piece of articular cartilage, is termed a ***sleeve fracture***; it occurs in the skeletally immature patient.

D. Evaluation

1. History—A direct blow to the anterior knee or forced and rapid knee flexion against a contracted quadriceps, anterior knee pain, and an inability to forcibly extend the knee suggest the diagnosis.

2. Examination—Patients should be examined for an extensor lag or a palpable defect suggesting disruption of the extensor mechanism. The anterior knee soft tissues should be inspected, since they are frequently compromised after direct trauma. The knee and lower extremity should also be examined for any associated injury suggested by the mechanism of injury.

3. Imaging—The patella can be difficult to discern on anteroposterior (AP) radiographs. However, it is well visualized on lateral radiographs, and articular step-off and diastasis can be assessed. Tangential views can be useful for evaluating marginal or the rare vertical fracture. Bilateral films are useful when a bipartite (accessory ossification center) patella is suspected, since these rarely occur unilaterally (Fig. 9-2). Computed tomography (CT) is usually unnecessary. Magnetic resonance imaging (MRI) may be used to diagnose sleeve fractures. Bone scintigraphy may be useful for diagnosing occult fractures.

E. Treatment—Despite largely favorable results of both conservative and operative management of patellar fractures, some loss of knee flexion usually occurs; ***an increase of up to 40% in patellofemoral arthrosis may also occur***.

1. Nonoperative treatment—Nonoperative treatment is indicated for nondisplaced fractures, which are defined as less than 2 mm of step-off and less than 3mm of diastasis without an extensor lag. Treatment consists of a long leg cylinder cast, weightbearing as tolerated for 4 to 6 weeks, and then careful progressive range of motion with subsequent quadriceps

strengthening. Almost 90% of patients heal with normal or slightly impaired function.

2. Operative treatment—Operative treatment is indicated for displaced fractures with loss of extensor function. The goals of surgery should be preservation of patellar function and anatomic reduction of the articular surface. A longitudinal midline incision is recommended, as it is useful for other knee procedures in case they become necessary. A defect in the medial and lateral retinaculum is usually noted during exposure of the fracture, and it should be repaired with the fracture. The reduction should not be based on the anterior patellar cortex because significant plastic deformation can occur from the injury. Instead, the reduction of the articular surface can be inspected through a medial parapatellar mini-arthrotomy or with arthroscopic assistance. Additional injury to compromised soft tissues should be reduced by avoiding compressive dressings and prolonged contact with ice. Consideration should be given to aspiration of anterior hematomas if the skin is tense and surgery will be delayed. Several options for fixation are available (Fig. 9-3).

• Modified tension band wiring—Popularized by the AO/ASIF group, modified tension band wiring is indicated for distracted, transverse, and some comminuted fractures. It consists of provisional fixation of the fracture with two 2.0-mm Kirschner wires, followed by augmentation with an 18G wire passed around the Kirschner wires and across the anterior aspect of the patella to serve as the tension band component of the construct. The wire can be placed in a "figure-eight" or a circular fashion. The anterior tension wire then converts the distractive force across the anterior patella into compressive force on the articular side of the patella. This technique requires early motion to work properly. ***The most common technical error occurs when the tension wire is not brought into direct contact with the patellar poles.***

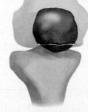 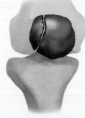 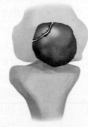

Lateral   Medial

Type I   Type II   Type III

FIGURE 9-2 Saupe's classification of accessory ossification centers of the patella. *Type 1*, inferior pole, 5%; T*ype II,* lateral margin, 20%; *Type III,* superolateral pole, 75%.

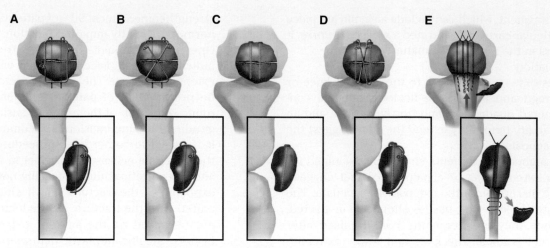

FIGURE 9-3 Techniques of patellar fracture fixation. **A.** Modified tension band wiring using a circular configuration. **B.** Modified tension band wiring using a figure-eight configuration. **C.** Lag-screw fixation. **D.** Combination cannulated lag screw and tension band wiring. **E.** Partial patellectomy. Note: The tendon is reapproximated at the level of the articular surface of the patella.

The intervening soft tissues gives way with loading, allowing the fracture to distract.

- Lag-screw fixation—Lag-screw fixation can be used to stabilize fragments in comminuted patellar fractures, thereby creating a fracture amenable to tension band wiring. It can be used as an alternative to tension band wiring, with comparable stability reported. There must be good quality bone for this technique to be used alone. There is concern that lag-screw fixation alone may be less able to withstand bending forces.

- Combination lag-screw fixation and tension band wiring—More recently, a technique combining cannulated lag-screw fixation and tension band wiring has been described. The fracture is initially stabilized with two 4.0- or 4.5-mm cannulated lag screws. An 18G wire is then passed through the center of the screw and across the anterior patella to act as a tension band. This technique results in a construct with a greater load to failure compared with either lag-screw fixation or tension band wiring alone.

- Partial patellectomy—Partial patellectomy is reserved for fragments not amenable to internal fixation. It usually consists of a comminuted distal pole and an intact proximal pole. The irreparable fragments can be resected, and the patellar tendon repaired with sutures through bony tunnels to the proximal fragment. *The tendon should be repaired close to the articular surface to minimize articular step-off and prevent patellar tilt in the sagittal plane.* A load-sharing wire passed through the patella and the tibial tubercle can be used to protect the repair. Problems with this technique include patella baja, altered patellar mechanics, weakened quadriceps, and decreased patient satisfaction rates.

- Total patellectomy—Total patellectomy may be the only alternative in severely comminuted displaced patellar fractures without any significant remaining articular fragments. The remaining defect can be repaired with a purse-string, vertical, or transverse closure. In addition, the repair may be reinforced with a quadriceps flap (Fig. 9-4). Loss of range of motion, extensor lag, quadriceps weakness, and discomfort after patellectomy are common.

F. Postoperative Management—Postoperative management includes initial immobilization and immediate weightbearing as tolerated. There is evidence that tensile forces across the patella are greater during attempts at nonweightbearing ambulation as the patient tries to keep the leg off the ground. Emphasis is placed on early range of motion (as the quality of fixation allows). Early range of motion is an essential principle in tension band fixation and is important in decreasing postoperative stiffness. The repair can be protected with the use of a locked hinge knee brace in which the amount of flexion is increased every 2 weeks (as the patient tolerates and as range of motion and quadriceps strength return).

G. Complications

1. Infection—Infection is rare. The risk may be increased by injury-compromised soft tissues and host factors.

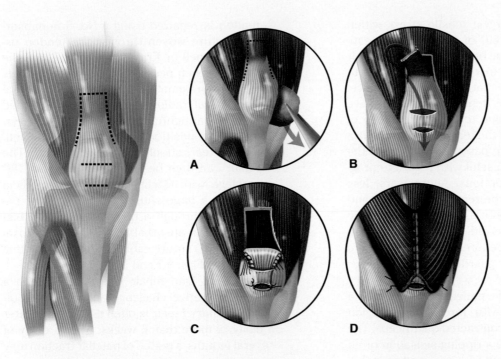

FIGURE 9-4 Miyakawa technique of patellectomy. **A.** Excision of the patella and outline of the incision in the quadriceps. **B.** Partial-thickness flap of the quadriceps tendon turned distally. **C.** Quadriceps flap passed through incisions in the area previously occupied by the patella. **D.** Proximal reconstruction with the vastus medialis obliquus and the vastus lateralis brought together over the quadriceps flap.

2. Loss of fixation—Loss of fixation may be secondary to underestimated fragment comminution most commonly involving the distal pole. If caught early, it can be treated with immobilization. If significant displacement occurs, partial patellectomy may be the best option.

3. Loss of range of motion—Slight loss of range of motion is common. The incidence can be reduced with secure internal fixation allowing early range of motion (within 1 or 2 weeks).

4. Posttraumatic arthrosis—Posttraumatic arthrosis is relatively common. One long-term study demonstrated a 70% incidence of arthrosis in patellar fracture compared with a 31% incidence in the contralateral, noninjured knee.

5. Nonunion—Nonunion was common when all patellar fractures were treated nonoperatively (up to 55%). With modern operative techniques, the nonunion rate is reported to be 1% or less.

6. Symptomatic Hardware—Symptomatic hardware is common secondary to the subcutaneous location of the patella.

II. Patellar Tendon Rupture

A. Overview—Patellar tendon rupture is an uncommon injury and in contrast to quadriceps tendon rupture, typically ***occurs in younger patients (younger than age 40)***. Thought to be the result of recurrent microtrauma and chronic tendon degeneration, patellar tendon rupture is associated with jumping sports (e.g., basketball), hence the term jumper's knee. In face, in one large study, 97% of biopsy specimens from ruptured patellar tendons demonstrated degenerative changes such as mucoid degeneration and calcific tendinopathy. Most commonly, ruptures occur at the proximal insertion of the patellar tendon. Most often, they are unilateral but can occur bilaterally, especially in patients with impaired collagen strength (e.g., rheumatoid arthritis, systemic lupus erythematosus, diabetes mellitus, and chronic renal failure) and patients on systemic corticosteroid therapy. They also occur after local steroid infiltration. Another common mechanism for patellar tendon rupture may be direct trauma. In one study of 35 patellar tendon ruptures, 27 occurred in motorcycle accidents. Finally, patellar tendon rupture can occur as a complication of total knee arthroplasty, patellar tendon harvest for ligament reconstruction, and devascularization after lateral retinacular release procedures.

B. Anatomy—The patellar tendon is approximately 4 mm thick at the midsubstance and 5 to 6 mm thick as its insertion on the tibial tubercle. It narrows slightly from proximal to distal. The distal expansions of the vastus medialis and vastus lateralis form the medial and lateral retinacula, respectively. Some 70% to 80% of the dry weight of the patellar tendon is collagen, of which 90% is Type I and approximately 10% is Type III. The blood supply originates from the medial and lateral geniculate arteries and the recurrent tibial artery, which branches through the fat pad and retinaculum to enter the tendon at its proximal and middle portion. The proximal and distal insertions, being relatively avascular, are also the most common sites of rupture.

C. Biomechanics—The largest tensile stress within the tendon occurs at 60° of flexion and is estimated to be 3.2 times the body weight during stair climbing. Strain at the insertion sites is three to four times greater than that at the midsubstance.

D. Classification—Patellar tendon ruptures have been classified according to the morphology of the tear, the location of the tear, and temporal factors. One classification, based on the age of the tears, was found to be useful with regard to prognosis and treatment options. Acute tears, less than 2 weeks old, can be repaired primarily and have an excellent prognosis. In contrast, chronic tears, more than 2 weeks old, tend to require more extensive surgical procedures for repair and are associated with a more guarded prognosis.

E. Evaluation
   1. History—Acutely, the patient usually gives a history consistent with forced knee flexion against a maximally contracted quadriceps. The patient may describe a ripping sensation or an audible pop associated with pain and an inability to immediately bear weight. Chronically, the patient may complain of weakness, instability, and an inability to fully extend the leg.
   2. Examination—Acutely, a hemarthrosis, a palpable defect, patella alta, and either a partial or a complete active extension loss may be found. Chronically, the defect may be filled with organized reparative tissue; in addition, the patient may have significant quadriceps atrophy and a gait abnormality characterized by forward flinging of the affected leg during the swing phase.
   3. Imaging—Plain radiographs are helpful, with the lateral view being most diagnostic because it can demonstrate patella alta (Fig. 9-5). The use of ultrasonography in the diagnosis of chronic tears of tendinitis has been described, but is operator dependent. MRI may be useful when another intraarticular injury is suspected or if the diagnosis is in question.

F. Treatment and Treatment Rationale—The treatment of patellar tendon rupture is surgical. Nonoperative treatment cannot restore complete extensor function.
   1. Acute repair—Acute repair is most desirable because the tendon can usually be repaired primarily. This treatment is associated with the best restoration of function and overall outcome.
      • Surgical technique—A midline longitudinal skin incision is used for the surgical approach and is extended to fully expose the rupture and either the patella or tibial tubercle depending on the site of rupture. The dissection is carried medially and laterally to expose the retinacular tears. The

tendon is repaired using a No. 5 nonabsorable suture woven through the tendon using a Bunnell or Krakow technique, and the suture is then passed through bone tunnels at the approximate site (Fig. 9-6). Intraoperative lateral radiographs are recommended before final tightening of the sutures to verify proper position of the patella. The retinacular tears should be repaired as well. The repair can then be reinforced using an 18G cerclage wire (McLaughlin wire), umbilical tape, or a large suture proximal to the patella and through a bone hole in the tibial tubercle. An absorbable, braided polydioxanone (PDS) suture cable is preferred for this purpose (Figs. 9-7 and 9-8).
   2. Late repair—Late repair is associated with a greater operative challenge and a worse outcome. Primary repair is often not possible after a delay of more than 6 weeks. After a delay of several months, a period of patellar traction may be needed to combat a chronic quadriceps contraction. With time, degenerative changes may occur within the patellofemoral articulation, and the ruptured tendon becomes contracted and bound in scar. Reconstructive choices include primary repair with hamstring or fascial lata autograft augmentation or in salvage cases, extensor mechanism allografts (Fig. 9-8 and 9-9).

G. Postoperative Management—Postoperative management includes immediate gentle passive range of motion followed by gentle active flexion at 2 weeks after surgery and active extension at 3 weeks. Initial toe-touch, protected weightbearing progresses to full weightbearing by 6 weeks. During this time, the repair is protected in a hinged knee brace, which is progressively opened as range of motion returns. Unrestricted activity is allowed after 4 to 6 months, when complete healing has occurred and quadriceps strength is within 90% of the unaffected extremity.

H. Complications—Knee stiffness and quadriceps weakness are the most common complications after patellar tendon repair. They can be combated with a well-supervised rehabilitation program emphasizing range of motion and quadriceps strengthening. Other complications include persistent hemarthrosis, rerupture, and patella baja.

III. Quadriceps Tendon Rupture
A. Overview—Quadriceps rupture, as opposed to patellar tendon rupture, *typically occurs in older patients, over 40 years old (average 47 years)*, and is typically associated with preexisting tendinopathy. This condition results from repetitive microtrauma associated with jumping sports (e.g.,

A

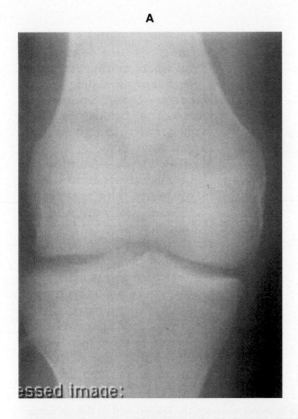

B

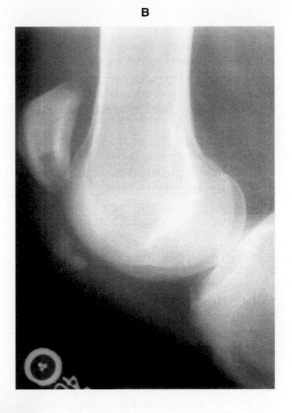

C

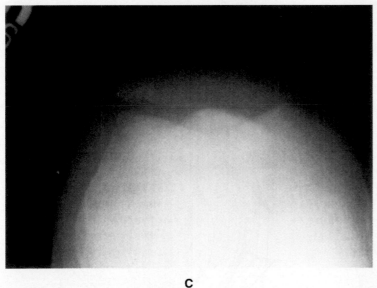

FIGURE 9-5   **A** and **B.** AP and lateral radiographs demonstrating a high-riding patella consistent with a patellar tendon rupture. Note the distal pole avulsion fragment. **C.** Sunrise view of the same knee. Note the absence of the patella in the trochlear groove.

basketball). The level of the tear is also associated with age. In one study, rupture at the tendon-bone junction occurred in 75% of patients over the age of 40, whereas midsubstance tears occurred in 71% of patients younger than 40 years. Bilateral ruptures have been reported in association with anabolic steroid use and chronic metabolic disorders such as diabetes mellitus, inflammatory arthropathies, and chronic renal failure.

B. Anatomy—The quadriceps tendon is a layered structure formed by the convergence of the quadriceps aponeurosis. The rectus femoris tendon broadens distally to insert on the proximal pole of the patella and forms the most superficial layer of the tendon. In addition, a layer extends anterior to the patella to become contiguous with the patellar tendon. The aponeuroses of the vastus lateralis and vastus medialis insert into the superolateral border and superomedial border of the patella, respectively, forming the middle layer of the tendon. The vastus intermedius aponeurosis merges with the deep surface

A   **B**

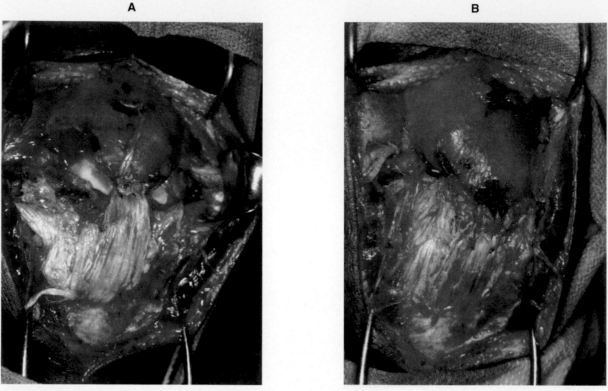

FIGURE 9-6 Patellar tendon repair. **A.** A midline longitudinal incision exposes the frayed end of the proximal patellar tendon stump and the medial and lateral retinacular tears. **B.** The tendon has been reapproximated to the distal pole of the patella using a large, nonabsorbable suture through bone tunnels in the patella.

A   **B**

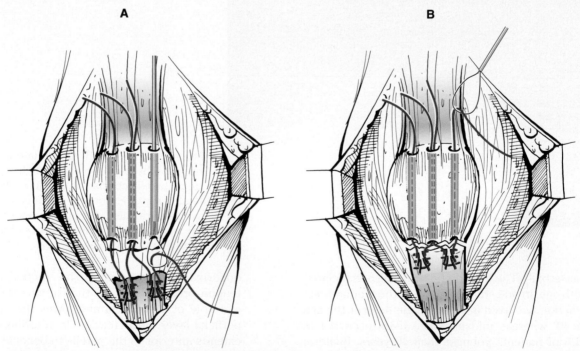

FIGURE 9-7 Suture technique of patellar tendon repair. **A.** A suture passer is used to guide the core sutures through the drill holes. **B.** The suture is retrieved and tied at the superior margin of the patella. (From Bedi A, Karunakar MA. Patella fractures and extensor mechanism injuries. In: Bucholz RW, Court-Brown CM, Heckman, JD, et al, eds. *Rockwood and Green's Fractures in Adults*. 7th ed. Philadelphia, PA: Lippincott Williams & Wilkins, 2010, with permission.)

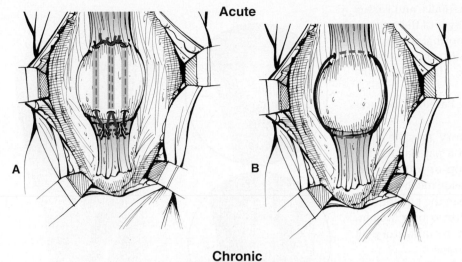

Acute

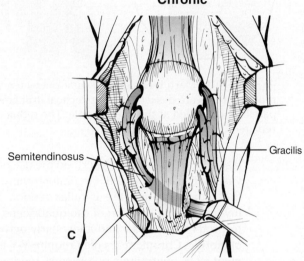

Chronic

Semitendinosus — Gracilis

FIGURE 9-8 Patella tendon repair. **A.** Direct repair to the inferior pole of the patella through three parallel drill holes. **B.** Addition of a cerclage wire for protection of the tendon repair. **C.** Chronic rupture reconstructed using semitendinosus-gracilis graft.

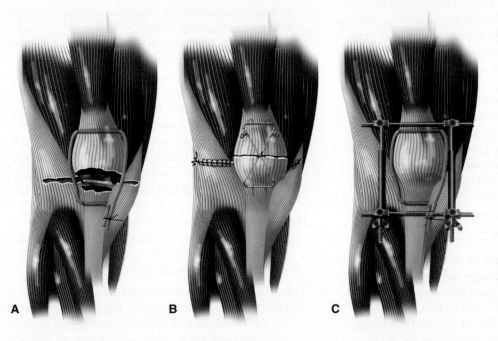

FIGURE 9-9 A. Neglected rupture reconstructed with a semitendinosus-gracilis autograft woven through the patella and the tibial tubercle. **B.** Use of a patellar tendon allograft, with attached patellar and tibial bone blocks, for end-to-end repair of a chronic rupure with inadequate local tissue. **C.** Use of an external fixator made of two Steinmann pins and a Charnley clamp connecting the patella and tibial tubercle. This may be added to prevent proximal patellar migration while protecting the reconstruction of a neglected rupture.

of the rectus femoris, vastus medialis, and vastus lateralis, forming the deepest layer of the tendon. The layered appearance of a normal quadriceps tendon can be delineated on MRI; approximately 10% have four layers, 60% have 3 layers; and 30% have 2 layers.

C. Biomechanics—See section on Patellar Fracture.

D. Evaluation

1. History—The patient's history may be similar to that of a patient with a patellar tendon rupture: a sensation of a pop or a tear when applying stress to the extensor mechanism of the knee. With a complete tear, the patient may report an immediate inability to bear weight. Rupture may be preceded by a history of chronic inflammatory symptoms.

2. Examination—Acutely, quadriceps tendon rupture presents with generalized swelling about the knee and tenderness on palpation at the proximal pole of the patella. Flexing the knee demonstrates (asymmetric) patella baja because the patellar tendon is intact. The patient is unable to maintain knee extension against gravity. A massive hematoma and preservation of knee extension through an intact extensor (patella) retinaculum may obscure the clinical diagnosis.

3. Imaging—In complete ruptures, plain radiographs demonstrate distal displacement of the patella. Tendon calcification, proximal patellar enesthesiopathy, or elongation of the proximal pole is often present, suggesting chronic inflammation and tendon degenerations as the etiologic factors. Periosteal reaction on the anterior surface of the patella is the so-called **tooth sign** and also represents long standing inflammation. Bony avulsion fractures may also be present. MRI or ultrasonography may be helpful when the diagnosis is in question.

E. Treatment and Treatment Rationale—Like the treatment for patellar tendon rupture, the treatment for a complete quadriceps tendon rupture is operative to restore full, active extension and quadriceps function. Nonoperative treatment is reserved for partial tears and strains. Long-term results are often compromised by persistent pain from quadriceps tendinitis. Results can also be compromised by preexisting patellofemoral chondromalacia.

F. Surgical Technique—Repair usually involves suturing of the tendon back to the proximal patella with large, nonabsorbable sutures through bony tunnels (Fig. 9-10). *Care must be taken to repair the tendon close to the articular surface to prevent "snowplowing" of the patellar into the trochlear groove*. The repair may be augmented with biologic grafts such as a flap of rectus femoris aponeurosis, as in the Scuderi technique (Fig. 9-11), or

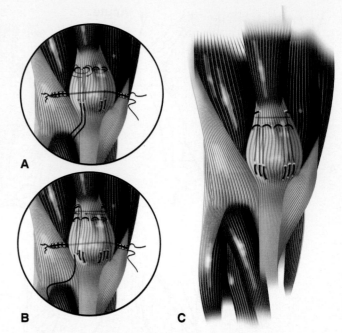

FIGURE 9-10 Marti technique for quadriceps tendon repair. Sutures are passed through vertical drill holes in the patella and are tied at the inferior pole. The retinaculum is repaired directly.

fascia lata. One author described the use of Dacron vascular grafts, passed circumferentially around the repair through the patellar tendon and the myocutaneous junction of the quadriceps tendon, to protect the repair and allow early active range of motion. Chronic tears may require V-Y advancement of a contracted quadriceps tendon with a partial-thickness turn-down aponeurotic flap to augment the repair (Codvilla tendon-lengthening technique). A delay in repair is associated with a less satisfactory outcome.

G. Postoperative Management—A cylinder cast or a locked brace is worn for 5 to 6 weeks. Non-weightbearing is continued for 3 weeks, after which weightbearing as tolerated is allowed in the cast. Afterward, the patient is placed in a hinged knee brace opened up to 50°. The brace is subsequently opened 10° to 15° weekly until 90° of motion and sufficient quadriceps strength are achieved for ambulation. An aggressive quadriceps-strengthening program is important for good functional recovery.

H. Complication—Complications include postoperative hemarthrosis, rerupture, persistent quadriceps atrophy (75%), quadriceps weakness (53%), and loss of knee range of motion.

IV. Tibial Tubercle Fracture (In Children)

A. Overview—Tibial tubercle fractures represent 1% to 3% of all physeal injuries. These injuries typically are seen most commonly in athletic

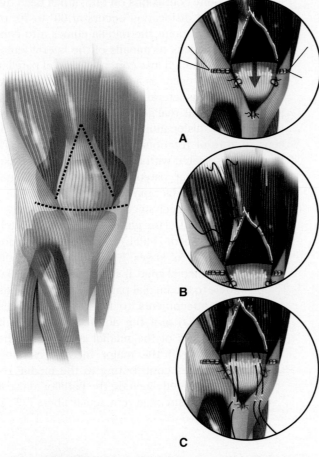

TABLE 9-1

Classification of Fibial Tubercle Avulsion Fractures According to Ogden

Type 1A	Fracture line leads through the ossification center of the tubercle without displacement
Type 1B	The fragment is displaced anteriorly and proximally
Type 2A	Fracture line leads through the junction of the ossification of the proximal end of the tibia and the tubercle
Type 2B	The tubercle fragment is comminuted
Type 3A	Fracture line extends to the joint and is associated with discontinuity of the joint surface
Type 3B	The tubercle fragment is comminuted

FIGURE 9-11 Scuderi technique for the repair of quadriceps tendon ruptures. **A.** A partial-thickness triangular flap of quadriceps tendon is turned down to reinforce the surgical repair. **B.** Bunnell pullout sutures and wires are placed on the medial and lateral portions of the tendon. **C.** Sutures and wires are pulled down and tied over padded buttons.

males from 14 to 16 years of age near skeletal maturity. The mechanism of injury typically involves a violent contraction of the quadriceps during extension, as in jumping. The injury may also occur with acute passive flexion of the knee against a contracting quadriceps, such as with landing after a jump or a fall. Predisposing factors include patella baja, tight hamstrings, pre-existing Osgood-Schlatter disease, and disorders with physeal anomalies.

B. Anatomy and Biomechanics—The tibial tubercle physis, which is continuous with the tibial plateau, is most vulnerable between the ages of 14 and 16 years when it closes from posterior to anterior. The ossification centre of the tibial tuberosity is connected to the metaphysis by fibrocartilage, which during skeletal maturation is gradually replaced by more fragile columnar cartilage, which is weak in resisting traction.

C. Classification—Description based on the displacement of the avulsed fragment of bone.

1. Watson-Jones classification—Type I: Small fragment is avulsed and displaced proximally. Type II: Secondary ossification center already coalesced with proximal tibial epiphysis; fracture is at this junction. Type III: Fracture line passes proximally through the tibial epiphysis and into the joint.

2. Ogden classification—Modification of the Watson-Jones classification (described above); subdivides each type into A and B categories to account for the degree of displacement and comminution (Table 9-1).

D. Evaluation—Patients typically present with a limited ability to extend the knee, as well as an extensor lag. Because the insertion of the medial retinaculum extends beyond the proximal tibial physis into the metaphysis, limited active extension of the knee is still possible after tibial tubercle fracture, although patella alta and extensor lag are present. Swelling and tenderness over the tibial tubercle are typically present, often with a palpable defect. Hemarthrosis is variable. Patella alta may be observed if severe displacement has occurred. Anteroposterior and lateral views of the knee are sufficient for the diagnosis; a slight internal rotation view best delineates the injury, as the tibial tubercle lies just lateral to the tibial axis.

E. Treatment and Treatment Rationale

1. Nonoperative treatment—Nonoperative treatment is indicated for Type IA fractures. Treatment consists of manual reduction followed by immobilization in a long-leg cast with the knee extended and patellar molding. The cast is continued for 4 to 6 weeks at which time the patient may be placed in a posterior splint for an additional 2 weeks. Gentle active range-of-motion exercises and quadriceps strengthening exercises are instituted and advanced as the symptoms decrease.

2. Operative treatment—Operative treatment is indicated for Type IB, II, and III fractures. A vertical midline approach is used to access the fractured tubercle, which may be addressed with smooth pins (more than 3 years from skeletal maturity), screws, threaded Steinmann pins, or tension bands. Cancellous screws placed horizontally through the tubercle into the metaphysis afford stable fixation. Some have recommended the use of 4.0-mm cancellous screws rather than larger implants, such as 6.5-mm screws, to lessen the incidence of bursitis that may develop over prominent screw heads. Washers may be helpful to prevent the screw head from sinking below the cortical surface. The patellar ligament and avulsed periosteum is also repaired. If severe comminution is present, a tension-holding suture may be necessary to secure the repair. Postoperatively, the patient is placed in a long-leg cast in extension with patellar molding for 4 to 6 weeks at which time the patient may be placed in a posterior splint for an additional 2 weeks. Gentle active range-of-motion exercises and quadriceps strengthening exercises are instituted and advanced as the symptoms decrease.

F. Complications

1. Genu recurvatum—This is secondary to premature closure of the anterior physis and is rare because the injury typically occurs in adolescent patients near skeletal maturity.

2. Knee stiffness—Loss of flexion may be related to scarring or postoperative immobilization. Loss of extension may be related to nonanatomic reduction and emphasizes the needs for operative fixation of Type IB, II, and III fractures.

3. Patella alta—This may occur if reduction is insufficient.

4. Osteonecrosis of fracture fragment—This is rare due to the soft-tissue attachments and the related blood supply.

5. Compartment syndrome—Although this is rare, it may occur with concomitant tearing of the anterior tibial recurrent vessels that retract into the anterior compartment when torn.

V. Patellar Dislocation

A. Overview—Patellar dislocation can occur during soccer, baseball, gymnastics, karate, track, and other sports. The mean age at injury is in the mid-20s and occurs in women slightly more often than in men. The mechanism of injury is a valgus load applied to a flexed, weightbearing, externally rotated knee, and the injury can occur with pivoting on a planted foot that results in a laterally dislocated patella. Based on physical examination under anesthesia and the

location of bony contusions on MRI, it has been hypothesized that dislocation occurs at 60° to 70° of flexion, at which point the patella comes into contact with the sulcus terminalis of the lateral femoral condyle. Although less common, medial patellar dislocation may occur as a postoperative complication (overzealous lateral release, medial reefing, or following a distal realignment procedure). Rarely, intraarticular dislocation associated with quadriceps rupture or rotational dislocation in the sagittal plane associated with degenerative joint disease (locking of patellar osteophytes on the proximal femoral articular ridge) may occur.

B. Anatomy and Biomechanics

1. Medial restraints of the patella—The medial patellofemoral ligament (MPFL) is a distinct structure in the majority of knees. Located in the second layer of the medial knee, it spans from the medial epicondyle to the medial patella (Fig. 9-12). It has additional attachments to the vastus medialis obliquus (VMO) and the adductor tubercle. It contributes 53% of the medial restraint to the patella, making it the major medial restraint. Other structures contributing to the medial restraint of the patella include the patellomeniscal ligament and associated retinacular fibers (22%).

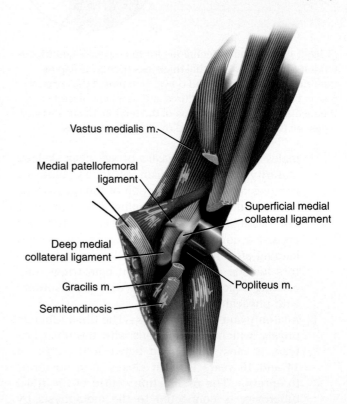

Vastus medialis m.

Medial patellofemoral ligament

Superficial medial collateral ligament

Deep medial collateral ligament

Gracilis m.

Popliteus m.

Semitendinosis

FIGURE 9-12 The first layer and the part of the second layer anterior to the superficial medial collateral ligament (MCL) are reflected forward to expose the underlying medial patellofemoral ligament (MPFL) and the underlying capsule. *VMO,* Vastus medialis obliquus.

C. Evaluation—Acutely, the patient may give a history similar to that of a rupture of the anterior cruciate ligament, reporting giving way, an audible pop, rapid swelling, and an initial inability to ambulate without assistance. If the knee is visualized immediately after injury, the patient may localize the dislocation to the medial aspect of the knee because they are misled by the prominence of the medial femoral condyle. Chronically, patients complain of various degrees of recurrent patellar subluxation and dislocation.

1. Examination—Acutely, approximately 80% of knees have an effusion, 40% have a positive apprehension sign with the knee flexed at 30°, and 70% have tenderness on palpation over the medial retinaculum, posterior medial soft tissues, and the adductor tubercle (Bassett's sign). Reflexive quadriceps inhibition and weakness may be caused by the acute hemarthrosis. Anatomic findings that may indicate a predisposition to patellar dislocation and instability include a Q angle greater than 20° (normal is 10° in men and 15° in women), genu valgus, patella alta, a shallow patellofemoral sulcus angle, VMO dysplasia, generalized ligamentous laxity, and pes planus. Other physical findings include an increased lateral patellar tilt and an increased ability to laterally displace the patella at 30° of knee flexion (as compared with the contralateral side). Medial mobility less than one quadrant indicates a tight lateral retinaculum and correlates with an abnormal passive patellar tilt test. Conversely, lateral mobility greater than three quadrants indicates insufficient medial restraints (Fig. 9-13).

2. Imaging
   • Plain films—AP, lateral, tunnel, and Merchant views should be obtained on the involved side. AP, lateral, and tunnel views are useful for ruling out fractures and evaluating for patella alta. Merchant views are useful for ruling out marginal fractures and evaluating lateral tilt and displacement and the femoral sulcus angle. Bilateral Merchant views are very useful for comparison. Several radiographic angles and ratios have been used to assess patellofemoral instability.

   (a) Patellofemoral sulcus angle—The Patellofemoral sulcus angle is measured on a Merchant view taken with the knee flexed 30° to 35°. Two lines are drawn along the slopes of the medial and lateral femoral condyles. An angle greater than 144° formed between the two lines is associated with patellar instability.

   (b) Congruence angle of Merchant—The congruence angle of Merchant is measured on a Merchant view taken as previously described, and the Patellofemoral Sulcus Angle is drawn as previously described. This angle is then bisected. A fourth line is then drawn from the apex of the patellofemoral sulcus angle through the lowest portion the medial ridge of the patella. If this last line falls medial to the bisector, the angle formed between the bisector and this line is expressed as negative degrees (it is expressed as positive degrees if it falls lateral to the bisector) (Fig. 9-14).

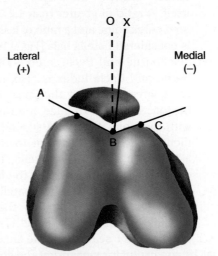

FIGURE 9-14 Congruence angle of Merchant. Line *BO* is the bisector of angle *ABC*. Line *BX* passes through the lowest point on the median ridge of the patella. Angle *OBX* is the congruence angle. If line *BX* falls to the medial side of line *BO*, the angle is expressed as negative degrees. If it falls to the lateral side of line *BO*, it is expressed as positive degrees.

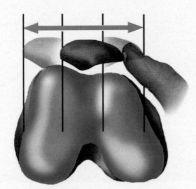

FIGURE 9-13 Assessment of patellar mobility medially and laterally. The patellofemoral joint can be divided into quadrants, and patellar mobility can be assessed in both directions.

A

B

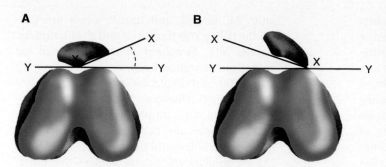

FIGURE 9-15 Measure of the lateral patellofemoral angle. Line *YY* is drawn across the most anterior portions of the femoral trochlea in the axial view of this left knee. Line *XX* follows the slope of the lateral patellar facet. **A.** Normal angle in which the angle opens laterally. **B.** Abnormal angle with the angle open medially.

A congruence angle of −6° to −8° is normal; greater than +16° is abnormal.

(c) Lateral patellofemoral angle—The lateral patellofemoral angle is also measured on a Merchant view. A line is drawn connecting the most anterior portions of the femoral condyles. A second line is drawn along the slope of the lateral patellar facet. Normally, the angle formed opens laterally. A neutral angle or one that opens medially is abnormal (Fig. 9-15).

(d) Blumensaat's line—With the knee flexed 30°, the distal pole of the patella should lie on a line extended from the roof of the intercondylar notch (Blumensaat's line) on the lateral radiograph. The location of the distal pole of the patella above and below this line is considered patella alta and baja, respectively.

(e) Insall-Salvati index—The Insall-Salvati index is measured on a lateral view at 30° of knee flexion. The index is the ratio of the patellar tendon length to the length of the patella itself. A ratio of greater than 1.2 is considered patella alta, and a ratio of less than 0.8 is considered patella baja (Fig. 9-16).

(f) Blackburne and Peele index—The Blackburne and Peele Index is also measured on a lateral view of the knee at 30° of flexion. A line is extended anteriorly level with the tibial plateau. A second perpendicular line is then drawn to the distal articular margin of the patella. The ratio of the length of this line to the length of the articular surface of the patella is normally 0.8. A ratio of greater than 1.0 is considered patella alta (Fig. 9-17).

• CT—Bilateral CT scans with the knees flexed at 10° are useful for measuring and comparing lateral patellar tilt. Three types of subluxation have been described (Fig. 9-18): Type I, lateral subluxation without patellar tilt; Type II, subluxation with lateral tilt; and Type III, lateral tilt without subluxation. In addition,

lateralization of the tibial tubercle can be evaluated with CT. Lateralization of the tibial tubercle greater than 9 mm has been closely associated with patellar malalignment.

• MRI—MRI may be useful for evaluating the integrity of the MPFL and for assessing associated chondral injuries. Proximal retraction of the VMO is consistent with disruption of the MPFL from the medial femoral epicondyle. In one study, the incidence of findings on MRI in the setting of acute patellar dislocation was as follows; effusion, 100% avulsion of the MPFL from the medial epicondyle, 87%; signal change in the VMO, 78%; lateral femoral condyle bone contusion, 87%; and medial patellar bone contusion, 30%.

D. Associated Injuries—Devastating osteochondral injuries can occur to the medial patellar facet or the lateral condylar ridge as the patella laterally

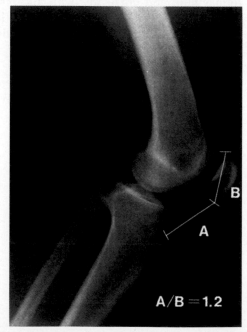

FIGURE 9-16 Lateral view of the knee with the Insall-Salvati index lines indicating a normal ratio (patellar tendon length to the patellar length of 1.2.

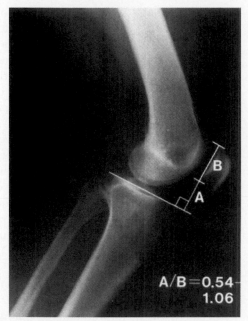

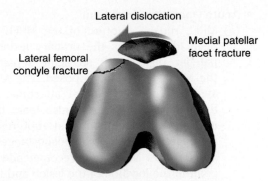

FIGURE 9-19   Osteochondral fracture of the lateral femoral condyle and medial patella in association with lateral patellar dislocation.

FIGURE 9-17   Lateral view of the knee with the Blackburne and Peele measurements indicating a normal ratio (height above the tibial plateau line *[A]* divided by the patellar articular surface length *[B]*).

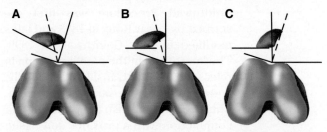

FIGURE 9-18   Three types of abnormal findings on axial CT scan as described by Fulkerson and associates. **A.** Type I, lateral subluxation without patellar tilt. **B.** Type II, subluxation with lateral tilt. **C.** Type III, lateral tilt without subluxation.

dislocates or relocates into the trochlear groove (Fig. 9-19). Osteochondral injuries involving either the patella or the lateral femoral condyle have been found in 68% of patients with acute patellar dislocations. The lateral condylar lesion is located just anterior to the sulcus terminalis. The patella contacts the sulcus terminalis at approximately 70° to 80° of flexion. Because of this, it has been suggested that patellar dislocation occurs in this 70° to 80° degree range of flexion. Attempts should be made to repair osteochondral injuries if feasible. Another injury associated with patellar dislocation is avulsion of the MPFL from the medial femoral epicondyle (94% in one study), which is discussed below.

E. Treatment and Treatment Rationale—Whether nonoperative or operative, early treatment is associated with better results. A poorer prognosis is associated with late presentation, inadequate prior treatment, bilateral injury, and female gender. Aspiration of a large hemarthrosis should be considered for pain relief, and evaluation for fat globules (suggesting occult osteochondral fracture) should be performed.
   1. Nonoperative treatment
      • Immobilization and rehabilitation—Immobilization and rehabilitation involves 6 weeks of strict immobilization in a cylinder cast or immobilizer, followed by aggressive physical therapy to regain motion and strength. Published data have reported a recurrent instability rate of greater than 40% with this protocol and 50% to 60% unsatisfactory results overall. Other reported problems include persistent muscular (quadriceps) atrophy, prolonged disability, and patellofemoral problems. There are also theoretical disadvantages to immobilization as a treatment in regards to ligament strength and cartilage integrity.
      • Functional treatment—Functional treatment involves early range of motion with patellar support bracing. Good results (66%), patient satisfaction rates (73%), and decreased rates of recurrent instability (26%) have been reported with this technique.
   2. Operative treatment—In general, the indications for operative intervention have been dislocation associated with fractures or loose osteochondral fragments as well as recurrent patellar subluxation or dislocation following nonoperative management. More recently, because of the high rate of recurrent instability with nonoperative management, there is now a trend towards acute operative intervention and repair of the primary pathologic lesion.

- Acute Operative Treatment
  - (a) MPFL repair—Rupture of the MPFL has been identified as the primary lesion in patellar dislocation, so acute repair of the MPFL has been proposed. The MPFL avulses from its femoral attachment in the majority of cases. It also tears from its patellar attachment and ruptures or attenuates within its midsubstance. A preoperative MR scan is recommended to confirm the location of the lesion and thus define the operative approach. A diagnostic arthroscopy is performed initially to document and address associated injuries and remove loose bodies. If the MPFL has been avulsed from its femoral insertion, an approach is made over the medial epicondyle, the distal margin of the VMO is elevated, and the proximal edge of the MPFL is identified and secured back to the medial epicondyle with suture anchors. Before and after the repair, patellar tracking may be evaluated arthroscopically via the superior medial portal. Initial reports of this procedure have been encouraging; there was no incidence of recurrent dislocation after 34 months of follow-up in one study.
- Operative treatment of chronic cases
  - (a) Proximal soft tissue procedures
    - Lateral retinacular release—The indications for lateral retinacular release include a patient with a tight lateral retinaculum (neutral or negative tilt) and minimal or no subluxation, whose symptomatic condition has failed to respond to conservative management. The procedure may also be performed in conjunction with realignment procedures for chronic subluxation or recurrent dislocation. A passive medial patellar tilt of 60° to 90° (the turn-up test) is the goal at the completion of the procedure (Fig. 9-20).

- Proximal "tube" realignment of the patella—A lateral release is performed initially. The vastus medialis is then freed and advanced laterally and distally and secured to the free edge of the lateral release. This creates a tube of tendon anterior and proximal to the patella.
- VMO advancement—Several techniques of VMO advancement have been described. The technique of Madigan involves the transfer of a division of the VMO laterally and suturing of the division to the patella and the quadriceps tendon. More commonly, a simple medial reefing of the VMO and medial retinaculum is combined with a lateral release (Fig. 9-21).
  - (b) Distal procedures—Considered reconstructive, distal procedures are associated with unpredictable changes in patellofemoral contact pressures and are associated with late degenerative changes. These procedures are not recommended in the presence of a normal Q angle (<15°).
    - Roulx-Goldthwait procedure—The Roux-Goldthwait Procedure was first described by Cesar Roux in 1888 and later modified by Joel Goldthwait in 1899. The lateral half of the patellar tendon is released distally, transferred medially, and secured at the sartorial insertion. This procedure is usually performed in conjunction with a proximal soft tissue procedure.
    - Hauser procedure—First described in 1938, the Hauser Procedure involves the direct medial transfer of the tibial tubercle. However, this results in posterior displacement of the tubercle as a result of the posterior medial slope of the proximal tibia. This is turn leads

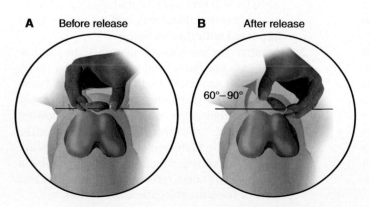

A Before release **B** After release

60°–90°

FIGURE 9-20 Turn-up test. At the completion of the lateral retinacular release, passive patellar tilt is performed to achieve a goal of 60° to 90° of medial tilt.

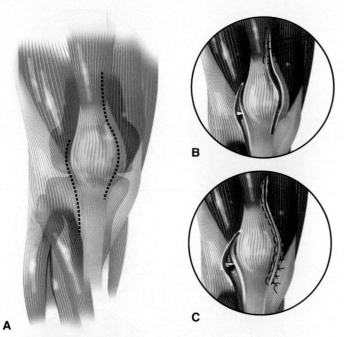

FIGURE 9-21 Proximal patellar realignment includes both a lateral release and medial reefing. **A.** Planned incisions. **B.** Procedure. **C.** Final result.

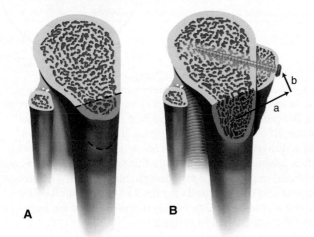

FIGURE 9-22 Transfer of the tibial tuberosity according to the Hauser technique. Because of the triangular shape of the proximal tibia, medial displacement *(a)* causes a posterior displacement *(b)* as well. This in turn decreases the lever arm of the patellar tendon and increases the compressive forces on the patellofemoral joint, predisposing it to degenerative changes.

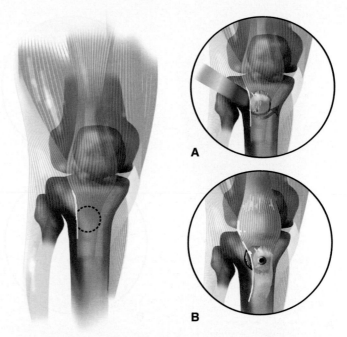

FIGURE 9-23 Elmslie-Trillat procedure. A lateral retinacular release is performed first. **A.** An osteotome is inserted in the retropatellar bursa from the lateral side and directed distally and medially. Care is taken to produce a 4- to 6-cm osteotomy and to preserve the integrity of the distal pedicle. **B.** The fragment is fixed with a single screw in the desired position. A medial plication may be added if sufficient stability is not restored after the distal transfer.

to increased patellofemoral contact forces and a predisposition to articular degeneration (Fig. 9-22).

- Elmslie-Trillat procedure—The Elmslie-Trillat Procedure is a modification of the Hauser Procedure. The tibial tubercle is left attached to a periosteal hinge distally and is rotated medially. The intact periosteal hinge limits the amount of posterior and distal displacement of the tibial tubercle (Fig. 9-23).
- Fulkerson procedure (anteromedial tibial tubercle transfer)—The Fulkerson Procedure is a modification of the Elmslie-Trillat Procedure. Using a long, oblique osteotomy, the surgeon medializes and anteriorly displaces the tibial tubercle, which corrects the Q angle and unloads the patellofemoral joint (Fig. 9-24).
- Hughston procedure—This is essentially an Elmslie-Trillant Procedure with a proximal realignment. The Hughston Procedure combines a lateral release, a distal tibial tubercle transfer, and a medial plication (Fig. 9-25).
- Galleazzi procedure—After a lateral release, the semitendinosus tendon is released proximally and then passed through the patella and sutured to itself. This technique is applicable in skeletally immature patients.

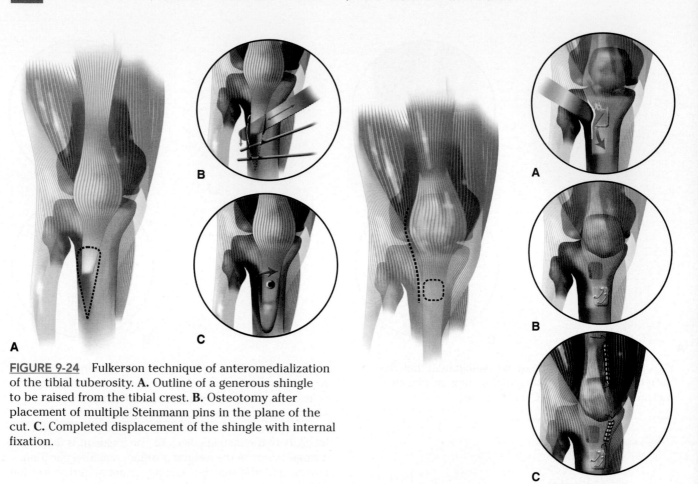

FIGURE 9-24 Fulkerson technique of anteromedialization of the tibial tuberosity. **A.** Outline of a generous shingle to be raised from the tibial crest. **B.** Osteotomy after placement of multiple Steinmann pins in the plane of the cut. **C.** Completed displacement of the shingle with internal fixation.

FIGURE 9-25 Hughston technique to realign the extensor apparatus. A lateral release is performed first. **A.** In knees with an increased Q angle, the tibial insertion of the patellar tendon is detached with a thin wafer of bone. **B.** Displacement in a distal and medial direction as required and fixed with a Stone stable. **C.** The VMO is then advanced in line with its fibers a few millimeters and sutured in place with nonabsorbable sutures. The smooth movement of the patella is checked every stitch or two, and if any abnormality is noted, the stitches are removed and the advancement redone.

(c) Patellectomy—A patellectomy is a last-resort salvage procedure. The results are described in the section on Patellar Fractures.

F. Complications—Complications from patellar dislocation undergoing nonoperative treatment include recurrent instability (40%), loss of knee range of motion, and symptomatic patellofemoral degenerative changes. Such treatment usually results in overall low satisfaction rates. Complications from operative treatment include overcorrection (with medial dislocation or adverse alteration in patellofemoral mechanics leading to early degenerative changes), nonunion, wound complications, and compartment syndrome (following distal procedures).

VI. Quadriceps Contusion

A. Overview—The quadriceps has a broad attachment to and lies directly over the femur. The position of the quadriceps renders it susceptible to crushing injuries between an external force and the underlying bone. A quadriceps contusion is an injury to the quadriceps mechanism sustained by a direct blow that damages the muscle but does not eliminate its function completely.

B. Classification—A quadriceps contusion is classified into three grades of severity 24 to 48 hours after initial hemorrhage and swelling cease. A mild contusion is characterized by local tenderness, ability to flex the knee more than 90°, and the ability to perform a deep knee bend. The average time of disability is 13 days. A moderate contusion is characterized by tenderness and swelling, ability to flex the knee more than 45° but less than 90°, and inability to perform a deep knee bend or rise from a chair without significant pain. The average time of disability is 19 days. A severe contusion is characterized by marked tenderness and swelling that obscures the contour of the muscle, inability to flex the knee more than 45°, and a severe limp. Often, there is a sympathetic effusion of the ipsilateral knee. The average time of disability is 21 days.

C. Evaluation—If a quadriceps rupture is suspected on clinical examination, plain films, MRI, and ultrasound may all be useful as discussed in the section on quadriceps tendon rupture. Myositis ossificans may be diagnosed as early as 2 to 4 weeks with plain films and usually involves the middle third of the thigh.

D. Treatment and Treatment Rationale—Quadriceps contusions should be observed closely until hemorrhage and edema have ceased. Although rare, thigh compartment syndrome after quadriceps contusion has been reported. With the exception of a compartment syndrome, treatment is nonoperative and is divided into three phases.

1. Phase I—The goal of Phase I treatment is to limit hemorrhage. This phase consists of rest, the application of ice, elevation, and immobilization with the hip and knee flexed to tolerance. A circumferential Ace bandage may be wrapped around the thigh for gentle compression. Massage, heat, diathermy, and range-of-motion exercises are avoided. Progression to Phase II occurs when there is stabilization of the thigh girth, pain at rest has ceased, and the patient is able to flex the knee to 90°.

2. Phase II—The goal of Phase II treatment is restoration of motion. This phase consists of the application of ice, use of a whirlpool, and well-leg, gravity-assisted range-of-motion exercises with an emphasis on flexion. The patient may begin isometric exercises and advance to weightbearing and ambulation as tolerated. Progression to Phase III occurs when the patient has more than 120° of active range of motion and equal thigh girth bilaterally.

3. Phase III—The goal of Phase III treatment is functional rehabilitation. Range of motion, strength, and endurance are emphasized. The patient progresses through static cycling with increasing resistance, walking, jogging (pool and surface), and finally, running. The patient is returned to full activity when full pain-free range of motion and function have been achieved. A thigh girdle with a thick pad is recommended for contact sports for 3 to 6 months.

E. Complications—In one study, the following risk factors were associated with the development of myositis ossificans: knee flexion less than 120° at the time of classification, occurrence of the injury while playing football, a history of previous quadriceps injury, the presence of a sympathetic knee effusion, and a delay in treatment of longer than 3 days. In the same study, in those patients who developed myositis ossificans it was attached to the femur by either a narrow stalk or a broad-based attachment or was separated from the femur by a narrow line of tissue. Usually, a distinct history of trauma and zoning of the lesion (peripheral maturation) makes the diagnosis of myositis ossificans clear, so no further workup is necessary. Rarely is the heterotopic bone of any functional significance and the initial treatment is conservative and includes active stretching. However, it should be remembered that synovial sarcoma, parosteal osteosarcoma, and periosteal osteosarcoma might each be mistaken for myositis ossificans.

SUGGESTED READINGS

Classic Articles

Bostrom A. Fracture of the patella. A study of 422 patellar fractures. *Acta Orthop Scand Suppl.* 1972;143:1.

Conlan T, Garth WP Jr, Lemons JE. Evaluation of the medial soft-tissue restraints of the extensor mechanism. *J Bone Joint Surg.* 1993;75A(5):682–693.

Fulkerson JP, Becker GJ, Meane JA. Anteromedialization of the tibial tuberosity for patellofemoral malalignment. *Clin Orthop.* 1983;177:176–181.

Hawkins RJ, Bell RH, Anisete G. Acute patellar dislocations: the natural history. *Am J Sports Med.* 1986;14:117–120.

Jackson DW, Feagin JA. Quadriceps contusions in young athletes. *J Bone Joint Surg.* 1973;55A(1):95–105.

Larsen E, Lund PM. Ruptures of the extensor mechanism of the knee joint: clinical results and patellofemoral articulation. *Clin Orthop.* 1986;213:150–153.

Marder RA, Swanson TV, Sharkey NA, et al. Effects of partial patellectomy and reattachment of the patellar tendon on patellofemoral contact areas and pressures. *J Bone Joint Surg.* 1993;75A(1):35–45.

McLaughlin HL, Francis KC. Operative repair of injuries to the quadriceps extensor mechanism. *Am J Surg.* 1956;91:651–653.

Ogden JA, Tross RB, Murphy MJ. Fractures of the tibial tuberosity in adolescents. *J Bone Joint Surg Am.* 1980;62:205–215.

Rasul AT Jr, Fischer DA. Primary repair of quadriceps tendon ruptures: results of treatment. *Clin Orthop.* 1993;289:205–207.

Ryan JB, Wheeler JH, Hopkinson WJ, et al. Quadriceps contusions: west point update. *Am J Sports Med.* 1991;19(3):299–304.

Siwek CW, Rao JP. Ruptures of the extensor mechanism of the knee joint. *J Bone Joint Surg.* 1981;63A(6);932–937.

Weber MJ, Janecki CJ, McLeod P, et al. Efficacy of various forms of fixation of transverse fractures of the patella. *J Bone Joint Surg.* 1980;62A(2):215–220.

Recent Articles

Maenpaa H, Lehto MUK. Patellar dislocation. *Am J Sports Med.* 1997;25(2):213–217.

Sallay PJ, Poggi J, Speer KP, et al. Acute dislocation of the patella: a correlative pathoanatomic study. *Am J Sports Med.* 1996;24(1):52–60.

Mosier SM, Stanitski CL. Acute tibial tubercle avulsion fractures. *J Pediatr Orthop.* 2004;24(2):181–184.

Review Articles

Boden, BP, Pearsall AW, Garrett WE, et al. Patellofemoral instability: evaluation and management. *J Am Acad Orthop Surg.*
1997;5(1):47–57.

Carpenter JE, Matthews LS. Fractures of the patella. *J Bone
Joint Surg.* 1993;75A(10):1550–1561.

Cramer KE, Moed BR. Patellar fractures: contemporary approach
to treatment. *J Am Acad Orthop Surg.* 1997;5(6):323–331.

Kettelkamp DB, DeRosa GP. Surgery of the patellofemoral joint.
Instru Course Lect. 1976;25:27–60.

Matava MJ. Patellar tendon ruptures. *J Am Acad Orthop Surg.*
1996;4(6):287–296.

Stefancin JJ, Parker RD. First-time traumatic patellar dislocation: a systematic review. *Clin Orthop Relat Res.*
2007;455:93–101.

CHAPTER 10

Tibial Plateau Fractures

Mark R. Brinker, Daniel P. O'Connor,
and Roman Schwartsman

I. Overview
   A. Mechanism of Injury—The fracture is usually a result of a compressive force: a direct axial compressive force, an indirect coronal compressive force, or a combined axial and coronal compressive force. The most common cause is a fall or a motor-vehicle accident.
   B. Factors Influencing Fracture Patterns
      1. Position of the leg relative to the direction of force application and degree of knee flexion at the time of force application.
         • Medial plateau fractures—Medial plateau fractures result from a combination of compression and varus stress.
         • Lateral plateau fractures—Lateral plateau fractures result from a combination of valgus stress and a force applied from the lateral side of the joint.
      2. Bone quality and the patient's physiologic age.
         • Young patients—Because of the good quality of their bone, young patients are prone to ligamentous injuries in combination with simple split fractures.
         • Older patients—Older patients are more likely to have depression-type or split-depression fracture without associated ligamentous injury.

II. Evaluation
   A. History
      1. Knee pain—Clinical suspicion for a tibial plateau fracture should be high whenever a patient complains of pain about the knee after sustaining an injury.
      2. Hemarthrosis with extension of the hematoma into the soft tissues—The presence of a hemarthrosis with extension of the hematoma into the soft tissues, particularly at the sites of ligamentous attachments, should heighten clinical suspicion for a tibial plateau fracture.
      3. Mechanism of injury—The mechanism of injury and any other influencing factors should be determined from the history.
   B. Physical Examination
      1. Inspection—The skin condition of the extremity should be noted. Specifically, internal degloving as well as open wounds should be noted. All open wounds must be examined to rule out communication with the joint. The joint should be injected with 50 mL of sterile saline under sterile conditions to determine whether any suspicious wounds communicate with the joint.
      2. Palpation—The neurovascular status of the extremity should be assessed.
         • Compartment syndrome—Compartment syndrome, although a rare entity with these types of fractures, must always be ruled out. Direct measurement of compartment pressures should be carried out if the clinical assessment is unreliable.
         • Pulses—The presence or absence of popliteal, dorsalis pedis, and posterior tibial pulses must be documented. Doppler studies or arteriograms are indicated if these pulses are absent.
         • Ligamentous injury—*A strong suspicion for ligamentous injury should be maintained* on examination because as many as 30% of these fractures may have an associated ligamentous injury. For example, pain and swelling over the medial collateral ligament (MCL) with a displaced lateral plateau fracture should be strongly suspicious for an associated MCL tear.
         • Meniscal injuries—Meniscal injuries are an associated finding in as many as 50% of tibial plateau fractures. The initial clinical examination is unreliable for diagnosing meniscal injuries in patients with tibial plateau fractures.

C. Radiographic Evaluation
   1. Initial radiographic series—The knee trauma series, the initial radiographic series, should include an anteroposterior view, a lateral view, two oblique views, and a 15° caudal tilt view. These films should be evaluated for shaft extension, articular depression, bone avulsions, and widening of the joint space. The 15° caudal view provides a more accurate assessment of joint depression than the anteroposterior view, since it accounts for the posterior slope of the tibial plateau.
   2. Varus/valgus stress views—Varus/valgus stress views can be obtained as a supplement to the knee trauma series and may aid in the identification of associated ligamentous injuries. A collateral ligament disruption is suggested when the medial or lateral clear space is widened by more than 1 cm compared with that of the contralateral limb stressed in the same way.
   3. Computed tomography (CT)—CT serves as an adjunct to plain radiographs in preoperative planning. The degree of articular displacement is best evaluated on a CT scan with sagittal and coronal reconstructions.
   4. Magnetic resonance imaging—Magnetic resonance imaging does not yet have a clear role in the evaluation of tibial plateau fractures, although it may serve as an adjunct to plain radiographs in certain cases and it may aid in identifying associated meniscal and ligamentous injuries.

III. Classification
   A. Schatzker Classification—The Schatzker classification (Fig. 10-1) is the most widely used and accepted system of classifying tibial plateau fractures.
      1. Type I fractures are a split of the lateral plateau. They occur predominantly in the young patients with strong bone and may be associated with a trapped meniscus at the fracture site. There is a high risk of ligamentous injury with these fractures.
      2. Type II fractures are split-depressions of the lateral plateau. An axial load caused by the femoral condyle first splits the plateau and then depresses its edge.
      3. Type III fractures are pure central depressions of the lateral plateau. They are more likely the result of a low-energy injury, and they occur predominantly in older patients. There is a low risk of ligamentous injury associated with these fractures.
      4. Type IV fractures involve the medial tibial plateau. They are usually high-energy injuries. There may be an associated traction lesion of the peroneal nerve.

   5. Type V fractures are bicondylar (Fig. 10-2). Typically, these fractures involve a split of both the medial and the lateral plateaus without any associated articular depression.
   6. Type VI fractures are characterized by the presence of an associated proximal tibial shaft fracture (i.e., metaphyseal-diaphyseal separation). They are almost always high-energy injuries with extensive comminution. There may be an associated popliteal artery disruption.
B. AO/OTA Classification (Fig. 10-3)
   1. Advantages and disadvantages—The advantage of the AO/OTA classification is that it is a unified, consistent approach to the classification of fractures that appears to have good intraobserver reliability. The disadvantage is that it is a cumbersome system that is impractical to apply to the acute clinical setting. The AO/OTA classification distinguishes fractures by type, group, and subgroup.
   2. Correspondence to the Schatzker classification—The AO/OTA type B fractures correspond to Schatzker Types I to IV. The AO/OTA Type C fractures correspond to Schatzker Types V and VI.

IV. Associated Injuries
   A. Meniscal Tears—Meniscal tears occur in as many as 50% of tibial plateau fractures. Meniscal tears that cannot be repaired should be excised at the time of definitive surgical treatment. Peripheral meniscal tears identified at the time of open reduction should be repaired with suture just before closure.
   B. Ligamentous Injuries—Associated ligamentous injuries are noted in as many as 30% of tibial plateau fractures. Treatment should be individualized according to the injury. The need for repair remains controversial since it is not entirely clear which combinations of ligament injury and fracture result in knee joint instability.
      1. Collateral ligament repair—Collateral ligament repair in the acute setting requires an undesirable amount of soft tissue stripping. Evidence in the literature supports the nonoperative management of MCL injuries since most heal satisfactorily.
      2. Repair of avulsions of the intercondylar eminence—Avulsions of the intercondylar eminence should be repaired, reattaching the cruciate ligament with a bone block.

V. Treatment and Treatment Rationale
   A. Indications—The specific indications for operative vs. nonoperative management remain controversial.

Schatzker type I   Schatzker type II   Schatzker type III

Schatzker type IV   Schatzker type V   Schatzker type VI

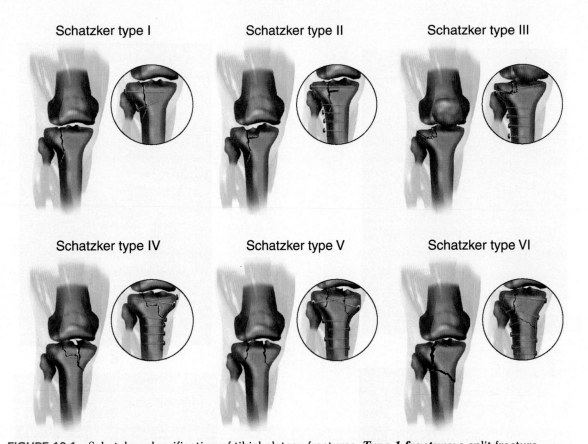

FIGURE 10-1   Schatzker classification of tibial plateau fractures. ***Type 1 fracture:*** a split fracture of the lateral plateau without any joint depression. More or less displacement may be present. Even if displacement is slight, there may be an associated peripheral tear of the lateral meniscus, which can be incarcerated in the fracture. Arthroscopy may be required to exclude a meniscus injury. Type I fractures can be fixed with lag screws (often with washers) if the bone is of good quality. In older, osteoporotic patients, a buttress plate may be advisable. ***Type II fracture***: a split-depression fracture. The depressed fragment may undergo severe fragmentation. These injuries generally occur in patients with decreased bone density. With a Type II fracture, the lateral plateau is exposed beneath the meniscus, and depressed articular surface fragments are carefully elevated en masse by opening the peripheral fracture defect. Sufficient bone graft is inserted into the remaining metaphyseal void. Then the split fragment is reduced and fixed with a buttress plate and lag screws. Allograft may be used in elderly patients. ***Type III fracture***: a pure depression fracture. The depressions vary in size and degree and may be central, or less commonly, peripheral. Instability may not be present when the depressed area is small or centrally located. An examination under anesthesia may be required to assess the stability of a knee with a Type III fracture. If instability is present in a Type III fracture, the depressed portion of the tibial plateau is elevated via an appropriately placed window in the metaphysis. Bone graft is packed into the resulting defect. If a large window is required, the cortex must be buttressed with a plate to prevent a split fracture. ***Type IV fracture***: a fracture of the medial plateau, which is frequently associated with a fracture of the intercondylar eminence. This high-energy injury may be associated with neurovascular or other significant soft tissue injury. Definitive fixation of Type IV (medial plateau) fractures usually requires a medial buttress plate to supplement the lag screws. Lag screws or a wire suture may be needed to anchor an intercondylar eminence fragment. ***Type V fracture***: a bicondylar fracture that may involve the articular surface. Occasionally, the fracture lines are so close to the intercondylar eminence that the weightbearing surfaces of the plateaus are not affected. The fracture lines may resemble an inverted Y. Lag screws with medial and lateral buttress plating provides optimal fixation for Type V plateau fractures. Buttress plates are important in preventing axial collapse. Hallmark of a ***Type VI fracture***: separation of the metaphysis from the diaphysis. Usually, the lateral plateau has a depressed or comminuted area, whereas the medial plateau tends to be more intact. Such impaction may involve both plateaus. Two plates are required for optimal fixation of a Type VI fracture. Both act as buttresses, but one (a DCP-type plate) must reconnect the metaphysis to the diaphysis, supplementing lag-screw fixation if possible. Thus this plate is used for either compression or neutralization.

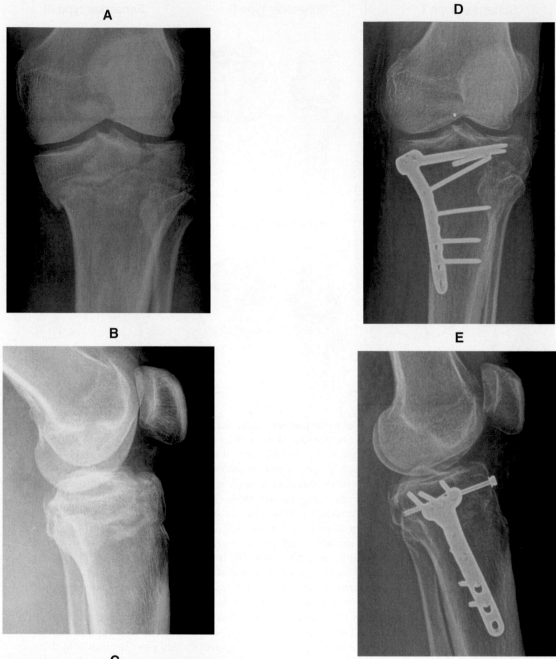

FIGURE 10-2 This 49-year-old man injured his leg while playing softball. The anteroposterior **(A)** and lateral **(B)** radiographs and computed tomography (CT) scan **(C)** revealed a Schatzker Type V fracture, with bicondylar involvement, an anterior fragment, and medial translation of the medial plateau. The condylar components of the fracture were treated using a medial locking plate, and the anterior fragment was stabilized using a lag screw **(D** and **E)**. At 4 months after surgery, the patient was pain-free, full weightbearing, and had full extension and flexion to 100°.

Type B1   Type B2   Type B3

Type C1   Type C2   Type C3

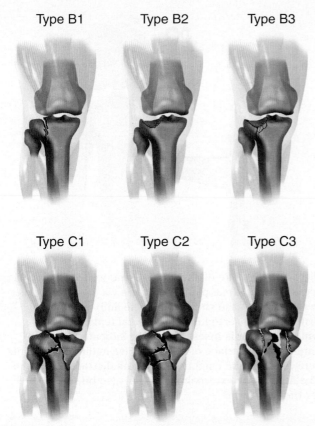

FIGURE 10-3 AO classification of fractures of the long bones, tibia/fibula, proximal segment. *B1*, partial articular fracture, pure split. *B2*, partial articular fracture, pure depression. *B3*, partial articular fracture, split depression. *C1*, complete articular fracture, articular simple, metaphyseal simple. *C2*, complete articular fracture, articular simple, metaphyseal mulifragmentary. *C3*, complete articular fracture, multifragmentary.

1. Articular surface displacement—Some authors advocate nonoperative management for fractures with as much as 1 cm of articular surface depression. Advocates of operative treatment are willing to accept only minimal displacement (≤2 mm) of the articular surface.
2. Varus/valgus instability—There is general consensus that varus/valgus instability (with the knee in extension) of 10° or more, relative to the contralateral knee, is an indication for operative management of the fracture.
   - Split fractures—Split fractures are likely to be unstable, since they involve the rim of the tibial plateau.
   - Split-depression fractures—Split-depression fractures carry a higher risk of instability.
   - Pure depression fractures—Pure depression fractures are generally stable because the intact cortical rim provides varus/valgus stability.

   - Plateau fractures with an associated shaft fracture—Plateau fractures with an associated tibial shaft fracture are inherently unstable and do not lend themselves to nonoperative treatment.
3. Injuries requiring emergent surgery—There is no controversy regarding the requirement for emergent surgical management of open fractures, fractures with an associated vascular injury, or those with an associated compartment syndrome.

B. Nonoperative Treatment—Nonoperative treatment is reserved for stable, minimally displaced plateau fractures.
   1. Protected mobilization—Protected mobilization in a hinged cast brace with partial weightbearing for 8 to 12 weeks is recommended. Full weightbearing can begin later as tolerated. Unrestricted activity is allowed at 16 to 26 weeks.
   2. Exercises—Progressive knee range-of-motion exercises and isometric quadriceps and hamstring exercises are initiated during the protected-weightbearing stage.

C. Operative Treatment
   1. Preoperative planning—Preoperative planning gives the surgeon insight into the "personality" of the fracture. A radiograph of the contralateral extremity may be used as a template. Traction radiographs allow for better visualization of the individual fracture fragments.
   2. Timing of surgery—The timing of surgery is influenced by the condition of the soft tissues. The soft tissues may become edematous within 8 to 12 hours of injury to the point where it may be judicious to let the swelling subside. The limb can be immobilized in a bulky Jones splint or with a knee-spanning temporary external fixator during this time. In high-energy injuries, it may take up to two weeks for the soft tissue swelling to subside.

VI. Anatomic Considerations and Surgical Techniques
   A. Limited Open-Reduction Techniques, Indirect-Reduction Methods, and Fluoroscopy—The use of limited open-reduction techniques, indirect-reduction methods, and fluoroscopy, rather than direct joint visualization, to assess articular surface congruence is advocated in cases of soft tissue compromise. This approach provides good visualization in the treatment of split fractures (Schatzker Types I, IV, and V). With depressed fracture fragments, visualization on the image intensifier is limited by the remaining plateau.
   B. Arthroscopy—Arthroscopy can serve as a less invasive method of assessing articular surface reduction. It is advocated by some authors for the

treatment of split fractures because of the theoretical possibility of the meniscus being trapped in the fracture at the time of indirect reduction. It is most useful for the treatment of central depression fractures (Schatzker Type III). There is the potential danger of compartment syndrome from fluid extravasation. High-pressure inflow is to be avoided. The compartments should be evaluated frequently during arthroscopic surgery in patients with tibial plateau fractures.

C. Surgical Treatment of Split Fractures (Schatzker Types I, IV, and V)

1. Fragment reduction—A tenaculum clamp may be used to reduce fractures displaced only medially or laterally.

2. Ligamentotaxis—In fractures in which there is a split, ligamentotaxis with a femoral distractor (Fig. 10-4) attached on the same side as the fragment may be used as a reduction aid. (This requires intact soft tissue attachments.)

3. Bone grafting—Bone grafting is typically not necessary in these types of fractures, and may, in fact, hinder reduction.

4. Fixation—Definitive fixation is accomplished with either screws or buttress plates, depending on bone quality.

D. Surgical Treatment of Depression Type Fractures (Schatzker Type III)

1. Fragment elevation—The depressed fragment can be elevated with a bone tamp through a fenestration of the cortex.

2. Bone grafting—The resultant metaphyseal defect should be filled with graft material to prevent articular collapse.

3. Fixation—Percutaneous large-fragment screws should be inserted parallel to the joint and just below the graft to stabilize and support the construct.

E. Surgical Treatment of Split Depression Fractures and Fractures with Metaphyseal-Diaphyseal Separation (Schatzker Types II and VI)

1. Open reduction and internal fixation techniques—Open reduction and internal fixation techniques provide the best means of establishing an anatomic reduction of the joint surface, restoring axial alignment, and instituting an early functional knee range-of-motion program.

2. Femoral distractor—The femoral distractor (see Fig. 10-4) can be used as a supplemental reduction aid in these types of fractures. The distractor is placed on the ipsilateral side of the fracture. Two femoral distractors may need to be used in Schatzker Type VI fractures.

3. Surgical approach
   • Incision

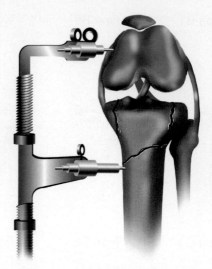

FIGURE 10-4 Use of a femoral distractor to aid in the reduction of a tibial plateau fracture via ligamentotaxis. In the sample case shown here, one limb of the AO distractor is inserted into the medial femoral condyle while the other is inserted into the subcutaneous anteromedial surface of the tibia. Five-millimeter Schantz screws should be used to anchor the distractor to bone. The AO tubular external fixator can also be substituted for the distractor.

   (a) Midline—A midline incision facilitates later knee arthroplasty or arthrodesis.
   (b) Dual incision—Anterolateral and posteromedial approaches advocated by some authors, particularly for Schatzker Type VI injuries.
   • Coronary ligament—The coronary ligament is incised horizontally to create the arthrotomy (Fig. 10-5).
   • Additional joint visualization—Additional joint visualization can be obtained by partially sectioning the iliotibial band.
   • Z-plasty—If even more visualization is necessary, a Z-plasty of the patellar tendon should be considered. (The tendon should be protected with a tension band after the repair.)

4. Specific techniques for Schatzker Type II fractures
   • Fragments—The fragments should be hinged outward like the pages of a book to preserve their soft tissue attachments. Depressed articular fragments should be elevated from below as large cancellous blocks.
   • Bone grafting—Bone grafting of the metaphyseal defect can either precede or follow reduction and stabilization of the split fragment at the discretion of the surgeon.

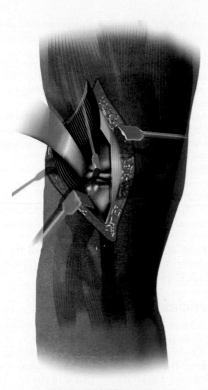

FIGURE 10-5   The arthrotomy should be made by incising the coronary ligament transversely below the meniscus.

- Stabilization—Definitive stabilization of the fracture is accomplished using large, cancellous lag screws inserted parallel to the joint line and a metaphyseal buttress plate of appropriate size.
5. Specific techniques for Schatzker Type VI fractures
   - Medial plateau fragment—The medial plateau fragment is usually the larger of the two and lends itself as a starting place for attachment of the lateral fragments and the tibial shaft.
   - Metaphyseal fracture components—The metaphyseal components should be reduced first, followed by reduction and stabilization of the metaphysis to the diaphysis. This can be accomplished by either:
      (a) Dual plates—Low profile plates inserted with minimal dissection are preferred.
      (b) Single plate—A single plate is sufficient in cases in which the fracture line is transverse.
      (c) Single plate with a contralateral external fixator—A single plate with a contralateral external fixator is used to neutralize shear forces when oblique fracture lines are present.

      (d) Circular thin wire (Ilizarov) external fixation—Ilizarov fixation is recommended for fractures in which the level of separation between the tibial shaft and metaphysis is very proximal. It is alternatively recommended as a means of definitive fixation in open fractures. Circular external fixation has been reported to have similar clinical outcomes as ORIF with fewer and less severe complications.
      (e) Circular thin wire external fixation combined with minimal internal fixation—Several recent reports have advocated that limited internal fixation using minimally invasive techniques may be used to reduce and stabilize the articular surface with external fixation used to stabilize the remaining fragments in high-energy, highly comminuted fractures.

VII. Complications of the Injury
   A. Posttraumatic Arthritis—Posttraumatic arthritis can occur either as a result of residual joint incongruity or as a result of cartilage damage sustained at the time of the initial injury.
   B. Loss of Meniscal Tissue—Loss of meniscal tissue contributes to excessive load bearing by the underlying articular surfaces, also leading to premature posttraumatic arthritis.
   C. Loss of Joint Motion—Loss of joint motion occurs as a result of periarticular soft tissue injuries and can be exacerbated by prolonged immobilization.
   D. Rare Complications—Rare complications include compartment syndrome, peroneal, neuropathy, popliteal artery injuries, deep vein thrombosis, and avascular necrosis.

VIII. Complications of Treatment
   A. Infection—Infection is a potentially devastating complication that occurs in as many as 12% of tibial plateau fractures. Infection may be related to either the initial condition of the fracture or the surgical intervention.
   B. Skin Slough—Skin slough at the fracture site, the result of poor surgical timing, poor soft tissue technique, or the used of bicondylar plates, is a major risk factor for later infection.
   C. Peroneal Neuropathy—Peroneal neuropathy can occur iatrogenically as a result of surgery or casting.
   D. Malunions and Nonunions—Malunions and nonunions are relatively rare complications. An increasing number of malunions and nonunions have been noted in Schatzker Type VI fractures treated by "hybrid" external fixation.

SUGGESTED READINGS

Classic Articles

Burri C, Bartzke G, Coldeway J, et al. Fractures of the tibial plateau. *Clin Orthop Relat Res.* 1979;138:84–93.

Marsh JL, Smith ST, Do TT. External fixation and limited internal-fixation for complex fractures of the tibial plateau. *J Bone Joint Surg Am.* 1995;77:661–673.

Rasmussen PS. Tibial condylar fractures: Impairment of knee joint instability as an indication of surgical treatment. *J Bone Joint Surg Am.* 1973;55:1331–1350.

Schatzker J, McBroom R, Bruce D. The tibial plateau fracture: the Toronto experience, 1968–1975. *Clin Orthop Relat Res.* 1979;138:94–104.

Tscherne H, Lobenhoffer P. Tibial plateau fractures—management and expected results. *Clin Orthop Relat Res.* 1993;292:87–100.

Waddell JP, Johnston DWC, Neidre A. Fractures of the tibial plateau—a review of 95 patients and comparison of treatment methods. *J Trauma.* 1981;21:376–381.

Watson JT. High-energy fractures of the tibial plateau. *Orthop Clin North Am.* 1994;25:723–752.

Recent Articles

Barei DP, Nork SE, Mills WJ, et al. Functional outcomes of severe bicondylar tibial plateau fractures treated with dual incisions and medial and lateral plates. *J Bone Joint Surg Am.* 2006;88:1713–1721.

Canadian Orthopaedic Trauma Society. Open reduction and internal fixation compared with circular fixator application for bicondylar tibial plateau fractures. Results of a multicenter, prospective, randomized clinical trial. *J Bone Joint Surg Am.* 2006;88:2613–2623.

Catagni MA, Ottaviani G, Maggioni M. Treatment strategies for complex fractures of the tibial plateau with external circular fixation and limited internal fixation. *J Trauma.* 2007;63:1043–1053.

Chan YS, Chiu CH, Lo YP, et al. Arthroscopy-assisted surgery for tibial plateau fractures: 2- to 10-year follow-up results. *Arthroscopy.* 2008;24:760–768.

Katsenis D, Dendrinos G, Kouris A, et al. Combination of fine wire fixation and limited internal fixation for high-energy tibial plateau fractures: functional results at minimum 5-year follow-up. *J Orthop Trauma.* 2009;23:493–501.

Kayali C, Ozturk H, Altay T, et al. Arthroscopically assisted percutaneous osteosynthesis of lateral tibial plateau fractures. *Can J Surg.* 2008;51:378–382.

Levy BA, Herrera DA, Macdonald P, et al. The medial approach for arthroscopic-assisted fixation of lateral tibial plateau fractures: patient selection and mid- to long-term results. *J Orthop Trauma.* 2008;22:201–205.

Rossi R, Bonasia DE, Blonna D, et al. Prospective follow-up of a simple arthroscopic-assisted technique for lateral tibial plateau fractures: results at 5 years. *Knee.* 2008;15:378–383.

Stevens DG, Beharry R, McKee MD, et al. The long-term functional outcome of operatively treated tibial plateau fractures. *J Orthop Trauma.* 2001;15:312–320.

Toro-Arbelaez JB, Gardner MJ, Shindle MK, et al. Open reduction and internal fixation of intraarticular tibial plateau nonunions. *Injury.* 2007;38:378–383.

Weigel DP, Marsh JL. High-energy fractures of the tibial plateau. Knee function after longer follow-up. *J Bone Joint Surg Am.* 2002;84-A:1541–1551.

Review Articles

Berkson EM, Virkus WW. High-energy tibial plateau fractures. *J Am Acad Orthop Surg.* 2006;14:20–31.

Mahadeva D, Costa ML, Gaffey A. Open reduction and internal fixation versus hybrid fixation for bicondylar/severe tibial plateau fractures: a systematic review of the literature. *Arch Orthop Trauma Surg.* 2008;128:1169–1175.

Musahl V, Tarkin I, Kobbe P, et al. New trends and techniques in open reduction and internal fixation of fractures of the tibial plateau. *J Bone Joint Surg Br.* 2009;91:426–433.

Textbooks

Browner BD, Levine AM, Jupiter JB, et al, eds. *Skeletal Trauma: Basic Science, Management, and Reconstruction.* Philadelphia, PA: WB Saunders; 2003.

Bucholz RW, Heckman JD, Court-Brown CM, et al, eds. *Rockwood and Green's Fractures in Adults.* Philadelphia, PA: Lippincott Williams & Wilkins; 2001.

Rüedi TP, Murphy WM, eds. *AO Principles of Fracture Management.* New York, NY: Thieme Medical Publishers; 2001.

Wagner M, Frigg R, eds. *AO Manual of Fracture Management: Internal Fixators.* New York, NY: Thieme Medical Publishers; 2006.

CHAPTER 11

Tibial Shaft Fractures

Catherine A. Humphrey and John T. Gorczyca

I. Introduction—Tibial shaft fractures are one of the most common diaphyseal fractures treated by orthopaedic surgeons. The majority of these fractures heal without complication and most patients return to their preinjury level of functioning. Specific types of tibial shaft fractures are more prone to complication and require the expertise of a well-trained orthopaedist to avoid complication and optimize functional outcome.

II. Evaluation
   A. History and Physical Examination
      1. History—Patients with tibial shaft fractures experience pain in the leg after sustaining a low- or high-energy injury. Information about the nature and timing of the accident, any reduction or manipulation performed on the extremity and the patient's significant medical history should be obtained.
      2. Visual examination—All clothing should be removed from the extremity. The overall appearance of the extremity should be noted for open wounds, alignment, contusions, swelling, and color. Wounds should be assessed for size, location, degree of contamination, and severity of tissue injury.
         • Deformities—Often a significant deformity is present at the level of the fracture. Contusions may indicate the point where a force was applied to the leg to create the fracture, or they may be incidental. The location of a significant contusion is important because it can necessitate a change in the treatment plan to avoid incising through badly traumatized tissue.
         • Comparison to the contralateral leg—Comparison of the injured leg to the contralateral leg usually reveals a large amount of swelling. This swelling progresses with time. The amount of swelling present should serve as a preliminary index of the severity of injury to the tissues.
         • Color—The color of the extremity reveals essential information about a limb's perfusion. A pinkish color indicates oxygenated blood in the capillaries of the skin but reveals little about the deep circulation. A gray or dusky color, however, indicates circulatory compromise and a potential for limb loss if proper treatment is not provided promptly.
         • Movement—After visually inspecting the leg, the physician should observe what the patient can do with the leg before the physician palpates or manipulates it. Attention should be directed at flexion and extension of the knee, ankle, and toes. Occasionally, the patient is too uncomfortable to comply with this part of the examination.
      3. Palpation
         • Pulses—An effort should be made to feel for pulses of the popliteal, dorsalis pedis, and posterior tibial arteries. If strong pulses are not appreciated, Doppler ultrasound should be used to evaluate the dorsalis pedis and posterior tibial arteries. If triphasic pulses are not present on Doppler ultrasound and the leg is deformed, traction should be applied to the extremity and the pulses re-evaluated. If the pulses remain abnormal, emergent arteriography and/or consultation with a vascular surgeon should be obtained.
         • Direct palpation—Occasionally, the injured leg appears fairly normal, and the results of the neurovascular exam are unremarkable. Direct palpation of the fracture, however, elicits pain and possible crepitation, which are indicative of a tibial shaft fracture.

4. Compartment syndrome—After ruling out vascular injury, the physician must evaluate for compartment syndrome. If the patient can actively flex and extend the ankle and toes without severe pain, compartment syndrome is not likely to be present at that time. Compartment syndrome can, however, evolve with time; thus serial examination and attention to the patient's symptoms are necessary.

• Signs and symptoms—The alert patient commonly has a significant amount of pain from the fracture, and so ruling out compartment syndrome becomes more difficult. *Pain out of proportion to the injury should make the physician suspicious. The most sensitive sign on physical examination is pain on passive stretch of the muscles in the involved compartment*. Other significant signs are tight compartments, decreased sensation, and muscle weakness, although these signs may not always be present. Examination of the pulses is misleading since pulses may be palpable when compartment syndrome is present.

• Compartment Pressure—Evaluation of the compartments in the unconscious, intoxicated, or otherwise mentally impaired patient is more difficult because the patient has an altered response to pain. If there is any suspicion of compartment syndrome, then slit-catheter measurement of pressure in all four compartments is necessary to confirm or rule out the diagnosis. The exact pressure at which compartment syndrome occurs is variable. In general, *a compartment-diastolic pressure difference of less than 30 mm Hg in any compartment is an indication for emergent four-compartment fasciotomy*.

5. Open fractures—It must be assumed that open wounds in the vicinity of a tibial shaft fracture communicate with the fracture, and urgent irrigation and debridement should be planned (Fig. 11-1). Open wounds a distance away from the fracture may communicate with the fracture. Probing or inspection of extremity wounds for communication with the fracture should be performed in the operating room after sterile preparation and draping of the extremity.

B. Radiographic Evaluation—Radiographic evaluation of a tibial shaft fracture requires anteroposterior and lateral X-ray films. These X-ray films must include the entire tibia in addition to the distal femur and ankle, since associated fractures may be present and could alter the treatment plan. Computed tomography is occasionally helpful in

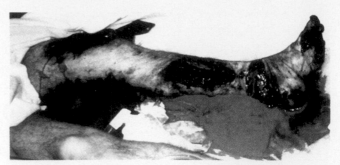

FIGURE 11-1 Clinical photograph of a young man involved in a coal mining accident showing severely contaminated wounds overlying his tibia fracture. Because of the significant tissue destruction this is a Gustilo type IIIb open tibia fracture.

delineating subtle fracture extension in very distal and very proximal shaft fractures. Stress fractures of the tibial shaft may not be visible on plain X-ray films. In this instance, an MRI scan or a three-phase bone scan assists in making the diagnosis.

III. Classification

A. Fracture—Several classification systems exist for the tibial shaft fracture. The importance of any system is its ability to differentiate fractures into treatment groups and its ability to predict outcome. For the closed tibial shaft fracture, the classification of Johner and Wruhs is straightforward and simple (Fig. 11-2). This classification system is based on the fracture location, the mechanism of injury, and the amount of energy dissipated in the fracture (i.e., the fracture comminution). The Arbeitsgemeinshaft für Osteosynthesfragen (AO) or Orthopaedic Trauma Association (OTA) classification is somewhat similar in scope but more detailed and complex. This classification is probably best used for accurately classifying fractures for research purposes because it allows for meaningful evaluation and comparison of fractures in different patients from different studies.

B. Open Fracture—Open fractures are best described using Gustilo's grading system. Type I open fractures have small (<1 cm), clean wounds; minimal injury to the musculature; and no significant stripping of periosteum from bone. Type II open fractures have larger (>1 cm) wounds but no significant soft-tissue damage, flaps or avulsions. Type III open fractures have larger wounds and are associated with extensive injury to the integument, muscle, periosteum, and bone. Gunshot injuries and open fractures caused by a farm injury are special categories of Type III open fractures on account of their higher risk of complications, particularly infection. Type IIIa injuries have extensive contamination and/or injury to

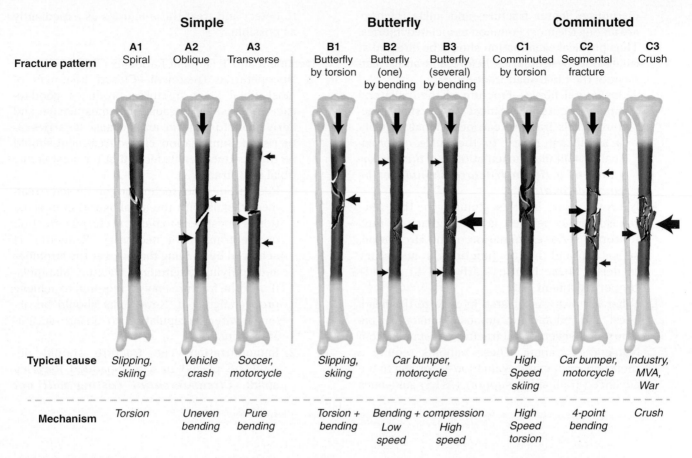

	Simple			Butterfly			Comminuted		
	A1 Spiral	**A2** Oblique	**A3** Transverse	**B1** Butterfly by torsion	**B2** Butterfly (one) by bending	**B3** Butterfly (several) by bending	**C1** Comminuted by torsion	**C2** Segmental fracture	**C3** Crush
Fracture pattern									
Typical cause	*Slipping, skiing*	*Vehicle crash*	*Soccer, motorcycle*	*Slipping, skiing*	*Car bumper, motorcycle*		*High Speed skiing*	*Car bumper, motorcycle*	*Industry, MVA, War*
Mechanism	*Torsion*	*Uneven bending*	*Pure bending*	*Torsion + bending*	*Bending + compression* *Low speed*	*High speed*	*High Speed torsion*	*4-point bending*	*Crush*

Fracture by torsion *(A1, B1, C1): One spiral fracture line, the others ± longitudinal fibular fracture are usually at a different level*

Fracture by bending *(A2, A3, B2, B3, C2): Transverse on tension side (i.e., opposite fulcrum). Fibular fracture is usually at the same level*

Fracture by crushing *(C3)*

<u>FIGURE 11-2</u>   Johner and Wruh's classification system for tibial shaft fractures.

the underlying soft tissue, but adequate viable soft tissue is present to cover the bone and neurovascular structures without a muscle transfer. Type IIIb injuries have such an extensive injury to the soft tissues that a rotational or free muscle transfer is necessary to achieve coverage of the bone and neurovascular structures. These injuries usually have massive contamination. Type IIIc injuries are any open fractures with an associated vascular injury that requires an arterial repair. Often, what appears to be a Type I or Type II open fracture on initial examination in the emergency room is noted to have significant periosteal stripping and muscle injury at the time of operative debridement and may require muscle transfer for coverage with serial debridements. Thus there is a tendency for the Gustilo classification type to increase with time.

C. Soft-Tissue Injury—Tscherne has classified closed fractures according to the severity of the soft-tissue injury. Grade 0 injuries have negligible soft tissue injury. Grade 1 closed fractures have superficial abrasions or contusions of the soft tissues overlying the fracture. Grade 2 closed fractures have significant contusion to the muscle and/or deep contaminated skin abrasions. The bony injury is usually severe in these injuries. Grade 3 closed fractures have a severe injury to the soft tissues, with significant degloving, crushing, compartment syndrome, or vascular injury. The influence of the soft-tissue injury on treatment is discussed later.

IV. Associated Injuries
   A. Fractures—Most tibial shaft fractures result from low-energy trauma and do not have associated injuries. As the severity of the tibial fracture increases, the incidence of associated injuries increases to greater than 50%. Injuries to the ipsilateral extremity, including knee ligament

disruption, femur fracture, and ankle fracture, are among the most common associated injuries. Thus physical examination should be directed at ruling out these injuries before and after treatment of the tibial shaft fracture.

    1. Ipsilateral fibula—Fracture of the ipsilateral fibula occurs with most tibial shaft fractures. This fracture can occasionally signify a significant injury to the ankle or proximal tibiofibular articulation, so *the importance of a fibula fracture should not be underestimated*.

  B. Neurovascular Injuries—Injury to the neurovascular structures is also common; thus thorough serial examination of the circulation, sensation and motor function is necessary to detect these injuries early and to provide proper treatment.

  C. Other Injuries—Associated injuries to the head, chest, and abdomen occur most commonly in patients with severe tibial fractures sustained from high-energy trauma. These patients require a thorough, systematic evaluation according to the advanced trauma life support (ATLS) guidelines to detect and treat these injuries as expediently as possible.

V. Treatment and Treatment Rationale (Table 11-1)

  A. Nonoperative Treatment—Closed treatment of most tibial shaft fractures produces good-to-excellent results. Because it is inexpensive and fairly quick to perform, and because it carries little risk of complication, closed treatment should be the treatment considered first for most stable tibial shaft fractures.

    1. Reduction—The technique of closed treatment begins with the administration of sedation or anesthesia to perform closed reduction of the fracture, if necessary. Reduction is achieved by hanging the leg over the stretcher and applying longitudinal traction. Manipulation of the fracture may be required to achieve proper alignment. X-ray films should be obtained after manipulation to ensure acceptable reduction.

    2. Immobilization—The fracture should initially be placed in a well-padded long leg splint. *Circumferential casting will not*

TABLE 11-1

Treatment Options for Tibial Shaft Fractures

Treatment Method	Advantages	Disadvantages	Best Uses
Casting	Noninvasive nature Inexpensive procedure	Difficulty in maintaining alignment Compromise in mobility	Minimally displaced closed fractures Sedentary patients
Standard external fixation	Minimally invasive nature Quick procedure Avoidance of traumatized tissue	Pin loosening with time Difficulty in maintaining alignment Patient dissatisfaction	Severely contaminated open fractures Life- or limb threatening conditions requiring rapid skeletal stabilization
Ring external fixation	Minimally invasive nature Wires that are less likely to loosen Ability to stabilize fractures in proximity to joints	Technically challenging procedure Patient dissatisfaction High incidence of pin tract infection	Complex high energy closed fractures Tibial shaft fractures extending into or near a joint
Open reduction with internal fixation	Achievement of stable fixation Early joint motion	Incision in area of trauma Strength of fixation not as good as with intramedullary nailing	Tibial shaft fractures extending to the metaphysis
Intramedullary nailing	Ease of alignment Strength of fixation Avoidance of traumatized tissue	Limited fixation strength with metaphyseal fractures	Displaced tibial shaft fractures (open or closed)

accommodate swelling and can lead to increasing pain and parasthesias subsequent to reduction. If a cast is applied, it must be bivalved to allow for soft-tissue swelling. The long leg splint or cast can be changed to a patella-tendon bearing (PTB) cast when soft callus has formed at the fracture site, at which time the fracture site will not have tenderness when pressure is applied. This may take as little as 8 to 10 days or, with some fractures, as long as 3 to 4 weeks. X-ray studies in the PTB cast are essential to confirm proper alignment. At this point, the patient may begin to bear weight on the extremity.

3. Alignment—There is considerable controversy regarding how much malalignment of a tibia fracture can be tolerated. Certainly, anatomic alignment with no angulation on the anteroposterior and lateral X-ray films is the goal, but this is not always achieved. Angulation in the sagittal plane is tolerated better than angulation in the coronal plane. This increased tolerance is due to the fact that the knee and ankle move in the sagittal plane, so this motion "makes up for" some angulation. Coronal plane angulation, however, results in varus or valgus malalignment, which produces asymmetric loading of the ankle and knee joints.

   - Angulation—It is not clear how much angulation is required to produce osteoarthritis, since multiple factors influence the progression of osteoarthritis, including the location of the fracture and the age of the patient. *In general, angulation of more than 10° in the sagittal plane and more than 5° in the coronal plane are significant enough to warrant remanipulation of the fracture or wedging of the cast. On the other hand, some surgeons argue that a tibia fracture that heals with as much as 20° angulation can be tolerated by most patients.* (The authors do not agree with these surgeons.)
   - Shortening—Shortening of 1 cm or less is rarely symptomatic, and shortening of 2 or 3 cm can be made tolerable with a 1.25 cm (0.5 in) shoe insert.
   - Rotational malalignment—The amount of rotational malalignment that can be tolerated varies from patient to patient. In general, if the rotational malalignment affects gait or causes knee or ankle symptoms, operative correction should be considered.

4. Assessment of healing—The patient in a patella-tendon bearing cast should have radiographic evaluation of the fracture every 6 or 8 weeks. When the healing appears complete on X-ray films and the patient has clinical evidence of healing (i.e., no motion or pain with force applied across the fracture), then the cast is no longer required. This may be as early as 8 weeks after the injury but most commonly occurs 12 to 16 weeks after the injury. At this point, a rehabilitation program, including gait training, ankle rehabilitation, and strengthening of the quadriceps and gastrocsoleus muscles, quickens the return to normal function.

B. Operative Treatment

   1. Indications
      - Absolute—There are several absolute indications for operative stabilization of tibial shaft fractures. **Open fractures** should have stabilization of the fracture to provide a stable environment for soft-tissue healing and to facilitate wound care. Fractures with a *vascular injury* require skeletal stabilization to protect the vascular repair. Fractures with **compartment syndrome** should have skeletal stabilization to provide a stable environment for the injured tissues. Stabilization of the tibia should be performed in tibial shaft fractures in *patients with multiple injuries* to improve patient mobility, minimize pain, and possibly reduce the release of pro-inflammatory mediators.
      - Relative—Relative indications for operative stabilization include significant shortening of the fracture on initial X-ray studies, significant comminution, a tibia fracture with an intact fibula (Fig. 11-3), and a displaced tibia fracture with a fibula fracture at the same level. In each of these fractures, there is a high incidence of malunion or nonunion with nonoperative treatment.

   2. External fixation
      - Standard—External fixation of a tibial shaft fracture is a quick and technically easy way to achieve fracture stability. For this reason, it is useful in a patient with multiple injuries who is hemodynamically unstable ("damage control") or in a patient who would benefit from quick fracture stabilization before emergent repair of an arterial injury. It also can be used if an open fracture wound is severely contaminated and the surgeon has reservations about putting hardware in the wound. An external fixator can be applied

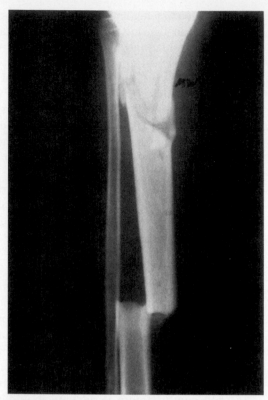

FIGURE 11-3 Anteroposterior X-ray film of a leg demonstrating a segmental tibia fracture with an intact fibula, a very unstable fracture.

through small incisions, thus avoiding additional trauma to tissues that may lack the ability to heal.

- Ring fixators—Ring fixators, including Ilizarov and hybrid fixators (which use half-pins on one side of the fracture and rings with wires on the other side), offer the same advantages of traditional external fixators. These fixators obtain fixation with wires passed through bone. The wires are then placed on tension and attached to a ring. The ring is then attached to the external fixation frame, which may consist of a single bar or multiple, smaller threaded rods. The bars are secured to half-pins inserted into the bone. The advantage of wires and rings is that they provide a relatively noninvasive means of fracture fixation, and obtain good fixation strength, particularly with metaphyseal proximal or distal tibia fractures. Ring fixators require more expertise than traditional external fixators do, but can be used to fix fractures that are more complex and fractures with intraarticular extension without spanning the associated joint (Fig. 11-4). Furthermore, the wires of these fixators do not loosen as quickly as the half-pins used with traditional external fixators,

so these fixators are useful for treating fractures that are likely to heal slowly.

3. Open reduction with internal fixation (ORIF)—ORIF is an excellent means by which to achieve stable fixation of a tibial shaft fracture and allow early postoperative motion. Successful healing is usually the rule. The chief risk of the procedure is wound-healing problems. In fractures with significant injury to the soft tissues of the leg, the use of a plate and screws may not be appropriate because the risk of wound-healing problems with this treatment may be too high. ***Severely traumatized legs with open tibial fractures (Gustilo type III) have a high incidence of wound-healing complications and deep infection when treated with ORIF.***

- Fracture fragments—When ORIF of a tibial fracture is performed, the surgeon must respect the biology and physiology of all of the tissues. ***It is unnecessary and unwise to attempt to reduce and stabilize every fracture fragment, since attempts to do this often require extensive dissection and periosteal stripping***. The result will be an attractive postoperative X-ray film of a tibia that lacks the ability to heal. It is preferable to obtain proper alignment and secure fixation of the proximal and distal tibia. The intervening bone fragments should be gently reduced with a dental pick, leaving their soft-tissue attachments alone so that they maintain their capacity to heal.

- Postoperative treatment—After ORIF of a tibial fracture, the incision should be closed over a suction drain and the leg splinted in neutral position to protect the soft tissues in the early healing phase. In 3 to 5 days, active motion of the knee and ankle should be initiated. Weightbearing should be prohibited until in the judgment of the surgeon, sufficient healing has occurred and the bone-plate construct can tolerate this. Often, a tibial fracture that has been treated with ORIF heals with minimal fracture callus (primary cortical healing). In these patients, a useful radiographic sign of fracture healing is "fading" or "blurring" of the fracture lines as new bone grows across the fracture line (Fig. 11-5) Weightbearing should begin with a protective orthosis, from which the patient can be weaned as healing nears completion and the patient becomes more comfortable.

A   B   C

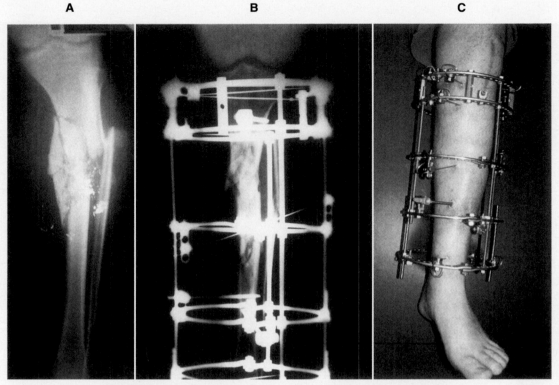

FIGURE 11-4   **A.** Anteroposterior X-ray film of a multifragmentary tibial shaft fracture caused by a gunshot wound. **B.** Postoperative X-ray film demonstrating excellent alignment achieved with an Ilizarov external fixator. **C.** Clinical photograph demonstrating minimal dissection of the skin in the fracture region.

- Minimally Invasive Plate Osteosynthesis (MIPO)—Techniques and devices have been developed that allow plate and screw fixation of tibial shaft fractures through small incisions and with limited dissection. This technique has the advantage of minimizing disruption of the peripheral blood supply to the bone, and potentially decreases wound healing problems. However, acceptable fracture reduction and stable fixation must be achieved if this technique is to be successful.
4. Intramedullary nailing
   - Advantages—Intramedullary nailing has emerged as the most popular method for stabilizing displaced tibial shaft fractures. The advantages of intramedullary nailing are that proper alignment of the fracture is not difficult to achieve and the intramedullary location of the nail makes it more resistant to fixation failure (Fig. 11-6). Intramedullary nails are inserted through incisions near the knee, so badly traumatized tissues in the mid-leg can be avoided. Placement of interlocking screws can be performed percutaneously through small incisions. The use of proximal and distal interlocking screws maintains proper length and rotation of even an unstable, comminuted fracture until healing has occurred.
   - Disadvantages—The main concern with intramedullary nailing is that placement of the nail in the intramedullary canal disrupts the endosteal circulation to the cortical bone. Certainly, this occurs, but its effect is short-lived (2 to 3 weeks), and it is probably not clinically significant.
   - Reaming
   (a) Advantages—Intramedullary reaming can be performed to enlarge the intramedullary canal and allow placement of a nail with a larger diameter. This achieves stronger fixation and may allow placement of interlocking screws with a larger diameter. This can be a very important step, since the interlocking screws of small diameter nails are the weak link in the fixation. Reaming before intramedullary nailing of closed tibia fractures reduces the rate of nonunion.
   (b) Disadvantages—Reaming of the tibial canal has raised concerns for two reasons.

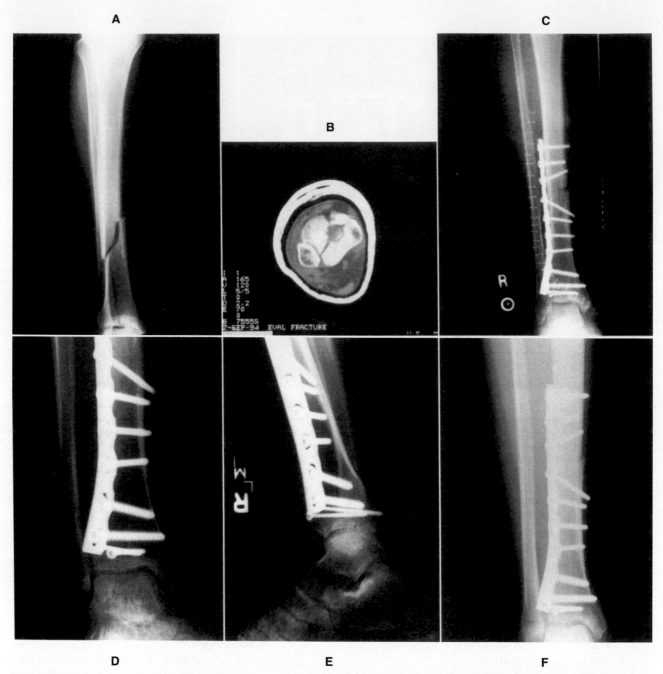

FIGURE 11-5   Anteroposterior X-ray film **(A)** demonstrating a tibial shaft fracture with extension into the weightbearing articular surface of the distal tibia. CT scan **(B)** demonstrating depression of the articular surface of the distal tibia. X-ray film **(C)** demonstrating good alignment of the tibia after ORIF. Anteroposterior **(D)** and lateral **(E)** X-ray films at 2 months show fading of the fracture lines, indicative of the healing process. Anteroposterior X-ray film **(F)** at 6 months shows complete healing of the tibial fracture in good alignment.

- Disruption of endosteal circulation—Reaming of the canal disrupts the endosteal circulation to a greater extent than passage of a smaller nail without reaming. Thus injuries that have already caused significant trauma to the periosteal (extramedullary) circulation such as the type IIIb open tibial fracture are at risk for suffering more damage to the circulation of the bone. There is animal study evidence that reamed intramedullary nailing causes more harm (***50% to 80% central cortical necrosis***) to the bony circulation than unreamed intramedullary nailing (***30% to 50% central cortical necrosis***). A practical compromise between strength of fixation and preservation of the osseous

A   B

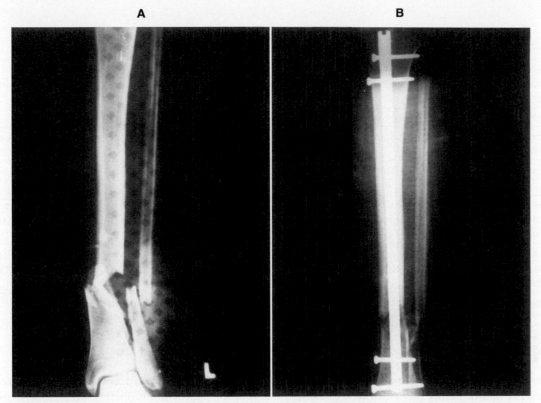

FIGURE 11-6   **A.** Anteriorposterior X-ray film demonstrating a displaced distal tibial shaft fracture. **B.** Postoperative X-ray film demonstrating good alignment after intramedullary nailing. The stability of the fixation is limited in this example because the intramedullary nail is much smaller than the distal intramedullary canal. This leg should be protected from weightbearing until significant healing has occurred.

circulation is "limited" reaming, whereby the reaming is performed to allow placement of a slightly larger-diameter nail and is discontinued when interference from the hard cortical bone ("chatter") occurs.

- Compartment syndrome—There has been concern that when reaming is performed within 2 or 3 days of injury, it increases the risk of compartment syndrome. There are several cases in which this has been reported, but is not clear whether the compartment syndrome resulted from prolonged intraoperative traction or from intramedullary reaming (if it is the result of either of these). The reported association, however, underlies the importance of postoperative examination of the extremity to detect and treat this complication as quickly as possible.

5. Amputation—Amputation is a consideration for a severe tibia fracture with associated neurologic, vascular and soft-tissue compromise. The LEAP study is a large-scale multi-centered prospective cohort study that compared function and psychological outcomes for those

patients with limb threatening leg injuries. The findings of the LEAP study are summarized in Table 11-2. The 2- and 7-year outcomes for patients treated with either limb reconstruction or amputation are similar. Significant disability occurs in most patients, whether they have been treated by limb salvage or by amputation. The LEAP study ***does not*** provide support for the concept that early primary amputation of a mangled extremity results in an improvement in patient function. Unless a patient is hemodynamically unstable secondary to his leg injury and amputation is a life-saving measure, immediate amputation should be avoided and a definitive treatment plan should be formulated only after thorough discussion with the patient and his family.

6. Flap coverage—Flap coverage becomes necessary if there is inadequate soft tissue to cover the bone, tendons, nerves, vessels, and orthopaedic hardware. The type of flap used depends on the location of the injury. ***Soft-tissue defects in the proximal third of the leg can be covered with a medial gastrocnemius muscle flap. Defects of the middle third of the leg***

TABLE 11-2

Findings of LEAP Study

When compared to population norms, patients who present to Level I trauma centers with mangled lower extremities are more extroverted, less agreeable, more likely to drink alcohol, more likely to smoke cigarettes and more likely to be blue collar, uninsured, neurotic and poor.
No injury severity scoring system provides valid predictive data for when to amputate.
The absence of plantar foot sensation on presentation is not predictive of function of the extremity or presence of foot sensation at 2 yr follow up.
Patients who sustain a mangled extremity have poor outcomes at 2 yr.
Patients continue to worsen between 2 yr and 7 yr follow up. Factors most associated with poor outcomes include older age, female gender, nonwhite race, lower level of education, current or previous smoking, living in a poor household, low self-efficacy, poor health status before the injury and involvement in the legal system for the purpose of obtaining disability.
Patients who underwent below knee amputation including those with free flap coverage functioned better than above knee amputations. Thru knee amputations had the poorest functional outcomes and required the highest energy expenditure to ambulate.
Patients treated with limb salvage have results comparable to patients treated with amputation.

can be covered with a soleus muscle flap. Defects of the distal third of the leg require a free vascularized muscle flap. A free vascularized flap may also be necessary for proximal or middle-third defects if the soleus or gastrocnemius muscles are injured and inappropriate for transfer. Alternatively, distally based sural island pedicle flaps can be tunneled subcutaneously to provide full-thickness coverage of small or medium sized tissue defects of the distal leg without necessitating suture anastomosis of the vessel or significant donor site morbidity. *Flap coverage should not be performed at the first debridement but in general should be performed within 1 week of injury.*

7. Negative Pressure Wound Therapy (NPWT)—Use of the VAC® or another negative pressure device to temporarily cover traumatic wounds allows controlled use of sub-atmospheric pressure (typically 125 mm Hg below ambient pressure) to a large surface of the wound, resulting in removal of hematoma and exudate, reduction of edema, and perhaps early granulation. In other parts of the body, NPWT has been associated with earlier wound closure, decreased infection, and fewer free flaps to cover wounds.

C. Antibiotics—Surgical treatment of closed tibial shaft fractures warrants antibiotic prophylaxis consisting of a first-generation cephalosporin administered intravenously before surgery and for 24 to 48 hours after surgery.

1. Gustilo type I and II open fractures—Gustilo type I and II open tibial shaft fractures require the same prophylaxis as closed tibial fractures treated surgically but the administration of antibiotics begins as soon as possible in the emergency room.

2. Gustilo type III open fractures—Type III open fractures require intravenous administration of a first-generation cephalosporin aimed at Gram-positive cocci, and an aminoglycoside or fluoroquinolone aimed at Gram-negative rods, beginning as soon as possible. Duration of postdebridement antibiotic prophylaxis is undergoing increased scrutiny, and recommendations range from 24 to 72 hours after debridement. The pre- and postoperative antibiotics are administered each time the patient undergoes operative debridement of the wound.

3. Contaminated or dirty fractures—If the open fracture occurs on a farm or if it is contaminated with dirt, intravenous penicillin should be added for prophylaxis against anaerobes. A patient who has sustained an open fracture in a swamp or another large body of water should be treated with a third generation cephalosporin to minimize the risk of *Aeromonas* infection.

4. Antibiotic-impregnated polymethylmethacralate (PMMA) beads—Some surgeons have reported excellent experience with antibiotic-impregnated PMMA beads, which are placed

in the traumatic wound after initial debridement and removed at the final debridement. This allows one to achieve a higher level of antibiotic (tobramycin or vancomycin) in the injured region than one could safely tolerate systemically (with intravenous antibiotics) and may lower the infection rate after open fracture. Antibiotics-impregnated PMMA beads should not be used alone in treating open fractures, since intravenous prophylaxis is still the gold standard.

D. Biologics—Research into the role of biologics to augment healing of tibia fractures has exploded over the last several years. Both osteoconductive and osteoinductive agents are available to fill segmental defects. **BMP-7 has been reported to be equivalent to autogenous bone grafting in the treatment of tibial nonunions**. However, no product on the market has been shown to be superior to autogenous bone grafting. In a large-scale clinical trial, BMP-2 was applied at the time of wound closure to open tibia fractures. It proved to decrease re-operation rates when used with unreamed tibial nails. In another study that combined data from new patients with patients from a previous study, there was no demonstrated benefit when applied in conjunction with reamed nailing.

VI. Anatomic Considerations and Surgical Techniques
A. External Fixation
1. Standard—Placement of external fixator half-pins should be performed perpendicular to the anteromedial surface of the tibia (i.e., at 45° to the sagittal plane) to obtain bicortical purchase and to avoid "burning" of the dense cortical tibial bone with the drill bit. The skin should be incised, and the subcutaneous tissues should be spread with a small clamp to avoid injury to the superficial structures, particularly the greater saphenous vein, which can be injured with placement of pins in the distal tibia. Predrilling the tract is strongly recommended before insertion of the external fixator pin.
2. Stability—The stability of fixation achieved with an external fixator can be increased by allowing the fracture ends to contact (the most important factor), increasing the diameter of the half-pins (the next most important factor, since stiffness is proportional to the fourth power of diameter), decreasing the distance between the bar and the bone (the stiffness of each pin is inversely proportional to the third power of the bone-to-bar distance), increasing

the distance between pins in each fragment of bone, and increasing the number of half-pins.
- Lag screws—Lag screws should not be used to supplement the external fixator because this will increase the risk of nonunion and refracture, probably as a result of the devitalization of bone performed in the process of reduction and screw fixation.
3. Hybrid fixation—The use of a ring fixator allows the placement of pins and wires in the metaphyseal bone of the tibial plateau and plafond. Precise knowledge of the local cross-sectional anatomy is necessary to prevent injury to the neurovascular structures.
4. Healing—Assessment of fracture healing in a patient treated in an external fixator is often very difficult. One clinical sign of fracture healing is painless weightbearing on the affected extremity, but this sign can be misleading. When in doubt, it is safest to "dynamize" the external fixator, which will result in higher axial load with weightbearing, and thus may stimulate further healing. Alternatively, the fixator can be removed and the patient prohibited from bearing weight until further healing has occurred.
B. ORIF
1. Timing—When ORIF is considered as a treatment option, careful assessment of the soft tissues is necessary to avoid incising through badly traumatized skin. Swelling of the leg increases for 2 or 3 days after the injury, so surgical timing is also critical. If ORIF cannot be performed within 6 to 8 hours after injury, it is best to wait until the swelling has subsided. Occasionally, one must wait 7 to 10 days, until the swelling and inflammation have subsided.
2. Approach—The incision should be longitudinal and approximately 1 cm lateral to the spine of the tibia. In the event of significant swelling during surgery, this incision allows tension-free approximation of the medial dermis to the tibialis anterior muscle, thereby providing coverage of the plate, neurovascular structures, and bone.
- Plate placement—If the surgeon chooses to place the plate on the lateral side of the tibia, the anterior compartment fascia should also be incised 1 cm lateral to the spine and the tibialis anterior muscle should be bluntly freed from the lateral tibial surface. The plate can also be placed on the anteromedial surface of the tibia, but medial plates cause more symptoms after the fracture has healed and require

elevation of the thin subcutaneous tissue layer from the tibia, which carries a risk of wound complications.

- Extension of the incision—The incision can be extended proximally, continuing just lateral to the tibial tuberosity, and even farther proximally as the lateral approach to the femur. For distal extension, the incision crosses the anteromedial ankle and continues to curve posteromedially along the medial malleolus, allowing exposure of the tibial plafond and medial malleolus. The extensor tendons will be visualized, but the tenosynovium should not be violated and should be repaired with suture if they are injured. Otherwise, in the event of a wound breakdown, the tendons will be exposed to the environment and will be less resistant to bacterial contamination and infection.

3. Technical details

- Contouring—Proper contouring of the plate is essential to achieve proper alignment of a tibial shaft fracture. The majority of the lateral surface is straight, but its distal surface rotates anteriorly. Thus the plate may require a twist distally to match the tibial surface and to avoid the distal tibiofibular articulation. The medial surface is flared proximally and distally; if this is not taken into consideration with proper plate contouring, the tibia will be stabilized in valgus malalignment.

- Large-fragment screws and plates—ORIF of tibial shaft fractures should be performed using large-fragment (4.5-mm cortical and 6.5 mm cancellous) screws and plates. The narrow plates have sufficient strength for the tibia. At least six cortices of screw purchase are necessary on each side of the fracture to achieve stable fixation and permit early postoperative knee and ankle motion.

- Lag screws—Lag-screw placement to achieve interfragmental compression is useful with simple fractures if it can be performed without significant elevation of the periosteum from the bone. Multifragmentary fractures, however, should not be treated with lag screws because the additional trauma to the osseous circulation far outweighs the benefit of the additional fixation. Multifragmentary tibial shaft fractures treated with ORIF should be reduced with traction and the comminuted pieces then gently reduced with a dental pick, taking care to preserve all soft-tissue attachments to the bone. The plate is then secured

proximally and distally, leaving the intervening fragments free and "loose" but with the best capacity to heal.

- Locked plating—Fixed angle plates should be used judiciously in the tibial diaphysis. **Osteoporotic fractures** benefit from the additional fixation strength afforded by the plate with locking screws, which function as a fixed angle device. Fractures with a zone of **segmental comminution** are effectively stabilized using a locked plate applied in a bridge fashion.

C. Intramedullary Nailing

1. Approach—Intramedullary nailing can be performed with the nail placed medial or lateral to the patella tendon, or through a patella tendon splitting incision. Placement of the nail with the patella tendon-splitting approach is straightforward and fairly easy, but one should avoid this temptation, since it could contribute to patella tendon symptoms. Whichever position for nail placement is chosen, the approach is through a midline or parapatellar incision. As the incision is extended through the subcutaneous tissue, the margin of the patella tendon should be noted and the retinaculum incised next to this. An awl or a guide wire is then inserted in the center of the proximal tibia at the "corner" where the anterior border of the tibia meets the plateau. Anteroposterior and lateral radiographic (fluoroscopic) confirmation of correct positioning and aim is helpful before proceeding. Next, the awl, a drill, or a cannulated cutting tool is used to create a hole in the proximal tibia. This is performed most easily if the knee is flexed 90° or more, which can be achieved with a bolster, with a metallic triangle designed for this purpose, or with a fracture table.

2. Reaming—If reaming is to be performed, a ball-tipped guide wire must be advanced across the fracture before reaming. Passage of the guide wire is easiest if the fracture can be reduced to anatomic alignment. If anatomic reduction of the fracture is difficult to achieve by closed methods, then placement of a curve near the tip of the wire will make wire passage easier. The wire should be advanced to the center of the distal tibial metaphysis, as confirmed by fluoroscopy. **A tourniquet should not be used during the reaming process because this may allow the reamer to burn the bone.** Reaming is performed with successively larger reamers until the interference of

the cortical bone occurs, which is evident by a "chattering" sound. Reaming beyond this point is seldom necessary and may result in thermal necrosis of the bone. The tibial nail diameter should be 1.5 to 2 mm smaller than the diameter of the last reamer. The length of the tibial nail is best determined before surgery by using fluoroscopy and a radiopaque ruler on the contralateral extremity. Alternatively, one may measure the length of the guide wire that protrudes from the intramedullary canal and subtract this figure from the length of the guide wire to determine nail length. The latter technique, however, can be misleading if the fracture has many fragments and is shortened.

3. Unreamed nailing—The surgeon may choose to insert the intramedullary nail without reaming. If a cannulated nail is available, a smooth guide wire is passed across the fracture and into the center of the distal tibial metaphysis and the nail is advanced over the wire. Maintaining manual reduction of the fracture will facilitate advancement of the nail into the distal fragment. Solid (noncannulated) nails require vigilant surveillance as the nail is advanced into the distal tibia to ensure that it passes in the center of the bone. Otherwise a "nail tunnel" is created in the incorrect position, complicating subsequent attempts at nail passage and decreasing the stability of fixation.

4. Interlocking screws—Placement of proximal interlocking screws is best achieved using the drill guides attached to the nail assembly. Distal interlocking screws can be placed using a variety of methods. The "free-hand" technique is very versatile but requires a sharp drill bit and a steady hand. The first step is to adjust the position of the leg and the beam of the fluoroscope until the beam passes through the center of the hole, which is confirmed by the presence of "perfect circle" on the fluoroscope. At the medial aspect of the distal tibia, a small, longitudinal incision is made centered at this point. The subcutaneous tissues are dissected bluntly with a small clamp. *If the saphenous vein is cut, it should be ligated or repaired*. Next, the tip of the drill bit is placed on the bone and the position adjusted until it is in the center of the circle by fluoroscopy. Without moving the tip of the drill bit from this point, the surgeon then aims the drill in the axis of the fluoroscope ray and drills through the near cortex.

At this point, the surgeon should detach the drill from the drill bit and confirm proper direction of the drill bit using fluoroscopy. The drill bit is then advanced through the nail and through the far cortex. The drill is removed and a depth gauge inserted through the holes to determine screw length. Fluoroscopic confirmation that the depth gauge actually passes through the nail should be obtained before screw placement. Next, the appropriate-sized screw is advanced across the bone, and the proper position is again confirmed before a second screw is placed in the same manner.

5. Proximal and distal fractures—Juxta-articular fractures present a technical challenge. Fractures of the proximal tibial shaft are notorious for resisting proper reduction. Typically, the fracture has apex-anterior angulation with a large anterior step (translation) at the anterior cortex. Valgus malalignment is also common. Multiple techniques exist to attempt to address this deformity. A more lateral entry point (i.e., lateral parapatellar) can be used in order to prevent valgus positioning of the reamers. The leg may be maintained in a semi-extended position over the course of reaming to maintain an anterior trajectory for the nail. Metadiaphyseal tibial shaft fractures that have been treated by intramedullary nailing often have marginal fixation strength, since the nail itself offers little resistance to motion from the large, cancellous proximal tibial canal. Some authors have reported excellent alignment of these fractures after using a small fragment plate and screws to obtain provisional reduction and stabilization of the fracture and then placing the intramedullary nail.

If a proximal tibia shaft fracture has been nailed and the reduction is unacceptable, the alignment can be improved by removing the proximal drill guide assembly from the nail, and applying an extension and varus force to the leg to correct the alignment. The proximal interlocking screws are then placed with the freehand technique.

Others have described the use of *Poller or blocking screws* to reestablish an intramedullary canal that better fits the nail. This technique requires thoughtful placement of screws to block the nail from following an undesirable trajectory (Fig. 11-7). Additional reduction aids include drilling schantz pins into the metaphyseal fragment to provide percutaneous control of the fragment.

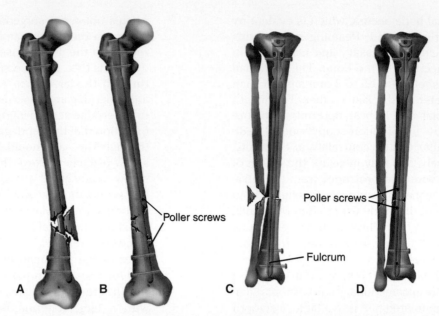

<u>FIGURE 11-7</u> With the aid of Poller screws malalignments can be prevented or corrected, while stability is simultaneously increased. **A.** Example of a distal femoral fracture: Due to the large discrepancy between medullary canal and nail diameter, the intramedullary nail may move a few millimeters sideways along the interlocking screws, which results in varus or valgus deformity. **B.** Placement of one (distal) or two (distal and proximal) Poller screws prevents malalignment and increases stability. **C.** Example of a distal tibial fracture: Despite the presence of an AP screw, displacement in the coronal plane can occur in cases of short distal fragments or poor bone stock. The AP screw acts as a fulcrum in these cases. **D.** Closed reduction and either unilateral or bilateral support with Poller screws placed bicortically in the sagittal plane prevents angulation in the coronal plane. (Redrawn with permission from Rüedi TP, Buckley RE, Moran CG. *AO Principles of Fracture Management.* Dübendorf, Switzerland: AO Foundation Publications; 2007.)

If operative assistance is limited, a femoral distractor can be applied to maintain the fracture reduction while instrumentation proceeds.

Proximal tibial shaft fractures that have been treated by intramedullary nailing often have marginal fixation strength, as the nail itself receives little resistance to motion from the large, cancellous proximal tibial canal. In these cases, the fracture should be protected with a hinged knee brace or knee immobilizer when the patient is not performing active knee range-of-motion exercises.

VII. Complications of the Injury
  A. Compartment Syndrome—Perhaps the most significant complication of a tibial shaft fracture is compartment syndrome. As discussed earlier, it is essential to rule this out early and to perform serial physical examinations. If compartment syndrome is diagnosed, emergent four-compartment fasciotomy should be performed and delayed wound closure planned. There are several means by which fasciotomy of the four leg compartments can be carried

out. The two-incision technique uses a medial longitudinal incision 1.5 cm posterior to the posteromedial crest of the tibia and a lateral longitudinal incision 1.5 cm anterior to the fibula. ***Through the medial incision, the deep posterior and superficial posterior compartments can be incised through their entire length. The lateral incision allows release of the anterior and lateral compartments of the leg.*** Some surgeons favor performing release of all four leg compartments through a single lateral incision, which is technically more difficult but preserves the medial skin.
  B. Deep Infection—The incidence of deep infection should be less than 1% with closed fractures but is higher in open fractures and can be as high as 25% to 50% with Gustilo type IIIb open tibial fractures. Treatment can be extremely complex and time consuming but is based on ***debridement*** of nonviable bone and tissue, ***dilution*** of bacteria with successive irrigations and debridements in the operating room, maintenance of the ***stability*** of the bone, and eradication of bacteria with long-term intravenous ***antibiotics*** directed at the causative organisms. ***Secondary closure***

of the wound is necessary to cover the bone, metallic implants, and neurovascular structures with healthy tissue. Rotational flaps or vascularized pedicle flap grafts are used for coverage if necessary. Bony reconstructive procedures are performed when the infection is cleared.

C. Vascular Injury—Tibial fractures with associated vascular injuries can result in widespread necrosis of the extremity tissue, necessitating amputation of the extremity if the arterial injury is not recognized and treated quickly.

D. Malreduction/Malalignment—Malreduction of a fracture treated nonoperatively can usually be predicted based on the initial X-ray films of the leg. *Tibial fractures with significant displacement, shortening, comminution, or an intact fibula are prone to malunions when treated nonoperatively. Operative management of these fractures decreases the risk of malunion*. Likewise, tibial fractures with associated fibular fractures at the same level are highly unstable. Maintaining anatomic alignment may be extremely difficult or impossible with these fractures. Thus a thorough assessment of the patient's needs and the fracture characteristics is essential to determine how much angulation can be accepted and to determine which fractures will benefit from surgical stabilization.

VIII. Complications of Treatment

A. Knee Pain—*The most common complication of intramedullary nailing of the tibia is anterior knee pain*. As many as 57% of patients complain of some knee discomfort in long term follow up. Careful assessment of the starting point and protection of the soft tissues during reaming minimizes trauma to the patella tendon and fat pad. Always *confirm appropriate nail position with a lateral fluoroscopic view at the knee to ensure that the nail is not protruding from the bone*.

B. Wound-Healing Problems—Problems with wound healing can be a devastating consequence of a tibial shaft fracture. Thorough assessment of the condition of the skin and soft tissues before making any incision is necessary to minimize the occurrence of this complication. If there is any concern about the healing capacity of the tissues due to significant contusion, fracture blisters, or decreased capillary perfusion, an incision should not be made and stabilization, if necessary, should be performed using external fixation. Wound-healing problems are treated locally with soft-tissue debridement and dressing changes until healing has

occurred. If the bone, a metallic implant, or a neurovascular structure lacks soft-tissue coverage in the wound, flap coverage is necessary. Tendons exposed in the wound may be treated with negative pressure wound therapy or dressing changes if the tenosynovium is intact and viable.

C. Osteomyelitis—Osteomyelitis is an uncommon but severe complication that can occur from operative stabilization of a tibial fracture. The incidence is approximately 1% with closed fractures but can be as high as 25% to 50 % with type IIIb open fractures. Treatment requires thorough debridement of all devitalized soft tissue and bone, maintenance of stability with internal or external fixation, soft-tissue coverage, and long-term (4- to 8-week) administration of appropriate intravenous antibiotics.

D. Compartment Syndrome—Compartment syndrome has been described as a complication of reamed intramedullary nailing of tibial shaft fractures. This complication has been reported after prolonged intraoperative traction applied to a leg with a fracture table. Compartment syndrome may also result from the underlying trauma, regardless of the operative intervention performed. In any event, routine postoperative clinical examination is necessary to detect and treat this complication early. *Epidural anesthesia during surgery may compromise the patient's clinical findings postoperatively, thereby making compartment syndrome more difficult, if not impossible, to diagnose by the patient's symptoms and clinical examination*.

IX. Nonunions—Like most other complications of tibial shaft fractures, nonunion occurs more frequently as the severity of the fracture increases. *Transverse fractures, open fractures, fractures with more than 3 mm of distraction after intramedullary nailing, and fractures with less than 50% cortical contact after stabilization have higher rates of reoperation to achieve union*.

Consensus has not been reached for the definition of *nonunion*, but a practical definition is a tibial fracture that in the judgment of the treating Orthopaedic Surgeon has not healed and lacks the ability to heal without specific intervention. There are several common scenarios in which nonunion occurs, and it is important to identify the scenario so that correct treatment can be delivered.

A. Infected Nonunion—Before performing surgery for any tibial nonunion, the treating orthopaedist must consider and rule out infection. The preoperative studies should include a white blood cell count, erythrocyte sedimentation rate and C reactive protein. When these laboratory indices are evaluated in combination, they have the highest sensitivity in detecting bone infections. The practical importance is that a formal irrigation and debridement must be performed if infection is present. Bone graft and bone graft substitute should not be implanted until the infection is treated.

B. Inadequate Stability—If gross motion is present, bone will have difficulty in bridging across a fracture. This scenario most often presents as a hypertrophic nonunion, with bone forming on each side of the fracture but not uniting the fracture. These fractures require mechanical stability to heal. Of course, infection must be ruled out, and the surgery that is undertaken to provide stability should not devitalize the bone. Most hypertrophic nonunions do not require bone grafting to heal, but if a large bony defect is present, bone grafting should be considered in order to decrease the healing time.

C. Poor Capacity to Heal—An atrophic nonunion is a fracture nonunion in which the bone ends produce minimal, if any, bone. This may result from significant devitalization of tissue as a result of the injury (e.g., highly comminuted fractures), poor perfusion of the tissues (e.g., peripheral vascular disease), or poor patient health. These nonunions require bone grafting to supplement the patient's deficient fracture healing capacity and require a stable environment as well. It may be recognized early in the treatment of a fracture that it has a poor capacity to heal. Early prophylactic bone grafting of these "impending nonunions," when performed judiciously, decreases the healing time of complex fractures. *Most surgeons wait until 6 weeks after the injury before performing prophylactic bone grafting of high-energy open tibial shaft fractures*.

D. Nonunion after External Fixation—Nonunions of tibial shaft fractures that have been treated with external fixators represent an interesting dilemma. The strongest means of fixation for these fractures is intramedullary nailing, but this has been associated with an unacceptably high infection rate, particularly when the external fixator has been in place for more than 2 weeks and when the external fixation has been complicated by a pin tract infection. A better alternative is ORIF (plate and screw fixation) with bone grafting when necessary, which has been associated with an excellent healing rate (>90%) and a low infection rate (3% to 6%).

Nonunion presenting as plate breakage is the most common serious complication of this procedure.

E. Nonunion after Intramedullary Nailing—Nonunions of tibial shaft fractures that were initially treated with intramedullary nailing can be managed in a number of ways. Removing proximal or distal interlocking screws to "dynamize" a nail (increase the transmission of force across a fracture) is frequently used. This is a low-risk procedure, but the scientific evidence showing a benefit to this procedure does not exist. When a hypertrophic nonunion is present, the optimal treatment is "exchange nailing," in which the nail is removed, the tibia is reamed, and a larger and stiffer intramedullary nail is placed. The fracture benefits from the improved stability of the larger nail and perhaps from the bone graft created and the "stimulation" to healing created by the reaming.

X. Deformities
A. Malunion—Malunion refers to a fracture that has healed in an unacceptable position. A tibial malunion can have an unacceptable position in the coronal plane (varus/valgus), the sagittal plane (recurvatum, procurvatum), axial length (shortening/distraction), axial rotation (internal/external rotation), or any combination of these. The patient's tolerance for deformity varies, depending on activity level, associated deformities, ability to compensate, and individual expectations. A symptomatic malunion is one that affects a patient's walking ability or that causes pain in an associated joint. Coronal plane, sagittal plane, axial rotation, and axial lengthening malunion can be corrected with an osteotomy and stabilization using internal fixation, intramedullary nailing, or external fixation (Fig. 11-8). Symptomatic axial shortening can be corrected with an osteotomy and distraction using an external fixator. Predictably better healing can be achieved with an osteotomy and shortening of the contralateral extremity, but this may be unacceptable to some patients.

XI. Special Considerations
A. Periprosthetic Fractures—Closed treatment or ORIF is the most viable treatment option for tibial shaft fractures distal to a total knee arthroplasty. Treatment depends on the needs of the patient and the requirements of the fracture. External fixation, in general, should be avoided because it has a fairly high risk of pin tract infection, which theoretically could spread infection to the prosthetic joint. Tibial shaft fractures in the proximity

A   B   C

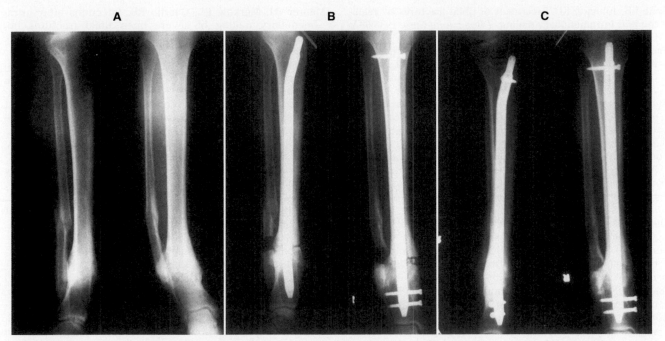

FIGURE 11-8 **A.** Lateral and anteroposterior X-ray films of a tibia following an open fracture that has healed in more than 20° of varus malalignment, causing ankle pain. **B.** After partial excision of the fibula and a tibial osteotomy, this fracture was stabilized with an intramedullary nail. A portion of the excised fibula was used as bone graft. **C.** Lateral and anteroposterior X-ray film 8 months after surgery, demonstrating excellent alignment and healing. The patient is now asymptomatic.

of a loose prosthetic joint can, in certain cases, be treated with a long-stem revision arthroplasty, with the stem of the prosthesis stabilizing the fracture. This treatment, however, is more acceptable for tibial metaphyseal fractures than for tibial shaft fractures.

B. Floating Knee—Ipsilateral femur and tibia fractures are commonly referred to as a **floating knee**. When treated nonoperatively, these injuries result in an unacceptable rate of malunion and knee stiffness. The femur fracture demands operative stabilization. Although many of the associated tibial fractures would heal nicely with nonoperative treatment, it is best to stabilize the tibia at the time of femur fracture stabilization (if the patient's medical condition will safely tolerate both procedures). If only one bone can be stabilized because of the patient's medical condition, the femur should be stabilized to facilitate mobilization (therefore the surgeon always begins by fixing the femur first in case the operation must be terminated prematurely as a result of intraoperative medical complications). Stabilization of both the femur and the tibia improves patient comfort and eliminates the need for long leg immobilization of the extremity, thereby facilitating knee rehabilitation and improving patient mobility.

C. Pathologic Fractures—Pathologic fractures of the tibial shaft are uncommon. If after obtaining a tissue diagnosis, the surgeon believes that limb amputation is not necessary, the fracture should be stabilized. Intramedullary nailing is the strongest and most practical fixation method, and should be used if possible. Postoperative radiation therapy or chemotherapy can be initiated when sufficient skin healing has occurred, which is generally 5 days after surgery.

SUGGESTED READINGS

Classic Articles

Bach AW, Hansen ST Jr. Plates versus external fixation in severe open tibial fractures: a randomized trial. *Clin Orthop.* 1989;241:89–94.

Behrens F, Johnson W. Unilateral external fixation: method to increase and reduce frame stiffness. *Clin Orthop.* 1989;241:48–56.

Behrens F, Johnson WD, Koch TW, et al. Bending stiffness of unilateral and bilateral fixator frames. *Clin Orthop.* 1983;178:103–110.

Blick SS, Brumback RJ, Lakatos R, et al. Early prophylactic bone grafting of high-energy tibial fractures. *Clin Orthop.* 1989;240:21–41.

Blick SS, Brumback RJ, Poka A, et al. Compartment syndrome in open tibial fractures. *J Bone Joint Surg.* 1986;68A:1348–1353.

Bone LB, Johnson KD. Treatment of tibial fractures by reaming and intramedullary nailing. *J Bone Joint Surg.* 1986;68A: 877–887.

Brumback RJ, Jones AL. Interobserver agreement in the classification of open fractures of the tibia: the results of a survey of two hundred and forty-five orthopaedic surgeons. *J Bone Joint Surg.* 1994;76A:1162–1166.

Burgess AR, Poka A, Brumback RJ, et al. Management of open grade III tibial fractures. *Orthop Clin North Am.* 1987;18:85–93.

Caudle RJ, Stern PJ. Severe open fractures of the tibia. *J Bone Joint Surg.* 1987;69:801–807.

Connolly JF, ed. *Tibial Nonunion.* Park Ridge, IL: American Academy of Orthopaedic Surgeons; 1991.

Court-Brown CM, Keating JF, McQueen MM. Infection after intramedullary nailing of the tibia: Incidence and protocol for management. *J Bone Joint Surg.* 1992;74B:770–774.

Ellis H. The speed of healing after fracture of the tibial shaft. *J Bone Joint Surg.* 1958;40B:42–46.

Gershuni DH, Mubarck SJ, Yaru NC, et al. Fracture of the tibia complicated by acute compartment syndrome. *Clin Orthop.* 1987;217:221–227.

Godina M. Early microsurgical reconstruction of complex trauma of the extremities. *Plast Reconstr Surg.* 1986;78:285–292.

Gordon L, Chiu EJ. Treatment of infected non-unions and segmental defects of the tibia with staged microvascular transplantation and bone-grafting. *J Bone Joint Surg.* 1988;70A:377–386.

Harmon PH. A simplified posterior approach to the tibia for bone-grafting and fibula transference. *J Bone Joint Surg.* 1945;27A:496.

Heckman JD, Ryaby JP, McCabe J, et al. Acceleration of tibial fracture-healing by non-invasive, low-intensity pulsed ultrasound. *J Bone Joint Surg.* 1994;76A:26–34.

Helfet DL, Jupiter JB, Gasser S. Indirect reduction and tension-band plating of tibial non-union with deformity. *J Bone Joint Surg.* 1992;74A:1279–1285.

Holbrook JL, Swiontkowski MF, Sanders R. Treatment of open fractures of the tibial shaft: ender nailing versus external fixation—A randomized prospective comparison. *J Bone Joint Surg.* 1989;71A:1231–1238.

Hooper GJ, Keddell RG, Penny ID. Conservative management or closed nailing for tibial shaft fractures: a randomised prospective trial. *J Bone Joint Surg.* 1991;73B:83–85.

Howard PW, Makin GS. Lower limb fractures with associated vascular injuries. *J Bone Joint Surg.* 1990;72B:116–120.

Johansen K, Helfet DH, Howey T, et al. Objective criteria accurately predict amputation following lower extremity trauma. *J Trauma.* 1990;30:568–572.

Johner R, Wruhs O. Classification of tibial shaft fractures and correlation with results after rigid internal fixation, *Clin Orthop.* 1983;178:7–25.

Johnson EE, Marder RA. Open intramedullary nailing and bone-grafting for non-union of tibial diaphyseal fracture. *J Bone Joint Surg.* 1987;69A:375–380.

Karlstrom G, Olerud S. Fractures of the tibial shaft: a critical evaluation of treatment alternatives. *Clin Orthop.* 1974;105:82–115.

Kettelkamp D, Hillberry BM, Murrish DE, et al. Degenerative arthritis of the knee secondary to fracture malunion, *Clin Orthop.* 1988;234:159–169.

Klemm KW, Borner M. Interlocking nailing of complex fractures of the femur and tibia. *Clin Orthop.* 1986;212:89–100.

Lange RH, Bach AW, Hansen ST Jr, et al. Open tibial fractures with associated vascular injuries: prognosis for limb salvage. *J Trauma.* 1985;25:203–208.

Maurer DJ, Merkow RL, Gusrilo RB. Infections after intramedullary nailing of severe open tibial fractures initially treated with external fixation. *J Bone Joint Surg.* 1989;71A:835–838.

McGraw JM, Lim EV. Treatment of open tibial-shaft fractures: external fixation and secondary intramedullary nailing. *J Bone Joint Surg.* 1988;70A:900–911.

McQueen MM, Christie J, Court-Brown CM. Compartment pressures after intramedullary nailing of the tibia. *J Bone Joint Surg.* 1990;72B:395–397.

Nicoll EA. Fractures of the tibial shaft: a survey of 705 cases. *J Bone Joint Surg.* 1964;46B:373–387.

Ostermann PA, Seligson D, Henry SL. Local antibiotic therapy for severe open fractures: a review of 1085 consecutive cases. *J Bone Joint Surg.* 1995;77B:93–97.

Paley D, Catagni MA, Argnani F, et al. Ilizarov treatment of tibial nonunions with bone loss. *Clin Orthop.* 1989;241: 146–165.

Paré A. The classic: compound fracture of the leg. Paré's personal care. *Clin Orthop.* 1983;178:3–6.

Patzakis MJ, Wilkins J, Tillman MM. Considerations in reducing the infection rate in open tibial fractures. *Clin Orthop.* 1983;178:36–41.

Patzakis MJ, Wilkins J, Wiss DA. Infection following intramedullary nailing of long bones: diagnosis and management. *Clin Orthop.* 1986;212:182–191.

Puno RM, Teynor JT, Nagano J, et al. Critical analysis of results of treatment of 201 tibial shaft fractures. *Clin Orthop.* 1987;212:213–219.

Rhinelander FW. Tibial blood supply in relation to fracture healing. *Clin Orthop.* 1974;105:34–81.

Rüedi TH, Webb JK, Allgöwer M. Experience with a dynamic compression plate (DCP) in 418 recent fractures of the tibial shaft. *Injury.* 1976;7:252–257.

Sarmiento A, Gersten LM, Sobol PA, et al. Tibial shaft fractures treated with functional braces: experience with 780 fractures. *J Bone Joint Surg.* 1989;71B:602–609.

Sarmiento A, Sobol PA, Sew Hoy AL, et al. Prefabricated functional braces for the treatment of fractures of die tibial diaphysis. *J Bone Joint Surg.* 1984;66A:1328–1339.

Sarmiento A. A functional below-the-knee brace for tibial fractures. *J Bone Joint Surg.* 1970;52A:295–311.

Schwartsman V, Martin SN, Ronquist RA, et al. Tibia fractures: the Ilizarov alternative. *Clin Orthop.* 1992;278:207–216.

Segal D, Brenner M, Gorczyca J. Tibial fractures with infrapopliteal arterial injuries. *J Orthop Trauma.* 1987;1:160-169.

Sledge SL, Johnson KD, Henley MB, et al. Intramedullary nailing with reaming to treat non-union of the tibia. *J Bone Joint Surg.* 1989;71A:1004–1019.

Takami H, Doi T, Takahashi S, et al. Reconstruction of a large tibial defect with a free vascularized fibular graft. *Arch Orthop Trauma Surg.* 1984;102:203–205.

Teitz CC, Carter DR, Frankel VH. Problems associated with tibial fractures with intact fibulae. *J Bone Joint Surg.* 1980;62A:770–776.

Tornetta P 3rd, Bergman M, Watnik N, et al. Treatment of grade-IIIb open tibial fractures: a prospective randomised comparison of external fixation and non-reamed locked nailing. *J Bone Joint Surg.* 1994;76B:13–19.

Veith RG, Winquist RA, Hansen ST Jr. Ipsilateral fractures of the femur and tibia: a report of fifty-seven consecutive cases. *J Bone Joint Surg.* 1984;66A:991–1002.

Weiland AJ, Moore JR, Hotchkiss RN. Soft tissue procedures for reconstruction of tibial shaft fractures. *Clin Orthop.* 1983;178:42–53.

Whittle AP, Russell TA, Taylor JC, et al. Treatment of open fractures of the tibial shaft with the use of interlocking nailing without reaming. *J Bone Joint Surg.* 1992;74A:1162–1171.

Wiss DA, Johnson DL, Miao M. Compression plating for nonunion after failed external fixation of open tibial fractures. *J Bone Joint Surg.* 1992;74A:1279–1285.

Yaremchuk MJ, Brumback RJ, Manson PN, et al. Acute and definitive management of traumatic osteocutaneous defects of the lower extremity. *Plast Reconstr Surg.* 1987;80:1–14.

Recent Articles

Brinker MR, Caines MA, Kerstein MD, et al. Tibial shaft fractures with an associated infrapopliteal arterial injury: a survey of vascular surgeons' opinions on the need for vascular repair. *J Orthop Trauma.* 2000;14(3):194–198.

Brinker MR, Cook SD, Dunlap JN, et al. Early changes in nutrient artery blood flow following tibial nailing with and without reaming: a preliminary study. *J Orthop Trauma.* 1999;13(2):129–133.

Brinker MR, O'Connor DP. Exchange nailing of ununited fractures. *J Bone Joint Surg Am.* 2007;89:177–188.

Felix NA, Stuart MJ, Hanssen AD. Periprosthetic fractures of the tibia associated with total knee arthroplasty. *Clin Orthop.* 1997;345:113–124.

Heckman JD, Ryaby JP, McCabe J, et al. Acceleration of tibial fracture-healing by non-invasive, low-intensity pulsed ultrasound. *J Bone Joint Sarg.* 1994;76A:26–34.

Hupel TM, Aksenov SA, Schcmitsch EH. Effect of limited and standard reaming on cortical blood flow and strength of union following segmental fracture. *J Orthop Trauma.* 1998;12:400–406.

Keating JF, O'Brien PI, Blachut PA, et al. Reamed interlocked intramedullary nailing of open fractures of the tibia. *Clin Orthop.* 1997;338:182–191.

Konrath G, Moed BR, Watson TJ, et al. Intramedullary nailing of unstable diaphyseal fractures of the tibia with distal intraarticular involvement. *J Orthop Trauma.* 1997;3:200–205.

Leunig M, Hertel R. Thermal necrosis after tibial reaming for intramedullary nail fixation: a report of three cases. *J Bone Joint Surg.* 1996;78B:584–587.

Moed BR, Kim EC, van Holsbeeck M, et al. Ultrasound for die early diagnosis of tibial fracture healing after static interlocked nailing without reaming: histologic correlation using a canine model. *J Orthop Trauma.* 1998;12:200–205.

Moed BR, Subramian S, van Holsbeeck M, et al. Ultrasound for the early diagnosis of tibial fracture healing after static interlocked nailing without reaming: clinical results. *J Orthop Trauma.* 1998;12:206–213.

Takami H, Takahashi S, Ando M, et al. Vascularized fibular grafts for the reconstruction of segmental tibial defects. *Arch Orthop Trauma Surg.* 1997;116:404–407.

Review Articles

Brumback RJ. Open tibial fractures: current orthopaedic management. *Instr Course Lect.* 1992;41:101–117.

Gustilo RB, Merkow RL, Templeman D. Current concepts review: the management of open fractures. *J Bone Joint Surg.* 1990;72A:299–303.

Littenberg B, Weinstein LP, McCarren M, et al. Closed fractures of the tibial shaft: a meta-analysis of three methods of treatment. *J Bone Joint Surg.* 1998;80A:174–183.

Melvin JS, Dombroski DG, Torbert JT, et al. Open tibial shaft fractures: I. Evaluation and initial wound management. *J Am Acad Orthop Surg.* 2010;18(1):10–19.

Melvin JS, Dombroski DG, Torbert JT, et al. Open tibial shaft fractures: II. Definitive management and limb salvage. *J Am Acad Orthop Surg.* 2010;18(2):108–117.

Textbooks

Chapman MW. Fractures of the tibia and fibula. In: Chapman MW, ed. *Operative Onhopaedics.* Philadelphia, PA: JB Lippincott; 1988.

Shuler FD, Obremskey WT. Tibial shaft fractures. In: Stannard JP, Schmidt AH, Kregor PJ, eds. *Surgical Treatment of Orthopaedic Trauma.* New York, NY: Thieme Medical Publishers, Inc.; 2007.

The American College of Surgeons Committee on Trauma. Biomechanics of injury. In: *Advanced Trauma Life Support for Doctors: Instructor Course Manual.* 6th ed. Chicago: First Impression; 1997:411–438.

Tile M. Fractures of the tibia. In: Schatzker J, Tile M, eds. *The Rationale of Operative Fracture Care.* New York, NY: Springer-Verlag; 1996.

Trafton PG. Tibial shaft fractures. In: Browner BD, Jupiter JB, Levine AM, et al, eds. *Skeletal Trauma.* Philadelphia, PA: WB Saunders; 1998.

Tschcrne H, Gotzen L. *Fractures Associated with Soft Tissue Injuries.* New York, NY: Springer-Verlag; 1984.

CHAPTER 12

Fractures of the Tibial Plafond

Mark R. Brinker and Daniel P. O'Connor

I. Overview
   A. Definition—Intraarticular fracture of the distal end of the tibia, also known as a ***tibial pilon*** fracture, involves disruption of the distal tibial weightbearing articular surface. It represents a wide spectrum of injury severity and accounts for approximately 5% to 7% of all tibia fractures and less than 1% of all lower-extremity fractures. These injuries are distinctly different from ankle fractures. Anatomic areas injured include the weightbearing articular surface of the distal tibia (epiphysis) and the distal tibial metaphysis, as well as the distal fibula (injured in approximately 75% of cases) and, sometimes, diaphyseal extension into the tibial shaft.
   B. Mechanism of Injury—Most commonly, the mechanism of injury is axial loading, but it may be rotation (shear loading) or a combination of axial loading and rotation. Axial loading injuries generally result in greater disruption of the articular surface (than rotational injuries) and commonly occur as a result of a fall from a height or a motor-vehicle accident; pure rotational injuries are lower-energy injuries that result in a lesser degree of articular cartilage disruption. (These injuries commonly occur as a result of a ski accident.) The direction of force applied to the distal tibia and the position of the foot and ankle at the time of injury determine the injury pattern.
      1. Axial loading while the ankle is plantar flexed—Posterior articular comminution predominates.
      2. Axial loading while the ankle is dorsiflexed—Anterior articular comminution predominates.
      3. Shear forces (rotational)—Shear forces result in a wide array of injury patterns.

II. Evaluation
   A. Clinical Presentation—Signs and symptoms include an inability to bear weight, marked pain, marked swelling, and evidence of soft tissue injury.
   B. Physical Examination
      1. Neurovascular examination—The neurovascular examination includes evaluation of the distal pulses and capillary refill, a motor examination, and a sensory examination.
      2. Soft tissues
         • Closed fractures—Closed fractures may be classified using the method of Tscherne.
         • Open fractures—Open fractures may be classified using the method of Gustilo.
   C. Imaging
      1. Plain radiographs—Plain radiographs show the extent of damage to the weightbearing articular surface. Anteroposterior (AP), lateral, and mortise views of the ankle are taken. AP and lateral views of the tibial shaft are obtained to assess for diaphyseal extension. Complementary views of the opposite ankle may also be helpful for comparisons.
      2. CT scanning (Fig. 12-1)
         • Evaluation of the injury—CT provides further evaluation of the extent of articular disruption, including the size and location of the articular fragments, the extent of metaphyseal injury, the location and orientation of die punch articular fragments, and the orientation of the fracture lines that extend into the diaphysis.
         • Preoperative planning—CT helps determine the orientation in which the hardware, including interfragmentary screws and transosseous implants of thin wire circular external fixators, should be placed. It also helps determine open surgical approaches.
      3. Plain tomography

III. Injury Classifications
   A. Overview—The variation in classification schemes reported in the literature makes the

A

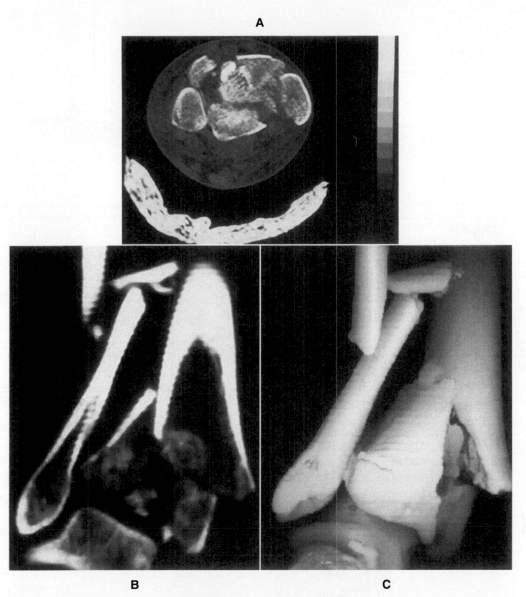

B   **C**

<u>FIGURE 12-1</u>   CT scan demonstrating a comminuted high-energy tibial plafond fracture. **A.** CT cross-sectional image. **B.** CT coronal reconstruction. **C.** CT three-dimensional reconstruction.

comparison of clinical series very difficult. The key distinctions between the various injury patterns and classifications are rotational (usually low-energy) versus axial loading (usually high-energy) mechanisms and the extent of injury of the articular surface of the distal tibia.

B. Specific Classifications Systems

   1. Rüedi and Allgöwer (1979)—The system of Rüedi and Allgöwer (Fig. 12-2) is perhaps the most widely used classification of tibial plafond fractures reported in the literature.

     • Type I—It involves a cleavage fracture of the distal tibia without major displacement of the articular surface.

     • Type II—It involves significant displacement of the joint surface without comminution.

     • Type III—It involves impaction and comminution of the articular surface.

   2. Kellam and Waddell (1979)

     • Type A—***Rotational fractures*** consist of minimal or no cortical comminution of the tibia, two or more large tibial articular fragments, and usually a transverse or short oblique fracture of the fibula above the plafond.

     • Type B—A compressive fracture pattern from ***axial loading*** demonstrates marked cortical comminution of the anterior tibia, multiple tibial fracture fragments, superior migration of the talus, and narrowing of the ankle joint seen on the X-ray film.

   3. Ovadia and Beals (1986)

     • Type I— It involves a nondisplaced articular fracture.

Type I

Type II

Type III

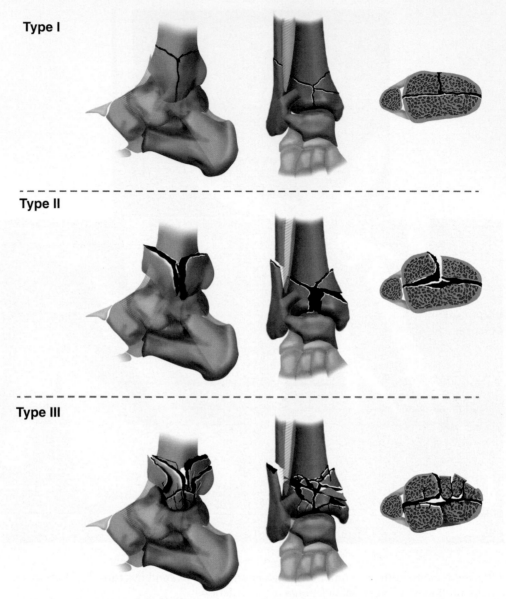

<u>**FIGURE 12-2**</u> The Rüedi and Allgöwer classification for pilon fractures. Type I is undisplaced with splitting fracture lines. Type II has displacement of the articular surface, with split type fractures. Type III is a crush or impacted injury with comminution and displacement of the articular surface.

- Type II—It involves a minimally displaced articular fracture.
- Type III—It involves a displaced articular fracture with several large fragments.
- Type IV—It involves a displaced articular fracture with multiple fragments and a large metaphyseal defect.
- Type V—It involves a displaced articular fracture with severe comminution.
4. AO/ASIF and the Orthopaedic Trauma Association (OTA) (1996)
   - Types
     (a) Extra-articular (43-A)

(b) Partial articular (43-B)
(c) Complete articular (43-C)
- Groups and subgroups
  (a) Metaphyseal simple (43-A1)
    - Spiral (43-A1.1)
    - Oblique (43-A1.2)
    - Transverse (43-A1.3)
  (b) Metaphyseal wedge (43-A2)
    - Posterolateral impaction (43-A2.1)
    - Anteromedial wedge (43-A2.2)
    - Extending into diaphysis (43-A2.3)
  (c) Metaphyseal complex (43-A3)
    - Three intermediate fragments (43-A3.1)

- More than three intermediate fragments (43-A3.2)
- Extending into diaphysis (43-A3.3)
  (d) Pure split (43-B1)
  - Frontal (43-B1.1)
  - Sagittal (43-B1.2)
  - Metaphyseal multifragmentary (43-B1.3)
  (e) Split depression (43-B2)
  - Frontal (43-B2.1)
  - Sagittal (43-B2.2)
  - Of the central fragment (43-B2.3)
  (f) Multifragmentary depression (43-B3)
  - Frontal (43-B3.1)
  - Sagittal (43-B3.2)
  - Metaphyseal multifragmentary (43-B3.3)
  (g) Articular simple, metaphyseal simple (43-C1)
  - Without impaction (43-C1.1)
  - With epiphyseal depression (43-C1.2)
  - Extending into diaphysis (43-C1.3)
  (h) Articular simple, metaphyseal multifragmentary (43-C2)
  - With asymmetric impaction (43-C2.1)
  - Without asymmetric impaction (43-C2.2)
  - Extending into diaphysis (43-C2.3)
  (i) Articular multifragmentary (43-C3)
  - Epiphyseal (43-C3.1)
  - Epiphysiometaphyseal (43-C3.2)
  - Epiphysiometaphysiodiaphyseal (43-C3.3)
  - Fibula
  (a) Fibula intact
  (b) Simple fracture of fibula
  (c) Multifragmentary fracture of fibula
  (d) Bifocal fracture of fibula
  C. Assessment of Classification Systems
  1. Martin et al. (1997)
  - The AO/ASIF classification has *good interobserver and intraobserver agreement at the type level.*
  - The AO/ASIF classification has *poor interobserver and intraobserver agreement at the group level.*
  - The Rüedi and Allgöwer classification has worse interobserver and intraobserver agreement than the AO/ASIF method when the classification is by type but better agreement than when the AO/ASIF classification is by group.
  - CT scanning does not improve agreement on classification but does improve agreement on articular surface involvement.

IV. Associated Injuries
  A. Skeletal
  1. Other injuries—Injuries that commonly result from axial loading include calcaneus fractures,

lumbar spine fractures, vertical shear pelvic fractures, and other long bone fractures.
  B. Soft-Tissue Injuries
  1. Open fractures
  2. Closed fractures—Because tibial plafond fractures may result from a high-energy injury, there may be a massive soft-tissue injury despite the absence of an open wound.
  C. Neurovascular Injuries
  D. Injuries to Other Body Parts—Injuries (those related to high-energy trauma) can occur to the head, thorax, abdomen, and other parts.

V. Treatment and Treatment Rationale
  A. Treatment Goals—Treatment goals include anatomic restoration of the distal tibial articular surface and early ankle range of motion.
  B. Treatment Options
  1. Nonsurgical—Cast and splints may be used to manage nondisplaced fractures but result in unacceptable outcomes for displaced tibial plafond fractures.
  2. Surgical—Displaced tibial plafond fractures require surgical reconstruction.
    (a) Historical methods—Pins and plaster, calcaneal traction (as a definitive treatment), and transarticular pin fixation are no longer used because of poor results.
    (b) Modern methods—Current methods include open reduction with internal fixation (ORIF) and external fixation with or without limited internal fixation, including bridging external fixation and thin wire circular external fixation (Ilizarov).
  C. Bony Considerations
  1. Tibia
    (a) Comminution—Lower-energy injuries with a small number of large articular fragments may be amenable to ORIF. *High-energy injuries with a large number of small articular fragments are best treated with external fixation (with or without limited internal fixation).*
    (b) Diaphyseal extension—Typically the epiphyseal and metaphyseal portions of the fracture heal more rapidly than the diaphyseal portion of the fracture. (Cancellous bone heals more rapidly than cortical bone.) The use of interfragmentary diaphyseal screws is associated with an increased rate of refracture.
  2. Fibula—Although the classic teaching of Rüedi and Allgöwer in the treatment of the tibial plafond fracture is to begin with open plating of the fibula, it must be remembered that *the most important treatment goal is to restore and*

maintain tibial length and alignment. There is no consensus on the indications for the various types of treatments for fibular fracture in the setting of a pilon fracture. Treatment options for fixation of the fibula include ORIF with plates and screws (the classic teachings), intramedullary pin or nail fixation (maintains reduction of alignment of the fibula with minimal soft-tissue dissection as compared with plates and screws, but does not control rotation of the fibula), and nonoperative treatment, most commonly used in cases in which the tibia is treated with external fixation.

D. Soft-Tissue Considerations—Although the injury to bone is immediately obvious in a tibial plafond fracture, the injury to the soft tissues may take days to weeks to manifest. The extent of bone injury and comminution is a good indication of the energy transmitted to the limb and is therefore a good indication of the extent of injury to the soft tissues.

1. Low-energy injuries—A lesser injury to the soft tissues may be amenable to ORIF.
2. High-energy injuries—Both open and closed high-energy fractures are best treated initially with external fixation with or without limited internal fixation.

E. Timing of Surgery
1. ORIF of closed tibial plafond fractures—The timing of ORIF is a critical issue in high-energy tibial plafond fractures and their associated soft tissue and bone injuries. ORIF may be performed in the first 6 to 12 hours after injury. After 12 hours, ORIF may be hazardous because of profound swelling. *If the soft tissues are such that the surgeon believes ORIF may be associated with a high risk of complication, a staged approach using calcaneal pin traction or an external fixator may be applied as temporary measures.* At 7 to 10 days (or more) after injury, the soft-tissue swelling may have subsided, and ORIF may be contemplated. *Waiting longer than 10 days to perform ORIF reduces risk of wound complications, but otherwise has no effect on outcome.*
2. Open fractures—Open fractures require emergent irrigation and debridement in the operating room.
3. External fixation—Surgical timing for the placement of an external fixator is much less of an issue than the timing for ORIF.

F. Results of Treatment (Table 12-1)

TABLE 12-1

Review of the Literature on Tibial Plafond Fractures

Author (Year)	No. of Cases	Findings/Conclusions
Rüedi and Allgöwer (1969)	84	The four operative principles for ORIF of tibial plafond fractures were outlined. ORIF with bone grafting was recommended (74% good or excellent results)
Rüedi (1973)	54	At 9-yr average follow-up after ORIF of comminuted intra-articular tibial plafond fractures, good or excellent results were seen in 70% of cases
Kellam and Waddell (1979)	26	The results of operative treatment of Kellam and Waddell Type A and B tibial plafond fractures were superior to those of nonoperative treatment. Acceptable results after operative treatment were seen in 84% of Type A injuries and 53% of Type B injuries
Rüedi and Allgöwer (1979)	75	At 6-yr average follow-up after ORIF of tibial plafond fractures, 70% of cases had a good or excellent result
Bourne et al. (1983)	42	Rüedi and Allgöwer Types I and II tibial plafond fractures did well after ORIF (>80% satisfactory results). Type III fractures did poorly after ORIF (only 44% had a satisfactory result)
Dillin and Slabaugh (1986)	11	"Internal fixation (of tibial plafond fractures) should be considered only when anatomic reduction and rigid fixation are goals that appear realistic after evaluation of the degree of comminution and soft-tissue injury. Otherwise, the results of closed reduction and immobilization are preferable to the serious complications that are risked with ill-advised internal fixation"

TABLE 12-1   *(continued)*

Review of the Literature on Tibial Plafond Fractures

Author (Year)	No. of Cases	Findings/Conclusions
Ovadia and Beals (1986)	145	Rigid ORIF produced the best results in this series of tibial plafond fractures
Etter and Ganz (1991)	41	At 8-yr average follow-up after ORIF of tibial plafond fractures, 90% of cases had a good or fair result
Murphy et al. (1991)	5	This study reported the results of a small series of tibial plafond injuries treated with the Monticelli-Spinelli circular external fixator
McFerran et al. (1992)	52	The overall local complication rate in treating tibial plafond fractures was 54% (88% of cases were treated with ORIF)
Bonar and Marsh (1993)	21	In the treatment of tibial plafond fractures using unilateral external fixation (15 cases also had limited internal fixation), 19 out of 21 fractures healed and 2 went on to nonunion. The authors reported few complications and advocated this technique
Bone et al. (1993)	20	There were favorable results with a low complication rate when external fixation with ORIF of severely comminuted and open tibial plafond fractures was used. Open fractures were managed with a Delta-framed external fixator across the ankle joint with screw or plate and screw fixation; closed fractures were treated with a Delta-framed external fixator across the ankle joint with ORIF at 3–7 days after the injury
Leone et al. (1993)	15	The authors concluded, "This retrospective study (of tibial plafond fractures) has demonstrated that primary closure of the medial wound, followed by delayed primary closure, or primary or delayed split-thickness skin grafting of the fibular wound in the presence of skin tension, is a judicious and responsible means to treat these delicate periarticular tissues"
Saleh et al. (1993)	12	The authors advocated articulated distraction (via a bridging unilateral external fixator) with limited internal fixation (during the same operative setting) for Rüedi and Allgöwer Type II and III tibial plafond fractures
Teeny and Wiss (1993)	60	In this review of the results of tibial plafond fractures treated with ORIF, 25% had good or excellent results, 25% had fair results, and 50% had poor results. There were no infections in Rüedi and Allgöwer Type I and II fractures, but there was a 10% ankle fusion rate. Type III fractures had a 37% infection rate and a 26% ankle fusion rate
Tornetta et al. (1993)	26	In the treatment of tibial plafond fractures using combined internal and external fixation, all fractures healed (11 required bone grafting.) Results were judged to be good or excellent in 81% of cases (69% of Rüedi and Allgöwer Type III injuries)
Helfet et al. (1994)	34	In this review of high-energy tibial plafond fractures (26 Rüedi and Allgöwer Type II injuries and 8 Rüedi and Allgöwer Type III injuries), 28 had ORIF and 6 had external fixation. Fracture healing was uneventful in 88% of cases; there were two delayed unions, one below-the-knee amputation, and one hardware failure. Excellent functional results were reported in 65% of Type II injuries and 50% of Type III injuries
Crutchfield et al. (1995)	38	This study compared the results of three different treatments of tibial plafond fractures: external fixation only (13 cases), external fixation with limited internal fixation (11 cases), and internal fixation only (14 cases). Clinical results by treatment type were as follows: external fixation only—23% excellent, 23% good, 54% poor; external fixation and limited internal fixation—27% excellent, 18% good, 55% poor; and internal fixation only—57% excellent, 29% good, 14% poor
Marsh et al. (1995)	49	In the treatment of tibial plafond fractures using an articulated external fixator (40 cases also had interfragmentary screw fixation and 14 had bone grafting), all fractures healed; the average duration of external fixation was 12 wk. There were no infections over the tibial incision or wound; there were two wound infections over the fibula

continued

TABLE 12-1 *(continued)*

Review of the Literature on Tibial Plafond Fractures

Author (Year)	No. of Cases	Findings/Conclusions
Barbieri et al. (1996)	34	In the treatment of tibial plafond fractures using hybrid external fixation combined with limited internal fixation, the average time to healing was 4.6 mo (range, 2.5–15 mo), and all fractures united. Good or excellent results were seen in 62% of cases; fair or poor results were seen in 38% of cases
DiChristina et al. (1996)	9	In a small series of high-energy tibial plafond fractures treated with an articulated external fixator, the union rate was 100%. All nine patients had complications associated with the external fixator. (Seven had drainage from the calcaneus half pins, and two had instability of the fracture in the frame.)
Gaudinez et al. (1996)	14	In the treatment of high-energy (Rüedi and Allgöwer Type II and III) tibial plafond fractures using hybrid external fixation (Monticelli-Spinelli), good or excellent subjective results were seen in 64% of cases, and good or excellent objective results were seen in 71% of cases. The authors concluded, "On the basis of these early results, by limiting additional trauma to the soft and bony tissues and allowing early ankle range of motion, indirect reduction and application of a hybrid external fixator is useful, particularly if the fracture fragments are so comminuted that anatomic reduction cannot be expected despite surgical intervention"
Griffiths and Thordarson (1996)	16	In the treatment of tibial plafond fractures using limited internal fixation and hybrid external fixation, all fractures healed, and fixators were removed at an average of 15.5 wk (range, 9–28 wk). Major complications were seen in 12% of cases, and minor complications were seen in 25% of cases. Ankle range of motion was good or excellent in 50% of cases and fair or poor in 50% of cases
McDonald et al. (1996)	13	Ilizarov external fixation is an effective treatment option for tibial plafond fractures
Rommens et al. (1996)	28	These authors recommended a step-wise reconstruction of AO Types C2 and C3 tibial plafond fractures to avoid soft-tissue complications and infection Step 1: Primary bridging external fixation Step 2: Secondary internal fixation when the soft tissues are stable
Wyrsch et al. (1996)	39	In this randomized, prospective study that compared the results of two methods of operative stabilization of tibial plafond fractures, 19 patients (group I) had ORIF of the tibia and fibula through two separate incisions. (One of these patients only had fixation of the tibia as the fibula was intact.) A total of 20 patients (group II) had external fixation with or without limited internal fixation. Complications (such as infection or amputation) were more frequent and more severe in the group treated with ORIF
Babis et al. (1997)	67	This study compared the results of three different treatments of tibial plafond fractures: 50 fractures were treated with ORIF (using the AO principles), 9 had limited internal fixation, and 8 had external fixation. Patients treated with ORIF (performed using the AO principles) had the final outcome at an average follow-up of 8.1 yr. A better reduction achieved at surgery was associated with a more favorable clinical result
Kim et al. (1997)	21	In the treatment of tibial plafond fractures using a ring fixator and arthroscopy, good results were seen in 71% of cases, fair results were seen in 19%, and poor results were seen in 10%
Sands et al. (1998)	64	In ORIF of tibial plafond fractures, complications included deep infection (5%), iatrogenic nerve injury (2%), malunion (6%), failure of fixation (6%), delayed union (5%), and nonunion (2%)
Williams et al. (1998)	54	Routine plating of the fibula was unnecessary in tibial plafond fractures treated with external fixation that spans the ankle joint

TABLE 12-1   *(continued)*

Review of the Literature on Tibial Plafond Fractures

Author (Year)	No. of Cases	Findings/Conclusions
Court-Brown et al. (1999)	24	In patients with AO Type A or C plafond fractures, results of half-ring external fixation with half-pins were comparable with small wire fixators when interfragmentary screw fixation was used for the articular component of the fractures. 75% of the patients had good or excellent results
Patterson et al. (1999)	21	Patients with Type C3 plafond fractures underwent fibular fixation and placement of a medial spanning external fixator, followed by removal of the external fixator and ORIF at an average of 24 days. Union rate was 95% at an average of 4.2 mo, with 77% good results, 73% had anatomic reduction, and there were no infections or soft-tissue complications. The ultimate arthrodesis rate was 9%
Pugh et al. (1999)	60	This retrospective review comparing half-pin external fixation, single-ring hybrid external fixation, and ORIF reported no statistically significant difference in complication rates but a higher malunion rate with external fixation
Sirkin et al. (1999)	56	This retrospective study evaluated AO Type C plafond fractures which had been treated with a staged protocol involving ORIF of the fibula within 24 hours of injury and spanning external fixation. Once soft-tissue swelling had diminished, the articular surface was reconstructed using ORIF. Time to ORIF of the tibia ranged from 4 to 31 days. Three patients (5%) developed deep infections; there were no other major complications
Blauth et al. (2001)	51	This retrospective study compared 15 cases of primary ORIF in 15 patients; 28 cases of reconstruction of the articular surface and external fixation for at least 4 wk; and 8 cases of a two-stage procedure involving minimally invasive reduction and reconstruction of the articular surface and temporary external fixation followed by definitive medial plate stabilization. Of the 23% who ultimately required arthrodesis, none had undergone the two-stage technique. The authors recommended the two-stage procedure
Letts et al. (2001)	8	This review of eight pediatric (ages, 13–17 yr) plafond fractures treated by ORIF found good to excellent outcomes in 63% of cases at an average of 16 mo after injury; two patients had posttraumatic osteoarthritis and one patient had physeal arrest
Manca (2002)	22	Type C fractures (16 closed, 2 Gustilo I, 3 Gustilo II, 1 Gustilo III) were treated by routing a Kirschner wire down the tibial intramedullary canal to reduce the articular surface under fluoroscopy, followed by percutaneous screw fixation and hybrid external fixation. 21 out of 22 cases healed at an average of 16 wk, 14 patients had excellent or good results, and 1 case later required arthrodesis for posttraumatic arthritis
Mitkovic et al. (2002)	28	Closed reduction and dynamic external fixation was used to treat Type C3 plafond fractures. The mean time to fracture union was 14 wk; there were no nonunions or deep infections. At a minimum of 2 yr after surgery, three cases had deformity, and 19 cases had excellent or good outcomes
Conroy et al. (2003)	32	Open plafond fractures were treated with debridement, immediate ORIF, and vascularized muscle flap. Two cases required amputation; none of the remaining required arthrodesis. Physical function at a minimum of 1 yr after injury was below that of the healthy population, but better than patients with lower extremity amputations
Lin et al. (2003)	30	The authors reviewed 22 closed, 3 Gustilo I, and 5 Gustilo II fractures treated using minimally invasive ORIF. At follow-up ranging from 17 to 39 mo, satisfactory results were reported in 83.3% of cases. There was one nonunion and one deep infection

continued

TABLE 12-1   *(continued)*

Review of the Literature on Tibial Plafond Fractures

Author (Year)	No. of Cases	Findings/Conclusions
Marsh et al. (2003)	35	In an investigation of long-term (5–12 yr after injury) consequences of plafond fracture treated with monolateral hinged external fixation and screw fixation of the articular surface reported that general health and ankle function was lower than the respective age-matched populations. 26 patients had grade 2 or 3 osteoarthritis of the ankle, and 27 patients reported being unable to run, although 25 patients reported their ankle function as excellent or good
Pollak et al. (2003)	80	This study of the health outcomes associated with plafond fracture at an average of 3 yr after injury reported that general health, ankle function, and employment were adversely affected by the injury. Other health conditions, being married, low income, less education, and treatment with external fixation were associated with lower outcomes
Okcu and Aktuglu (2003)	44	This retrospective study compared 24 cases of nonspanning Ilizarov external fixation with 30 cases of ankle-spanning monolateral articulated external fixation in the treatment of plafond fracture; limited ORIF was concomitantly performed when necessary. At 3–9 yr after injury, functional outcomes, radiographic results, and complication rates were similar in the two groups, the Ilizarov group had better ankle motion
Sirkin et al. (2004)	46	This retrospective study included 29 closed and 17 open fractures treated with immediate ORIF of the fibula, application of temporary spanning external fixation, and open reconstruction after soft-tissue swelling subsided. All patients were followed for at least 12 mo. There were three deep infections, one resulting in amputation, and no other substantial wound problems
Syed and Panchbhavi (2004)	7	Patients with closed plafond fractures were treated with closed reduction and percutaneous cannulated screw fixation. Subjective functional outcomes were good to excellent at an average follow-up of 30.6 mo
Williams et al. (2004)	32	In a study of determinants related to outcomes at 24–129 mo after plafond fracture, the presence of radiographic posttraumatic arthritis was associated with injury severity and accuracy of reduction. None of these variables was related to the clinical ankle score, SF-36 scores, or return to work status. These outcomes were associated with socioeconomic factors such as education and work-related injury
Kapukaya et al. (2004)	12	Patients with open tibial plafond fractures (eight Type III, 2 Type IVA, 2 Type IVB) were treated with a circular external fixation, including bone transport for Type IVB fractures; postoperative articular reduction was fair in eight patients and poor in four. At an average follow-up period of 55 mo, seven cases had grade 2 arthritis and four cases had grade 3 arthritis. AOFAS scores ranged from 28 to 90. Poor joint reduction appears to have negative impact on clinical and patient outcomes
Aggarwal and Nagi (2006)	21	Patients with plafond fractures were treated by debridement (if open) and hybrid external fixation. At 12–67 mo after injury, 16 cases had good to excellent subjective outcomes, 3 had fair outcomes, and 2 had poor outcomes
Harris et al. (2006)	79	This retrospective study compared the results of ORIF vs. limited open reduction and external fixation in patients with high-energy plafond fractures (43 OTA Type 43-C3, 5 Type 43-B1, 4 Type 43-B2, 2 Type 43-B3, 15 Type 43-C1, and 10 Type 43-C2); 71% underwent a staged procedure. At 24–38 mo after injury, there were two nonunions (3%), four malunions (5%), and 31 cases with posttraumatic arthritis (39%). Complications and lower Foot Function Index scores and MFA scores were more common after open injuries, which were more likely to be treated by external fixation, possibly indicating a bias toward treating more severe injuries with external fixation

TABLE 12-1 *(continued)*

Review of the Literature on Tibial Plafond Fractures

Author (Year)	No. of Cases	Findings/Conclusions
Marsh et al. (2006)	41	This multicenter randomized trial compared fixed to mobile-hinge ankle-spanning external fixation in the treatment of plafond fractures. At 1 and 2 yr after injury, there were no differences between groups with respect to ankle motion, pain, disability, or patient-reported health-related quality of life, although the sample size may have limited the ability to detect clinically relevant differences
Vidyahara et al. (2006)	21	Eight patients with Type B and 13 with Type C plafond fractures were treated with the Ilizarov external fixator. At 2 yr after injury, there were no nonunions and the AOFAS scores were excellent in 11 patients, good in five, fair in four, and poor in one
Bahari et al. (2007)	42	Patients treated with the AO distal tibia locking plate and minimally invasive percutaneous plate osteosynthesis were followed for an average of 20 mo after injury. All fractures healed in acceptable alignment. Physical health status and function were good to excellent, 89% reported returning to their preinjury functional level, and 95% returned to work
Chen et al. (2007)	128	At a mean follow-up of 10 yr for patients with Rüedi-Allgöwer Type I ($n = 39$), Type II ($n = 62$), and Type III ($n = 27$) injuries, Type III injuries had lower reduction and functional outcome scores, Types II and III had more ankle arthritis, and open fractures had lower outcomes in general. Fixation of a fractured fibula was associated with higher outcomes
Grose et al. (2007)	44	Patients were treated with delayed ORIF using a lateral approach. Anatomic or near-anatomic reduction was achieved in most (93%) cases. There were two deep infections (4.5%) and four nonunions (9%). The authors concluded that the lateral approach was a viable technique for internal fixation of plafond fractures
Koulouvaris et al. (2007)		This retrospective study compared three treatments for plafond fracture: half-pin, spanning external fixation, ankle-sparing hybrid external fixation, and staged internal fixation. The average follow-up ranged from 38 to 132 mo. Spanning external fixation resulted in longer time to union and a lower rate of return to activities; these associations were present even after stratifying by fracture type
Salton et al. (2007)	19	Patients were treated with limited incision percutaneous plate fixation using either a single procedure or a staged protocol. One patient went on to nonunion, and another had malunion, neither requiring surgical treatment. Four patients underwent late symptomatic hardware removal
Bacon et al. (2008)	42	AO Type C plafond fractures were treated either by temporary external fixation followed by ORIF ($n = 28$) or by Ilizarov external fixation ($n = 14$). ORIF resulted in a longer time to union, but lower rates of nonunion, malunion, and infection, although these differences did not reach statistical significance
Gardner et al. (2008)	10	Patients with open AO Type C3 plafond fractures were treated using a three-stage protocol: debridement and external fixation; ORIF and antibiotic bead placement at 1–3 wk after injury; and bone grafting several months after injury. Two cases had deep infection after bone grafting, and one required amputation. The other nine cases healed at an average of 24 wk

A   B

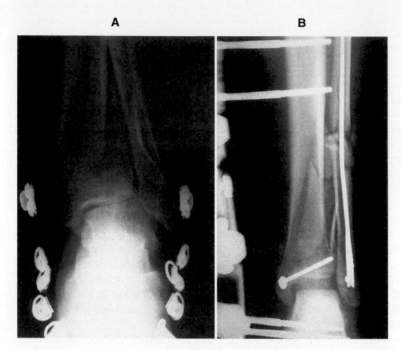

FIGURE 12-3 **A.** Injury film of a high-energy tibial plafond fracture. **B.** The fracture has been stabilized with a unilateral external fixator that spans the ankle joint. Note that the fibula has been stabilized with an intramedullary nail.

VI. Anatomic Considerations and Surgical Techniques
   A. ORIF—Rüedi and Allgöwer's four classic principles are:
     1. Reconstruct the fibula (restore fibula length).
     2. Reconstruct the articular surface of the tibia.
     3. Perform cancellous bone grafting of the distal tibial metaphysis.
     4. Stabilize the medial aspect of the tibia (medial buttress plate).

B. External Fixation
   1. Types
     • Unilateral external fixation (Fig. 12-3)—Unilateral external fixation spans the ankle joint. Fixation is performed proximally in the tibia and distally in the talus and calcaneus.
     • Ilizarov external fixation (Fig. 12-4)—Ilizarov external fixation consists of fine wires (1.8 mm) for interfragmentary fixation. It

A   B   C

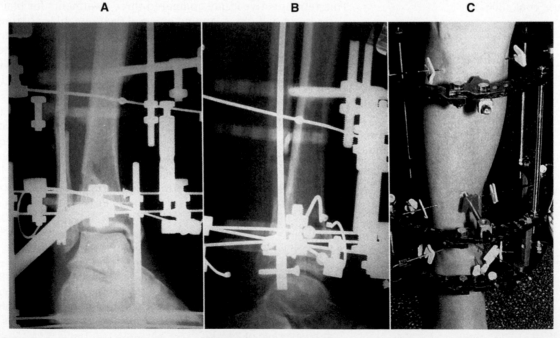

FIGURE 12-4 **A.** Early postoperative AP view after Ilizarov external fixation of the high-energy tibial plafond fracture shown in Figure 12-1. Note that thin wire fixation was used in the calcaneus for added stability (the ankle joint was immobilized), and the patient began full weightbearing as tolerated on the first postoperative day. **B.** Lateral X-ray film at 4 week after the injury, showing anatomic restoration of the articular surface of the distal tibia. Note that the foot fixation has been removed and the patient began ankle range of motion exercises. **C.** Clinical photograph of the patient ambulating in the frame.

allows early weightbearing and early ankle joint range of motion.

- Hybrid external fixation—In hybrid external fixation, a ring with wires distally at the articular fragments is connected to bars attached to half pins in the proximal fragment.

C. Soft Tissues—The skin bridge between the tibia incision and the fibula incision should be a minimum of 7 cm (Fig. 12-5). Careful soft-tissue handling and limited periosteal stripping are essential. Tension-free closure is important. If one of the wounds must be left open (because of an inability to close both wounds), it is preferable to leave the lateral wound open. (The medial wound is closed.)

D. Ligamentotaxis—When traction is applied across the ankle joint (via a traction pin in the calcaneus or an external fixator), the intra-articular fragments may be reduced by the pull of the capsule and ligamentous structures. This technique may be used in conjunction with ORIF or external fixation. Centrally depressed fragments generally do not reduce using this technique.

VII. Complications of the Injury and Treatment—Complications include soft-tissue slough, infection,

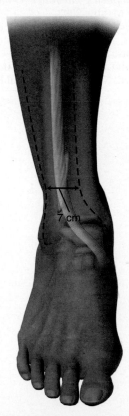

FIGURE 12-5 The AO/ORIF incisions for repair of a tibial plafond fracture. At least a 7-cm bridge must be maintained between the anteromedial and posterolateral incisions. Soft-tissue injury or fracture configuration may require modifications of these incisions.

neurovascular injury, malalignment or malreduction of the ankle joint, amputation, malunion, nonunion, decreased ankle joint range of motion, chronic edema, and posttraumatic arthritis.

SUGGESTED READINGS

Classic Articles

Bourne RB, Rorabeck CH, Macnab J. Intra-articular fractures of the distal tibia: the pilon fracture. *J Trauma.* 1983;23(7):591–596.

Kellam JF, Waddell JP. Fractures of the distal tibial metaphysis with intra-articular extension: the distal tibial explosion fracture. *J Trauma.* 1979;19(8):593–601.

Maale G, Seligson D. Fractures through the distal weight-bearing surface of the tibia. *Orthopedics.* 1980;3(6):517–521.

Ovadia DN, Beals RK. Fractures of the tibial plafond. *J Bone Joint Surg.* 1986;68A(4):543–551.

Rüedi T. Fractures of the lower end of the tibia into the ankle joint: results 9 years after open reduction and internal fixation. *Injury.* 1973;5(2):130–134.

Rüedi TP, Allgöwer M. Fractures of the lower end of the tibia into the ankle-joint. *Injury.* 1969;2:92–99.

Rüedi TP, Allgöwer M. The operative treatment of intra-articular fractures of the lower end of the tibia. *Clin Orthop Rel Res.* 1979;138:105–110.

Shenck M. Treatment of comminuted distal tibial fractures by combined dual-pin fixation and limited open reduction. *J Bone and Joint Surg.* 1965;47A(8):1537–1553.

Recent Articles

Anderson DD, Mosqueda T, Thomas T, et al. Quantifying tibial plafond fracture severity: absorbed energy and fragment displacement agree with clinical rank ordering. *J Orthop Res.* 2008;26:1046–1052.

Bacon S, Smith WR, Morgan SJ, et al. A retrospective analysis of comminuted intra-articular fractures of the tibial plafond: open reduction and internal fixation versus external Ilizarov fixation. *Injury.* 2008;39:196–202.

Blauth M, Bastian L, Krettek C, et al. Surgical options for the treatment of severe tibial pilon fractures: a study of three techniques. *J Orthop Truama.* 2001;15:153–160.

Bozic V, Thordarson DB, Hertz J. Ankle fusion for definitive management of non-reconstructable pilon fractures. *Foot Ankle Int.* 2008;29:914–918.

Bozkurt M, Ocguder DA, Ugurlu M, et al. Tibial pilon fracture repair using Ilizarov external fixation, capsuloligamentotaxis, and early rehabilitation of the ankle. *J Foot Ankle Surg.* 2008;47:302–306.

Chen L, O'Shea K, Early JS. The use of medial and lateral surgical approaches for the treatment of tibial plafond fractures. *J Orthop Trauma.* 2007;21:207–211.

Chen SH, Wu PH, Lee YS. Long-term results of pilon fractures. *Arch Orthop Trauma Surg.* 2007;127:55–60.

Dirschl DR, Ferry ST. Reliability of classification of fractures of the tibial plafond according to a rank-order method. *J Trauma.* 2006;61:1463–1466.

Dunbar RP, Barei DP, Kubiak EN, et al. Early limited internal fixation of diaphyseal extensions in select pilon fractures: upgrading AO/OTA type C fractures to AO/OTA type B. *J Orthop Trauma.* 2008;22:426–429.

Gardner MJ, Mehta S, Barei DP, et al. Treatment protocol for open AO/OTA type C3 pilon fractures with segmental bone loss. *J Orthop Trauma.* 2008;22:451–457.

Grose A, Gardner MJ, Hettrich C, et al. Open reduction and internal fixation of tibial pilon fractures using a lateral approach. *J Orthop Trauma.* 2007;21:530–537.

Harris AM, Patterson BM, Sontich JK, et al. Results and outcomes after operative treatment of high-energy tibial plafond fractures. *Foot Ankle Int.* 2006;27:256–265.

Howard JL, Agel J, Barei DP, et al. A prospective study evaluating incision placement and wound healing for tibial plafond fractures. *J Orthop Trauma.* 2008;22:299–305; discussion 305–306.

Kapukaya A, Subasi M, Arslan H, et al. Non-reducible, open tibial plafond fractures treated with a circular external fixator (is the current classification sufficient for identifying fractures in this area?). *Injury.* 2005;36:1480–1487.

Koulouvaris P, Stafylas K, Mitsionis G, et al. Long-term results of various therapy concepts in severe pilon fractures. *Arch Orthop Trauma Surg.* 2007;127:313–320.

LeBus GF, Collinge C. Vascular abnormalities as assessed with CT angiography in high-energy tibial plafond fractures. *J Orthop Trauma.* 2008;22:16–22.

Marsh JL, Muehling V, Dirschl D, et al. Tibial plafond fractures treated by articulated external fixation: a randomized trial of postoperative motion versus nonmotion. *J Orthop Trauma.* 2006;20:536–541.

Marsh JL, Weigel DP, Dirschl DR. Tibial plafond fractures: how do these ankles function over time? *J Bone Joint Surg Am.* 2003;85:287–295.

Orthopaedic Trauma Association Committee for Coding and Classification: Fracture and dislocation compendium. *J Orthop Trauma.* 1996;10(suppl. 1):1–154.

Pollak AN, McCarthy ML, Bess RS, et al. Outcomes after treatment of high-energy tibial plafond fractures. *J Bone Joint Surg Am.* 2003;85:1893–1900.

Ristiniemi J. External fixation of tibial pilon fractures and fracture healing. *Acta Orthop Suppl.* 2007;78(326):3, 5–34.

Salton HL, Rush S, Schuberth J. Tibial plafond fractures: limited incision reduction with percutaneous fixation. *J Foot Ankle Surg.* 2007;46:261–269.

Scott AT, Owen JR, Khiatani V, et al. External fixation in the treatment of tibial pilon fractures: comparison of two frames in torsion. *Foot Ankle Int.* 2007;28:823–830.

Topliss CJ, Jackson M, Atkins RM. Anatomy of pilon fractures of the distal tibia. *J Bone Joint Surg Br.* 2005;87:692–697.

Vidyadhara S, Rao SK. Ilizarov treatment of complex tibial pilon fractures. *Int Orthop.* 2006;30:113–117.

Review Articles

Barei DP, Nork SE. Fractures of the tibial plafond. *Foot Ankle Clin.* 2008;13:571–591.

Brumback RJ, McGarvey WC. Fractures of the tibial plafond, *Orthop Clin North Am.* 1995;26(2):273–285.

Mast JW, Spiegel PG, Pappas JN. Fractures of the tibial pilon, *Clin Orthop Rel Res.* 1988;230:68–82.

Marsh JL, Borrelli J Jr, Dirschl DR, et al. Fractures of the tibial plafond. *Instr Course Lect.* 2007;56:331–352.

Papadokostakis G, Kontakis G, Giannoudis P, et al. External fixation devices in the treatment of fractures of the tibial plafond: a systematic review of the literature. *J Bone Joint Surg Br.* 2008;90:1–6.

Tarkin IS, Clare MP, Marcantonio A, et al. An update on the management of high-energy pilon fractures. *Injury.* 2008;39:142–154.

Textbooks

Browner BD, Jupiter JB, Levine AM, et al, eds. *Skeletal Trauma: Basic Science, Management, and Reconstruction.* 4th ed. Philadelphia, PA: Saunders; 2009.

Canale ST, ed. *Campbell's Operative Orthopaedics.* 10th ed. Philadelphia, PA: Mosby; 2003.

Bucholz RW, Heckman JD, Koval KJ, et al, eds. *Rockwood and Green's Fractures in Adults.* Philadelphia, PA: Lippincott Williams & Wilkins, 2005.

Wagner M, Frigg R. *AO Manual of Fracture Management: Internal Fixators.* New York, NY: Thieme Medical Publishers; 2006.

CHAPTER 13

Injuries of the Ankle

Donald S. Stewart II and William C. McGarvey

I. Bony Injuries of the Ankle
  A. Anatomy and Biomechanics (Figs. 13-1 to 13-3)—The normal ankle is a three-bone articulation stabilized on both sides by ligamentous structures. The tibia joins the fibula and houses the talus in a mortise configuration held fast by four syndesmotic ligaments and the interosseous membrane. The medial malleolus yields the deltoid ligament, which is divided into two layers: the superficial layer, and the shorter, stouter, stronger, deep layer. The fibula gives rise to the three components of the lateral collateral ligamentous complex: the anterior talofibular ligament (ATFL), the calcaneofibular ligament (CFL) *(the strongest lateral ankle ligament)*, and the posterior talofibular ligament (PTFL). The talus is wider anteriorly and causes widening and deepening of the mortise in dorsiflexion to enhance stability of the joint. Motion is predominantly sagittal but not purely hinged because dorsiflexion also yields slight external rotation, whereas plantar flexion also causes internal rotation of the talus with respect to the tibia. The articulation between the tibial roof (plafond) and the talar dome is not flat, but demonstrates a shallow bicondylar appearance dorsally with corresponding indentations on the plafond. This configuration is rather stable, but subtle shifts in the articulation lead to extreme decreases in contact area and corresponding increases in contact stress. *A 1 mm talar shift can reduce the contact surface 42%.* This effect can be quite extraordinary because the normal joint reaction force in a one-legged stance can be as high as four times the body weight, with only 6% to 16% of this being borne on the fibula and the remainder absorbed through the tibiotalar articulation.
  B. Fracture Types—Ankle fractures can be subdivided into several categories: those that involve the malleolar projections and those involving the tibial plafond.
    1. Malleolar fractures—Malleolar fractures can include bimalleolar, trimalleolar, or isolated medial or lateral malleolar fractures.
      • Examination—There is a history of a twisting injury or a low-energy fall, local swelling, ecchymosis, occasional deformity, or rare neurovascular compromise (the risk increases with higher-energy injuries).
      • Classification—The fractures are classified based on radiographic findings. Two popular systems exist. The *Danis-Weber (AO/ASIF)* classification is based on the level of the fibular fracture. The *Lauge-Hansen classification* (older and more complex) is based on the position of the foot at the time of the injury, combined with the applied deforming forces; it describes the initial point of injury and the path it will take. Both classifications are commonly used, but neither is universally accepted, although they overlap somewhat. A Weber A type fracture corresponds to a Lauge-Hansen supination-adduction injury, whereas a Weber B is the equivalent of a Lauge-Hansen supination-external rotation or a pronation-abduction injury. A Weber C type fracture corresponds to a Lauge-Hansen pronation-external rotation type injury (Fig. 13-4).
      • Treatment—Treatment is based on the amount of distortion of the anatomic structures and articular incongruity. Goals include the restoration of proper anatomy, articular congruity, and biomechanical function.
        (a) Isolated lateral malleolar fractures—In the absence of a medial injury, isolated lateral malleolar fractures do not alter tibiotalar mechanics and therefore can

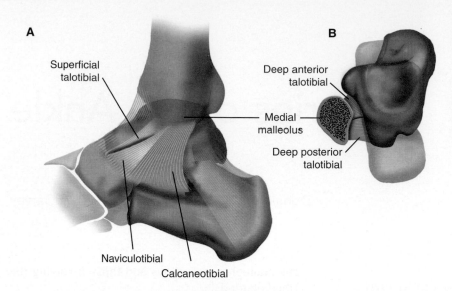

A

Superficial
talotibial

Medial
malleolus

Naviculotibial

Calcaneotibial

B

Deep anterior
talotibial

Deep posterior
talotibial

FIGURE 13-1 The medial collateral (deltoid) ligament of the ankle includes both superficial and deep components. **A.** The superficial components include the superficial talotibial, naviculotibial, and calcaneotibial components. **B.** The deep deltoid ligament fibers run transversely from the posterior colliculus of the tibia to the talus.

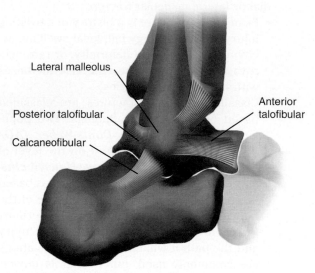

Lateral malleolus

Posterior talofibular

Calcaneofibular

Anterior
talofibular

FIGURE 13-2 The lateral ankle ligaments include the anterior talofibular (the most important stabilizer and the most commonly injured), the calcaneofibular, and the posterior talofibular.

be treated with protected weightbearing in a walking cast or brace as soon as symptoms allow. Ligamentous structures and medial stability prevent displacement of the fracture and more important, lateral shift of the mortise. Care must be taken to rule out the possibility of a medial ligamentous or syndesmotic injury (Fig. 13-5).

(b) Isolated medial malleolar fractures— Isolated medial malleolar fractures have a relatively high risk of nonunion (5%

to 15%) with over 2 mm of displacement. ***Therefore all but nondisplaced fractures should be treated with open reduction with internal fixation (ORIF).*** Vertically oriented fracture lines are more unstable and are associated with stress fractures. (Strong considerations should be given to operative management of vertically oriented fractures as they tend to be stress fractures and may fall into varus with casting. Two cancellous screws or one screw and a K-wire are required to control rotation in addition to applying a compressive force across the fracture site.

(c) Bimalleolar fractures and equivalents— ***Bimalleolar fractures*** and equivalents create loss of both medial and lateral support (with a fractured distal fibula and either a fracture of the medial malleolus or a deltoid ligament rupture). These are unstable fractures, and therefore there is poor control of reduction with nonoperative treatment. ***ORIF of both fragments is the treatment of choice. Bimalleolar equivalents*** are Weber B fracture patterns (aka SER- IV equivalents) with an associated deltoid ligament injury. Clues to a bimalleolar equivalent are medial hindfoot ecchymosis, medial ankle tenderness, bone flecks off the distal tip of the medial malleolus, and a widened medial clear space. Stress views should be performed to evaluate opening of the

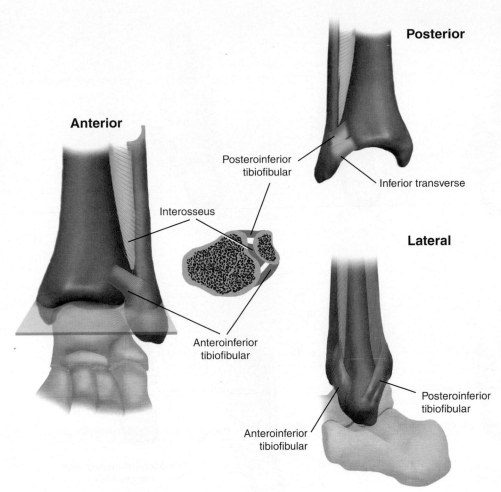

Anterior

Posteroinferior
tibiofibular

Interosseus

Anteroinferior
tibiofibular

Posterior

Inferior transverse

Lateral

Posteroinferior
tibiofibular

Anteroinferior
tibiofibular

FIGURE 13-3 The syndesmotic ligaments include the anteroinferior tibiofibular ligament (*AITFL*), the posteroinferior tibiofibular ligament (*PITFL*), the inferior transverse ligament (*ITL*), and the interosseous ligament (*IOL*).

medial clear space and a medial clear space greater than 4 mm is an indication for surgery. Magnetic resonance imaging (MRI) may be helpful to evaluate the deltoid if stress views are unclear. It is unnecessary to repair the deltoid ligament in a bimalleolar equivalent; anatomic reduction of the fibular yields restoration of the mortise in about 90% of cases. In the remaining 10% of cases a medial arthrotomy is required for extraction of an incarcerated deltoid ligament. Occasionally, the tibialis posterior tendon is interposed between the medial fragments; this is sometimes suggested radiographically by a posteromedial flake of bone on the injury films. Nonoperative care is acceptable when there is no injury to the deltoid ligament and no talar shift (one can accept up to 2 mm of fibular displacement). *A high fibular fracture suggests a syndesmotic ligament injury.* These are stable after repair of both malleoli.

However, with a bimalleolar equivalent, syndesmotic fixation should be incorporated when the fibular fracture is more than 4.5 cm from the joint line and when the deltoid ligament is not repaired. Recent studies have shown that fracture pattern does not reliably predict a syndesmotic injury. Intraoperative stress testing should be performed after definitive fixation of ankle fractures. Intraoperative radiographs at the time of surgery help assess medial stability after fibular fixation to determine the need for syndesmotic screw fixation, *but the most reliable indication is attempting manual displacement of the fibula from the tibia while under direct visualization.* Careful attention should be paid to proper replacement of the fibula in the tibial groove posterior to the midline to avoid malreduction while applying syndesmotic fixation. Contralateral ankle films and possible open repair of the

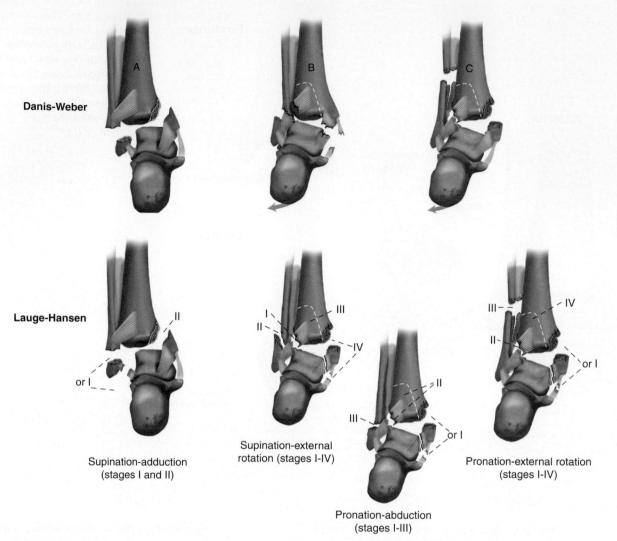

Danis-Weber

Lauge-Hansen

Supination-adduction
(stages I and II)

Supination-external
rotation (stages I-IV)

Pronation-abduction
(stages I-III)

Pronation-external rotation
(stages I-IV)

FIGURE 13-4   Danis-Weber (AO/ASIF) and Lauge-Hansen classifications of ankle fractures.

syndesmosis may be necessary. Because of the shape of the talus, the ankle should be maximally dorsiflexed before placement of a syndesmotic screw; failure to do this results in limited ankle dorsiflexion. Syndesmotic screws have been shown to alter the mechanics of the distal tibiofibular joint *(especially external rotation),* so they should be removed but no sooner than 8 to 12 weeks to allow for ligamentous healing. Weightbearing may begin after 6 weeks if the screw has captured three cortices.

(d) Trimalleolar fractures—Trimalleolar fractures represent a bimalleolar fracture combined with a bony injury to the posterior tibial plafond (posterior malleolus). ORIF is necessary because these injuries are unstable. The principles are the same as those for bimalleolar fractures. The posterior fragment frequently maintains its attachment to the fibula by the posteroinferior tibiofibular ligament (PITFL) and therefore reduces once the lateral malleolus is repaired. *The posterior malleolar fragment should be fixed if over 25% of the posterior distal tibial articular surface is involved on the lateral radiograph and the fragment is still more than 2 mm displaced after reduction of the fibula.* Contact stresses at the ankle do not increase until 25% to 40% of the posterior joint surface is removed. Anterior or posterior surgical approaches for ORIF are acceptable.

2. Pilon fractures—Higher-energy injuries involving the tibial plafond are discussed in detail in Chapter 12.

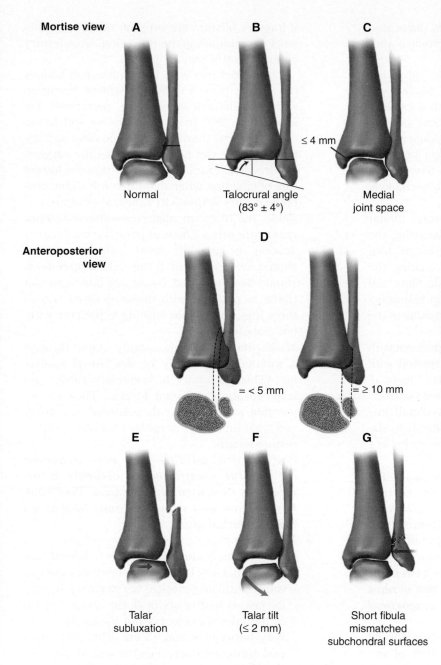

Mortise view

A Normal

B Talocrural angle (83° ± 4°)

C Medial joint space

≤ 4 mm

Anteroposterior view

D

= < 5 mm = ≥ 10 mm

E Talar subluxation

F Talar tilt (≤ 2 mm)

G Short fibula mismatched subchondral surfaces

FIGURE 13-5 Restoration of the ankle mortise requires anatomic reduction of the lateral malleolus so that its articular surface is congruous with the reduced talus. **A.** On a mortise radiograph, the condensed subchondral bone should form a continuous line around the talus, and there should be no proximal displacement, malrotation, or angulation of the lateral malleolus. **B** and **C.** A proper talocrural angle and normal joint space width also indicate normality. On the mortise view, the medial joint space should be less than or equal to 4 mm, and the superior joint space should be within 2 mm medially of its width laterally. **D.** Adequate tibiofibular overlap on the anteroposterior view indicates a proper syndesmotic relationship. The space between the medial wall of the fibula and the incisural surface of the tibia should be less than 5 mm. The anterior tubercle of the tibia should overlap the fibula by at least 10 mm. **E** and **F.** Talar malalignment is indicated by the talus's lateral displacement or tilt into valgus. **G.** Although the talus may be reduced by external pressure, its alignment is not maintained by a shortened, malrotated lateral malleolus, as shown.

3. Open ankle fractures—Treatment depends on the soft tissue injury. ***Gustilo Type I, II, and sometimes IIIA open injuries can be treated by the same principles as described for closed injuries as long as thorough and extensive debridement is performed.*** Closure or coverage is preferable within 5 days. More severe soft-tissue injuries are frequently associated with greater bony destruction as well. These often necessitate a combination of internal and external fixation and multiple debridements with secondary soft tissue coverage such as a muscle pedicle flap. Antibiotics should be given for at least 48 hours after closure.

C. Techniques for Fixation of Ankle Fractures—The technique used for the fixation of ankle fractures depends on the type of fracture sustained. Fixation usually begins with lateral stabilization because, usually, this is simpler and provides enough fixation to hold the mortise reduced. ***Care should be taken to avoid the superficial peroneal nerve and less commonly the sural nerve.*** Lag-screw fixation of the fibular fracture is incorporated when possible. Liberal use of intraoperative radiographs is a must to assess reduction.

Fracture dislocations should undergo emergent reduction followed by immediate internal fixation, splinting with very close follow up, or a spanning external fixator. Fractures that remain dislocated or subluxated can lead to skin compromise and/or further cartilaginous injury.

1. Difficult repairs in osteoporotic fibulae—Difficult repairs in osteoporotic fibulae are sometimes better approached with a posteriorly applied antiglide plate. This can obviate the need for screws in the distal fragment by acting as a buttress and preventing proximal migration of the fibula. It appears that a locking plate offers at least the same biomechanical strength as a conventional plate.

2. Severe fibular comminution—Severe fibular comminution may be treated by reducing the distal fragment to the talus with K-wire fixation, applying a plate, and bone grafting the resultant defect. Contralateral ankle films and preoperative templating can prevent malreduction, which is most commonly shortening of the fibula.

3. Seriously ill patients—Seriously ill patients with isolated fibular fractures may be treated with intramedullary rods (e.g., Rush rods). The obvious limitation is the lack of rotational control.

4. Small medial malleolar fragments—Small medial malleolar fragments may be difficult to stabilize with screws, and tension band wiring is a useful alternative.

5. Syndesmotic fixation—Syndesmotic fixation is obtained with a 30° anteriorly directed cortical screw *(a positioned screw, not a lag screw). The ankle should be maximally dorsiflexed, and clamped, and a set screw placed. A lag screw should not be placed across the syndesmosis. The optimal position is 2 cm proximal to the joint and 3.5 or 4.5 mm screws may be used in a bicortical or unicortical fashion.*

D. Associated Injuries—Any open reduction should be accompanied by direct visualization of the joint because osteochondral lesions are common. Also, plafond extension or lateral ligament disruption should be addressed if encountered.

E. Complications

1. Soft tissue problems—Fracture blisters are managed by delaying treatment until it is reasonable and safe to proceed with surgery. Pneumatic compression is sometimes helpful in reducing edema and decreasing the time to surgery. *Clear fracture blisters* are relatively safe and may be debrided at the time of surgery. *Blood-filled blisters* should be avoided for their high risk of necrosis and slough. The risk of slough is also increased as much as 10% to 20% by delaying closed reduction of a dislocated ankle.

If fracture blisters are present, or there is difficulty in maintaining the reduction, a temporary external fixator may be placed.

Open fractures with inadequate soft tissues for closure pose a difficult problem. Irrigation and debridement should be performed followed by a VAC prior to definitive soft tissue coverage. VAC therapy continued after soft tissue coverage can further increase the survival of a free flap. Fractures tend to have the lowest rate of infection when definitive soft tissue coverage occurs within 5 to 7 days after injury.

2. Ankle fractures in diabetes—*The clinician must rule out a Charcot process;* if a Charcot process is present, *total contact casting* should be considered. If this fails, *arthrodesis* should be performed. Healing of bone and soft tissue in patients with diabetes takes two to three times as long as healing in patients without diabetes.

3. Malunions—Malunions usually occur through a rotational deformity of the lateral malleolus. (This deformity is frequently subtle and leads to abnormal joint forces.) They are repairable with a fibular derotational osteotomy and sometimes an interpositional bone graft to restore length.

4. Posttraumatic arthritis—*The best treatment for painful posttraumatic arthritis is arthrodesis in neutral dorsiflexion, 5° of hindfoot valgus, and rotation equal to that on the unaffected side.*

5. Nerve injury
   • Lateral malleolus—The direct lateral approach has the highest incidence of injury to the superficial peroneal nerve (SPN). It exits its fascial hiatus about 9 cm above the tip of the lateral malleolus but its location may vary between 4 and 13 cm. The posterolateral approach decreases the risk of injury to the SPN but increases the risk of injury to the sural nerve.
   • Medial malleolus—The saphenous nerve is a very consistent structure and runs with the saphenous vein about 1 cm anterior to the medial malleolus. A direct medial approach can minimize injury to the nerve.

6. Return to function—A return to normal automobile braking time following ORIF of an ankle fracture is about 9 weeks.

II. Soft-Tissue Injuries of the Ankle

A. Ankle Sprains—The most common ligamentous injury in the human body is an ankle sprain; it accounts for 15% of all athletic injuries. Some

20% to 40% of all ankle sprains proceed to chronic instability. Peroneal tendon weakness is the number one cause of recurrent ankle sprains in ballet dancers.

1. Anatomy—The ankle is stable when loaded and unstable when unloaded. Ankle ligaments include the deltoid ligament medially (see Fig. 13-1), and the ATFL (**which is intracapsular**), CFL, and PTFL laterally (see Fig. 13-2). Subtalar ligaments include the lateral talocalcaneal ligament, cervical ligament, interosseous talocalcaneal ligament (**between the middle and the posterior calcaneal facets**), CFL (spans both the ankle and subtalar joint), and inferior extensor retinaculum. Syndesmotic ligaments include the interosseous membrane, the anteroinferior tibiofibular ligament (AITFL), posteroinferior tibiofibilar ligament (PITFL), the interosseous ligament, and the inferior transverse ligament (ITL) (see Fig. 13-3).

2. Lateral ligament sprains—The ATFL is the most common injury of the lateral ankle ligaments (about 70% of cases). The mechanism of injury is usually a **rollover of a plantar-flexed inverted foot**; the talus is in its most vulnerable position, so **the ATFL is at risk for injury**.
   - Physical examination—The lateral ankle is tender and ecchymotic. A positive anterior drawer sign is diagnostic of an ATFL injury. A positive talar tilt (best tested with the foot in the neutral position) is diagnostic of a CFL injury.
   - Radiography—There is no consensus in the literature regarding the most important radiographic findings. Stress X-ray studies are helpful only with contralateral views. The talar tilt should be considered abnormal if there is a difference of 10° or more from the normal side. The anterior drawer is abnormal radiographically if there is a difference of more than 3 mm from the normal side. **Occasionally, ligaments may avulse a small piece of bone in the subfibular region, which may be visualized on radiographs.**
   - Classification
     (a) Grade I involves an ATFL sprain.
     (b) Grade II involves an ATFL rupture and a partial CFL tear.
     (c) Grade III involves a complete ATFL and CFL tear.
   - Treatment—Some 95% of acute sprains respond well with appropriate therapy.
     (a) Grade I injuries are treated with rest, ice, compression, and elevation (RICE). Early weightbearing and rehabilitation focusing on proprioception and peroneal strengthening are useful.
     (b) Grade II and III injuries require functional bracing or short-term immobilization in a cast in dorsiflexion (2 to 6 weeks), followed by gradual return to activity. Rehabilitation is instituted, as previously described.

3. Deltoid ligament sprains—Isolated sprains of the deltoid ligament are rare. They are more commonly seen in conjunction with a syndesmotic injury. Isolated injuries are treated with 6 to 8 weeks of casting, with a gradual return to normal activity.

4. Syndesmosis sprains—Syndesmosis sprains account for 10% of all ankle ligament injuries.
   - History and physical examination—There is a history of a twisting injury; pain occurs with dorsiflexion and eversion. The results of the **squeeze test** (ankle pain on compressing the mid-tibia and fibula together) are positive. Check for a Maisonneuve injury with palpation of the fibular neck and X-rays of the proximal tibia and fibula if clinically appropriate. Inability to perform a single leg hop is the best indicator for a syndesmotic sprain without diastasis at the initial point of injury. Other findings may not present until a day later.
   - There are four ligaments involved in the syndesmosis.
     (a) Anterior inferior tibiofibular ligament (AITFL)—This is the ligament most commonly involved in syndesmotic external rotation injuries.
     (b) Posterior inferior tibiofibular ligament (PITFL).
     (c) Interosseous ligament (IOL).
     (d) Transverse osseous ligament (TOL).
   - Radiography (see Fig. 13-5)—Radiographs can appear normal; often, there are subtle abnormalities. More than 5 mm of tibiofibular clear space is abnormal. More than 4 mm of medial joint space is abnormal. Late findings demonstrate calcification of the interosseous membrane in 90% of cases.
   - Classification
     (a) Type I involves straight lateral talar subluxation.
     (b) Type II is a type I injury plus plastic deformation of the fibula.
     (c) Type III involves posterior rotary displacement of the fibula and talus.
     (d) Type IV involves complete diastasis with migration of the talus superiorly between the tibia and fibula.

- Treatment
  - (a) Stable injuries—***Stable injuries (less than 5 mm of medial joint space) are treated with RICE and return to weightbearing as tolerated with activity modification.***
  - (b) Unstable nondisplaced injuries—Unstable injuries with spontaneous reduction as seen on radiographs are treated with casting for 4 to 6 weeks and protected weightbearing thereafter. These injuries take twice as long to heal as a typical lateral ankle sprain.
  - (c) Unstable displaced injuries—***Unstable displaced injuries require syndesmotic reduction and screw fixation followed by cast immobilization for 4 to 6 weeks.*** Irreducible injuries may even necessitate opening the joint medially to remove an incarcerated deltoid ligament. With type II injuries, a fibular osteotomy is necessary because the plastic deformation of the fibula results in inability to reduce the ankle mortise. ***ORIF may be performed up to 1 year from the time of injury, provided that there is no radiographic evidence of arthritis.***

5. Chronic lateral ankle instability—Chronic lateral ankle instability is characterized by persistent lateral ankle pain, giving way, weakness, and recurrent sprains.
   - Diagnosis—The diagnosis is made via a history, physical examination, and radiographic studies (MRI and ultrasound). Conservative treatment with bracing and therapy is effective in 50% of cases.
   - Treatment—Treatment involves surgery when conservative treatment has failed. It is imperative to rule out a varus hindfoot or a cavovarus deformity; if these are present, osteotomies are required at the time of soft tissue reconstruction to prevent recurrence.
     - (a) Anatomic procedures
       - Modified Broström procedure—The most anatomic procedure is the modified Broström procedure, which is direct ATFL and CFL repair, including augmentation with the inferior extensor retinaculum to augment and control the subtalar joint. This procedure has a greater than 90% success rate.
       - Free tissue graft—Allograft or autograft semitendinosus may be used for

attenuated ligaments or following a failed Broström procedure.
     - (b) Nonanatomic procedures
       - Peroneal "sacrificing" procedures—Peroneal sacrificing procedures include those of Larsen, Watson-Jones, Chrisman-Snook, and Evans. These procedures sacrifice half or all of the peroneus brevis to reconstruct the lateral ligaments (provides a checkrein). Limitations of this type of repair are that it can easily be overtightened and is nonanatomic. The Evans is sometimes used for augmentation in "unskilled" positions in athletics or in very heavy athletes.

6. ***Thickening of the AITFL (with soft-tissue impingement) as a result of an inversion ankle injury***—The thickened AITFL rubs over the anterolateral tibia.
   - ***Diagnosis—There is persistent pain at the ankle joint line (especially the lateral joint line) without instability.*** The pain is usually relieved by injection of steroids. This problem is not well visualized on imaging studies.
   - Treatment—The injection of steroids is occasionally therapeutic. Arthroscopic debridement is often required.

B. Peroneal Tendon Dislocations
   1. Anatomy—Normally, the peroneal tendons course in a groove behind the fibula; the peroneus brevis is anterior to the peroneus longus. ***The tendons are kept in place by the superior peroneal retinaculum. It originates from the posterolateral rim of the fibula and inserts into the lateral calcaneus.***
   2. Mechanism of injury—Hyperdorsiflexion and eversion occur; 75% of cases occur as a result of snow skiing.
   3. Examination—Examination findings of a peroneal tendon dislocation differ from those of an ankle sprain because the pain is more posterior. Occasionally, the examiner can provoke a dislocation with resisted dorsiflexion and eversion from a plantar flexed and inverted position. Plain X-ray films show a lateral flake of bone in 15% to 50% of cases (***Rim Fracture of the fibula***). MRI is useful for defining the intratendinous pathologic process.
   4. Treatment
      - ***Nonsurgical management—Is the correct treatment for most cases, but has only a 50% success rate.***

- *Surgical management is the treatment of choice for patients needing a quick return to activity. This consists of acute repair of the superior peroneal retinaculum and possible fibular groove deepening.*

5. Chronic dislocations—Chronic dislocations require surgical treatment. Multiple operative procedures have been described. Fibular groove deepening with a retinacular repair has the best success rate with the fewest complications.

C. Subtalar Injuries—Subtalar injuries can mimic an ankle sprain. They are diagnosed by physical examination. *There should be a high index of suspicion for a subtalar injury in the patient with persistent lateral ankle pain and tenderness in the sinus tarsi.* The treatment principles are the same as those for a true ankle sprain.

D. Achilles Tendon Rupture—Achilles tendon rupture is the third most common of the major tendon disruptions.

1. Mechanism of injury—The mechanism of injury is severe force and acceleration/deceleration secondary to forceful dorsiflexion of the plantar-flexed ankle. The rupture usually occurs 2 to 6 cm from the insertion site of the Achilles tendon. Prerupture tendinosis sometimes exists; possible causes include overuse, chronic steroids, gout, and fluoroquinolones.

2. Diagnosis
   - History—The patient relates a history of a pop, a snap, and the feeling of being hit in the back of the heel. *Adolescents and young adults are at increased risk of spontaneous Achilles tendon rupture if taking fluoroquinolones with an increased relative risk of 3.7.*
   - Examination—There is heel cord tenderness and a palpable defect. *Thompson's test* (lack of full plantar flexion in response to a calf squeeze with the patient prone) is positive.
   - Radiography—Ultrasound and MRI are the studies of choice if the diagnosis is in question.

3. Treatment
   - Nonoperative—Nonoperative treatment is popular in Europe. The technique involves gradually reapproximating the tendon ends by plantar flexing the ankle, gradually bringing the foot to neutral position over 2 to 3 months. Progression to healing may be followed with ultrasound studies. This treatment is good for nonactive and elderly patients and those with compromised skin or poor wound-healing ability (i.e., patients with peripheral vascular disease or diabetes) and patients being treated with steroids or chemotherapy. *Nonoperative treatment is associated with a higher incidence of rerupture (18%).*
   - Operative—Operative treatment is generally considered more effective by US surgeons. Operative treatment is a better choice for active athletic patients who are reliable and strong. *Operative treatment is associated with a higher incidence of infection but a lower incidence of rerupture (2%).*
     - (a) Treatment goal—The goal is to restore the anatomy of the Achilles tendon.
     - (b) Wound slough and nerve injury—Careful soft tissue technique helps avoid risks of wound slough and sural nerve injury. *The sural nerve is the nerve at greatest risk during percutaneous repair of the Achilles tendon. Casting the patient in 20° of plantarflexion allows for the greatest tissue perfusion. Perfusion of the skin decreases with increased dorsiflexion or plantarflexion.*
     - (c) Suture technique—End-to-end repair using a locked suture technique (Krakow) is stronger than other suture techniques (Bunnel, Kessler).
     - (d) Plantaris tendon—The repair may be augmented with the plantaris tendon if it is present. Some 70% to 80% of patients have a plantaris tendon.
     - (e) Acute repair—An acute repair may be performed up to 3 months after the injury with good results.
   - Chronic tears—Injuries neglected longer than 3 to 6 months usually require reconstruction (rather than a direct repair).
     - (a) Treatment options—Treatment options for the reconstruction of chronic tears include the use of the flexor hallucis longus (strongest), the flexor digitorum longus, the peroneus brevis, free grafts, or a turn-down procedure.
       - *Gaps less than 4 cm can be reconstructed with a V–Y advancement*
       - *Gaps greater than 5 cm should be reconstructed with a turndown and FHL transfer for augmentation.*
     - (b) Skin slough—There is a relatively high risk of skin slough as a result of retraction of the posterior soft tissues and

poor local vascularity (preoperative tissue expanders should be considered).
- Laceration—The patient should undergo immediate (<8 hours) irrigation and debridement. Repair of the Achilles tendon may be performed as previously outlined.

III. Ankle Dislocations and Fracture Dislocations
A. Mechanism of Injury—Ankle dislocations and fracture-dislocations usually result from high-energy trauma.
B. Diagnosis—Usually, there is an obvious deformity. There may be open or tenting skin over a fracture fragment. The articular surface is at risk because the talus often abuts the edge of the distal tibia, creating a focal pressure point.
C. Treatment—The primary goal is to reestablish the normal architecture of the ankle joint via closed manipulation. This reduces the risk of full-thickness skin necrosis by relieving skin tension and relieves pressure on the articular surface. The reduction must be performed with relative urgency (should not be left until the next day). In fact, it can be done in the emergency department under regional anesthetic block.
1. Open dislocation or fracture-dislocation—If the dislocation or fracture-dislocation is open, reduction of the joint is better performed in combination with irrigation and debridement in the operating room. (If a delay exists, the reduction may be performed in the emergency department after the joint has been washed out; the ankle joint should be redislocated later in the operating room for a formal irrigation and debridement.)
2. Fracture-dislocations—The treatment of the fracture portion of a fracture-dislocation is similar to the treatment of ankle fractures.

SUGGESTED READINGS

Classic Articles

Ahlgren O, Larsson S. Reconstruction for lateral ligament injuries of the ankle. *J Bone Joint Surg.* 1989;71B:300–303.

Alexander AH, Lichtman DM. Surgical treatment of transchondral talardome fractures (osteochondritis dissecans): long-term follow-up. *J Bone Joint Surg.* 1980;62A:646–652.

Amendola A. Controversies in diagnosis and management of syndesmosis injuries of the aside. *Foot Ankle.* 1992;13:44–50.

Anderson IF, Crichton KJ, Grattan-Smith T, et al. Osteochondral fractures of the dome of the talus. *J Bone Joint Surg.* 1989;71A:1143–1152.

Ashton-Miller JA, Ottaviani RA, Hutchinson C, et al. What best protects the inverted weightbearing ankle against further inversion? Evertor muscle strength compares favorably with shoe height, athletic tape, and three orthoses. *Am J Sports Med.* 1996;24:800–809.

Bahr R, Lian O, Bahr IA. A twofold reduction in the incidence of acute ankle sprains in volleyball after the introduction of an injury prevention program: a prospective cohort study. *Scand J Med Sci Sports.* 1997;7:172–177.

Beauchamp CG, Clay NR, Thexton PW. Displaced ankle fractures in patients over 50 years of age. *J Bone Joint Surg.* 1983;65B:329–332.

Belcher GL, Randomisli TE, Abate JA, et al. Functional outcome analysis of operatively treated malleolar fractures. *J Orthop Trauma.* 1997;11:106–109.

Berndt AL, Harty M. Transchondral fractures (osteochondritis dissecans)of the talus. *J Bone Joint Surg.* 1959;41A:988–1020.

Boden SD, Labropoulos PA, McCowin P, et al. Mechanical considerations for the syndesmotic screw: a cadaver study. *J Bone Joint Surg.* 1989;71A:1548–1555.

Boytim MJ, Fischer DA, Neumann L. Syndesmotic ankle sprains. *Am J Sports Med.* 1991;19:294–298.

Bray TJ, Endicott M, Capra SE. Treatment of open ankle fractures: immediate internal fixation versus closed immobilization and delayed fixation. *Clin Orthop.* 1989;240:47–52.

Brown TD, Hurlbut PT, Hale JE, et al. Effects of imposed hindfoot constraint on ankle contact mechanics for displaced lateral malleolar fractures. *J Orthop Trauma.* 1994;8:511–519.

Brumback RJ, McGarvey WC. Fractures of the tibial plafond: evolving treatment concepts for the pilon fracture. *Orthop Clin North Am.* 1995;26:273–285.

Bulucu C, Thomas KA, Halvorson TL, et al. The contribution of the lateral ankle ligaments. *Foot Ankle.* 1991;11:389–393.

Burns WC 2nd, Prakash K, Adelaar R, et al. Tibiotalar joint dynamics: indications for the syndesmotic screw—a cadaver study. *Foot Ankle.* 1993;14:153–158.

Callaghan MJ. Role of ankle taping and bracing in the athlete. *Br J Sports Med.* 1997;31:102–108.

Canale ST, Belding RH. Osteochondral lesions of the talus. *J Bone Joint Surg.* 1980;62A:97–102.

Canale ST, Kelly FB Jr. Fractures of the neck and talus. *J Bone Joint Surg.* 1978;60A:143–156.

Cawley PW, France EP. Biomechanics of the lateral ligaments of the ankle: an evaluation of the effects of axial load and single plane motions on ligament strain patterns. *Foot Ankle.* 1991;12:92–99.

Cierny G 3rd, Byrd HS, Jones RE. Primary versus delayed soft tissue coverage for severe open tibial fractures: a comparison of results. *Clin Orthop.* 1983;178:54–63.

Clarke HJ, Michelson JD, Cox QG, et al. Tibiotalar stability in bimalleolar ankle fractures: a dynamic in vitro contact area study. *Foot Ankle.* 1991;11:222–227.

Coltart WD. Aviator's astragalus. *J Bone Joint Surg.* 1952;34B:545–566.

Colville MR, Marder RA, Boyle JJ, et al. Strain measurements in lateral ankle ligaments. *Am J Sports Med.* 1990;18:196–200.

Conlin FD, Johnson PG, Sinning JE Jr. The etiology and repair of rotary ankle instability. *Foot Ankle.* 1989;10:152–155.

Curtis MJ, Michelson JD, Urquhart MW, et al. Tibiotalar contact and fibular malunion in ankle fractures: a cadaver study. *Acta Orthop Scand.* 1992;63:326–329.

deSouza LJ, Gustilo RB, Meyer TJ. Results of operative treatment of displaced external rotation-abduction fractures of the ankle. *J Bone Joint Surg.* 1985;67A:1066–1074.

Diamond JE. Rehabilitation of ankle sprains. *Clin Sports Med.* 1989;8:877–891.

Dimon JH 3rd. Isolated displaced fracture of the posterior facet of the talus. *J Bone Joint Surg.* 1961;43A:275–281.

Earll M, Wayne J, Brodrick C, et al. Contribution of the deltoid ligament to ankle joint contact characteristics: a cadaver study. *Foot Ankle*. 1996;17:317–324.

Eiff MP, Smith AT, Smith GE. Early mobilization versus immobilization in the treatment of lateral ankle sprains. *Am J Sports Med*. 1994;22:83–88.

Eisele SA, Sammarco GJ. Fatigue fractures of the foot and ankle in the athlete. *J Bone Joint Surg*. 1993;75A:290–298.

Franklin JL, Johnson KD, Hansen ST Jr. Immediate internal fixation of open ankle fractures: report of thirty-eight cases treated with a standard protocol. *J Bone Joint Surg*. 66A–1349–1356, 1984.

Greene TA, Hillman SK. Comparison of support provided by a semirigid orthosis and adhesive ankle taping before, during, and after exercise. *Am J Sports Med*. 1990;18:498–506.

Hamilton WG, Hamilton LH. Foot and ankle injuries in dancers. In: Coughlin MJ, Mann RA, eds. *Surgery of the Foot and Ankle*. 7th ed. Philadelphia, PA: Mosby; 1999:1225–1256.

Hamilton WG, Thompson FM, Snow SW. The modified Brostrom procedure for lateral ankle instability. *Foot Ankle*. 1993;14:1–7.

Harper MC, Keller TS. A radiographic evaluation of the tibiofibular syndesmosis. *Foot Ankle*. 1989;10:156–160.

Harper MC. The stabilizing role of the medial, lateral, and posterior ankle structures. *Clin Orthop*. 1990;257:177–183.

Hartford JM, Gorczyca JT, McNamara JL, et al. Tibiotalar contact area: contribution of posterior malleolus and deltoid ligament. *Clin Orthop Relat Res*. 1995;320:182–187.

Hennrikus WL, Mapes RC, Lyons PM, et al. Outcomes of the Chrisman–Snook and modified Brostom procedures for chronic lateral ankle instability: a prospective, randomized comparison. *Am J Sports Med*. 1996;24:400–404.

Hockenbury RT, Johns JC. A biomechanical in vitro comparison of open versus percutaneous repair of tendon Achilles. *Foot Ankle Int*. 1990;11:67–72.

Hopkinson WJ, St Pierre P, Ryan JB, et al. Syndesmosis sprains of the ankle. *Foot Ankle*. 1990;10:325–330.

Johnson EE, Davlin LB. Open ankle fractures: the indications for immediate open reduction and internal fixation. *Clin Orthop*. 1993;292:118–127.

Joy G, Patzakis MJ, Harvey JP Jr. Precise evaluation of the reduction of severe ankle fractures. *J Bone Joint Surg*. 1974;56A:979–993.

Kannus P, Renstrom P. Treatment for acute tears of the lateral ligaments of the ankle: operation, cast, or early controlled mobilization. *J Bone Joint Surg*. 1991;73A:305–312.

Karlsson J, Bergsten T, Lansinger O, et al. Reconstruction of the lateral ligaments of the ankle for chronic lateral instability. *J Bone Joint Surg*. 1988;70A:581–588.

Karlsson J, Lansinger O, Faxen E. Nonsurgical treatment of chronic lateral insufficiency of the ankle joint. *Acta Orthop Scand*. 1990;61(suppl. 239):93.

Karlsson J, Lansinger O. Lateral instability of the ankle joint. *Clin Orthop*. 1992;276:253–261.

Konradsen L, Holmer P, Sondergaard L. Early mobilizing treatment for grade III ankle ligament injuries. *Foot Ankle*. 1991;12:69–73.

Lantz BA, McAndrew M, Scioli M, et al. The effect of concomitant chondral injuries accompanying operatively reduced malleolar fractures. *J Orthop Trauma*. 1991;5:125–128.

Lassiter TE Jr, Malone TR, Garrett WE Jr. Injury to the lateral ligaments of the ankle. *Orthop Clin North Am*. 1989;20:629–640.

Lauge–Hansen N. Fractures of the ankle. II. Combined experimental-surgical and experimental-roentgenologic investigations. *Arch Surg*. 1950;60:957–985.

Limbird RS, Aaron RK. Laterally comminuted fracture-dislocation of the ankle. *J Bone Joint Surg*. 1987;69A:881–885.

Lindsjo U. Operative treatment of ankle fracture-dislocations: a follow-up study of 306/321 consecutive cases. *Clin Orthop*. 1985;199:28–38.

Liu SH, Baker CL. Comparison of lateral ankle ligamentous reconstruction procedures. *Am J Sports Med*. 1994;22:313–317.

Liu SH, Jacobson KE. A new operation for chronic lateral ankle instability. *J Bone Joint Surg*. 1995;77B:55–59.

Marti RK, Raaymakers EL, Nolte PA. Malunited ankle fractures: the late results of reconstruction. *J Bone Joint Surg*. 1990;72B:709–713.

Matsen FA 3rd, Winquist RA, Krugmire RB Jr. Diagnosis and management of compartmental syndromes. *J Bone Joint Surg*. 1980;62A:286–291.

McCullough CJ, Burge PD. Rotary stability of the load-bearing ankle: an experimental study. *J Bone Joint Surg*. 1990;72B:709–713.

McLennan JG. Treatment of acute and chronic luxations of the peroneal tendons. *Am J Sports Med*. 1980;8:432–436.

Michelson JD, Magid D, Ney DR, et al. Examination of the pathologic anatomy of ankle fractures. *J Trauma*. 1992;32:65–70.

Michelson JD, Magid D, Ney DR. Examination of the pathologic anatomy of ankle fractures. *J Trauma*. 1992;32:65–70.

Miller CD, Shelton WR, Barrett GR, et al. Deltoid and syndesmosis ligament injury of the ankle without fracture. *Am J Sports Med*. 1995;23:746–750.

Miller SD. Late reconstruction after failed treatment for ankle fractures. *Clin Orthop North Am*. 1995;26:363–373.

Myerson MS. Achilles tendon ruptures. *Instr Course Lect*. 1999;48:219–230.

Needleman RL, Skrade DA, Stiehl JB. Effect of the syndesmotic screw on ankle motion. *Foot Ankle*. 1989;10:17–24.

Nielsen JO, Dons–Jensen H, Sorensen HT. Lauge–Hansen classification of malleolar fractures: an assessment of the reproducibility in 118 cases. *Acta Orthop Scand*. 1990;61:385–387.

Nigg BM, Skarvan G, Frank CB, et al. Elongation and forces of ankle ligaments in a physiological range of motion. *Foot Ankle*. 1990;11:30–40.

Ogilvie–Harris DJ, Reed SC, Hedman TP. Disruption of the ankle syndesmosis: bio mechanical study of the ligamentous restraints. *Arthroscopy*. 1994;10:558–560.

Phillips WA, Schwartz HS, Keller CS, et al. A prospective, randomized study of the management of severe ankle fractures. *J Bone Joint Surg*. 1985;67A:67–78.

Raatikainen T, Puutkonen M, Puranen J. Arthrography, clinical examination, and stress radiograph in the diagnosis of acute injury to the lateral ligaments of the ankle. *Am J Sports Med*. 1992;20:2–6.

Ramsey P, Hamilton W. Changes in tibiotalar contact caused by lateral talar shift. *J Bone Joint Surg*. 1976;58-A:356–357.

Renstrom PA, Konradsen L. Ankle ligament injuries. *Br J Sports Med*. 1997;31:11–20.

Renstrom PAFH. Persistently painful sprained ankle. *J Am Acad Orthop Surg*. 1994;2:270–280.

Rosenbaum D, Becker HP, Sterk J, et al. Long-term results of the modified Evans repair for chronic ankle instability. *Orthopedics*. 1996;19:451–455.

Rovere GD, Clarke TJ, Yates CS, et al. Retrospective comparison of taping and ankle stabilizers in preventing ankle injuries. *Am J Sports Med*. 1988;16:228–233.

Rowley DI, Norris SH, Duckworth T. A prospective trial comparing operative and manipulative treatment of ankle fractures. *J Bone Joint Surg*. 1986;68B:610–613.

Sammarco GJ, Carrasquillo HA. Surgical revision after failed lateral ankle reconstruction. *Foot Ankle*. 1995;16:748–753.

Schaffer JJ, Manoli A 2nd. The antiglide plate for distal fibular fixation: a biomechanical comparison with fixation with a lateral plate. *J Bone Joint Surg.* 1987;69A:596–604.

Stanton-Hicks M, Janig W, Hassenbusch S, et al. Reflex sympathetic dystrophy: changing concepts and taxonomy. *Pain.* 1995;63:127–133.

Stuart PR, Brumby C, Smith SR. Cmparative study of functional bracing and plaster casts treatment of stable lateral malleolar fractures. *Injury.* 1989;20:323–326.

Tunturi T, Kemppainen K, Patiala H, et al. Importance of anatomical reduction for subjective recovery ankle fracture. *Acta Orthop Scand.* 1983;54:641–647.

van der Linden PD, van de Lei J, Nab HW. Achilles tendonitis associated with fluoroquinolones. *Br J Pharmacol.* 1999;48:433–437.

van Dijk CN, Mol BW, Lim LS, et al. Diagnosis of ligament rupture of the ankle joint: physical examination, arthrography, stress radiography and sonography compared in 160 patients after inversion trauma. *Acta Orthop Scand.* 1996;67:566–570.

Vangsness CT Jr, Carter V, Hunt T, et al. Radiographic diagnosis of ankle fractures. Are three views necessary? *Foot Ankle Int.* 1994;15:172–174.

Veltri DM, Pagnani MJ, O'Brien SJ, et al. Symptomatic ossification of the tibiotalar syndesmosis in professional football players: a sequela of the syndesmotic ankle sprain. *Foot Ankle.* 1995;16:285–290.

Vosburgh C, Gruel CR, Herndon WA, et al. Lawn mower injuries of the pediatric foot and ankle: observations on prevention and management. *J Pediatr Orthop.* 1995;15:504–509.

Ward AJ, Ackroyd CE, Baker AS. Late lengthening of the fibula for malaligned ankle fractures. *J Bone Joint Surg.* 1990;72:714–717.

Whitelaw GP, Sawka MW, Weltzler M, et al. Unrecognized injuries of the lateral ligaments associated with lateral malleolar fractures of the ankle. *J Bone Joint Surg.* 1989;71A:1396–1399.

Wuest TK. Injuries to the distal lower extremity syndesmosis. *J Am Acad Orthop Surg.* 1997;5:172–181.

Xenos JS, Hopkinson WJ, Mulligan ME, et al. The tibiofibular syndesmosis: evaluation of the ligamentous structures, methods of fixation, and radiographic assessment. *J Bone Joint Surg.* 1995;77A:847–856.

Yablon IG, Heller FG, Shouse L. The key role of the lateral malleolus in displaced fractures of the ankle. *J Bone Joint Surg.* 1977;59A:169–173.

Yablon IG, Leach RE. Reconstruction of malunited fractures of the lateral malleolus. *J Bone Joint Surg.* 1989;71A:521–527.

Yde J, Kristensen KD. Ankle fractures: supination–eversion fractures of stage II—primary and late results of operative and nonoperative treatment. *Acta Orthop Scand.* 1980;51:695–702.

Yde J, Kristensen KD. Ankle fractures: supination-eversion fractures of stage IV—primary and late results of operative and nonoperative treatment. *Acta Orthop Scand.* 1980;51:981–990.

Recent Articles

Chao KH, Wu CC, Lee CH. Corrective Elongation osteotomy without bone graft for old ankle fracture with residual diastasis. *Foot Ankle Int.* 2004;25:123–127.

Clare MP, Fitzgibbons TC, McMullen ST. Experience with the vacuum assisted wound closure negative pressure technique in the treatment of non-healing diabetic and dysvascular wounds. *Foot Ankle Int.* 2002;23:896–901.

Clanton TO, Paul P. Syndesmosis injuries in athletes. *Foot Ankle Clin.* 2002;7:529–549.

Egol KA, Sheikhazadeh A, Mogatederi S. Lower extremity function for driving an automobile after operative treament of ankle fracture. *Bone Joint Surg Am.* 2003;85:1185–1189.

Kim T, Ayturk UM, Haskell A, et al. Fixation of osteoporotic distal fibula fractures: a biomechanical comparison of locking versus conventional plates. *J Foot Ankle Surg.* 2007;46(1):2–6.

Nielson JH, Sallis JG, Potter HG, et al. Correlation of interosseous membrane tears to the level of the fibular fracture. *J Orthop Trauma.* 2004;18:68–74.

Nussbaum ED, Hosea TM, Sieler SD, et al. Prospective evaluation of syndesmosis ankle sprains without diastasis. *Am J Sports Med.* 2001;29:31–35.

Poynton AR, O'Rourke K. An analysis of skin perfusion over the Achilles tendon in varying degrees of plantarflexion. *Foot Ankle Int.* 2001;22:572–574.

Redfern DJ, Sauvé PS, Sakellariou A. Investigation of incidence of superficial peroneal nerve injury following ankle fracture. *Foot Ankle Int.* 2003;24:771–774.

Richardson EG, ed. *Orthopaedic Knowledge Update: Foot and Ankle 3.* Rosemont, IL: American Academy of Orthopaedic Surgeons; 2004:81–89.

Zalavras C, Thordarson D. Ankle syndesmotic injuries. *J Am Acad Orthop Surg.* 2007;15(6):330–339.

Review Articles

Bennett WF. Lateral ankle sprains. I. Anatomy, biomechanics, diagnosis, and natural history. *Orthop Rev.* 1994;23:381–387.

Marder RA. Current methods for the evaluation of ankle ligament injuries. *Instr Course Lect.* 1995;44:349–357.

Roberts CS, DeMaio M, Larkin JJ, et al. Eversion ankle sprains. *Orthopedics.* 1995;18:299–304.

St Pierre R, Allman F Jr, Bassett FH 3rd, et al. A review of lateral ankle ligamentous reconstructions. *Foot Ankle.* 1982;3:114–123.

Textbooks

Browner BD, Jupiter JB, Levine AM, et al. *Skeletal trauma: Fractures Dislocations. Ligamentous Injuries.* 2nd ed. Philadelphia, PA: WB Saunders; 1998.

Chapman MW, ed. *Operative Orthopaedics.* Philadelphia, PA: JB Lippincott; 1988.

Colville MR. Reconstruction of the lateral ankle ligaments. *Instr Course Lect.* 1995;44:341–348.

Coughlin MJ, Mann RA, eds. *Surgery of the Foot and Ankle.* 7th ed. St Louis, MO: Mosby; 1999.

Kozin SH, Berlet AC. *Handbook of Common Orthopaedic Fractures.* West Chester, PA: Medical Surveillance; 1990.

Mizel MS, Miller RA, Sciolo MW, eds. *Orthopaedic Knowledge Update Foot and Ankle: #2.* Rosemont, IL: American Academy of Orthopaedic Surgeons; 1998.

Muller ME, Allgower M, Schneider R. *Manual of Internal Fixation.* Berlin: Springer-Verlag; 1979.

Myerson MS, ed. *Current Therapy in Foot and Ankle Surgery.* St Louis, MO: Mosby; 1993.

Rockwood CA, Green SP, eds. *Fractures in Adults.* 3rd ed. Philadelphia, PA: JB Lippincott; 1991.

CHAPTER 14

Injuries of the Foot

Donald S. Stewart II and William C. McGarvey

I. Talus Fractures and Dislocations
 A. Anatomy
  1. Parts—The talus comprises three distinct parts: the head, which articulates with the navicular; the neck, which is nonarticular; and the body, which has articulations with the tibia above and the calcaneus below. Approximately 50% of the talus is covered by articular cartilage. The talus has no muscular or tendinous attachments. The talar dome is wider anteriorly. The posterior process of the talus contains the medial and the lateral tubercles, between which the flexor hallucis longus courses. The lateral tubercle is larger and may exist as a separate ossicle (the os trigonum), attached only by ligamentous structures.
  2. Blood supply—The talus receives its blood supply from two main sources: extraosseous and intraosseous (Fig. 14-1).
   • Extraosseous supply
    (a) Posterior tibial artery
     • Artery of the tarsal canal—The artery of the tarsal canal gives off a deltoid branch, which passes through the deltoid ligament and supplies the medial body of the talus.
     • Calcaneal branches
    (b) Anterior tibial artery (dorsalis pedis artery)
     • Medial tarsal branches
     • Anterolateral malleolar artery—The anterolateral malleolar artery contributes to the *artery of the tarsal sinus*.
    (c) Peroneal artery—The peroneal artery contributes to the artery of the tarsal sinus.
   • Intraosseous supply
    (a) Talar head

    • Superomedial half—The superomedial half is supplied by branches from the anterior tibial artery (dorsalis pedis artery).
    • Inferolateral half—The inferolateral half is supplied by the arteries of the tarsal sling (artery of the tarsal canal and artery of the tarsal sinus).
   (b) Talar body—The main blood supply is the anastomosis between the artery of the tarsal canal and the artery of the tarsal sinus.
 B. Injury Types
  1. Talar head fractures—Talar head fractures account for 5% to 10% of all talus fractures.
   • Mechanism of injury
    (a) Axial loading with the ankle in plantar flexion or compression of the head of the talus against the distal tibia with the ankle in dorsiflexion
    (b) Shear fracture of the navicular as it medially dislocates over the talar head during an inversion injury
   • Associated injuries—Metatarsal fractures are common associated injuries; midfoot instability is common.
   • Treatment
    (a) Nondisplaced fractures—Most fractures are nondisplaced because of the strong capsular and ligamentous attachments. Treatment involves a short leg cast and nonweightbearing for 4 to 8 weeks
    (b) Displaced fractures—No good evidence exists to guide treatment in regards to fragment excision versus open reduction and internal fixation. If the fragment is large enough, standard practice is to internally fix it and excise small fragments.

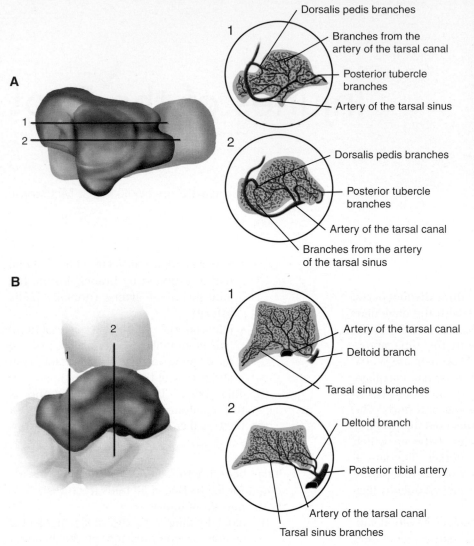

FIGURE 14-1 **A.** Sagittal sections through the talus in planes *1* and *2*. Note that the body of the talus is supplied mainly by branches from the artery of the tarsal canal and the posterior tubercle branches (*2*), whereas the head of the talus is supplied by branches from the dorsalis pedis and the tarsal sinus arteries (*1*). **B.** In the coronal plane, the lateral two-thirds of the talar body is supplied by branches from the artery of the tarsal canal and the medial one-third by the branches entering through the deltoid ligament insertion.

- Complications—Complications include arthritis due to malalignment, osteonecrosis (approximately 10% of cases), and osteochondral fractures.

2. Talar neck fractures—***Talar neck fractures are also called aviator's astragalus.***
    - Overview—Talar neck fractures are high-energy injuries usually occurring as a result of hyperdorsiflexion in which the talus impinges on the distal tibia. Approximately 15% to 20% of these injuries are open fractures. They are frequently associated with malleolar fractures (25% of cases); injury to the medial malleolus is more common. There is a high risk of soft-tissue injuries and compartment syndrome.
    - Classification—According to the Hawkins classification (Fig. 14-2), talar neck fractures are classified into four types.

    (a) Type 1 is nondisplaced.
    (b) Type 2 involves a displaced talar neck fracture and subluxation or dislocation of the subtalar joint.
    (c) Type 3 involves a displaced talar neck fracture and dislocation of both the ankle and subtalar joints.
    (d) Type 4 involves a displaced talar neck fracture and dislocation of the ankle and subtalar joints with a talonavicular dislocation.
    - Radiography—A foot and ankle series is obtained. The talar neck profile is best seen on the Canale view (maximum plantar flexion with 15° of pronation with the beam directed 75° cephalad from the horizontal).
    - Treatment—***Treatment is determined by the Hawkins type.*** The goal of treatment is anatomic reduction; historically, early

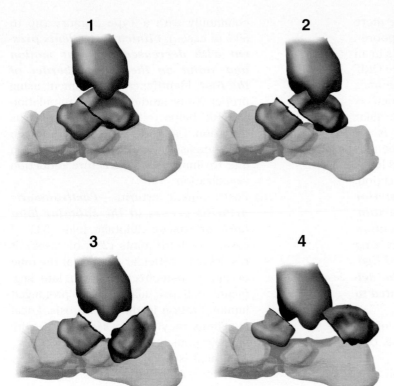

FIGURE 14-2 Hawkins (and Canale) classification of talar neck fractures. *(1)* Nondisplaced; *(2)* with subtalar subluxation or dislocation; *(3)* with talar body dislocation; and *(4)* with talar body and head dislocation.

reduction of displaced fractures was thought to reduce the risk of osteonecrosis. Recently, a study has shown that approximately 60% of orthopedic traumatologists find it acceptable to operate after 8 hours, and 46% find it acceptable to operate after 24 hours.

(a) Hawkins Type 1—Type 1 injuries are treated with 4 to 6 weeks of non weightbearing in a short leg cast, followed by 1 to 2 months in a walking cast. If joint stiffness or late fracture displacement is a concern, percutaneous fixation may be contemplated.

(b) Hawkins Type 2—Type 2 injuries constitute an orthopaedic emergency. Immediate manipulation of the fragments with traction and plantar flexion to realign the talar head fragment with the talar body is recommended. If the reduction is anatomic (reported to occur in approximately 50% of cases), the injury may be treated in the same manner as a Hawkins Type I injury. Residual deformity must be corrected to accept no more than 5 mm of displacement, with angulation of 5° or less. One study by Sangeorzan (1992) showed that as little as 2 mm of displacement of the talar neck significantly affects articular pressures. Most agree that

Type II fractures should undergo internal fixation to avoid late displacement. Open reduction may be carried out through an anterolateral (least vascular risk) or anteromedial arthrotomy, or through a posterolateral approach. Fixation is usually via screws placed across the talar neck. The surgical approach is determined by the location of the fracture fragments, open wounds, contused skin, and adjacent fractures. The anteromedial approach is the most frequently used, but carries the greatest risk of injury to the artery to the tarsal canal. Sometimes, both the anteromedial and anterolateral approaches are necessary to allow for cross screw fixation. ***The posteromedial approach should be avoided because of the high incidence of painful sequelae.*** Intraoperative radiographs are necessary to ensure proper bony reduction and avoid malalignment ***(especially a varus deformity of the talar neck). Posterior-to-anterior–directed screws demonstrate the largest strength of fixation compared with K-wires or anterior-to-posterior directed screws***.

(c) Hawkins Type 3—Treatment of Type 3 injuries is similar to that of Type 2 injuries.

However, soft-tissue problems are more frequent, and results are generally poorer. Manipulation less frequently results in an acceptable reduction, and therefore ORIF is more commonly required. Sometimes skeletal traction through the calcaneus is necessary to gain reduction of the talar body fragment. If the talar body is extruded, primary Blair fusion may be performed, as replacement of the talus leads to a notoriously high rate of infection. *The deltoid branch of the posterior tibial artery may be the only remaining blood supply to the talus. Attention must be directed toward minimizing soft-tissue stripping of the deltoid ligament. The talus may spin on the deltoid ligament and must be derotated to maintain the blood supply*.

(d) Hawkins Type 4—Type 4 is a rare injury. Treatment principles follow those outlined for a Type 2 injury.

- Complications—Patients report a high rate of dissatisfaction as a result of the numerous sequelae.

(a) Skin necrosis and infection—The dorsal skin envelope is particularly at risk for necrosis and infection. A delay in fracture reduction if it is tenting the skin increases the risk of ischemia. Osteomyelitis is common in open injuries and requires excision of infected bone and subsequent arthrodesis.

(b) Delayed union or nonunion
- Delayed union—Delayed union occurs in approximately 10% of cases and is defined as failure to heal after 6 months. It occurs secondary to the tenuous blood supply of the talus with slow revascularization. Weightbearing should be limited until bridging callus is seen.
- Nonunion—Frank nonunion is rare. The incidence of both nonunion and delayed union is reduced with immediate internal fixation. Fractures that have failed to unite 1 year after the injury should be treated with ORIF and bone grafting.

(c) Malunion—*Varus malunion is the most common malunion* and commonly results from closed manipulation without internal fixation. This deformity ultimately leads to degenerative arthritis of the subtalar joint and occurs most commonly with a Type 2 injury (up to 50% of cases). *Clinically, patients present with decreased subtalar motion and stand on the lateral border of the foot.* Identifying malalignment using proper X-ray studies after manipulation or ORIF helps reduce the risk of varus malunion. Using only a medial approach may increase the risk of a varus malunion due to limitations of fracture reduction visualization.

(d) Posttraumatic arthritis—*Posttraumatic arthritis occurs at the subtalar joint (50% of cases),* tibiotalar joint (33% of cases), or both joints (25% of cases). It results from articular damage at the time of injury, osteonecrosis with late segmental collapse, malunion, or prolonged immobilization leading to fibrosis. Local injections may be necessary to identify specific joint involvement. Conservative treatment is frequently effective, but if it is unsuccessful, arthrodesis may be the only alternative.

(e) Osteonecrosis—The incidence is related to injury type (Table 14-1). *"Hawkins sign"* (Fig. 14-3), if present, is seen on plain X-ray films at 6 to 8 weeks, and signifies revascularization and atrophic changes in the body of the talus. Hawkins sign appears as a subchondral luceny in the dome of the talus on the anteroposterior view. *Its presence signifies that osteonecrosis will not occur; its absence does not indicate that osteonecrosis will definitely occur.* MRI or nuclear medicine studies are sometimes helpful in determining this in equivocal cases. In cases of osteonecrosis, an increase in the radiographic density of the talar body is not seen for 3 months or more. If osteonecrosis is present, weightbearing

TABLE 14-1

Incidence of Osteonecrosis after Talar Neck Fractures

Hawkins Classification	Incidence
Type 1	Up to 13%
Type 2	20% to 50%
Type 3	Virtually 100%
Type 4	Virtually 100%

is controversial. Bony union of the fracture does not appear to be delayed by osteonecrosis. Weightbearing, however, should be delayed until union of the talar neck fracture. In cases with documented osteonecrosis, some injuries heal well as long as late segmental collapse is avoided. Offloading in a patellar tendon-bearing brace should be maintained until revascularization of the talus occurs (up

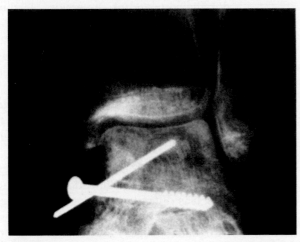

FIGURE 14-3 Hawkins sign. Note the atrophy in the subchondral area of the talus, which suggests vascularity. (This is a good prognostic sign for viability of the talus.) (Reprinted with permission from Mann RA, Coughlin MJ, Surgery of the foot and ankle, ed 6, St. Louis, 1993, Mosby).

to 36 months by creeping substitution). A late segmental collapse is a difficult problem from a management standpoint; tibiocalcaneal fusion, Blair fusion, and modified Blair fusion (maintaining the head and neck of the talus) are treatment options.

(f) Nerve injury
- Posterolateral approach—Damage to the sural nerve is most likely.
- Anteromedial approach—Damage to the saphenous nerve is most likely
- Anterolateral approach—Damage to the dorsal intermediate cutaneous branch of the superficial peroneal nerve is most likely.

3. Talar body fractures—Talar body fractures include fractures involving the superior articular surface or the trochlear region. *These fractures can occur in any plane and have a much poorer prognosis than talar neck fractures.* The classification (Fig. 14-4) is based on the plane of the fracture and fracture fragment displacement. Treatment involves surgery in all but those with minimal displacement. The medial surgical approach with a malleolar osteotomy gives wide exposure for fixation. The lateral approach carries less risk of vascular compromise. Fracture fixation may be achieved with cancellous screws, K-wires, or Herbert screws. The overall incidence of osteonecrosis is approximately 50% and in general is not

FIGURE 14-4   Fractures of the talar body.

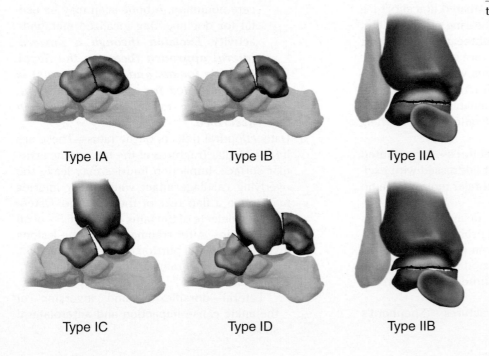

Type IA   Type IB   Type IIA

Type IC   Type ID   Type IIB

related to fracture type for talar body fractures. (The incidence of osteonecrosis is related to fracture type for talar neck fractures.) The treatment of osteonecrosis after a talar body fracture is similar to that for osteonecrosis after a talar neck fracture.

4. Talar process fractures
   - Lateral process fractures (Snowboarder's fracture)—*The mechanism of injury is dorsiflexion, inversion, external rotation, and axial loading.* The lateral process of the talus contains the attachments for the cervical, bifurcate, anterior talofibular, and lateral talocalcaneal ligaments.
     (a) Examination—The physical findings mimic those of a lateral ankle sprain. *A history of an inversion injury is characteristic. A high index of suspicion is needed to make the diagnosis.* Radiographs often demonstrate subtle or no obvious findings. Evaluation with computed tomography (CT) is often helpful.
     (b) Radiography
        - Plain films—AP view of the ankle and view with the leg internally rotated 20° are the views that best visualize the lateral process in order to look for a fracture.
        - CT—Coronal slices
     (c) Treatment—Treatment depends on the size of the fragment, displacement, and comminution.
        - Nondisplaced fractures—Nondisplaced fractures may be treated in a short leg cast (nonweightbearing) for 4 weeks, followed by weightbearing in a short leg cast for two more weeks.
        - Displaced fractures without comminution—Displaced fractures without comminution are amenable to ORIF with small fragment fixation or a Herbert screw.
        - Comminuted fractures—Comminuted fractures are best addressed with excision and early subtalar motion with no weightbearing.
     (d) Complications—A delay in diagnosis causes the greatest problems. Healed displaced fragments can give rise to subtalar arthritis. If excision does not provide relief, subtalar arthrodesis is the treatment of choice.
   - Posterior process fractures (Shepherd's fractures)

     (a) Diagnosis—There may be a history of trauma or pain of insidious onset. The pain may be vague and nonspecific and may localize to the posterior ankle. The pain is usually aggravated by forced equinus of the ankle. *Hallux motion may reproduce the painful symptoms as the flexor hallucis longus courses adjacent to the tubercles then through a groove under the sustentaculum tali.*
     (b) Mechanism of injury—Two mechanisms of injury have been proposed: hyperdorsiflexion and/or inversion, leading to tightening of the posterior talofibular ligament with avulsion of the lateral tubercle, and forced plantar flexion, causing compression of the lateral tubercle between the tibia and the calcaneus.
     (c) Stress fractures—*Stress fractures leading to failure of the lateral ossicle to unite may occur as a result of repetitive activity.*
     (d) Radiography—The lateral ankle view provides the best delineation of the fracture. It is difficult to distinguish between an acute fracture of the trigonal process (roughened edges) and discontinuity of the os trigonum (smooth edges). *A bone scan can be helpful.*
     (e) Treatment—Treatment involves a nonweightbearing cast for 4 weeks, followed by a walking cast for 2 weeks. Persistent pain is treated with further casting. Symptoms lasting over 6 months indicate nonunion. A bone scan may be useful for documenting localized metabolic activity. *Excision through a posterolateral approach (between the flexor hallucis longus and the peroneals) is recommended for cases of nonunion. Athroscopic excision has also been described.*

5. Osteochondral defects of the talus—These are intra-articular fractures of the talar dome articular surface. Impaction injuries may leave the overlying cartilage intact while shear injuries may cause a flap tear of the cartilage. Osteochondral defects of the talus occur in 6.5% of all ankle sprains. After trauma, 55% of the lesions involve the medial portion of the talus, and 45% involve the lateral talus.
   - Mechanism
     Lateral—dorsiflexion and inversion of the ankle cause impaction and anterolateral shear.

Medial—Plantar flexion and inversion cause the superomedial ridge of the talus to rub on the tibial plafond, resulting in a medial lesion.

- Diagnosis—Symptoms mimic those of an ankle sprain; this injury may have the sensation of a foreign body.
- Radiography—*A lateral lesion is usually flatter and more wafer-like as opposed to a medial lesion, which is deep and cup-shaped.* CT can help delineate the depth and size of the lesion, but MRI is more accurate in determining the overlying cartilage separation and dissociation of the fragment from its subchondral bed. MRI can also identify associated soft-tissue injuries.
- Classifications
  (a) Berndt and Harty classification—The Berndt and Harty classification (Table 14-2) is the original and most widely used classification.
  (b) Ferkel CT classification
  (c) Anderson MR classification
- Treatment (based on the Berndt and Harty classification)
  (a) Stage I and II lesions and medial Stage III lesions—Stage I and II lesions and medial Stage III lesions are treated by cast immobilization for 6 to 12 weeks. If symptoms persist over 4 to 6 months, injuries are treated surgically as described next.
  (b) Stage IV and lateral Stage III lesions—*Stage IV lesions and lateral Stage III lesions are treated surgically.* Smaller lesions are treated by surgical excision and drilling of the base of the lesion. This can be done either open or

arthroscopically. Larger lesions involving over one-third of the articular surface are treated with operative reduction and fixation of the fragment. The use of bone graft is controversial. Medial or lateral arthrotomies are usually satisfactory, but large posteromedial lesions may require a malleolar osteotomy. Nonweightbearing with aggressive range-of-motion exercises is continued for 8 to 12 weeks.

- Chronic lesions—Chronic lesions should be suspected in patients with persistent symptoms after appropriate conservative treatment for an ankle sprain. Symptoms are usually activity-related and include pain, locking, and swelling. These lesions may not be visible on plain X-ray films, and a bone scan, an MRI, or both modalities may be helpful. MRI can assess stability by demonstrating the presence or absence of a fibrous attachment or fluid in the base of the fragment and in the fragment bed. The treatment for unstable chronic lesions is similar to that for acute lateral Stage III and Stage IV lesions. Ankle stiffness and arthritis are common with chronic lesions.

6. Dislocations involving the talus—Talar dislocations are high-energy injuries; 10% to 15% of these injuries are open.
- Subtalar dislocation—These are relatively rare injuries accounting for about 1% of all injuries to the foot. Subtalar dislocations occur with dislocation of both the subtalar and talonavicular joint. They are usually high-energy injuries, but may occur after small injuries. It is important to distinguish subtalar dislocations based on energy (high or low) and direction of dislocation in terms of treatment and prognosis.
- Anatomic classification:
  (a) Medial subtalar dislocations occur with forceful inversion of the foot while in plantar flexion. These are the most common, and 40% have an open injury.
  (b) Lateral subtalar dislocations occur with forceful eversion of the foot while in plantar flexion. These are usually higher energy with higher incidence of open injuries with over half being open.
  (c) Posterior dislocations may occur with hyper plantar flexion
  (d) Anterior dislocations are very rare and may result from a traction injury.
- Radiographs—Plain radiographs including three views of the foot and ankle are required

TABLE 14-2

Berndt and Harty Classification of Osteochondral Lesions of the Talus

Classification	Description
Stage I	There is a small area of compressed subchondral bone.
Stage II	There is a partially detached osteochondral fragment.
Stage III	There is a completely detached osteochondral fragment that is located in the talar crater.
Stage IV	There is a completely detached osteochondral fragment that is loose within the joint.

for full evaluation. After reduction, plain films should be repeated to look for concentric reduction of the subtalar and talonavicular joint. Broden's views can demonstrate reduction at the subtalar joint. Postoperative plain films and CT scans can further assess for associated impaction fractures or osteochondral fractures that may occur at the talonavicular or subtalar joint or evaluation of incarcerated fragments.

- Treatment
  (a) Documentation of a complete neurovascular exam is crucial both pre- and postreduction.
  (b) Reduction consists of knee flexion, traction/countertraction at the foot, recreation of the injury force, and direct pressure to the talar head as the calcaneus is gently manipulated back into position. This should be done in a timely fashion to reduce tenting of the skin and possible skin necrosis.
  (c) Open injuries
    - Irrigation and debridment
    - Since lateral dislocations are higher-energy injuries, many require secondary grafting or flap procedures.
  (d) Irreducible joints—If the joint cannot be reduced closed, then open reduction must be performed through an anteromedial or anterolateral approach to the talus
    - Medial dislocations
      - Buttonholing of the talar head through the extensor retinaculum
      - Entrapment of the extensor digitorum brevis
      - Entrapment of the lateral branch of the deep peroneal nerve
      - Impaction of the navicular onto the talar head
    - Lateral dislocations
      - Impaction of the navicular onto the talar head
      - Entrapment of the talar head by the posterior tibial tendon or flexor digitorum longus
  (e) Postreduction
    - If the joint is stable and concentrically reduced then casting for at least 1 month is recommended with early range-of-motion exercises.
    - If the joint is incongruent, then again check for impediment to reduction or impaction fragments in the joint. This may require formal open reduction.

- Unstable joints are common with high-energy injuries. External fixation of the ankle and/or the subtalar joint may be required for at least 4 weeks. An alternative is Steinmann pin fixation of the subtalar joint and casting for 6 weeks.
  (f) Complications
    - Skin necrosis
    - Subtalar arthritis
    - Continued instability
    - Avascular necrosis
    - Infection
    - Neurovascular injury usually occurs in higher energy injuries (Usually involves the posterior tibial artery or tibial nerve)
    - Posterior tibial tendon injury
- Total talar dislocation—Total talar dislocation represents a rare injury; most are open. They are treated by reduction after irrigation and debridement, if possible. Occasionally, contamination is severe enough that complete talar extrusion may require talectomy. (Treatment, in such a case, is by primary tibiocalcaneal arthrodesis.)

II. Calcaneal Fractures and Subtalar Dislocations
  A. Historical Perspective—There is no consensus regarding the optimal treatment of calcaneal fractures. Management includes nonreduction, closed reduction, ORIF, and primary arthrodesis, and there are no formal indications or agreement on approach or outcome criteria.
  B. Anatomy—The calcaneus is the largest, most irregularly shaped bone in the foot; it contains a large amount of cancellous bone and has multiple processes. The tuberosity serves as the site of attachment for the broad, expansive Achilles tendon posteriorly and the plantar fascia inferiorly. The posterior facet is the largest articular surface and supports the lateral process and body of the talus. The sustentacular fragment houses the middle facet and the stout interosseous talocalcaneal ligament. The flexor hallucis longus runs in a groove just below the sustentaculum tali. The anterior process is protuberant just superior to the cuboid articulation, which contains the bifurcate ligament attachments to the navicular and cuboid. Approximately 60% of foot fractures involve the calcaneus. Approximately 2% of all fractures involve the calcaneus.
  C. Fracture Classification—No consensus regarding the optimal classification exists.
    1. Essex-Lopresti (Table 14-3)—The most commonly used classification is that of **Essex-Lopresti**. It

TABLE 14-3

Essex-Lopresti Classification of Calcaneal Fractures

Extra-articular calcaneal fractures (≈25% of cases)

Anterior process fractures

Tuberosity fractures

Medial process fractures

Sustentaculum tali fractures

Body fractures without involvement of the subtalar joint

Intra-articular calcaneal fractures (≈75% of cases)

Nondisplaced fractures

Joint depression fractures

Tongue-type fractures

Severely comminuted fractures

separates fractures into intra-articular (75% of cases) and extra-articular (25%).

2. Sanders (Fig. 14-5)—The **Sanders** system is a CT classification; it has become very popular and carries prognostic implications.

D. Associated Injuries—Calcaneal fractures are usually the result of a fall from a height or other high-energy mechanisms. Approximately 10% of these fractures are associated with a lumbar spine fracture, particularly of L1. Approximately 10% of calcaneal fractures are bilateral.

E. Specific Injury Types

1. Intra-articular fractures—Two general types of intra-articular fractures have been described (joint depression and tongue type).

   • Mechanism of injury—The mechanism of injury is most commonly axial loading. The lateral process of the talus acts as a wedge, creating a primary fracture line (vertical) and a secondary fracture line (more posteriorly directed), which determines the type of fracture.

   • Diagnosis—Tenderness, tremendous swelling at the heel, and ecchymosis occur; evidence of neural compromise (tarsal tunnel distribution) may also occur.

   • Radiography—Plain lateral X-ray films of the foot and an axial heel view usually demonstrate **shortening and widening of the calcaneus, usually with a varus orientation of the tuberosity.** Loss of Bohler's and Gissane's angles is also diagnostic. The primary and secondary fracture lines are sometimes well visualized. Broden's views demonstrate subtalar joint involvement and are used

to evaluate intraoperative posterior facet reduction.

• CT Scan—CT helps assess **involvement of the posterior facet** and the extent of comminution. CT is also useful for evaluating involvement of the calcaneocuboid joint. As previously described above, a CT classification has been described by Sanders (see Fig. 14-5). The CT cuts should be done perpendicular to the posterior facet, and sagittal cuts should be parallel to the plantar aspect of the foot. CT cuts should be 3 mm thick. CT helps demonstrate the typical **shortening, widening, and varus and medial displacement of the heel.**

• Soft-tissue management—Intra-articular fractures of the calcaneus are associated with tremendous swelling. Operative intervention is best performed within 12 hours of the injury or 1 to 2 weeks after the injury, when the swelling resolves. Sequential compression devices may be helpful in reducing edema. Fat pad explosion or atrophy can cause long-term problems. Tendons (flexor hallucis longus, peroneus longus) can be incarcerated within the fracture fragments or dislocated. Compartment syndrome is common and must be addressed by compartment pressure monitoring and fasciotomy. This occurs in the deep central compartment which houses the lateral plantar nerve and quadratus plantae. Clinical exam of pain out of proportion to exam is unreliable and compartmental pressure monitoring is recommended. In the "wrinkle test," the skin appears wrinkled, indicating that swelling has subsided; this test is used to determine surgical timing from the soft-tissue standpoint. Fractures should be reduced within 3 weeks if possible as fracture consolidation after 3 weeks can make reduction and fixation extremely difficult.

• Associated injuries—There is approximately a 10% incidence of lumbar spine injury and 25% incidence of other lower-extremity injury.

• Treatment—Treatment depends on the severity of the fracture and the extent of articular comminution.

(a) Nondisplaced articular fractures—Nondisplaced articular fractures are managed in a bulky (Robert-Jones) dressing. Once ankle control is restored and swelling subsides, active subtalar range of motion is instituted, but weightbearing

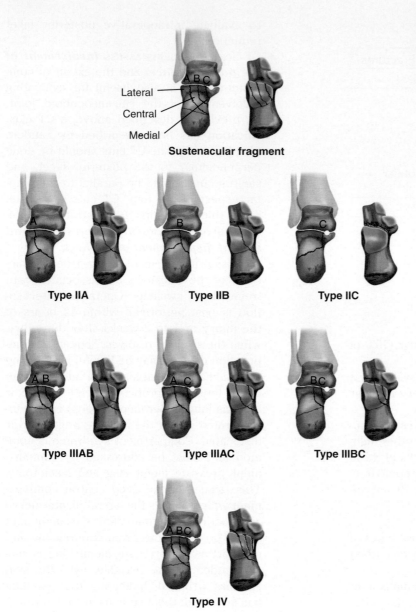

FIGURE 14-5 CT classification of intra-articular calcaneal fractures. It is important that the coronal section analyzed include the widest point of the articular surface (the sustenaculum tali).

is still prohibited. Usually, walking can start at about 8 to 12 weeks, depending on comminution.

(b) Displaced intra-articular fractures with large fragments—Displaced intra-articular fractures with large fragments should undergo ORIF when the soft tissues allow. The surgical approach is based on the surgeon's preference and familiarity.

Percutaneous fixation may be used in certain instances especially large tongue type fractures. An Essex Lopresti maneuver with the patient in the prone position may help unlock and reduce the tuberosity fragment.

The lateral extensile approach is the most popular, but a modified subtalar approach, a medial approach, or combined approaches are also acceptable. ***With the lateral approach, care must be taken to make full-thickness soft-tissue flaps and avoid the sural nerve.*** The lateral approach is made with the vertical limb 0.5 cm anterior to the Achilles. This extends to the junction of the lateral and plantar skin. The horizontal limb runs along the line formed by the lateral and plantar skin. The lateral calcaneal artery is critical in maintaining flap viability and runs 1.5 cm anterior to the Achilles in the vertical limb. The "constant fragment" is held reduced by the strong talocalcaneal ligament, and the joint can be reconstructed by using subcortical cancellous screw fixation. The next step is to correct the morphology of the calcaneus to restore height and width. Skeletal traction via a Steinmann pin in the tuberosity is sometimes helpful. The anterolateral fragment is usually superiorly displaced and may need to be rotated and depressed into position. This restores the angle of Gissane, and the anterolateral fragment can be provisionally pinned. Lateral buttress plating with fixation into the tuberosity joint fragment and anterior process usually hold the calcaneus in an appropriate position. Bone grafting is optional, but has not been shown to speed healing or alter results.

The medial approach provides better visualization of the sustentaculum tali. Articular reduction is performed using the sustentacular fragment as the key under direct visualization. The difficulty with the medial approach is how to address the posterior facet. A limited approach and potentially percutaneous elevation of the fragment are options. To successfully mobilize fragments with the medial approach, the fracture should be addressed within 1 week.

Use of a ring external fixator system is another alternative to difficult fractures or open fractures. McGarvey et al. recently reported outcomes using an Ilizarov fixator and limited incisions for displaced calcaneal fractures. Sanders Type II to IV fractures (both open and closed fractures) were included. Thirty-three fractures were evaluated and there was only one deep wound infection. There were no deep infections or wound complications in the open subgroup after initial wound management and free flaps if necessary. At an average 2-year follow up, no subsequent revision procedures had been performed.

(c) Displaced intra-articular fractures with severe comminution—*Increasing intra-articular comminution leads to less satisfactory results*. Therefore, although an initial attempt at ORIF may be reasonable, if the joint surface is not

reconstructible, and the likelihood of posttraumatic subtalar arthritis is high, primary arthrodesis is recommended. Attention should still be paid to restoring the heel width and height.

(d) Open fractures are especially problematic as they commonly arise from high-energy trauma. Up to 70% wound complications have been reported with greater than 50% incidence of osteomyelitis. Reports with early irrigation, IV antibiotics debridement, and provisional fixation with delayed reconstruction show better results with 10% to 20% incidence of infection, wound complication, or osteomyelitis.

• Complications
(a) Soft-tissue breakdown—Soft-tissue breakdown remains the most common and a severe complication, particularly related to the lateral extensile approach. Typically, it occurs at the apex of the incision and can occur as long as 4 weeks from injury. Systemic factors, such as diabetes mellitus, peripheral vascular disease, alcohol abuse, and smoking, contribute to wound complications.

(b) Local infection—Local infection is also common and should be addressed with early debridement and antibiotics. If the wound is infected with *Staphylococcus aureus* and there is early healing, then the treatment is hardware removal and irrigation and debridement.

(c) Subtalar arthrosis—Subtalar arthrosis continues to be problematic even after a good articular reduction. University of California at Berkley Laboratory-type orthotic devices may be helpful. Persistent pain that does not respond to conservative treatment is managed with subtalar arthrodesis. Factors associated with likelihood of late arthrosis and need for a subtalar arthrodesis are: work-related injury, Sanders Type IV fractures, initial Bohler's angle less than 0°, and initial nonoperative treatment.

(d) Anterior ankle impingement—Anterior ankle impingement may occur if the fracture has not been reduced and the talus settles. In these cases, *a bone block distraction arthrodesis* of the subtalar joint may be beneficial.

(e) Lateral impingement—Lateral impingement of the fibula on the peroneal tendons is also the result of inadequate reduction because the prominent lateral wall of the calcaneus abuts the fibula with weightbearing (causing compression of the peroneal tendons as they pass through the groove). In these cases, lateral wall exostectomy will be beneficial with possible tenolysis and repair or excision of peroneal tendon tears.

(f) Cutaneous neuromas—Cutaneous neuromas, particularly of the sural nerve, can arise after surgery using the lateral approach to the calcaneus. Treatment involves resection and burying of the nerve into the peroneal muscle belly.

(g) Heel pad pain is very common due to injury to the specialized plantar fat pad with resultant scarring and fibrosis. No good solutions exist and currently cushioned inserts are recommended.

• Results of the operative treatment of calcaneal fractures—The results are disappointing even in the best of hands. Calcaneal fractures account for a large number of days missed from work and require lengthy periods of rehabilitation. *Even with anatomic restoration of the posterior facet, subtalar stiffness continues to be troublesome. The most predictable outcome is restoration of heel height and width.* In a randomized prospective multicenter study, patients with operative treatment had an overall significantly better outcome than nonoperatively treated patients when worker's compensation patients were removed.

(a) Operative versus nonoperative complications of calcaneal fractures in order of frequency at 2-year follow up.
  • Nonoperative
    • Post traumatic arthrosis (16%)
    • Lateral ostectomies (0.8%)
    • Compartment syndrome (0.8%)
  • Operative
    • Wound slough (16%)
    • Malposition (6%)
    • DVT (1.2%)

2. Extra-articular fractures—*Extra-articular fractures are usually avulsion fractures of a process of the calcaneus.*
  • Types
    (a) Anterior process fractures of the calcaneus—The mechanism of injury is plantar flexion and inversion. The bifurcate ligament attaches to the anterior process of the calcaneus. These

fractures are often confused with lateral ankle sprains, but tenderness is more distal over the sinus tarsi. Radiographic findings can be subtle. The treatment of fractures with a small bony fragment is short leg casting for 4 to 6 weeks with weightbearing as tolerated. The treatment of fractures with a large bony fragment, a displaced fragment, or an injury involving a portion of the calcaneocuboid articular surface is ORIF. Fractures that were treated nonoperatively and that failed to unite may be excised if they are symptomatic.

(b) Tuberosity fractures of the calcaneus—Tuberosity fractures involve avulsion of a bony fragment when the Achilles tendon is loaded beyond the tensile strength of its attachment. Sometimes such a large fragment is avulsed that the articulation of the posterior facet becomes involved. Treatment is based on the degree of displacement. Nondisplaced or minimally displaced fractures are treated with immobilization in equinus for about 3 weeks. Displaced fractures require ORIF to restore the integrity of the Achilles tendon and reduce the potential for soft-tissue compromise, which can be caused by tenting of the fragment against the tenuous posterior skin. *Failure to repair the injury may lead to plantar flexion weakness.*

III. Injuries of the Midfoot
  A. Navicular Fractures—Injuries of the navicular are classified into four types: dorsal lip (cortical avulsion), tuberosity, body, and stress fractures.
    1. Dorsal lip fracture—Dorsal lip fractures are the most common type; they are usually mechanically insignificant. They occur with twisting and inversion. Treatment involves casting if the injury is symptomatic. If the fracture heals with exuberant callus with a dorsal exostosis, it can irritate the deep peroneal nerve, which courses directly above it. Treatment of an exostosis causing painful symptoms is shoe modification or excision of the prominence.
    2. Tuberosity fracture—A tuberosity fracture is usually an avulsion injury from a sudden forceful contraction of the tibialis posterior tendon. Because the insertion site of the tibialis posterior is broad, the displacement is usually minimal. Treatment involves short leg casting with an arch mold. This fracture should not be

confused with an accessory navicular (which is present in 12% of the population). Painful nonunion is rare, but if it occurs, resection of the ossicle with reattachment of the tibialis posterior tendon is usually successful. Advancement of the tendon in combination with excision (modified Kidner procedure) is usually unnecessary.

3. Body fracture—A body fracture usually occurs from axial loading of the navicular in plantar flexion. It involves the talonavicular and the naviculocuneiform joints. Inadequate management may lead to debilitating collapse and arthrosis.
   - Classification of Sangeorzan (Fig. 14-6):
     (a) Type I involves a transverse coronal fracture (<50% of the body).
     (b) Type II is the most common. The fracture courses dorsal lateral to plantar medial. The plantar medial fragment is often smaller and comminuted.
     (c) Type III involves central or lateral comminution, often with lateral displacement of the forefoot leading to an abduction deformity. Sometimes calcaneocuboid joint subluxation occurs.
   - Treatment
     (a) Nondisplaced fractures can be casted for 6 weeks in a short leg nonweight-bearing cast.
     (b) In displaced fractures, ORIF is indicated with strict attention to preserving medial column length and preventing abduction deformities of the forefoot that can lead to late arthrosis. Typically, open reduction is necessary, and internal fixation with cancellous screws is used for large fragments. Severe comminution requires interposition bone grafting and possibly external fixation to preserve length.
     (c) External fixation is also a good option when the soft tissues are too swollen for open reduction and internal fixation, when additional fixation is needed to augment internal fixation, and for ligamentotaxis of comminuted fractures.
     (d) Primary arthrodesis may be necessary for extremely comminuted fractures.
     (e) Often, late arthrodesis of the naviculocuneiform and talonavicular joints is necessary for symptomatic relief.

4. Stress fractures—Stress fractures are commonly found in athletes performing repetitive stressful activities; they often go unrecognized. Poor radiographic representation leads to delay in diagnosis (average, 4 months after symptoms begin).
   - Diagnosis—The diagnosis is suggested by a history of repetitive stress athletics (e.g., jumping, running) and focal tenderness. If plain X-ray films are negative or nondiagnostic, an MRI or a bone scan may be helpful. Plain radiographs characteristically show vertical fracture lucency in the central third of the navicular, but CT scanning should be performed to further characterize the fracture pattern.
   - Treatment—Treatment is based on the amount of displacement and CT can help determine this.
     (a) ***Nondisplaced fractures can be treated in a non-weightbearing short leg cast for 6 to 8 weeks***.
     (b) ***Displaced fractures require ORIF with grafting of the fracture site***, preferably from a lateral approach with lateral to medial screw fixation because the lateral fragment is most often smaller.

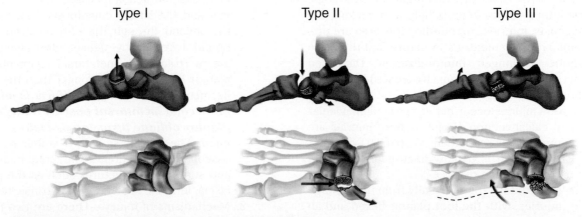

Type I   Type II   Type III

<u>FIGURE 14-6</u> Classification of navicular body fractures.

B. Cuboid Injuries
   1. Minimally displaced avulsion fractures of the cuboid—The majority of cuboid fractures are minimally displaced and insignificant. These usually result from inversion strain. The fracture is best visualized on the anteroposterior radiograph at the lateral border of the foot. Conservative treatment is 4 weeks of weightbearing in a hard-soled shoe.
   2. "Nutcracker fracture"—The nutcracker fracture is frequently missed.
      • Mechanism of injury—A high-energy abduction force leads to crushing of the cuboid with potential plantar extrusion of bone and lateral subluxation of the forefoot as a result of a shortened lateral column.
      • Treatment—Open reduction with bone grafting is usually necessary for preserving length. Occasionally an H-plate may be applied to support the length, but fixation is often difficult because of comminution; therefore, external fixation tends to be more reliable for the restoration of lateral column length.
      • Late sequelae—Arthrosis is common. Treatment is by calcaneocuboid arthrodesis. Fusion of the cuboid metatarsal joint should not be attempted because results are routinely poor; this joint tends not to be symptomatic. Interpositional arthroplasty may be effective as a salvage procedure.
   3. Calcaneocuboid subluxation—Calcaneocuboid subluxation is seen predominantly in dancers; it results from overuse. The injury is self-limited and is treated symptomatically with physical therapy and orthoses.
C. Cuneiform Fractures—Cuneiform fractures are rare, isolated injuries. They are usually found in conjunction with other high-energy injuries such as tarsometatarsal fracture-dislocations. Cuneiform fractures are frequently overlooked because of the more obvious adjacent pathologic condition. A bone scan is helpful in making the diagnosis. Injuries surrounding this area are predominantly ligamentous in nature and therefore require prolonged immobilization. Displaced fractures and dislocations are treated with ORIF.
D. Midtarsal Joint Injuries
   1. These injuries occur between the talonavicular and calcaneocuboid joints. These injuries are commonly missed initially in up to 30% of cases.
   2. Classification is usually anatomic and based on the direction of force.
      • Longitudinal force, usually from high-energy injuries, with the foot plantar flexed and an axially based force on the metatarsal heads.

This impacts the talonavicular and calcaneocuboid joints and leads to an array of injury patterns. Fracture lines usually extend vertically through the navicular based on a medial or middle column line of force.
   • Medial force results in a spectrum of injury patterns and may be the precursor to a full subtalar dislocation. A "medial swivel" injury occurs when the rotational force is around the talocalcaneal interosseous ligament causing dislocation of the talonavicular joint with an intact calcaneocuboid joint and subluxation of the subtalar joint.
   • Lateral force—an abduction injury to the midfoot leads to the classic "nutcracker" injury as described above. Another variant is the "lateral swivel" injury leading to talonavicular dislocation with an intact calcaneocuboid joint and subluxation of the subtalar joint. Look for the avulsed tuberosity of the navicular as a clue to these injury patterns.
   • Plantar force—hyperplantarflexion injuries may cause injury to the dorsal talonavicular joint complex. X-rays may show a dorsal fleck at the talonavicular joint capsule.
   • Crush—see crush injury section.
   3. Treatment—Early recognition is the key to a good outcome. If the joint is concentrically reduced, then 6 weeks of casting can be initiated. Irreducible dislocations require open reduction and possible excision versus internal fixation of fragments. Continued pain or instability may warrant future arthrodesis.
E. Tarsometatarsal (Lisfranc's) Fracture-Dislocations
   1. Anatomy of the tarsometatarsal joint (Fig. 14-7)—The tarsometatarsal joint comprises the bases of the first through the fifth metatarsals; the medial, middle, and lateral cuneiforms; and the cuboid. Joint stability is derived from the "keystone effect" at the base of the second metatarsal, which is recessed between the medial and the lateral cuneiforms. The bases of the second through the fifth metatarsals are bound together by dense interosseous ligaments (transverse metatarsal ligaments); the plantar ligaments are stronger than the dorsal ligaments. *The medial cuneiform is joined to the second metatarsal base by a large stout plantar oblique ligament, or Lisfranc's ligament.* The transverse arch is stabilized by the osseous configuration at the metatarsal bases and supporting structures such as the plantar fascia, intrinsic muscles, and extrinsic tendons.
   2. Mechanisms of injury—There are two mechanisms of injury: direct and indirect.

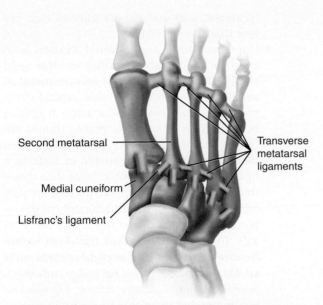

FIGURE 14-7 Tarsometatarsal articulation (plantar view). Note the "keystone effect" at the base of the second metatarsal.

Second metatarsal

Transverse metatarsal ligaments

Medial cuneiform

Lisfranc's ligament

- Direct forces—Direct forces are less common than indirect forces.
- Indirect forces
  (a) Axial loading and loading with the foot in a plantar-flexed position. Such forces lead to predictable patterns of injury. Continued loading leads to accentuation of the longitudinal arch and destruction of the weak dorsal tarsometatarsal ligaments with dislocation or avulsion fractures of the metatarsal bases.
  (b) A new mechanism of injury is arising in collegiate and professional athletics probably due to shoe and turf changes. With the foot planted and a rotational force applied, diastasis at the medial cuneiform and second metatarsal occurs. The energy then propagates between the medial and middle cuneiform. This is important to distinguish, as a screw should be placed through the Lisfranc ligament and between the cuneiforms.
3. Classification—The classification distinguishes the amount of rotation and force applied (Fig. 14-8).

FIGURE 14-8 Classification of tarsometatarsal fracture-dislocations. *L,* lateral; *M,* medial.

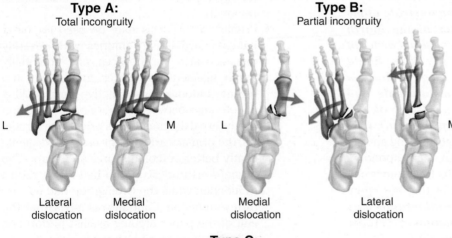

Type A:
Total incongruity

L   M

Lateral dislocation   Medial dislocation

Type B:
Partial incongruity

L   M

Medial dislocation   Lateral dislocation

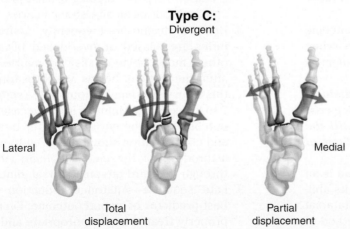

Type C:
Divergent

Lateral   Medial

Total displacement   Partial displacement

4. Associated injuries—Because of the position of the foot, it is common to see metatarsal neck fractures or metatarsophalangeal joint dislocations with indirect force injuries. ***Vascular injury is common and involves the perforating branch of the dorsalis pedis artery. This can occasionally cause a compartment syndrome.***

5. Diagnosis—Physical examination demonstrates tremendous swelling, tenderness of the midfoot, and ecchymosis. Abduction or pronation stress to the forefoot elicits pain at the midfoot in more subtle injuries. Motion of the second metatarsal head frequently elicits midfoot pain. Compartment syndrome is possible.

6. Radiography—High-energy Lisfranc's injuries are usually well demonstrated on plain radiographs. However, these injuries may be subtle. (There is a 20% reported incidence of missed diagnoses on review of plain X-ray films.) ***Attention should be directed toward the base of the second metatarsal to detect a bony avulsion, or "fleck sign," signifying ligamentous disruption. In addition, the medial border of the second metatarsal should align with the medial border of the middle cuneiform on the anteroposterior plain radiograph. Oblique films demonstrate alignment of the medial border of the fourth metatarsal paralleling the medial border of the cuboid. Lateral view X-ray films should reveal an unbroken line along the dorsum of the first and second metatarsals and the respective cuneiforms. Also, look for opening at the plantar aspect of the first tarsometatarsal joint.*** Weightbearing anteroposterior radiographs with corresponding contralateral foot radiographs for comparison often reveal the unstable joint that has spontaneously relocated. ***Stress radiographs may also be helpful in these instances.*** (Proper analgesia should be administered.)

7. Treatment—Because of the poor outcome associated with these injuries, even when properly fixed early, aggressive treatment is indicated.
    - ***Nondisplaced stable fracture-dislocations can be managed in a short leg cast with no weightbearing. ORIF is still the gold standard for more than 1 to 2 mm of displacement***.
    - Closed reduction and internal fixation is an option but controversy exists as to its ability to properly align the tarsometatarsal joints. This is a more reasonable method of treatment with low-energy injuries that are less than 1 week old.
    - Open reduction and internal fixation with solid or cannulated screws is the gold standard. The base of the second metatarsal should be reduced; this occasionally requires debridement of a bone fragment or extraction of an incarcerated tibialis anterior tendon (dorsal), peroneus longus tendon (plantar), or a portion of Lisfranc's ligament. Once Lisfranc's joint has been reduced, the remainder of the foot usually follows because of the attachments of the interosseous ligaments to the lesser metatarsals. ***(No intermetatarsal ligament exists between the first and second metatarsals so they must be reduced independently).*** Screw fixation (usually 3.5 or 4.0 mm) is recommended over pins to maintain proper position and prevent late loss of reduction, especially with pure ligamentous injuries, which require longer periods of healing. An exception to this rule is the lateral joint complex (metatarsals 4 and 5), which should have motion maintained and which is better treated with K-wires. Screws should be left in place for at least 16 weeks before removal.
    - Primary arthrodesis may be used for older patients, high-energy injuries with severely damaged articular surfaces, and potentially purely ligamentous injuries. In addition, in a recent randomized prospective study looking at outcomes between primary open reduction and internal fixation versus primary arthrodesis, the primary arthrodesis group had significantly better outcome scores at 2 years. The primary arthrodesis group had a 92% return to function while the ORIF group had 65% return to function. Caution was advised at the end of the paper arguing against performing an arthrodesis on all Lisfranc injuries.

8. Delayed diagnosis—Frequently, Lisfranc injuries are missed or overlooked because of other, more obvious skeletal injuries. Only after the patient begins weightbearing may this injury become symptomatic (sometimes 7 to 8 weeks after injury). In these cases, poor outcomes are the norm even after treatment, and consideration should be given to primary arthrodesis of the medial column (the first through the third tarsometatarsal joints).

9. Late sequelae—Anatomic reduction is the best predictor of a good outcome. Even when properly treated in an appropriate and timely

fashion, the results of the treatment of Lisfranc's injuries are poor, and there is a high rate of degenerative arthrosis (approximately 25%) and fixed deformity. Purely ligamentous injuries tend to have a worse outcome. After hardware removal, these injuries may "spring open." ***Arthrodesis is a useful and reliable procedure and should include all involved tarsometatarsal joints except those at the base of the fourth and fifth metatarsals, which tend not to fuse reliably and lead to long-term pain.*** Pain arises predominantly from the joints of the medial column, and this can be confirmed by selective injections.

- Post traumatic arthritis occurs in 25% of injuries
  - (a) Anatomical reduction is associated with a better radiographic and functional outcome
  - (b) There is a trend toward worse outcomes with purely ligamentous injuries

IV. Forefoot Injuries
  A. Metatarsal Fractures—The majority of metatarsal fractures are low-energy injuries, so an orthopaedic surgeon is frequently not consulted.
  1. Metatarsal neck and shaft fractures—Metatarsal neck and shaft fractures usually result from direct trauma but less commonly can occur as a stress fracture.
     - Diagnosis—The history is compatible with either direct trauma or pain from repetitive use. Traumatic injuries are often associated with focal swelling and tenderness that can increase significantly when there are multiple fractures, leading to compartment syndrome.
     - Radiography—The lateral foot radiograph is most important for detecting a sagittal plane deformity, which will be the most symptomatic.
     - Treatment
       (a) Nondisplaced fractures—The majority of nondisplaced fractures are treated conservatively with shoe wear modification, casts, or a hard-soled shoe, with activity modification advancing to weightbearing as tolerated. Overtreatment should be avoided. Protected immobilization or nonweightbearing can give rise to late sequelae such as osteopenia, atrophy, and reflex sympathetic dystrophy (RSD).
       (b) Displaced fractures—No absolute indications for operative intervention exist.

Surgical correction should be considered for angulation greater than 10° in any plane or displacement greater than 3 or 4 mm. Sagittal plane displacement is poorly tolerated. Plantar displacement can give rise to excessive metatarsal overload and may cause a painful plantar keratosis; excessive dorsal angulation may lead to a prominence that results in corns and shoe-wear problems. Transverse plane displacement is better tolerated, although if it is great enough, it can lead to intermetatarsal impingement and neuroma formation. Reduction of a displaced metatarsal neck or shaft fracture may be performed open or closed. Longitudinal traction may be applied (Chinese finger traps) and manipulation performed. If the fracture is stable, a cast may be applied, and management is the same as that for nondisplaced fractures. Unstable fractures are treated operatively.
       (c) Irreducible fractures—Irreducible fractures require open treatment. Direct exposure of the fracture is performed, and fixation is with crossed pins or mini fragment screws.
       (d) Multiple metatarsal fractures—Multiple metatarsal fractures are unstable injuries that generally occur as the result of higher-energy trauma. (Soft-tissue complications can occur.) Attempts at closed manipulation may be successful, and if they are, the fracture may be held with K-wire fixation. If it is not reducible using closed means, ORIF is performed with K-wires, mini fragment screws, or plate fixation.
       (e) Metatarsal fractures with bone loss—Maintenance of length is important, especially if there are multiple metatarsal fractures. Transfixation pins from the head of the involved metatarsal to the adjacent stable metatarsal head, or external fixation, are useful. Open bone grafting is performed when the soft tissues allow. Failure to maintain length can result in abnormal loading and the development of painful keratoses.
       (f) Nonunions—Nonunions generally occur in proximal metatarsal fractures. They are frequently hypertrophic and asymptomatic and therefore need no treatment. For symptomatic metatarsal

nonunions, open bone grafting is generally successful.

(g) First metatarsal fractures—The first metatarsal is integral in maintenance of the medial column and supports one-third of the forefoot's pressure. If malunion occurs then transfer metatarsalgia and further collapse of the medial column may occur. ***Therefore, displaced first metatarsal fractures should undergo ORIF.***

(h) Open metatarsal shaft fractures require open reduction and internal fixation usually with K-wires to allow stability for soft-tissue healing.

2. Metatarsal head fractures—Metatarsal head fractures are rare injuries and are usually the result of direct trauma.
   - Associated injuries—The clinician should rule out tarsometatarsal joint injuries and proximal metatarsal fractures.
   - Deforming forces—Displacement is usually plantar and lateral.
   - Treatment—Manipulation with traction is often successful; if the fracture is unstable, interosseous pinning may be necessary. Fractures devoid of soft-tissue attachments may require ORIF. ***Symptomatic osteochondral lesions may require open debridement.***
   - Complications and late sequelae—Stiffness and arthritis occur; osteonecrosis has not been reported.

3. ***Fractures of the proximal fifth metatarsal*** (Fig. 14-9):
   - Zone I—Avulsion fractures occur when the peroneus brevis contracts against a sudden inversion stress. Another theory is that the fracture occurs at the insertion of the ligament at the base of the fifth metatarsal, which acts as a tether. The fracture fragment is proximal to the tuberosity and is contained within the attachment of the peroneus brevis.
     (a) Treatment—***Treatment involves weightbearing as tolerated in a hard-soled shoe.*** These fractures typically are clinically healed by 3 to 4 weeks.
     (b) Nonunion—Nonunion is rare, but if symptomatic, it can be treated with excision of the fragment.
   - Zone II—Metaphyseal–diaphyseal junction fractures (***Jones fracture***) can arise as a result of acute trauma or chronic stress (more common). The fracture occurs in a watershed zone, which leads to a delay in healing or nonunion. It is important to distinguish between the acute and chronic Jones fracture. Radiographs of the foot will characterize the fracture. Bone scans may be important to evaluate for an impending stress fracture. The incidence of delayed union and nonunion is relatively high. Hypertrophic nonunions may be treated with intramedullary screw fixation if the medullary canal is still open. If the medullary canal is sclerotic or the nonunion is atrophic, open inlay bone grafting is necessary. Results are generally good.
     (a) Nonoperative treatment of acute fracture—A short leg nonweightbearing cast is worn for 6 to 8 weeks. The patient then may transition to a fracture boot. It is common for the fracture to take 3 months or more to heal.

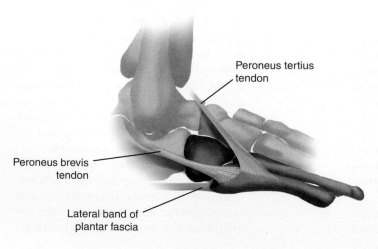

FIGURE 14-9 Lateral forefoot and the important soft-tissue-supporting structures inserting on the proximal fifth metatarsal.

Peroneus tertius tendon

Peroneus brevis tendon

Lateral band of plantar fascia

(b) Operative treatment of acute fracture—Highly competitive athletes are treated with single intramedullary screw fixation because inactivity is debilitating and the refracture rate is higher in this population.

- Zone III—Diaphyseal fractures (Dancer's fractures) result from a rotation injury. ***Treatment is with shoe-wear modifications or casting with weightbearing as tolerated in acute fractures.*** Union may take up to 20 weeks.

B. Toe Injuries

1. Phalangeal fractures—Phalangeal fractures occur most commonly in the proximal phalanx and most often in the fifth toe. The most common mechanism of injury is direct trauma (stubbing).

- Treatment
  (a) Nondisplaced fractures—Treatment consists of symptomatic management of pain and swelling and usually requires only shoe-wear modifications.
  (b) Displaced fractures—They tend to displace with plantar apex angulation. Displaced fractures are often amenable to manipulation; digital block is sufficient anesthesia. Once properly aligned, the toe is buddy-taped to the adjacent toe. Firm-soled shoes or sandals are used until symptoms abate.
  (c) Open fractures—Treatment involves local incision and drainage with primary closure and management as previously discussed.
  (d) Intra-articular fractures—Intra-articular fractures usually involve the condyle at the base of the phalanx. They may require open treatment and K-wire fixation. Failure to treat may lead to joint subluxation or painful arthrosis requiring resection arthroplasty.

2. Lesser toe dislocations

- Mechanism—A stubbing injury causes hyperdorsiflexion with a residual dorsal and lateral deformity. The plantar plate is injured, and the toe is displaced proximally.
- Treatment—Manual reduction is usually sufficient for simple dislocations. Buddy-taping is used for 1 to 2 weeks. ***Complex dislocations*** of the metatarsophalangeal joints occur when the plantar capsule (and plantar plate) and the deep transverse metatarsal ligament are displaced over the head of the metatarsal and become trapped between the flexor tendons laterally and the lumbricals medially. These injuries may require open reduction with division of the transverse metatarsal ligament and the plantar plate.

- Specific injuries
  (a) Metatarsophalangeal joint dislocations—The most common site of dislocation in the lesser toes is the metatarsophalangeal joint.
  (b) Recurrent, chronic metatarsophalangeal joint dislocations—Recurrent dislocation of the metatarsophalangeal joint requires a dorsal metatarsophalangeal joint capsulotomy and split flexor-to-extensor tendon transfer (Girdlestone-Taylor procedure). If arthrosis or plantar callusing is present, resection arthroplasty of the metatarsal heads or the base of the proximal phalanx is necessary.
  (c) Interphalangeal joint dislocations—Dislocations of the interphalangeal joint are rare; closed reduction and buddy-taping is usually successful. Chronic problems require resection arthroplasty, which may be combined with syndactylization.

3. Hallux interphalangeal dislocations—Hallux interphalangeal dislocations result from direct trauma or push-off. ***They are often irreducible.*** Treatment requires open reduction with removal of the entrapped plantar plate and the interphalangeal sesamoid if present. Joint stiffness is a common long-term sequela.

4. Turf toe injuries—Injury of the plantar plate and sesamoid complex (Fig. 14-10).

- Mechanism—Seen in push off sports with hyperextension of the first MTP. May also be seen with posterior axial force on the heel causing a hyperextension of the MTP
- Presentation—Painful, swollen first MTP joint with pain reproduced with passive hyperextension. May have increased anterior drawer of the first MTP.
- X-rays—Demonstrate concentric reduction of the joint. Significant findings are proximal migration of the sesamoids. Increased diastases of a bipartite sesamoid or a sesamoid fracture are common findings. Stress views will show a lag of the sesamoid as the toe extends.
- Treatment
  (a) Nonoperative—Plantar flexion taping. Rigid orthotic. Rest.
  (b) Operative—Excision or bone grafting of the sesamoid and repair of the plantar plate complex.

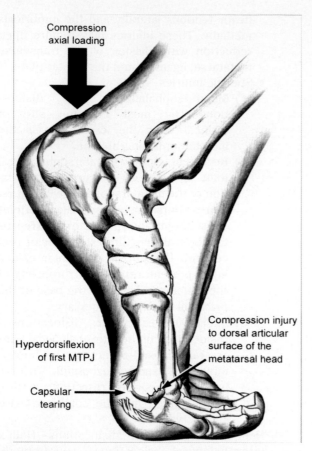

Compression
axial loading

Hyperdorsiflexion
of first MTPJ

Capsular
tearing

Compression injury
to dorsal articular
surface of the
metatarsal head

FIGURE 14-10 Turf toe injuries. (Reprinted with permission from Pedowitz WJ, Pedowitz DI. Hallux valgus in the athlete. In: Johnson DH, Pedowitz RA, eds. *Practical Orthopaedic Sports Medicine & Arthroscopy*. Philadelphia: Lippincott Williams & Wilkins, 2007: 922.)

C. Lawnmower Injuries—Lawnmower injuries usually occur when children play too close to a lawnmower or adults attempt to cut grass on an inclined wet surface. They usually result in much tissue destruction.
1. Treatment—***Aggressive debridement*** is imperative because these injuries tend to be highly contaminated. Multiple trips to the operating room and multiple procedures are often necessary. ***Early skin grafting*** is often helpful after bony stabilization.
2. Antibiotic coverage—A first-generation cephalosporin and an aminoglycoside should be administered. If the wound is contaminated with dirt (or other contaminants), a penicillin-class drug should be added.

V. Compartment Syndrome
A. Overview—Compartment syndrome results from increased tissue pressure within one or more of the tight osseofascial compartments of the body.

This section deals with compartment syndrome of the foot; however, many of the principles are the same as for compartment syndrome of other parts of the body. Compartment syndrome of the foot commonly results from a crush injury.
B. Anatomy—There are five major foot compartments: medial, lateral, central, interosseous, and calcaneal; at least nine have been reported using injection studies. Each compartment has separate and distinct boundaries. The calcaneal compartment communicates with the deep posterior compartment of the leg through an opening for tendinous and neurovascular structures behind the medial malleolus.
C. Diagnosis—Diagnosis is less specific than for compartment syndrome of the forearm and leg. (Symptoms of pain on passive stretch, pain out of proportion with the severity of injury, and dysesthesia are less reliable indicators.) A high index of suspicion is necessary in the patient with a tense swollen foot. Confirmation of the diagnosis may be made by compartment pressure measurement. (Abnormal values are the same as those for the other compartments of the body: pressure within 30 mm Hg of the systemic diastolic pressure.)
D. Treatment—Treatment involves fasciotomy. The technique and approach are determined by associated osseous or soft-tissue injuries. ***The classic description is two dorsal incisions and one medial incision.*** When associated with a Lisfranc injury or metatarsal fractures, two dorsal incisions along the second and fourth metatarsals allow access to all compartments. When no dorsal repair is required or trauma is limited to the hindfoot, a plantar medial approach provides access to all compartments. Fasciotomy incisions are initially left open for 5 to 7 days, and either a primary repair is performed or a split-thickness skin graft is used for coverage. ***Splint, do not cast compartment syndromes or one can compromise limb viability.***
E. Sequelae—Sequelae include late contractures; ***claw toes are the most common*** because of the loss of function of the intrinsic muscles. A cavus foot may also occur. Treatment is directed at the specific deformity. Reconstructive procedures are more reliable than simple soft-tissue releases.

VI. Complex Regional Pain Syndrome (Formerly RSD)
A. Definition—CRPS is a pain syndrome that occurs with trophic changes of the involved extremity. It is believed to be caused by inappropriate hyperactivity of the sympathetic nervous system. This section deals with CRPS of the foot; however,

many of the principles are the same as for CRPS of other parts of the body.

B. Clinical Syndrome—The classic presentation involves distal extremity pain associated with smooth, shiny skin; diffuse swelling; abnormal skin color and temperature; allodynia (hypersensitivity); and joint pain and tenderness. Radiographs demonstrate osteopenia (especially periarticular) and a moth-eaten appearance of the bone. Not all signs and symptoms are uniformly present. There are three stages.

1. Stage I (<3 months)—In Stage I, pain is out of proportion to the original injury; the skin temperature changes; and allodynia, guarding, and edema occur.

2. Stage II (3 to 9 months)—In Stage II, trophic changes lead to stiffness and abnormal posturing of the limb. Abnormal color and sweating may be present. Radiographs reveal osteopenia, and a bone scan demonstrates increased uptake, especially diffuse periarticular uptake.

3. Stage III (>1 year)—In Stage III, the limb becomes cool and undergoes skin color, texture, and temperature changes. Joint stiffness becomes more significant, and contractures are common.

C. Pathophysiology—The abnormal response to pain is caused by persistent sympathetic tone, which stimulates primary afferent nociceptors in normal and damaged peripheral tissues. An abnormal feedback cycle is initiated and expands to involve more normal tissues. Excessive sympathetic tone increases the amount of edema and causes impaired capillary flow, ischemia, and pain. It also prevents the removal of ischemic by-products from the injured site. This stimulates further sympathetic flow and an ever-increasing feedback loop.

1. Central nervous system involvement (gate theory)—Pain sensation is regulated in the spinal cord; small afferent Type C fibers transmit pain sensation, thus "opening the gate." These fibers can be inhibited by small cells in the substantia gelatinosa. Large afferent Type A fibers stimulate the substantia gelatinosa fibers that block central pain stimulators, thus "closing the gate." Modalities such as physical therapy, transcutaneous electrical stimulation, and massage stimulate Type A fibers.

2. Peripheral nervous system involvement—Experiments have shown that damaged nerves respond to sympathetic activity. Prostaglandin is released in response to norepinephrine release at sympathetic terminals.

D. Diagnosis—The clinical findings have been described above. They can occur after a relatively mild injury. Radionuclide studies may be helpful, particularly with the presence of diffuse periarticular uptake in the third phase of a triple-phase technetium bone scan. Sympathetic blockade is the diagnostic study of choice. The response is monitored based on pain sensation and pinprick, motor function, skin temperature, and blood pressure fluctuations. In true RSD, the response to the blockade outlasts the return of somatic sensation.

E. Treatment—***The best results occur when treatment is initiated early, so the key is a prompt diagnosis.*** The basis for treatment is to interrupt sympathetic nerve function. A multidisciplinary treatment regimen is vital and should address the psychologic components of the problem as well.

1. Pharmacologic therapy—Nonsteroidal anti-inflammatory drugs, calcium channel blockers, alpha- and beta-adrenergic blocking agents, serotonin antagonists, and antidepressants have all been used for symptom management. The best results for RSD of the foot are usually obtained by sympathetic blockade via a series of lumbar injections. If this treatment is ineffective, the diagnosis must be questioned. Regional blocks can also be effective. Sympathetic antagonists (e.g., reserpine, guanethidine, and phentolamine) are sometimes effective.

2. Physical therapy—***Physical therapy is the first-line treatment; it restores motion and increases pain tolerance.*** Tactile desensitization, gentle assistance with exercise, transcutaneous electric nerve stimulation, whirlpool, massage, and contrast baths are effective. Aggressive or forceful manipulation can aggravate the hypersensitivity. Compression stockings are helpful for edema control.

3. Surgical sympathectomy—Sympathectomy may be indicated when pharmacotherapy provides only transient but significant relief.

VII. Crush Injuries of the Foot—Crush injuries occur when extrinsic compressive or shear force is applied to the foot over a variable period. Persistent neuritis is the number one reason for a poor outcome following a crush injury.

A. Types—There are four types: compressive, contusion, shear/degloving, and mangling.

1. Compressive—A compressive injury involves fracture or dislocation with or without a break in the soft-tissue envelope.

2. Contusion—A contusion is a closed soft-tissue injury predominantly involving the skin and subcutaneous tissue without fracture or dislocation.

3. Shear/degloving—Shear/degloving involves a soft-tissue avulsion caused by the application of tangential force to the foot surface.

4. Mangling—Mangling involves marked disruption of the bones and soft tissues.

B. Evaluation—Neurovascular status is determined by physical examination, and osseous structures are evaluated via radiographic studies. The soft tissues are evaluated, and the compartment pressures are measured.

C. Treatment
   1. Appropriate and aggressive soft-tissue debridement
   2. Rigid fracture fixation
   3. Fasciotomies when there is compartment syndrome
   4. Early soft-tissue coverage, preferably within 48 hours
   5. Split-thickness skin excision (to treat and evaluate for acute soft-tissue necrosis)—Split-thickness skin excision is performed in the standard fashion; a dermatome is used to excise the involved area of skin. Subcutaneous and subdermal punctate bleeding defines areas of viable soft tissues. White and avascular areas are assumed to be necrotic. Necrotic areas are fully excised down to tendon, and the superficial skin layer is reapplied in a skin-graft fashion for coverage. This technique is helpful for immediate coverage as well as in the prevention of deep tissue necrosis.

VIII. Puncture Wounds of the Foot—Puncture wounds are usually caused by stepping on a nail or another impaling object. These injuries are frequently ignored or undertreated.

A. Diagnosis—A history is taken, and a physical examination is performed. (The puncture wound is usually plantar.) Radiographs occasionally show flecks of foreign material.

B. Treatment
   1. Initial presentation after the injury—Local wound care, tetanus prophylaxis, administration of oral antibiotics, and frequent follow-up are performed until the puncture wound is healed. ***The removal of a foreign body should be performed as necessary.***
   2. Established infection—Aggressive surgical irrigation and debridement with intravenous antibiotics for infecting organisms are

performed. The most common organism is *S. aureus; Pseudomonas aeruginosa* is the most characteristic organism.

3. Late sequelae—Late sequelae include osteomyelitis and gas gangrene.

4. Miscellaneous—It is important to look at the patient's overall health status as well as the mechanism. In a healthy person with a puncture wound, local debridment with antibiotic coverage is adequate. When the puncture occurs through the sole of a shoe beware of pseudomonas and treat appropriately. If the wound fails to respond then MRI is recommended to rule out osteomyelitis and a surgical debridment is performed. Diabetic patients often have a delayed presentation due to neuropathy. If seen in a delayed fashion an MRI is again recommended to rule out osteomyelitis or a deep abscess. If osteomyelitis is present, irrigation and debridement versus partial/complete amputation must be considered.

SUGGESTED READINGS

Classic Articles

Bibbo C, Anderson RB, Davis WH. Injury characteristics and the clinical outcome of subtalar dislocations: a clinical and radiographic analysis of 25 cases. *Foot Ankle Int.* 2003;24:158–163.

Boon AJ, Smith J, Zobitz ME. Snowboarder's talus fracture: mechanism of injury. *AJSM.* 2001;29:333–338.

Borelli J Jr, Lashgari C. Vascularity of the lateral calcaneal flap: a cadaveric injection study. *JOT.* 1999;13:73–77.

Buckley R, Tough S, McCormack R, et al. Operative compared with nonoperative treatment of displaced intra-articular calcaneal fractures: a prospective, randomized, controlled multicenter trial. *J Bone Joint Surg Am.* 2002;84:1733–1744.

DeLee JC, Curtis R. Subtalar dislocation of the foot. *J Bone Joint Surg Am.* 1982;64:433–437.

Ebraheim NA, Skie MC, Podeszwa DA, et al. Evaluation of process fractures of the talus using computed tomography. *J Orthop Trauma.* 1994;8:332–337.

Fulkerson E, Razi A, Tejwani N. Acute compartment syndrome of the foot. *Foot Ankle Int.* 2003;24:180–187.

Heier KA, Infante AF, Walling AK, et al. Open fractures of the calcaneus: soft tissue injury determines outcome. *JBJS Am.* 2003;5(12):2276–2282.

Kuo RS, Tejwani NC, DiGiovanni CW, et al. Outcome after open reduction and internal fixation of lisfranc joint. *J Bone Joint Surg Am.* 2000;82:1609.

Lawrence SJ, Botte MJ. The sural nerve of the foot and ankle: an anatomic study with clinical and surgical implications. *FAI.* 1994;15:490–494.

Leitner B. Obstacles to reduction in subtalar dislocations. *J Bone Joint Surg Am.* 1954;36:299–306.

Main and Jowett. Injuries of the midtarsal joint. *JBJS Br.* 1975;57–B(1):89.

Marsh, J, Saltzman C, Iverson M, et al. Major opentrauma of the talus. *J Orthop Trauma.* 1995;9:371–376.

Plewes LW, McKelvey KG. Subtalar dislocation. *J Bone Joint Surg Am*. 1944;26:585–588.

Sangeorzan BJ, Wagner UA, Harrington RM, et al. Contact characteristics of the subtalar joint: the effect of talar neck misalignment. *J Orthop Res*. 1992;10:544–551.

Swanson TV, Bray TJ, Holmes GB Jr. Fractures of the talar neck: a mechanical study of fixation. *JBJS*. 1992;74:544–551.

Thompson MC, Matthew A, Mormino MD. Injury to the tarsometatarsal joint complex. *J Am Acad Orthop Surg*. 2003;11:260–267.

Tucker DJ, Feder JM, Boylan JP. Fractures of the Lateral Process of the talus: two case reports and a comprehensive literature review. *FAI*. 1998;19:641–646.

Recent Articles

Aldridge JM, Easley, Nunley: Open calcaneal fractures. Results of operative treatment. *J Orthopedic Trauma*. 18:7–11, 2004.

Bibbo C, Robert B. Anderson M.D.; W. Hodges Davis M.D.. Injury Characteristics and the Clinical Outcome of Subtalar Dislocations: a Clinical and Radiographic Analysis of 25 Cases. *FAI*. 2003;(2):158–163.

Coetzee JC, Thuan V. Ly Surgical technique arthrodesis compared with open reduction and internal fixation. Treat- ment of primarily ligamentous lisfranc joint injuries: pri- mary. *J Bone Joint Surg Am*. 2007;89:122–127.

Milenkovic S, Radenkovic M, Mitkovic M. Open subtalar dislocation treated by distractional external fixation. *J Orthop Trauma*. 2004;18(9):638–640.

Patel R, Anthony Van Bergeyk MD, Stephen Pinney MD. Are displaced talar neck fractures surgical emergencies? *A Survey of Orthopaedic Trauma Experts*. 2005;(26):378–381.

Robinson TF. Arthrodesis as salvage for calcaneal avulsions. *FAC* 2002;7:107–120.

Review Articles

Ahmad J, Steven M. Raikin MD. Current concepts review: talar fractures. *Foot Ankle Int*. 2006;27:475–482.

Textbooks

Sarrafian SK. Anatomy of the Foot and Ankle Descriptive, Topographic, Functional. 2nd ed. Philadelphia: JB Lippincott 1993. p. 192

CHAPTER 15

Pelvic Ring Injuries

David J. Hak

PELVIC FRACTURES

I. Anatomy
  A. Ring Structure of Three Bones—Two innominate bones and the sacrum. Innominate bone is formed by fusion of three ossification centers—ilium, ischium, and pubis.
  B. Sacroiliac (SI) Joint is Comprised of Two Parts:
    1. Articular portion—Located anteriorly. Not a true synovial joint. Articular cartilage on sacral side. Fibrous cartilage on iliac side.
    2. Fibrous or ligamentous portion—Located posteriorly.
  C. Ligaments
    1. Posterior SI ligaments—Considered to be the strongest ligaments in the body (Fig. 15-1).
      • Short component—Oblique fibers that run from the posterior ridge of the sacrum to the posterosuperior and posteroinferior iliac spines.
      • Long component—Longitudinal fibers that run from the lateral sacrum to the posterosuperior iliac spines; merges with sacrotuberous ligament.
    2. Anterior SI ligaments—Runs from ilium across sacrum (Fig. 15-2).
    3. Sacrotuberous ligaments—Strong band running from posterolateral sacrum and dorsal aspect of the posterior iliac spine to the ischial tuberosity. Along with the posterior SI ligaments, these ligaments maintain vertical stability of the pelvis (Fig. 15-3).

  4. Sacrospinous ligament—Runs from the lateral edge of the sacrum and coccyx to the sacrotuberous ligament and inserts on the ischial spine. Triangular in shape. Separates the greater and lesser sciatic notches.
  5. Iliolumbar ligaments—Run from L4 and L5 transverse processes to the posterior iliac crest stabilizing the spine to pelvis.
  6. Lumbosacral ligaments—Run from L5 transverse process to the sacral ala.
  D. Pubic Symphysis
    1. Hyaline cartilage on medial (articular) aspect of pubis.
    2. Surrounded by fibrocartilage and a thick band of fibrous tissue.
  E. The iliopectineal line (pelvic brim) separates the false pelvis (above) from the true pelvis (below).
    1. False pelvis—Iliac wings and sacral ala; surrounds the intra-abdominal contents; contains iliacus muscle.
    2. True pelvis—Pubis, ischium and small portion of ilium; contains floor of true pelvis (coccyx, coccygeal and levator ani muscles, urethra, rectum, vagina) and obturator internus muscle.
  F. Neural Structures
    1. Sciatic nerve—Formed by roots from the lumbosacral plexus (L4, L5, S1, S2, S3). Exits the pelvis deep to the piriformis muscle.
    2. Lumbosacral trunk—Formed from anterior rami of L4 and L5, crosses the anterior sacral ala and SI joint. ***Fractures of the sacral ala or***

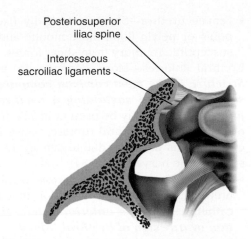

<u>FIGURE 15-1</u> Cross section through the sacroiliac joint, showing the direction of the interosseous sacroiliac ligaments.

Posteriosuperior iliac spine

Interosseous sacroiliac ligaments

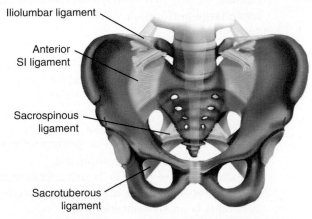

Iliolumbar ligament

Anterior SI ligament

Sacrospinous ligament

Sacrotuberous ligament

<u>FIGURE 15-2</u> Anterior view of the pelvis showing the anterior SI ligament and the sacrospinous ligaments that is a strong triangular ligament anterior to the sacrotuberous ligament.

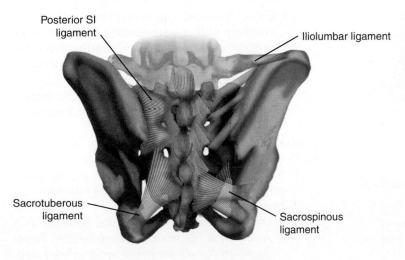

Posterior SI ligament

Iliolumbar ligament

Sacrotuberous ligament

Sacrospinous ligament

dislocations of the SI joint are most likely to injure the lumbosacral trunk.

   3. L5 nerve root—Exits below L5 transverse process and crosses the sacral ala 2 cm medial to the SI joint. ***May be injured during anterior approach to the SI joint.***

G. Vascular Structures

   1. Median sacral artery—Continuation of the aorta, which travels along the vertebral column. Small caliber and not of major significance.

   2. Superior rectal artery (hemorrhoidal artery)—Continuation of the superior mesenteric artery. Rarely involved in pelvic trauma.

   3. Common iliac artery—Divides into internal and external iliac arteries.

   4. Internal iliac artery (hypogastric artery)—***Major importance in pelvic trauma***.

     • Anterior division

       (a) Inferior gluteal artery—Exits the pelvis through the greater sciatic notch inferior to the piriformis (***between piriformis and superior gamelli***). Supplies the gluteus maximus.

       (b) Internal pudendal artery—Crosses the ischial spine and exits through the lesser sciatic notch. Commonly injured in pelvic fractures.

       (c) Obturator artery—May be disrupted in pubic rami fractures.

         • Superior vesical artery—A branch of the obturator artery that supplies the bladder.

       (d) Inferior vesical.

       (e) Middle rectal artery.

     • Posterior division

       (a) More prone to damage due to posterior pelvic displacement.

       (b) Superior gluteal artery—Largest branch of the internal iliac artery. Courses across

<u>FIGURE 15-3</u> Posterior view of the pelvis showing the posterior sacroiliac ligament, iliolumbar ligament, sacrospinous ligament and the sacrotuberous ligament.

the SI joint, and exits through the greater sciatic notch superior to the piriformis. Supplies gluteus medius, gluteus minimus, and tensor fascia lata muscles. Most commonly injured vessel in pelvic fractures with posterior ring disruptions. *Can be injured in obtaining a posterior iliac crest bone graft if you stray inferiorly*. Can also be injured when passing a gigli saw through the sciatic notch during a pediatric innominate osteotomy.

    (c) Iliolumbar artery.
    (d) Lateral sacral artery.

5. Corona mortis (Fig. 15-4)
- Common anastomosis between the obturator and external iliac systems. Incidence: venous anastomosis (70%), arterial anastomosis (34%), venous and arterial anastomosis (20%).
- Crosses the superior pubic ramus in a vertical orientation at an average of 6.2 cm (range, 3 to 9 cm) from the pubic symphysis.
- If accidentally cut, the vessels may retract inferiorly into the obturator foramen and cause serious bleeding.

6. Pelvic veins—Massive venous plexus that drain into the internal iliac vein. *Major source of hemorrhage in most pelvic fractures*.

H. Urethra
1. Anatomy
- Male urethra has three portions—Prostatic, membranous, and bulbous. Bulbous urethra is located inferior to the urogenital diaphragm; if ruptured retrograde urethrogram dye extravasates into the perineum.

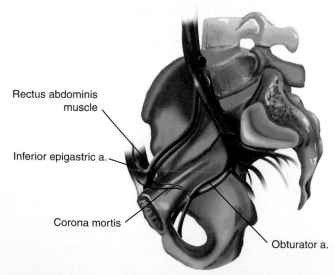

Rectus abdominis muscle

Inferior epigastric a.

Corona mortis

Obturator a.

FIGURE 15-4 Schematic drawing showing the arterial and venous anastomsis between the external iliac and obturator systems known as the corona mortis.

- Female urethra—Short, not rigidly fixed to pubis or pelvic floor, more mobile and less susceptible to injury from shear forces.

2. Urethral injuries—More common in males. *Stricture is the most common complication seen in patients sustaining a urethral injury*. Impotence may be present in 25% to 47% of patients with urethral rupture. Cause is uncertain but is probably due to damage to parasympathetic nerves (S2 to S4).
- Obtain *retrograde urethrogram* to rule out urethral injury prior to insertion of a Foley catheter if there is *anterior pelvic disruption or any sign of urethral injury*.
- Signs of urethral injury: (a) inability to void despite a full bladder, (b) blood at the urethral meatus (c) high-riding or abnormally mobile prostate, and (d) elevated bladder on IVP.
- *Absence of meatal blood or a high-riding prostate does not rule out urethral injury*.
- Passing a Foley may turn a small perforation into a large perforation.

I. Bladder
1. Anatomy
- Males—Bladder neck is attached to the pubis by puboprostatic ligaments and is contiguous with the prostate.
- Females—Bladder lies on the pubococcygeal portion of levator ani muscles.
- Superior and upper posterior portion of the bladder are covered by peritoneum.
- Remainder of the bladder is extraperitoneal and covered with loose areolar tissue. Space of Retzius is located anteriorly.

2. Bladder injuries
- May be caused by bony spicules from pubic rami fractures, blunt force injuries causing rupture, or shearing injuries.
- Intraperitoneal ruptures—Require operative repair.
- Extraperitoneal ruptures—Managed nonoperatively unless undergoing ex lap for other reasons or a bony spicule invading the bladder. Catheter drainage and broad-spectrum antibiotics. Cystogram prior to catheter removal to verify healing. About 87%, healed by 10 days. Virtually all healed by 3 weeks.

II. Evaluation
A. History
1. Mechanism of injury determines energy of injury and likelihood of associated injuries.
2. Low-energy injuries
- Occur in elderly osteoporotic patients as a result of a fall from standing height. Treatment: analgesia, weight bearing as tolerated.

- Stress fractures may occur without an identified fall. Bone scan is useful for diagnosis.
3. High-energy injuries
  - Common mechanisms are motor vehicle accidents (MVA), motorcycle accidents, pedestrian versus MVA, or fall from height.
  - Associated injuries are common.
  - High incidence of hemorrhage and hypovolemic shock.
  - Require emergent evaluation and treatment.
B. Physical Examination
  1. First priority is to assess for other life-threatening injuries using Advanced Trauma Life Support (ATLS) protocols.
  2. Bimanual compression and distraction of the iliac wings.
  3. Manual leg traction can aid in determination of vertical instability.
  4. Careful palpation of the posterior pelvis in awake patients can identify posterior pelvic injuries.
  5. Rectal examination—High-riding prostate may indicate urethral tear. Positive guaiac test may indicate visceral injury. Palpation of the sacrum for irregularity.
  6. Vaginal examination—Bleeding or lacerations indicating open fractures.
  7. Perineal skin—Lacerations may indicate open fracture. May be caused by hyperabduction of the leg.

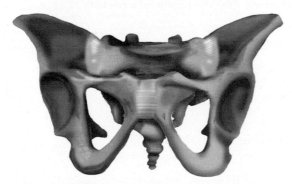

FIGURE 15-5   Anterior posterior view of pelvis.

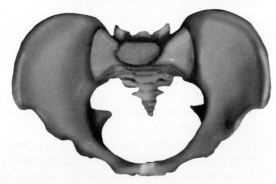

FIGURE 15-6   Inlet view of pelvis.

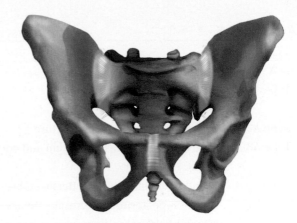

FIGURE 15-7   Outlet view of pelvis.

C. Radiographic Examination
  1. Anteroposterior pelvis (Fig. 15-5)—Part of the initial trauma series along with a chest and lateral cervical spine X-ray. Can identify up to 90% of pelvic injuries.
  2. Pelvic inlet view (Fig. 15-6)—40° to 45° caudal tilt. Shows **anterior–posterior displacement.**
  3. Pelvic outlet view (Fig. 15-7)—40° to 45° cephalad tilt. Shows **superior–inferior displacement** and visualizes the sacral foramen.
  4. CT scan—Provides **best visualization of the SI joint.** May identify sacral fractures not well visualized on plain films.
  5. Lateral sacral view—**Identifies transverse sacral fractures.**
D. Abdominal Injury Evaluation
  1. Computed tomography (CT) scan—Extravasation of contrast can also aid identification of associated arterial injuries.
  2. Ultrasound—Focused Abdominal Sonogram for Trauma (FAST)—Widely used to evaluate for intra-abdominal fluid and solid organ injuries.
  3. Diagnostic peritoneal lavage (DPL)—If a pelvic fracture is present the location should be supraumbilical to avoid a false positive result due to a pelvic hematoma.

III. Classification
  A. Tile Classification (Table 15-1 and Figs. 15-8 to 15-11)
    1. Combines mechanism of injury and stability
      - Type A: stable
      - Type B: rotationally unstable
      - Type C: vertically unstable
    2. Aids in determining prognosis and treatment options.
  B. Young and Burgess Classification (Table 15-2)
    1. Based on mechanism of injury
      - Anterior–posterior compression
      - Lateral compression

TABLE 15-1

Tile Classification

Type A	Stable pelvic fractures
Type A1	Typically an avulsion fracture
	Pelvic ring intact
Type A2	Nondisplaced pelvic ring fracture
Type A3	Transverse fractures of sacrum and coccyx
	Pelvic ring intact
Type B	Rotationally unstable, vertically stable
Type B1	Anterior–posterior compression injury
	"Open book" pelvic fractures
	Divided into three stages:
	Stage 1: Pubic symphysis diastasis <2.5 cm
	No involvement of posterior pelvic ring
	Stage 2: Pubic symphysis diastasis >2.5 cm
	Unilateral posterior pelvic ring injury
	Stage 3: Pubic symphysis diastasis >2.5 cm
	Bilateral posterior pelvic ring injuries
Type B2	Lateral compression injury—Ipsilateral
	The rami are commonly fractured anteriorly
	The posterior complex is crushed
Type B3	Lateral compression—Contralateral (bucket handle)
	The major anterior lesion is usually on the opposite side of the posterior lesion, but all four rami may be fractured anteriorly
	The affected hemi-pelvis rotates anteriorly and superiorly (like the handle of a bucket)
	Flexion of hemi-pelvis results in leg length discrepancy
	Reduction requires derotation of hemi-pelvis
	Usually caused by a direct blow on the iliac crest
Type C	Rotationally and vertically unstable
Type C1	Ipsilateral anterior and posterior pelvic injuries
Type C2	Bilateral hemi-pelvic disruptions
Type C3	Any pelvic fracture with an associated acetabular fracture

- Vertical shear
- Combined mechanism

2. A spectrum of associated injuries is produced based on the direction and magnitude of the injury force.
3. Alerts surgeon to potential resuscitation requirements and associated injury patterns.

C. Bucholz Classification—Based on severity of posterior pelvic ring injury.

1. Type I—Anterior ring injury, stable or intact posterior ring (may have a nondisplaced sacral fracture or injury to the anterior SI ligaments).
2. Type II—Anterior ring injury along with partial disruption of the SI joint, but the posterior SI ligaments remain intact.
3. Type III—Complete disruption of the SI joint (including the posterior SI ligaments) with displacement of the hemipelvis.

IV. Pelvic Stability

A. Decision Making (operative versus nonoperative, weight bearing status) is based on pelvic stability and degree of displacement.

1. Stable pelvis is defined as a pelvis that can withstand normal physiological forces without deformation.
2. Pelvic instability has two components—Rotational instability and vertical instability.
3. Associated bony injuries may mimic pure ligamentous injuries and lead to pelvic instability.

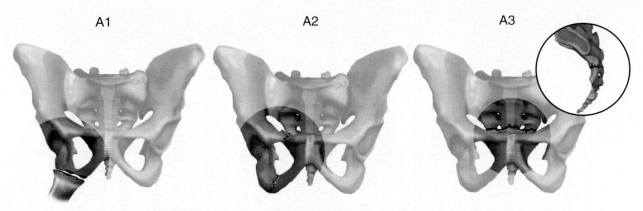

FIGURE 15-8   Tile classification of pelvic fracture. Type A1 avulsion fracture. Type A2 nondisplaced pelvic ring fracture. Type A3 transverse sacral or coccyx fracture.

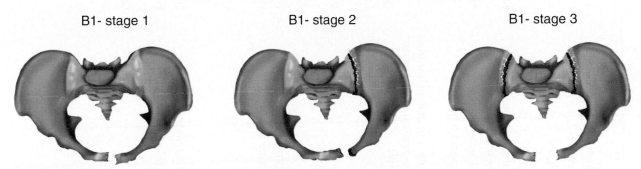

FIGURE 15-9   Tile classification of pelvic fracture. Type B1, stage 1 symphysis pubis disruption. Type B1, stage 2 symphysis pubis disruption. Type B1, stage 3 symphysis pubis disruption.

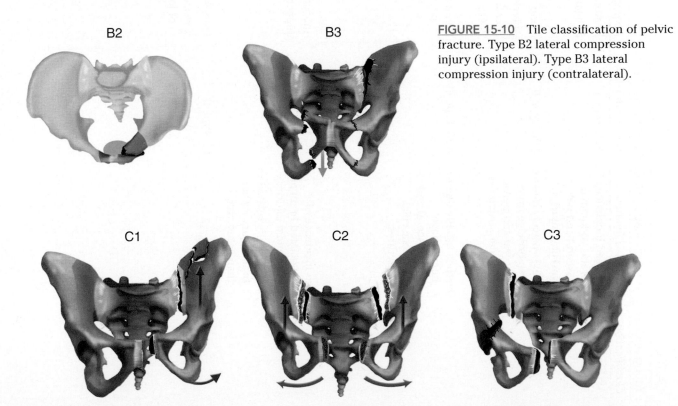

FIGURE 15-10   Tile classification of pelvic fracture. Type B2 lateral compression injury (ipsilateral). Type B3 lateral compression injury (contralateral).

FIGURE 15-11   Tile classification of pelvic fracture. Type C1 pelvic injury. Type C2 pelvic injury. Type C3 pelvic injury.

TABLE 15-2

Young and Burgess Classification of Pelvic Ring Injuries

Classification	Associated Injuries	Subclassification	Radiographic/Anatomic Features	Treatment/Comments
APC	Increased incidence of brain, abdominal, visceral and pelvic vascular injuries	APC Type I	Symphysis widened 1–2 cm SI ligaments intact	Usually treated nonoperatively 6.5% pelvic vascular injury
	Death is usually due to hemorrhage from visceral and pelvic vascular structures	APC Type II	Symphysis widened >2 cm Anterior SI ligaments disrupted Sacrotuberous ligaments ruptured Posterior SI ligaments intact	Emergent external fixator for hemodynamic instability May be definitively treated in external fixator or by symphysis plating 10% pelvic vascular injury
	Death is usually due to hemorrhage from visceral and pelvic vascular structures	APC Type III	Complete separation of hemipelvis from pelvic ring (no vertical displacement as seen in LC-III)	APC-III is the most common severe injury seen in pedestrians Greatest 24-h fluid resuscitation requirements Emergent external fixator for hemodynamic instability Definitive fixation requires both anterior and posterior fixation 22% pelvic vascular injury
LC	High incidence of associated brain and abdominal injuries	LC Type I	Anterior pelvic ring injury Impaction of sacrum on side of injury	Usually result from a MVA Usually treated nonoperatively—weight bearing on unaffected side
	Death usually related to brain injury rather than hemorrhage	LC Type II	Anterior pelvic ring injury "Crescent fracture" of iliac wing or near SI joint	Occasionally external fixator applied for hemodynamic instability or to permit early mobilization in polytrauma patient Usually result from a MVA Emergent external fixator for hemodynamic instability Definitive treatment with internal fixation 8% pelvic vascular injury

LC Type III	LC-I or LC-II on side of injury, with addition of open book type injury of SI joint on opposite side	LC-III injuries usually occurs as a result of a crush, and injuries are usually isolated to the pelvic region—brain, lung, spleen, or liver injuries are not seen or rare
	Pelvic ring internally rotated on injury side, opposite side is externally rotated	Emergent external fixator for hemodynamic instability
		Definitive treatment with internal fixation
		23% pelvic vascular injury
VS	Associated injuries similar to LC	Usually occurs as a result of a fall
	Vertical displacement of hemipelvis	Emergent external fixator for hemodynamic instability
	Usually occurs as rupture of SI joint, but occasionally occurs as fracture through sacrum or ilium	Traction acutely if patient hemodynamically stable
		Definitive treatment with internal fixation
		10% pelvic vascular injury
Combined Mechanism	Combination of LC and VS, or LC and APC	Emergent external fixator for hemodynamic instability
		Definitive treatment based on primary component of injury
		10% pelvic vascular injury

APC, Anterior–Posterior Compression; LC, Lateral Compression; VS, Vertical Shear.

4. Common radiographic signs of pelvic instability:
   - Displacement of the posterior SI complex greater than 5 mm in any plane
   - Presence of posterior fracture gap, rather than impaction
   - Avulsion of the L5 transverse process or the sacral ischial end of the sacrospinous process
5. Intraoperative traction/stress examination may occasionally be required to determine stability.

B. Ligament Sectioning Studies
   1. Sectioning of the pubic symphysis results in pubic diastasis less than 2.5 cm, but the intact sacrospinous ligaments prevents further displacement. The pelvis is rotationally and vertically stable.
   2. Sectioning of the pubic symphysis and sacrospinous ligaments results in pubic diastasis greater than 2.5 cm. Further external rotation of the hemipelvis is limited by the posterior iliac spine abutting the sacrum. The pelvis is rotationally unstable, but vertically stable.
   3. Section of the pubic symphysis, sacrospinous, sacrotuberous, and posterior SI ligaments causes the pelvis to become both rotationally and vertically unstable.

V. Associated Injuries
  A. High-Energy Injuries Commonly Have Associated Injuries
   1. Major central nervous system, chest and abdominal injuries
   2. Hemorrhage 75%
   3. Associated musculoskeletal injuries 60% to 80%
   4. Urogenital injuries 12%
   5. Lumbosacral plexus injuries 8%
   6. Mortality rate 15% to 25%
  B. Hemorrhage—Occurs in up to 75% of pelvic fractures.
   1. Hemorrhage is a leading cause of death in patients with pelvic fractures.
   2. Requires aggressive fluid resuscitation. Shock from hypovolemia is associated with the highest mortality rate following pelvic fractures.
   3. Three sources of bleeding—Osseous, vascular, and visceral.
   4. Intra-abdominal source of bleeding is present in up to 40% of cases.
   5. Arterial source of bleeding is present in only 10% to 15% of cases.
   6. Major source of bleeding is from venous plexus leading to large retroperitoneal hematoma.
   7. Retroperitoneal space can hold up to 4 L of blood.
   8. Location of arterial injuries can be predicted based on pelvic fracture pattern.

   - APC-III or Tile C injury—Superior gluteal artery is most commonly injured.
   - LC pattern—Obturator artery or a branch of the external iliac artery are most commonly injured.

C. Open pelvic fractures—High mortality rate (30% to 50%). Potential for major vascular injury with hemorrhage. High incidence of gastrointestinal and genitourinary injuries. May require diverting colostomy for intestinal injuries. Requires aggressive multidisciplinary treatment.

VI. Emergent Treatment
  A. Pelvic Binder—Commercial device that can be used for prehospital and emergent stabilization of pelvic fractures. *In APC ("open-book") fractures, use of a pelvic binder will close the ring and tamponade venous bleeding.* Prolonged use is associated with skin necrosis complications. An improvised binder can be made using a sheet to provide circumferential compression around the pelvis.
  B. Medical Antishock Trousers (MAST)—Commonly used in the past for prehospital stabilization—now mostly replaced by use of a pelvic binder.
     Complications include limited access for exam, decrease lung expansion, and *may contribute to lower extremity compartment syndrome*.
  C. Skeletal Traction—May be used to correct vertical displacement of the hemipelvis.
  D. Resuscitation of Patients in Hypovolemic Shock
   1. Two large bore intravenous lines (16G or larger) in the upper extremities. Lower extremity lines may be less efficient due to pelvic venous injuries.
   2. Administer at least 2 L of crystalloid solution over 20 minutes and determine response.
   3. If only a transient improvement or no response then begin blood administration. Universal donor O negative blood is immediately available for exsanguinating hemorrhage. Type specific blood is usually available within ten minutes. Fully crossmatched blood is preferred but takes approximately 1 hour to complete crossmatch.
   4. 50% to 69% of unstable pelvic fractures will require four or more units of blood; 30% to 40% will require 10 or more units.
   5. Platelets and fresh frozen plasma will be required with massive transfusions to correct dilutional coagulopathy.
   6. Avoid or correct hypothermia. Warm fluids, increase ambient temperature, and avoid heat loss. Hypothermia can lead to coagulation problems, ventricular fibrillation and acid–base disturbances.

7. Adequate volume replacement should produce urinary output of approximately 50 cc per hour in an adult (ATLS guidelines).

E. External Fixation
   1. Emergently placed in hemodynamically unstable patient who does not respond to initial fluid resuscitation.
   2. Function
      • Stabilizes pelvis preventing redisruption of clots
      • May decrease pelvic volume
   3. Anterior external fixation alone does not provide adequate posterior stabilization if the posterior ring is disrupted.
   4. Place skin incisions at right angles to the pelvic brim in line with the direction of the reduction (avoids the need for additional releasing incisions; pin travels along the incision line as the pelvis is reduced).
   5. Spinal needle or thin K-wire can assist in determining the orientation of the pelvic brim.
   6. Place bars far enough away from the abdomen to allow for abdominal distention.

F. Pelvic C-Clamps—In original design, points of clamp applied to posterior ilium in line with the sacrum. Requires fluoroscopy and technical expertise. Higher risk of iatrogenic injury than standard anterior external fixator. Newer designs can be applied to the trochanteric area decreasing potential complications from malposition.

G. Angiographic Embolization—Indicated for patients who remain hemodynamically unstable following resuscitation, application of external fixator, and after other sources of bleeding (abdomen, chest) are ruled out. Arterial source of bleeding is present in only 10% to 15% of patients.

H. Peritoneal Packing—Popularized in European trauma centers. Significantly reduces blood product transfusion and can decrease the need for emergent angiography.

VII. Definitive Surgical Treatment
A. External Fixation
   1. Temporary use for emergent stabilization and resuscitation.
   2. May be used definitively for "open book" (Tile type B1, Young and Burgess APC-II, Bucholz type II) injuries in which the posterior SI ligaments are intact.
   3. External fixation alone does not provide adequate stabilization if the posterior pelvic ring is disrupted.

B. Internal Fixation—Numerous techniques are available depending on fracture pattern. Fractures that are unstable posteriorly require posterior stabilization. Plating of a symphyseal dislocation should be performed first if the innominate bones are intact as it may help reduce displacement in the posterior pelvic ring; otherwise, the posterior reduction is usually performed first.

C. Anterior Pubic Symphysis Plating—Reduction and fixation of a simple pubic symphysis diastasis greater than 2.5 cm may be done acutely prior to or following laparotomy by extending the laparotomy incision distally, or in delayed manner using a Pfannenstiel incision. Identify the midline raphe and separate two bellies of rectus abdominis muscle. The insertion of the rectus may have been traumatically avulsed from the pubic ramus but otherwise does not need to be released.
   1. Reduction with a Weber tenaculum for "open book" type injuries (Fig. 15-12). Clamp is placed anteriorly through the rectus muscle. Points of the tenaculum are placed at the same level of the pubic body.
   2. If the hemipelvis is posteriorly displaced an anteriorly directed force may be obtained using a Jungbluth pelvic reduction clamp (Fig. 15-13).

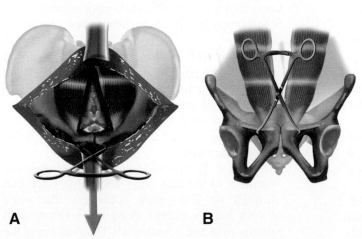

FIGURE 15-12 **A.** For reduction of a pubic symphysis diastasis, reduction is obtained using a Weber tenaculum placed anterior to the rectus muscles. The insertion of the rectus is not divided. **B.** The points of the clamp are placed at the same level on the pubic body so that with closure, any sagittal plane rotation of the symphysis is reduced.

A   **B**

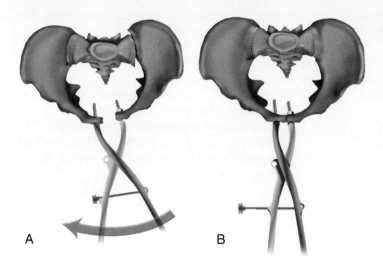

FIGURE 15-13 **A.** Jungbluth pelvic reduction clamp may be used to provide a strong anterior reduction force when the hemipelvis is posteriorly displaced. Screw cutout may be prevented with an anchoring plate and nut placed from inside the pelvis. **B.** Once the hemipelvis is reduced, the clamp is tightened and held while standard anterior fixation is applied.

Anchoring plate and nut may be placed behind the pubis to prevent clamp pullout.

3. Fixation hardware—Several different plate and screw options may be used. Matta recommends a six-hole, 3.5-mm curved reconstruction plate. Double plating has been described to improve stability if posterior fixation cannot be performed. Residual symphysis motion may lead to screw loosening or plate breakage.

D. Pubic Rami Fractures—Most are treated nonoperatively. Unstable fractures may be plated through an ilioinguinal approach. Another alternative is placement of a retropubic medullary superior pubic ramus screw.

E. Posterior Pelvic Ring Fixation
1. Displaced SI joint disruptions require open reduction. Nonanatomic SI reduction is associated with long-term pain. Vertically displaced malunions may result in leg length discrepancy and sitting imbalance.
   • Posterior approach—Prone position. Simpler exposure and secure fixation with iliosacral screws. Wound healing complications reported as high as 25% in some series but less than 3% in other series.
     (a) Matta angle jaw forceps can be used to obtain reduction—One tip placed in the sciatic notch, the other placed on outer ilium.
     (b) Cephalad displacement—Reduction may be achieved with Weber tenaculum, or a femoral distractor may be used by placing Shantz pins in the posterior iliac spines.
   • Anterior approach—Supine position. Higher risk of neurologic injury (L5 nerve root lies 2 cm medial to the SI joint). Fixation with

two parallel plates or special four-hole quad plate. Allows direct visualization of the joint but anterior plating may result in posterior joint opening. Fixation is not as secure as iliosacral screws. May allow primary SI joint fusion. Recommended when there is a severe posterior soft tissue injury.

2. Iliosacral screws—May be performed in the supine or prone position. Placed percutaneously along with closed reduction or following open reduction of SI joint or sacral fracture. Requires good C-arm visualization (Fig. 15-14). Use washers in older patients to prevent screw penetration through the cortex. Solid screws are stronger than cannulated and allow use of an oscillating drill that provides better proprioceptive feedback. One or two screws are placed depending on anatomy and stability.

3. Posterior transiliac plate—4.5 mm reconstruction plate tunneled subcutaneously securing fixation to both posterior iliac spines.

F. Crescent Fractures—Fracture dislocations of the SI joint may involve a portion of the sacrum or ilium.
1. Fixation with interfragmentary lag screws if the intact portion of the ilium is large and firmly attached to the sacrum (iliosacral screws not needed).
2. If the fragment is small or the posterior ligaments are injured then internally fix with iliosacral screws.

G. Iliac Wing Fractures—Displaced or unstable fractures of the iliac wing may require fixation through an ilioinguinal approach. Iliac wing is very narrow except along the crest or as it widens near the acetabulum. Fixation along the

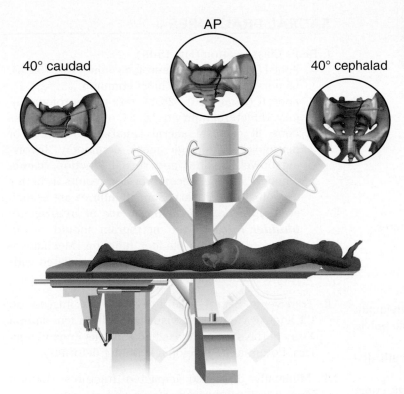

40° caudad

AP

40° cephalad

FIGURE 15-14 Patients may be positioned prone as shown here or supine for placement of iliosacral fixation screws. A long radiolucent board or table is required to allow positioning of the image intensifier to obtain anteroposterior, cephalad, and caudad projections.

crest with plates (on the inner or outer aspect of the ilium) or fixation with long 3.5 mm lag screws placed between the tables.

VIII. Nonoperative Treatment
  A. Stable nondisplaced or minimally displaced fractures may be treated nonoperatively. Lateral compression injuries (Young and Burgess LC-I, Tile B2) in which the sacral fracture is impacted are often stable and may be treated with weight bearing only on the unaffected side.
  B. Simple "open book" (Tile type B1 stage 1, Young and Burgess APC-II, Bucholz type II) injuries in which pubic diastasis is less than 2.5 cm can be treated nonoperatively.
  C. Nonoperative treatment of unstable or severely displaced fractures requires prolonged immobility and yields poor results.
  D. Early mobilization prevents complications related to prolonged bedrest.
  E. Vertically unstable fractures in which there is a contra-indication to operative treatment may be treated with skeletal traction.

IX. Complications of Injury and Treatment
  A. Nerve Injury—May occur from the initial injury as a result of tension or compression. Iatrogenic injury may occur from surgical manipulation, surgical approach, or misdirected drills or screws. Overall prevalence, 10% to 15%. Many recover

partially or completely. Permanent nerve injury has a major effect on patients' functional outcome.
  B. Thromboembolism
    1. Deep venous thrombosis—Incidence, 35% to 50%. Can occur in the pelvic or lower-extremity veins.
    2. Pulmonary embolism (PE)—Symptomatic PE incidence 2% to 10%. Fatal PE incidence 0.5% to 2%.
    3. Numerous prophylaxis and treatment options—Low dose heparin, low molecular weight heparin, Coumadin, mechanical compression devices, inferior vena caval filters.
    4. Diagnosis—Contrast venography, duplex ultrasound, magnetic resonance venography.
  C. Closed Internal Degloving Injuries—Morel Lavallée Lesions. Occurs as a result of a shear injury to the soft tissues in which the subcutaneous tissue is torn from the underlying fascia. Occurs most commonly over the greater trochanter, but also over the flank and thigh. Signs and symptoms include swelling, contour deformities, skin hypermobility and a loss of sensation over the affected area. May be colonized by bacteria. Treatment: Serial debridement.
  D. Hardware Failure
    1. ***Fatigue failure of hardware following symphyseal plating*** is common. In asymptomatic patients, treatment consists of only observation.

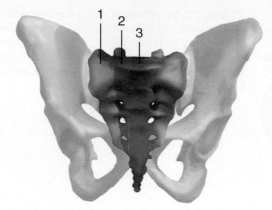

FIGURE 15-15 Denis classification of sacral fractures.

X. Nonunions and Malunions
  A. Occur most commonly as a result of inadequate initial treatment of displaced and unstable pelvic ring injuries.
  B. Cranial displacement—Results in leg length discrepancy and sitting imbalance.
  C. Treatment is complicated—Average OR time 7 hours (by highly experienced surgeon). Average blood loss: 1,977 cc. 19% complication rate. Risk of neurovascular injury.
  D. Three-stage reconstruction often required—(a) anterior approach—to release structures or perform osteotomies; (b) posterior approach—to release structures or perform osteotomies, followed by reduction and internal fixation; and (c) repeat anterior approach—for reduction and internal fixation. Depending on the deformity one may alternatively begin posteriorly.
  E. Nonunions or malunions are often resistant to correction of deformity due to soft tissue constraints. Normal internal fixation hardware may be inadequate to prevent loss of reduction. May require activity limitations for up to 5 months after surgical correction.

XI. Deformities and Other Sequelae
  A. Leg length discrepancy and sitting imbalance if the hemipelvis is displaced vertically
  B. Osteitis Pubis—Occurs following bladder neck suspension surgery. May be activity-induced overuse injury in athletes due to repetitive adductor and rectus abdominis muscle contractions. Bilateral uptake on bone scan, whereas tumors or stress fractures show unilateral uptake. Physical examination findings include tenderness over the symphysis pubis, pain on passive abduction of the hip. Normal sedimentation rate.

SACRAL FRACTURES

I. Denis Classification (Fig. 15-15)
  A. Zone I (alar region)—Neurologic injury rare (5.9%). L5 nerve root injury is most common.
  B. Zone II (foraminal)—28.4% rate of neurologic injury. Unilateral injury to L5, S1, or S2 nerve roots.
  C. Zone III (central sacral canal)—56.7% rate of neurological damage most commonly involving bowel, bladder and sexual function (cauda equina). Surgical decompression results in better neurological recovery. Zone III injuries are associated with the ***highest incidence of neurogenic bladder injury.*** Cystometrogram should be obtained to evaluate bladder function. Mechanism is frequently a fall from a height. Associated with thoracolumbar burst fractures.

II. Transverse Sacral Fractures—May be missed on CT and AP views. Best visualized with a true lateral X-ray of the sacrum. Classified as Denis Zone III injuries. Potential to develop a kyphotic deformity.

III. Minimally displaced impacted fractures (Lateral compression injuries)—Stable and may be treated nonoperatively unless nerve root decompression is required.

IV. Surgical Treatment—Displaced fractures are reduced under direct vision using the posterior spines to aid manipulation. If fracture is transforaminal, the loose bone fragment should be removed and the nerve roots visualized during reduction. Fully threaded iliosacral screws avoid overcompression of the fracture, which may cause nerve root compression in zone II transforaminal injuries.

SUGGESTED READINGS

Classic Articles

Borelli J Jr, Koval KJ, Helfet DL. The crescent fracture: a posterior fracture dislocation of the sacroiliac joint. *J Orthop Trauma.* 1996;10(3):165.

Burgess AR, Eastridge BJ, Young JWR, et al. Pelvic ring disruptions: effective classification system and treatment protocols. *J Trauma.* 1990;30(7):848.

Dalal SA, Burgess AR, Siegel JH, et al. Pelvic fracture in multiple trauma: classification by mechanism is key to pattern of organ injury, resuscitative requirements and outcome. *J Trauma.* 1989;29(7):981.

Denis F, Davis S, Comfort T. Sacral fractures: an important problem: retrospective analysis of 236 cases. *Clin Orthop.* 1988;227:67.

Matta JM, Dickson KF, Markovich GD. Surgical treatment of pelvic nonunions and malunions. *Clin Orthop.* 1996;329:199.

Matta JM, Tornetta P 3rd. Internal fixation of unstable pelvic ring injuries. *Clin Orthop.* 1996;329:129.

Montgomery KD, Geerts WH, Potter HG, et al. Thromboembolic complications in patients with pelvic trauma. *Clin Orthop.* 1996;329:68.

Routt MLC Jr, Simonian PT, Mills WJ. Iliosacral screw fixation: early complications of the percutaneous technique. *J Orthop Trauma.* 1997;11(8):584.

Simonian PT, Routt MLC Jr. Biomechanics of pelvic fixation. *Orthop Clin North Am.* 1997;28(3):351.

Tile M. Pelvic ring fractures: should they be fixed? *J Bone Joint Surg Br.* 1988;70(1):1.

Tile M. Acute pelvic fractures: I: causation and classification. *J Am Acad Orthop Surg.* 1996;4(3):143.

Tile M. Acute pelvic fractures: II: principles of management. *J Am Acad Orthop Surg.* 1996;4(3):152.

Recent Articles

Cothren CC, Osborn PM, Moore EE, et al. Preperitonal pelvic packing for hemodynamically unstable pelvic fractures: a paradigm shift. *J Trauma.* 2007;62(4):834–839.

Dyer GS, Vrahas MS. Review of the pathophysiology and acute management of haemorrhage in pelvic fracture. *Injury.* 2006;37(7):602–613.

Geeraerts T, Chhor V, Cheisson G, et al. Clinical review: initial management of blunt pelvic trauma patients with haemodynamic instability. *Crit Care.* 2007;11(1):204.

Giannoudis PV, Tzioupis CC, Pape HC, et al. Percutaneous fixation of the pelvic ring: an update. *J Bone Joint Surg Br.* 2007;89(2):145–154.

Grotz MR, Allami MK, Harwood P, et al. Open pelvic fractures: epidemiology, current concepts of management and outcome. *Injury.* 2005;36(1):1–13.

Harwood PJ, Grotz M, Eardley I, et al. Erectile dysfunction after fracture of the pelvis. *J Bone Joint Surg Br.* 2005;87(3):281–290.

Henry SM, Pollak AN, Jones AL, et al. Pelvic fracture in geriatric patients: a distinct clinical entity. *J Trauma.* 2002;53(1):15–20.

Holden CP, Holman J, Herman MJ. Pediatric pelvic fractures. *J Am Acad Orthop Surg.* 2007;15(3):172–177.

Kommu SS, Illahi I, Mumtaz F. Patterns of urethral injury and immediate management. *Curr Opin Urol.* 2007;17(6):383–389.

Krieg JC, Mohr M, Ellis TJ, et al. Emergent stabilization of pelvic ring injuries by controlled circumferential compression: a clinical trial. *J Trauma.* 2005;59(3):659–664.

Magnussen RA, Tressler MA, Obremskey WT, et al. Predicting blood loss in isolated pelvic and acetabular high-energy trauma. *J Orthop Trauma.* 2007;21(9):603–607.

Mehta S, Auerbach JD, Born CT, et al. Sacral fractures. *J Am Acad Orthop Surg.* 2006;14(12):656–665.

Olson SA, Burgess A. Classification and initial management of patients with unstable pelvic ring injuries. *Instr Course Lect.* 2005;54:383–393.

Raman R, Roberts CS, Pape HC, et al. Implant retention and removal after internal fixation of the symphysis pubis. *Injury.* 2005;36(7):827–831.

Templeman DC, Simpson T, Matta JM. Surgical management of pelvic ring injuries. *Instr Course Lect.* 2005;54:395–400.

Tornetta P III, Templeman DC. Expected outcomes after pelvic ring injury. *Instr Course Lect.* 2005;54:401–407.

Yoon W, Kim JK, Jeong YY, et al. Pelvic arterial hemorrhage in patients with pelvic fractures: detection with contrast-enhanced CT. *Radiographics.* 2004;24(6):1591–1605.

Recent Journal Symposiums

Goulet JA (Ed). Hip and Pelvic trauma. *Orthop Clinic North Am.* 2004; 35(4):431-504

CHAPTER 16

Fractures of the Acetabulum

Kyle F. Dickson

I. Introduction—Fractures of the acetabulum generally occur in younger individuals as a result of high-energy motor-vehicle accidents. Radiographic analysis and classification of displaced acetabular fractures by Letournel's classification allows the surgeon to choose better the appropriate surgical approach. Displaced fractures of the acetabulum require operative anatomic reduction. Incongruity of the acetabulum, even as small as 1 mm, results in posttraumatic arthritis characterized by erosion of the femoral head and loss of articular cartilage. This condition is often misdiagnosed as avascular necrosis, which is characterized by collapse of the femoral head with maintenance of the joint space.

II. Bony Anatomy—The acetabulum is part of the innominate bone and is formed by the ilium, ischium, and pubis. Letournel described the acetabulum as an inverted "Y" with anterior and posterior columns (Fig. 16-1). The anterior column includes the pelvic brim, anterior wall, superior pubic ramus, and anterior border of the iliac wing. The posterior column includes the greater and lesser sciatic notch, posterior wall, ischial tuberosity, and most of the quadrilateral surface.

III. Radiographic Evaluation
   A. Views and Radiographic Landmarks—Radiographic evaluation includes the following views: anteroposterior (AP) (Fig. 16-2A), 45° obturator oblique (Fig. 16-2B), and the 45° iliac oblique (Fig. 16-2C). Six radiographic lines on the AP radiograph represent the tangency of the X-ray beam to the pelvis, not necessarily the anatomic landmarks (Table 16-1). Disruption of the normal radiographic lines represents a fracture to that area of bone. The anatomic area responsible for each line is described in Table 16-1. For a fracture to be truly nondisplaced, no displacement of the radiographic landmark must be seen on at least two of the three radiographic views.

   B. The 45° Oblique Views—The 45° obturator oblique radiograph is taken with the fractured acetabulum rotated toward the X-ray beam, showing the obturator foramen and profiling the anterior column medially and the posterior wall laterally (Fig. 16-2B). The 45° iliac oblique radiograph is taken with the fractured acetabulum rotated away from the X-ray beam, showing the iliac wing and profiling the posterior column (greater and lesser sciatic notch) medially and the anterior wall laterally (Fig. 16-2C).

   C. Analysis of the Fractured Acetabulum
      1. Incongruency—Besides fracture displacement, congruency of the femoral head within the acetabulum is analyzed. Subtle anterior subluxation can be seen on the obturator oblique view, and subtle posterior subluxation can be seen on the iliac oblique view (medialization of the femoral head with respect to the dome of the acetabulum). Comparing the injured side with the unaffected side on the AP and 45° oblique views of the pelvis helps detect any incongruency. Minimally displaced fractures of the acetabulum can be diagnosed by detecting these subtle subluxations of the femoral head.
      2. Roof arc measurements—Roof arc measurements are defined as the angle formed by a line parallel to the patient passing through the center of the acetabulum and a line from the center of the acetabulum to the fractured area of the dome. The medial roof arc (MRA) measurement is made on the AP radiograph (Fig. 16-3), the anterior roof arc (ARA) measurement is made on the obturator oblique radiograph (Fig. 16-4), and the posterior roof arc (PRA) measurement is made on the iliac oblique radiograph (Fig. 16-5). Roof arc measurements of 45° correspond roughly to 10 mm of the dome on a

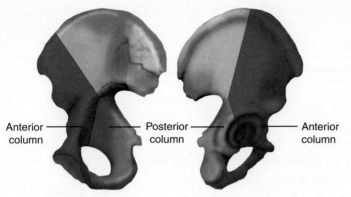

FIGURE 16-1 Delineation of the anterior and posterior columns of the acetabulum on the inner *(left)* and outer *(right)* aspects of the innominate bone.

computed tomography (CT) scan (Fig. 16-6). These roof arc measurements are used for making decisions for surgery and are important in T-shaped and transverse fractures (see Treatment section).

D. CT Scan—Congruency of the femoral head in the acetabulum and classification of the fracture type can usually be performed with plain radiographs alone. CT is useful in defining: posterior pelvic injuries (e.g., sacroiliac joint, sacral fractures), fractures of the quadrilateral surface, marginal impactions of the posterior wall, rotation of the articular pieces, and intraarticular free fragments. The CT scan is used to classify fractures by looking at the orientation of fracture planes. Vertical fracture planes on CT correspond to transverse or T-shaped fractures, and horizontal lines

correspond to column fractures (Fig. 16-7). Three-dimensional CT can provide a useful overall picture of the fracture configuration, but because of smoothing artifacts in the computer reconstructions, nondisplaced fractures and fractures in the plane of the CT scan can be missed. Computer systems that can remove the femoral head from the images are more useful for evaluation of the acetabulum.

IV. Classification—Letournel's classification of acetabular fractures (Fig. 16-8 and Table 16-2) separates the fractures into simple fractures (posterior wall, posterior column, anterior wall, anterior column, and transverse fractures) and complex associated fracture patterns that combine two of the simple patterns (associated posterior column and

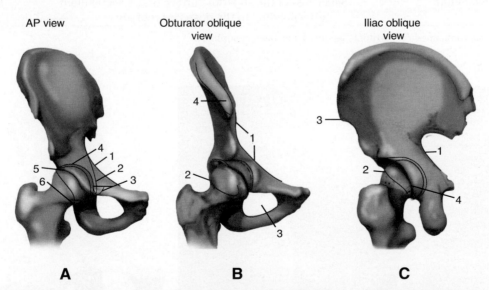

FIGURE 16-2 Normal radiographic landmarks of the acetabulum. **A.** AP radiographic view. 1, Iliopectineal line; 2, ilioischial line; 3, radiographic U, or teardrop; 4, acetabular roof; 5, anterior rim of the acetabulum; 6, posterior rim of the acetabulum. **B.** Obturator oblique view. 1, Iliopectineal line; 2, posterior rim of the acetabulum; 3, obturator foramen; 4, anterior superior iliac spine. **C.** Iliac oblique view. 1, Posterior border of the innominate bone; 2, anterior rim of the acetabulum, 3, anterior border of the iliac wing; 4, posterior rim of the acetabulum.

TABLE 16-1

Radiographic Views and Landmarks of the Acetabulum

Radiographic Views and Landmarks	Anatomic Representation	Column
AP View		
Iliopectineal line	Inferior three fourths: pelvic brim	Anterior
	Superior one fourth: superior quadrilateral surface and the greater sciatic notch	
Ilioischial line	Posterior portion of the quadrilateral surface and the Ischium	Posterior
Radiographic U, or teardrop	External limb: outer aspect of the cotyloid fossa	Usually anterior
	Internal limb: outer wall of the obturator canal, which merges with the quadrilateral surface	
Dome of the acetabulum	Small area of the superior surface of the acetabulum corresponding to the medial roof arc	Anterior and posterior
Anterior rim of the acetabulum	Lateral border of the anterior wall contiguous with the inferior margin of the superior pubic ramus	Anterior
Posterior rim of the acetabulum	Lateral border of the posterior wall contiguous with the inferior articular surface of the acetabulum	Posterior
Obturator Oblique (45°) View		
Iliopectineal line	Pelvic brim	Anterior
Posterior rim of the acetabulum	Lateral border of the posterior wall	Posterior
Dome of the acetabulum	Small area of the superior surface of acetabulum corresponding to the anterior roof arc	Anterior
Iliac Oblique (45°) View		
N/A	Posterior border of the innominate bone (greater and lesser sciatic notch)	Posterior
Anterior rim of the acetabulum	Lateral border of the anterior wall	Anterior
N/A	Anterior border of the iliac wing	Anterior
Dome of the acetabulum	Small area of the superior surface of the acetabulum corresponding to the posterior roof arc	Posterior

N/A, Not Applicable (no named radiographic landmark has been described).

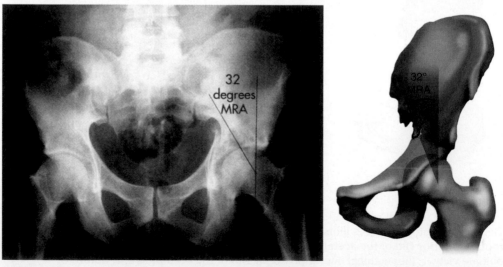

FIGURE 16-3 The medial roof arc angle is formed by a line passing through the center of the acetabulum parallel to the patient and another line from the center of the acetabulum medially to the fractured dome as seen on an AP radiograph. The angle in this case is 32°.

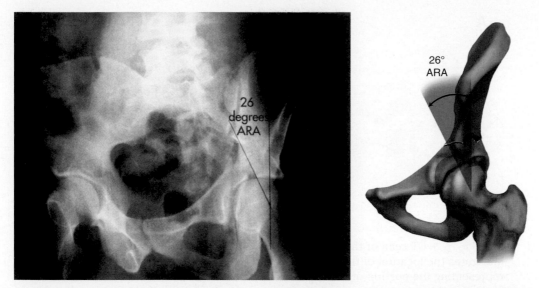

FIGURE 16-4 The anterior roof arc angle is formed by a line passing through the center of the acetabulum parallel to the patient and another line from the center of the acetabulum medially to the fractured dome as seen on the obturator oblique radiograph. The angle in this case is 26°.

posterior wall, associated transverse and posterior wall, T-shaped, associated anterior wall or column and posterior hemitransverse, and both column).

A. Simple Fractures

1. Posterior wall fractures (Figs. 16-8 and 16-9 and Table 16-2)—Posterior wall fractures involve various amounts of the articular and retroacetabular surfaces. Posterior wall fractures have displacement of the posterior rim line on both the AP and obturator oblique views. The fracture may involve the greater and lesser sciatic notch, but the ilioischial line on the AP view remains intact. Occasionally, a **gull sign** is present where the displaced posterior wall remains hinged medially, with superior and posterior displacement of the lateral aspect of the posterior wall giving the appearance of a gull wing (Fig. 16-9).

2. Posterior column fractures (Fig. 16-8 and Table 16-2)—Posterior column fractures involve

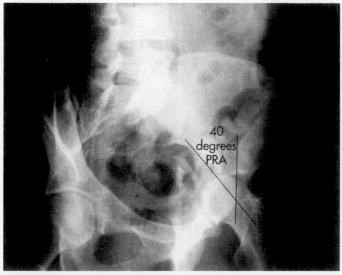
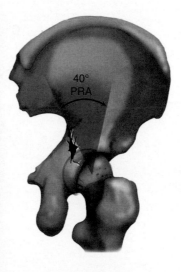

FIGURE 16-5 The posterior roof arc angle is formed by a line passing through the center of the acetabulum parallel to the patient and another line from the center of the acetabulum medially to the fractured dome as seen on the iliac oblique radiograph. The angle in this case is 40°.

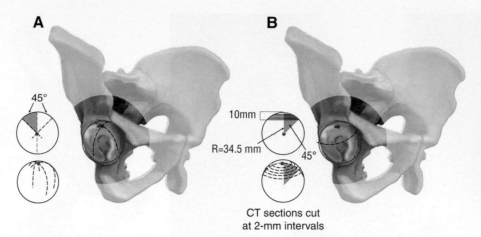

FIGURE 16-6 CT scan of the acetabular dome. **A.** This right acetabulum illustrates the location of the three acetabular roof arcs. These arcs are lines representing the portion of the subchondral bone tangent to the X-ray film in the AP, obturator oblique, and iliac oblique views. The anterior roof arc begins at the posterior lip of the acetabulum, crosses the vertex and extends to the anteroinferior articular surface. The medial and posterior arcs begin at the mid and anterior lip of the acetabulum, cross the vertex, and extend to the acetabular fossa and posteroinferior articular surface, respectively. The inset illustrates a globe with three arcs at 45° intervals, shown from above and obliquely. These lines are analogous to three lines of longitude on a globe 45° apart. **B.** The line shown in the acetabulum represents the level of the CT image 10 mm inferior to the vertex of the acetabulum. The circle along the subchondral bone 10 mm inferior to the vertex is equivalent to a fracture line for which all three roof arc measurements are 45° in almost all cases. The inset illustrates evaluation of the superior acetabulum by CT to 10 mm inferior to the vertex in 2-mm intervals.

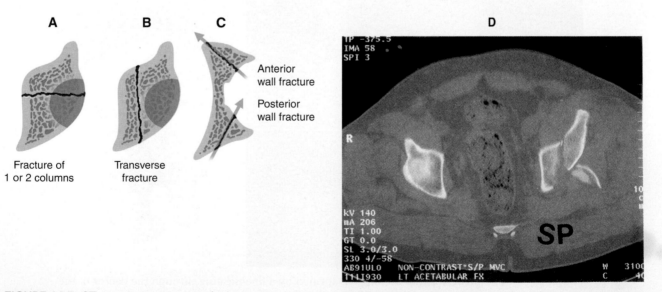

FIGURE 16-7 CT scan cross section. **A.** A transverse fracture plane represents a column-type fracture. **B.** A vertical fracture plane represents a transverse-type fracture. **C.** A 45° oblique fracture plane represents a wall-type fracture. **D.** CT scan demonstrating an associated transverse and posterior wall fracture.

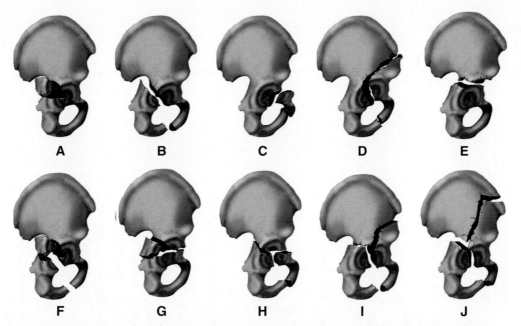

FIGURE 16-8 Classification of acetabular fractures according to Letournel. **A.** Posterior wall fracture. **B.** Posterior column fracture. **C.** Anterior wall fracture. **D.** Anterior column fracture. **E.** Transverse fracture. **F.** Associated posterior column and posterior wall fracture. **G.** Associated transverse and posterior wall fracture. **H.** T-shaped fracture. **I.** Associated anterior wall or column and posterior hemitransverse fracture. **J.** Both-column fracture.

the ischial retroacetabular surface. The fracture line exits the bone in the greater sciatic notch, traverses the articular surface, and usually exits through the obturator foramen and the inferior pubic ramus. Occasionally, the fracture line runs vertically, splitting the ischial tuberosity, without entering the obturator foramen.

Depending on the size of the posterior column fragment, the fracture may involve part of the teardrop or brim of the pelvis anteriorly.

3. Anterior wall fractures (Fig. 16-8 and Table 16-2)—Anterior wall fractures involve the central portion of the anterior column, disrupting the anterior rim of the acetabulum on the

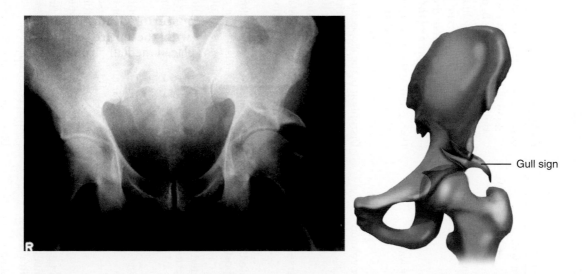

Gull sign

FIGURE 16-9 Gull sign. AP radiograph and drawing of a posterior wall fracture. The displaced posterior wall fracture remains hinged medially, with superior and posterior displacement of the lateral aspect of the posterior wall giving the appearance of a gull wing.

TABLE 16-2

Letournel's Classification of Acetabular Fractures

Fracture Pattern	Radiographic Features	Typical Surgical Approach	Cases with Good to Excellent Results (%)
Posterior wall	Disruption of the posterior rim; the fracture can extend to part of the greater and/or lesser sciatic notch; the ilioischial line remains intact on the AP radiograph; occasionally the *gull sign* is seen	Kocher-Langenbeck	82
Posterior column	Disruption of the ilioischial line and the posterior border of the innominate bone (greater and lesser sciatic notch); the obturator foramen is usually disrupted; the fracture can involve part of the teardrop and the anterior brim of the pelvis	Kocher-Langenbeck	91
Anterior wall	Disruption of the iliopectineal line on both the AP and obturator oblique views; disruption of the anterior rim of the acetabulum on the AP and iliac oblique views	Ilioinguinal	78
Anterior column	Disruption of the iliopectineal line on the AP and obturator oblique views; disruption of the anterior rim of the acetabulum on the AP and iliac oblique views; usually there is an inferior rami fracture; occasionally medial translation of the dome on the AP view is observed	Ilioinguinal	88
Transverse	Disruption of the ilioischial and iliopectineal lines; disruption of the anterior and posterior rims of the acetabulum; the obturator foramen is usually intact	Kocher-Langenbeck	98
Associated posterior column and posterior wall	Disruption of the posterior rim of the acetabulum and the ilioischial line (segmental disruption of the posterior rim of the acetabulum); usually disruption of the obturator foramen is observed	Kocher-Langenbeck	47
Associated transverse and posterior wall	Disruption of the iliopectineal and the ilioischial lines, also disruption of the anterior and posterior rims of the acetabulum (segmental disruption of the posterior rim of the acetabulum); the obturator foramen is usually intact	Kocher-Langenbeck (occasional use of an extended approach [see text])	74
T-shaped	Disruption of the iliopectineal and ilioischial lines, also disruption of the anterior and posterior rims of the acetabulum; the vertical component of this fracture usually disrupts the obturator foramen but may pass posteriorly, splitting the ischial tuberosity; the obturator foramen is usually disrupted	Kocher-Langenbeck (occasional use of an extended approach [see text])	77
Associated anterior wall or column and posterior hemitransverse	Disruption of the iliopectineal and the ilioischial lines, also disruption of the anterior and posterior rims of the acetabulum; the obturator foramen is disrupted	Ilioinguinal	88
Both column	Disruption of the iliopectineal and ilioischial lines; disruption of the anterior border of the iliac wing and posterior border of the innominate bone; the spur sign may be seen; the obturator foramen is disrupted	Ilioinguinal (occasional use of an extended approach [see text])	77

AP and iliac oblique views without disrupting the inferior pubic ramus. Disruption of the iliopectineal line occurs on the AP and obturator oblique views.

4. Anterior column fractures (Fig. 16-8 and Table 16-2)—Anterior column fractures can exit the bone very high (iliac crest) or very low (superior pubic rami). Disruption of the iliopectineal line on the AP and obturator oblique views occurs with these fractures. The fracture involves the inferior pubic ramus and may be associated with medial translation of the dome on the AP view.

5. Transverse fractures (Fig. 16-8 and Table 16-2)—Transverse fractures divide the acetabulum into two portions. The upper portion contains the roof of the acetabulum, and the lower portion contains a portion of the anterior and posterior wall and an intact obturator foramen (unless the obturator foramen is disrupted by an associated pelvic injury). Letournel subdivided transverse fractures based on where the fracture line traversed the acetabulum: (a) transtectal, the fracture line crosses the articular surface of the superior acetabulum; (b) juxtatectal, the fracture line crosses the junction of the articular surface and the superior cotyloid fossa; and (c) infratectal, the fracture line crosses through the cotyloid fossa. The transverse fracture line crosses both columns, but is not considered a both-column fracture. In transverse fractures, the two columns are not separated from each other. Transverse fractures have disruption of the anterior rim, posterior rim, iliopectineal line, and ilioischial line, but the obturator foramen is usually intact.

B. Complex Fractures—Complex or associated fractures usually combine two of the simple fracture patterns.

1. Associated posterior column and posterior wall fractures (Fig. 16-8 and Table 16-2)—The ilioischial line is displaced from the teardrop, and the iliopectineal line is intact. Even 1 mm of displacement can lead to severe arthrosis.

2. Associated transverse and posterior wall fractures (Fig. 16-8 and Table 16-2)—An associated transverse and posterior wall fracture involves a simple transverse pattern associated with a posterior wall fracture. The obturator foramen is usually intact.

3. T-shaped fractures (Fig. 16-8 and Table 16-2)—T-shaped fractures are transverse fractures that have an additional vertical fracture line separating the lower anterior column from the lower posterior column. The vertical line usually disrupts the obturator foramen, which differentiates the T-shaped fracture from the transverse fracture. The vertical fracture line occasionally descends more posteriorly, splitting the ischium, keeping the obturator foramen intact.

4. Anterior wall or column and posterior hemitransverse fractures (Fig. 16-8 and Table 16-2)—Anterior wall or column fractures associated with a posterior hemitransverse fracture combine either an anterior wall or an anterior column fracture with a transverse fracture through the posterior column. The difference between this fracture and the T-shaped fracture is often subtle. The difference is in the orientation of the fracture pattern anteriorly. T-shaped fractures have an anterior transverse fracture line that corresponds with a vertical orientation on the CT scan, whereas the anterior component of the anterior wall or anterior column fracture associated with a posterior hemitransverse fracture is horizontal for an anterior column fracture and approximately 45° for an anterior wall fracture (Fig. 16-7). Furthermore, an anterior column fracture often involves the crest, which does not occur in T-shaped fractures.

5. Both-column fractures (Figs. 16-8 and 16-10 and Table 16-2)—In both-column fractures, both the anterior and posterior columns are disrupted, as in the transverse fractures, associated transverse and posterior wall fractures, associated anterior wall or column and posterior hemitransverse fractures, and T-shaped fractures. The both-column fracture also has separation of the two columns similar to that in T-shaped fractures and the associated anterior wall or column and posterior hemitransverse fractures. However, in the both-column fracture, the articular surface has been completely separated from the posterior portion of the intact innominate bone. All the other fracture patterns have some articular surface that remains in its original anatomic position attached to the intact portion of the posterior ilium. Because the two columns (with the entire articular surface) are displaced medially from the intact portion of the posterior ilium, a radiographic **spur sign** can be seen best on the obturator oblique view and represents the intact portion of the posterior ilium that remains in its anatomic position (Fig. 16-10). This sign is pathognomonic of a both-column fracture.

C. Additional Fracture Patterns—In any classification system, there is some overlap in the fracture patterns. Furthermore, to reduce the number of fracture patterns to ten, some of the associated or

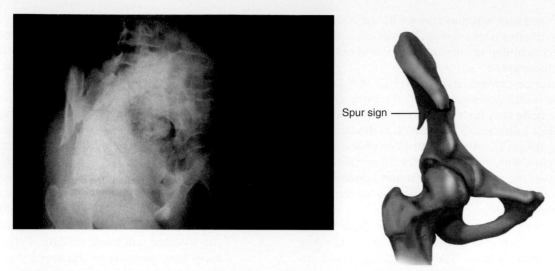

Spur sign

FIGURE 16-10 Spur sign. Obturator oblique radiograph and drawing of a both-column fracture. Note the medial translation of the dome of the acetabulum and the femoral head. The spur sign represents the intact portion of the iliac wing that remains in its anatomic position.

complex fracture patterns are put into one of the larger groups because their treatment is very similar to one of the simple fracture patterns; that is, associated anterior wall and column fractures are grouped with the anterior column fractures, and the associated posterior column and anterior hemitransverse fractures are grouped with the T-shaped fractures.

V. Treatment
  A. Operative Indications—Indications for operative treatment include displaced fractures (≥2 mm) of the acetabular dome (MRA < 45°, ARA < 35°, PRA < 65° in transverse and T-shaped fractures), posterior wall fractures causing hip instability (fractures involving anywhere between 20% and 65% of the posterior wall), and loss of congruency or parallelism between the curvature of the femoral head and the acetabular articular surface on any of the three views (AP, obturator oblique, iliac oblique). Closed reduction is not applicable for the treatment of displaced articular fractures of the acetabulum.
  B. Nonoperative Indications—Nonoperative treatment of acetabular fractures is indicated in patients with local or systemic infection, severe osteoporosis, nondisplaced fractures of the acetabulum, displaced fractures with a large portion of the acetabulum intact (intact superior 10 mm of the dome on CT or roof arc measurements of MRA < 45°, ARA < 65°, PRA < 35° in transverse and T-type fractures), or secondary congruence of the acetabulum and femoral head in both-column fractures. In both-column fractures only, the articular surface is completely dissociated from the intact

portion of the ilium. If the articular surface remains nondisplaced or minimally displaced and congruent around the femoral head, then secondary congruence exists, and nonoperative treatment can be considered. Relative contraindications to surgery include advanced age, associated medical conditions, and associated soft tissue and visceral injuries.
  C. Surgical Approaches—The choice of surgical approach depends on the fracture configuration. The Kocher-Langenbeck approach provides access to the posterior column, and the ilioinguinal approach provides access to the anterior column. Extended approaches (extended iliofemoral, triradiate, and simultaneous and sequential Kocher-Langenbeck and ilioinguinal approaches) are needed for some transtectal transverse fractures, T-shaped fractures, associated anterior wall or column and posterior hemitransverse fractures, and both-column fractures with significant displacement of both the anterior and posterior columns. Ideally, the surgeon chooses one approach that can be used to reduce and fix the entire fracture. If a combined anterior ilioinguinal and posterior Kocher-Langenbeck approach is required for the fracture, the author's choice is to perform them sequentially, not concurrently, because of some limited access of each approach if they are performed simultaneously. The surgical approaches that are performed about the hip are listed in Table 16-3 with their dissection intervals, structures at risk, complications, and anatomic considerations. Cross-sectional anatomy around the hip (CT scans and magnetic resonance images) is

TABLE 16-3

Surgical Approaches about the Hip

Approach	Surgical Interval	Structures at Risk	Complications	Anatomic Considerations
Kocher-Langenbeck	The gluteus maximus is split (distal to the branching and innervation by the inferior gluteal nerve)	*Sciatic nerve* (protected by the obturator internus) *Ascending branch of the medial femoral circumflex artery and the medial femoral circumflex artery* (taking down the quadratus femoris from the femur instead of the ischium or taking down the piriformis or obturator interims <1 cm from their insertion can damage these vessels) *Inferior gluteal artery* *Inferior gluteal nerve* (damaged when splitting the gluteus maximus too far proximally, midway between the greater trochanter and the PSIS) *Femoral nerve* (placement of a retractor on the anterior wall of the acetabulum) *Obturator artery* (during hip arthroplasty the obturator artery can be injured if a retractor is placed beneath the transverse acetabular ligament in the acetabulum) *Superior gluteal neurovascular bundle* (exits the greater sciatic notch and is injured with aggressive retraction of the abductors anteriorly and superiorly)	Sciatic nerve palsy 10% Heterotopic bone formation without prophylaxis 23% (8% incidence of heterotopic bone formation that causes a significant decrease in hip range of motion [i.e., <90° of flexion]) Infection 3%	The superior gluteal nerve exits superior to the piriformis, and the sciatic nerve exits inferior to the piriformis. The inferior gluteal nerve exits the pelvis below the piriformis through the greater sciatic notch
Ilioinguinal	There are *three windows:* (1) medial to the lymphatics and the external iliac artery and vein, (2) between the external iliac vessels and the iliopsoas, and (3) lateral to the iliopsoas	*Lateral femoral cutaneous nerve* (runs up to 3 cm from the ASIS deep to the inguinal floor)	Direct hernia 1%	A direct hernia is medial to the inferior epigastric artery; an indirect hernia is lateral to the inferior epigastric artery. The inferior epigastric artery is deep to the deep inguinal ring

(continued)

TABLE 16-3 (continued)

Surgical Approaches about the Hip

Approach	Surgical Interval	Structures at Risk	Complications	Anatomic Considerations
Ilioinguinal (continued)		Femoral artery (injured with a retractor in the second window) / Femoral vein (injured with a retractor in the second window and may lead to a deep vein thrombosis) / Femoral nerve (protected with the psoas muscle, although vigorous retraction of the psoas muscle may cause injury to the nerve) / Inferior epigastric artery (deep to the inguinal ligament and is the last branch of the iliac artery before it passes underneath the inguinal ligament) / Spermatic cord (vas deferens and testicular artery as a result of overretraction) / Bladder (lies behind the symphysis pubis)	Significant lateral femoral cutaneous nerve numbness 23% / External iliac artery thrombosis 1% / Hematoma 5% / Infection 2% / Heterotopic bone formation 4% (2% significant decrease in range of motion [<90° of hip flexion])	
Extended iliofemoral	*Proximal*—The interval is between the gluteus maximus and the abdominal muscles. *Distal* *Superficial*—The interval is between the sartorius (femoral nerve) and the tensor fascia lata (superior gluteal nerve). *Deep*—The interval is between the rectus femoris (femoral nerve) and the gluteus medius (superior gluteal nerve)	*Posterior branches of the lateral femoral cutaneous nerve* (are cut with the incision) / *Lateral femoral circumflex vascular bundle and the ascending branch of the lateral femoral circumflex artery* (must be ligated) / *Superior gluteal artery, vein, and nerve* (exiting from the greater sciatic notch, excessive anterosuperior retraction of the abductors)	Heterotopic bone formation without prophylaxis 70% (20% significant decrease in motion [<90° of hip flexion]) / Sciatic nerve palsy 1% / Hematoma 8% / Deep vein thrombosis 5% / Infection 1%	The gluteal muscle flap is based off both the superior and the inferior gluteal neurovascular bundles. The inferior gluteal nerve supplies the gluteus maximus. The superior gluteal nerve supplies the gluteus medius and minimus and the tensor fascia lata. The upper third of the blood supply of the gluteus maximus comes from the superior gluteal artery, and the lower two thirds comes from the inferior gluteal artery

Approach	Interval	Dangers	Complications	Anatomy
Combined Kocher-Langenbeck and ilioinguinal and triradiate exposures	See Kocher-Langenbeck and Ilioinguinal Approaches	See Kocher-Langenbeck and Ilioinguinal Approaches	See Kocher-Langenbeck and Ilioinguinal Approaches	See Kocher-Langenbeck and Ilioinguinal Approaches
Smith-Petersen (anterior approach)	*Superficial*—The interval is between the sartorius (femoral nerve) and the tensor fascia lata (superior gluteal nerve) *Deep*—The interval is between the rectus femoris (femoral nerve) and the gluteus medius (superior gluteal nerve)	*Lateral femoral cutaneous nerve* (especially if a retractor is placed superficial to the rectus) *Lateral femoral circumflex artery and the ascending branch of the lateral femoral circumflex artery* (need to be ligated)	Lateral femoral cutaneous nerve palsy 5% Infection 2% Femoral nerve palsy 1%	The lateral femoral cutaneous nerve pierces the sartorius approximately 2.5 cm below the ASIS and lies very close to the interval between the sartorius and the tensor fascia lata. The lateral femoral circumflex artery is deep to the rectus, lying in its sheath close to the femoral nerve. The lateral femoral circumflex artery has an ascending branch that lies within the psoas sheath. These arteries cross the gap between the muscles of the tensor fascia lata and the sartorius below the ASIS and must be ligated
Watson-Jones (anterolateral approach)	The interval is between the gluteus medius (superior gluteal nerve) and the tensor fascia lata (superior gluteal nerve). The superior gluteal nerve enters the muscles proximal to the incision	*Femoral nerve* (retract or placed anterior to the rectus or too-vigorous retraction) *Femoral artery and vein* (retraction on top of the rectus vs. deep to it) *Profunda femoris artery* (lies on the psoas muscle deep to the femoral artery and may be injured with a poorly placed retractor)	Abductor weakness (as a result of the abductors being taken down by a tenotomy or a greater trochanter osteotomy) Femoral shaft fracture (during dislocation in a total hip arthroplasty)	The profunda femoris artery branches from the femoral artery and passes deep to the femoral artery and lies on top of the psoas muscle

(continued)

TABLE 16-3 (continued)

Surgical Approaches about the Hip

Approach	Surgical Interval	Structures at Risk	Complications	Anatomic Considerations
Hardinge (lateral approach)	The gluteus medius (incision distal to the superior gluteal nerve innervation) and the vastus lateralis (well away from the more anterior and medial femoral nerve innervation) are split	*Femoral nerve, artery, and vein* (retractors) *Transverse branch of the lateral femoral circumflex artery* (cut when the vastus lateralis is released) *Gluteus medius* (abductors damaged through retraction) *Superior gluteal nerve* (too-proximal splitting of the gluteus medius)	Weakness of the hip abductors	—
Ludloff (medial approach)	The superficial interval is between the adductor longus (anterior division of the obturator nerve) and the gracilis (anterior division of the obturator nerve). Both muscles are proximally innervated, and therefore the interval is safe. The deep interval is between the adductor brevis (anterior and/or posterior divisions of the obturator nerve) and the adductor magnus (posterior division of the obturator nerve and the tibial portion of the sciatic nerve)	*Obturator nerve* (vigorous retraction) *Medial femoral circumflex artery* (lies on the medial side of the psoas tendon and can be injured when cutting the psoas tendon in children)	Obturator nerve palsy	The anterior division of the obturator nerve passes downward in front of the obturator externus and adductor brevis and behind the pectineus and adductor longus. It sends muscular branches to the gracilis, adductor brevis, adductor longus, occasionally to the pectineus, and to the articular branch of the hip joint. The posterior division of the obturator nerve pierces the obturator externus and passes downward behind the adductor brevis and in front of the adductor magnus. It sends muscular branches to the obturator externus, to the adductor part of the adductor magnus, and occasionally to the adductor brevis. Its terminal branch is to the knee joint

PSIS, Posterosuperior iliac spine; *ASIS,* anterosuperior iliac spine.

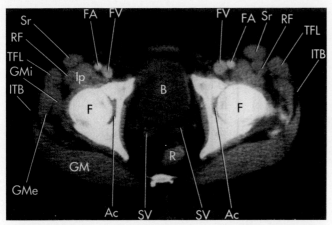

FIGURE 16-11 Anatomy of the hip as seen on CT scan. Ac, Acetabulum; B, urinary bladder; F, head of femur. FA, femoral artery; FV, femoral vein; GM gluteus maximus; GMe, gluteus medius; GMi, gluteus minimus; Ip, iliopsoas; ITB, iliotibial band; R, rectum; RF, rectus femoris; Sr; sartorius; SV, seminal vesicles; TFL, tensor fascia lata. (Reprinted with permission from Bo Wi, Wolfman NT, Krueger WA, et al. *Basic Atlas of Sectional Anatomy: With Correlated Imaging.* 3rd ed. Philadelphia, PA: WB Saunders; 1998.)

shown in Figures 16-11 and 16-12. The three main approaches for acetabular fractures include the Kocher-Langenbeck, the ilioinguinal, and the extended iliofemoral.

1. Kocher-Langenbeck approach—The Kocher-Langenbeck approach for acetabular fractures is different from that used in total hip arthroplasty.

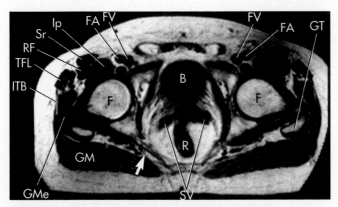

FIGURE 16-12 Anatomy of the hip as seen on magnetic resonance imaging. B, Urinary bladder; F, head of femur; FA, femoral artery; FV, femoral vein; GM, gluteus maximus; GMe, gluteus medius; GT, greater trochanter; Ip, iliopsoas; ITB, iliotibial band; R, rectum; RF, rectus femoris; Sr, sartorius; SV, seminal vesicles; TFL, tensor fascia lata; arrow, sacrospinous ligament. (Reprinted with permission from Browner BO, Jupiter JB, Levine AM, et al, eds. *Skeletal Trauma: Fractures, Dislocations, Ligamentous Injuries.* 2nd ed. Philadelphia, PA: WB Saunders; 1998.)

- Ascending branch of the medial femoral circumflex artery—Preserving the ascending branch of the medial femoral circumflex artery supplying the femoral head is very important for preventing avascular necrosis. The artery runs deep to the quadratus femoris and superficial to the obturator externus. It then runs deep to the conjoined tendon (gemellus superior and inferior and obturator internus) and piriformis tendon next to the greater trochanter before attaching to the femoral arterial ring at the base of the femoral neck.

- Patient positioning—The patient is usually positioned prone to help the femoral head reduce to the anterior wall of the acetabulum. This positioning allows easier reduction of posterior wall and column fractures. The Judet fracture table is used for traction and allows the knee to remain flexed at 60° to 90°, relaxing the sciatic nerve. If a Judet table is unavailable, the patient is placed in a lateral decubitus position with the entire leg draped free. In this position, medial subluxation of the femoral head, especially in transverse fractures, may cause difficulty with anatomic reduction.

- Incision and dissection (Fig. 16-13)—The incision starts 5 cm lateral to the posterior superior iliac spine (PSIS), proceeds to the greater trochanter, and then continues along the axis of the femur for 20 cm. The gluteus maximus is split along its fibers until the branches of the inferior gluteal nerve, which are approximately halfway between the greater trochanter and the PSIS, are identified. The fascia lata is split along the axis of the femur. The tendinous portion of the gluteus maximus insertion or sling is released 5 mm from the femur and reapproximated at the end of the procedure. A branch of the posterior circumflex artery is deep to the tendon and may be accidentally cut (retracting deep into the leg) if release of the tendon is too aggressive. The sciatic nerve is identified on the quadratus femoris and followed proximally below the piriformis to ensure that it is not caught in the fracture site. A branch of the inferior gluteal artery may lie lateral to the sciatic nerve and require coagulation or ligation. The tendons of the piriformis and obturator internus are separately tagged and cut sharply 1 cm from the greater trochanter. This ensures protection of the ascending branch of the medial femoral circumflex

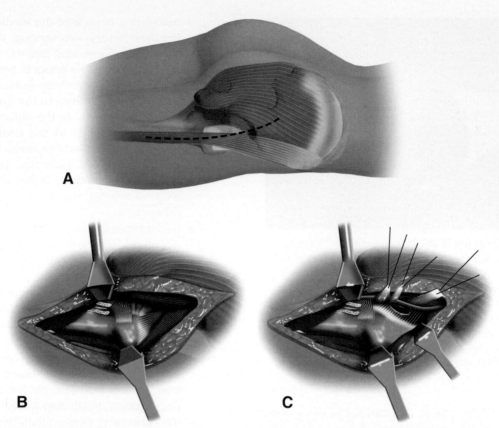

FIGURE 16-13 Kocher-Langenbeck approach. **A.** Skin incision. **B.** Splitting of the gluteus maximus muscle and transection of its tendon. The sciatic nerve is visible on the posterior aspect of the quadratus femoris. **C.** The completed exposure of the retroacetabular surface. Transection and reflection of the obturator internus tendon gives access to the ischial tuberosity and the lesser sciatic notch. A capsulotomy can be made at the acetabular rim.

artery. The tendons are retracted posteriorly, with the obturator internus tendon leading to the lesser sciatic notch, which protects the sciatic nerve. The piriformis leads to the greater sciatic notch. The joint capsule can be opened along the rim, protecting the labrum to visualize the hip joint. In posterior wall fractures, the capsule is reflected with the piece of the posterior wall, maintaining the blood supply to the fragments. A trochanteric osteotomy can be used for additional exposure of the joint and the superior acetabulum; the ascending branch of the medial femoral circumflex artery needs to be protected when the osteotomy is performed. Exposure of the quadrilateral surface through the greater sciatic notch allows palpation of the fracture lines that cross this surface and is used to assess reductions of transverse fractures. After reduction and fixation, the tendons are reattached anatomically, and a Hemovac is used deep to the fascia lata.

2. Ilioinguinal approach—The ilioinguinal approach allows full access to the anterior column and limited access to the posterior column. It is required for anterior column and wall fractures, most associated anterior wall or column and posterior hemitransverse fractures, and both column fractures.

- Patient positioning—The ilioinguinal approach is performed with the patient in the supine position with the hip flexed 20° to 30 on the Judet fracture table. Flexion of the hip relaxes the iliopsoas tendon. If a Judet table is not available, the entire leg is prepared and draped free to allow flexion of the hip to relax the iliopsoas tendon.

- Incision and dissection (Fig. 16-14)—The incision starts at the midline two fingerbreadths above the symphysis pubis, proceeds to the anterosuperior iliac spine (ASIS), and then continues along the iliac crest past its widest dimension. The abdominal muscles and iliacus muscle are released from the crest

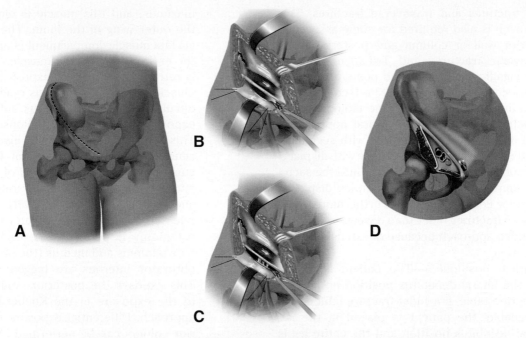

FIGURE 16-14 Ilioinguinal approach. **A.** Skin incision. **B.** Internal iliac fossa has been exposed, and the inguinal canal has been unroofed by distal reflection of the external oblique aponeurosis. **C.** An incision along the inguinal ligament detaches the abdominal muscles and transversalis fascia, giving access to the psoas sheath, the iliopectineal fascia, the external aspect of the femoral vessels, and the retropubic Retzius space. **D.** Oblique section through the lacuna musculorum and lacuna vascularum at the level of the inguinal ligament.

through their tendinous attachment, and the iliacus is mobilized from the internal iliac fossa to the sacroiliac joint and pelvic brim. Distally, the external oblique aponeurosis is split in line with the skin incision and is folded back, unroofing the inguinal canal. The spermatic cord or round ligament and the ilioinguinal nerve are isolated with a rubber drain. The floor of the inguinal canal is incised with caution, watching for the lateral femoral cutaneous nerve running distally up to 3 cm from the ASIS. The incision through the floor of the inguinal canal leaves 2 mm of tendon attached to the transverse abdominis and obliquus internus muscles for closure and prevention of a direct hernia. Medially, the rectus is released approximately 1 cm from lateral to medial, or alternatively the two heads of the rectus are split (similar to a Pfannenstiel approach) performing a modified Stoppa approach. The iliopectineal fascia separates the psoas muscle and femoral nerve from the external iliac artery and vein and lymphatics. This thick, fibrous sheath runs along the pelvic brim to the sacroiliac joint and separates the true pelvis from the false pelvis. Adequate exposure of the bone

requires complete division of this fascia. The obturator nerve and artery are visualized entering the obturator foramen. Anomalous branches or origin of the artery occurs in 50% of patients. The obturator artery usually originates from the internal iliac artery. Anomalous branches or origins may come from the external iliac or the inferior epigastric artery. In less than 5% of cases, this anomalous branch is the main obturator artery and needs to be ligated to prevent tearing during the procedure; (The anomalous branch is called the **corona mortis**, "crown of death"). The incision provides access to the innominate bone through three surgical windows: (1) the retropubic Retzius space (medial to the lymphatics and the external iliac artery and vein), (2) the quadrilateral surface and anterior wall (between the external iliac vessels and the iliopsoas muscle), and (3) the internal iliac fossa and the sacroiliac joint (lateral to the iliopsoas muscle).

3. Extended iliofemoral approach—The extended iliofemoral approach allows access to both the anterior and posterior columns simultaneously. The approach is required for some transtectal associated transverse and posterior

wall fractures and transverse fractures. This approach is also required for some associated anterior wall or column and posterior hemitransverse fractures and T-shaped fractures with significant anterior and posterior column displacement. Although most both-column fractures are repaired through the ilioinguinal approach, the extended iliofemoral approach is used in both column fractures with segmental greater sciatic notch pieces, those with displacement of fracture lines that enter into the sacroiliac joint, and those with complex displaced posterior column fractures. Furthermore, some of these fractures older than 3 weeks require an extended approach because of extensive callus formation.

- Patient positioning—The patient is placed in the lateral decubitus position on a Judet fracture table. If a Judet fracture table is not available, the patient is placed in the lateral decubitus position and the entire leg is draped free.
- Incision and dissection (Fig. 16-15)—The incision starts at the PSIS and follows the iliac crest to the ASIS and proceeds down the lateral side of the thigh for 20 cm toward the lateral border of the patella. The knee is flexed more than 60° to relax the sciatic nerve. The iliac crest incision is taken through the tendinous portion of the gluteus

maximus, and this muscle is elevated from the outer wing of the ilium. The tensor fascia lata muscle compartment is opened along the entire length of the muscle. The muscle is retracted posteriorly, exposing the rectus muscle fascia. This fascia is opened longitudinally, retracting the rectus anteriorly and exposing the fascia of the iliopsoas muscle. This fascia is carefully split, ligating the ascending branch of the lateral femoral circumflex vessels. The tendons of the gluteus minimus, gluteus medius, obturator internus, and piriformis are sequentially tagged and released. Alternatively, a greater trochanteric osteotomy is performed, releasing the gluteus minimus and medius (the piriformis and obturator internus are tagged separately). This exposes the posterior column, similar to the exposure in the Kocher-Langenbeck approach. Differential exposure to the anterior column can be performed by release of the rectus femoris from the anterior inferior iliac spine (AIIS), the sartorius muscle from the anterior superior iliac spine (ASIS), or the iliopsoas muscle from the iliac fossa. The surgeon must ensure that adequate soft-tissue attachments and vascular supply exists for all fracture fragments. After anatomic reduction and fixation of the acetabulum, the tendons are anatomically reattached.

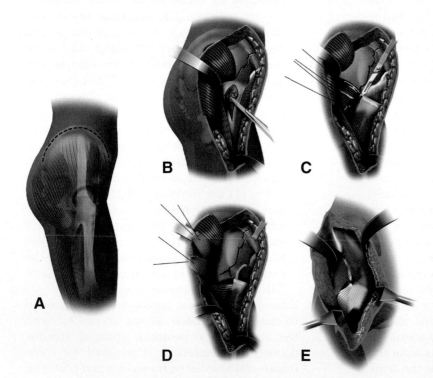

FIGURE 16-15 Extended iliofemoral approach. **A.** Skin incision. **B.** The gluteal muscles have been elevated from the iliac wing. The lateral femoral circumflex vessels are ligated and transected. **C.** The tendons of the gluteus minimus and medius are transected in midsubstance at their trochanteric insertions. **D.** The completed exposure of the external aspect of the bone with a capsulotomy along the acetabular rim. **E.** The completed exposure of the internal aspect of the bone.

D. Treatment of Specific Fracture Types—Reduction of the fractured acetabulum is one of the most challenging problems facing the orthopaedic surgeon. The reduction maneuvers are fracture dependent but are greatly facilitated by use of the Judet fracture table. Various reduction forceps may be used to reduce the acetabulum. Fixation is also individualized to the fracture type, but the most secure fixation is a combination of lag screws and buttress plating. Screw penetration of the joint must be avoided and can be checked with the C-arm at the end of the procedure. In a concave joint such as the acetabulum, only one view is needed to prove that the screw is not in the hip joint.

1. Posterior wall fractures—Posterior wall fractures are often associated with marginal articular impaction fractures next to the major fracture lines. The impacted articular pieces are elevated with 5 to 10 mm of cancellous bone to the reduced femoral head. Cancellous bone graft from the greater trochanter is packed behind the elevated fragments. Alternatively, an injectable calcium phosphate can be used behind the reduced marginal impaction. The cortical posterior wall is reduced and held with a ball spike. Initial fixation is with lag screws and is followed by a buttress plate. When comminuted or small bony fragments attached to the acetabular labrum are present, a spring plate (one-third tubular plate) under a reconstruction plate is used. The keys to successful surgery on posterior wall fractures are leaving as much of the capsule attachment (blood supply) to the posterior wall fragments as possible and performing an anatomic reduction of the fragments.

2. Posterior column fractures—Posterior column fractures have a rotational deformity of the posterior column around the femoral head as the head pushes medially. Reduction involves removing the hematoma and debris from the fracture line and placing reduction screws and occasionally a half-pin in the ischial tuberosity. The reduction screws are used with the pelvic reduction clamps (Farabeuf and Jungbluth). In addition, an angled reduction clamp can be placed with one tong on the quadrilateral surface, and the other on the supra-acetabulum on the anterior column. This clamp helps to de-rotate the posterior column. The reduction is checked both on the retroacetabular surface as well as on the quadrilateral surface. Fixation is performed with a combination of lag screws and a buttress reconstruction plate.

3. Anterior wall and anterior column fractures—Surgery is performed on anterior wall and anterior column fractures through the ilioinguinal approach. Reduction and fixation is similar to that of posterior wall and posterior column fractures. Around the pectineal eminence, the acetabulum is easily penetrated with screws; therefore, placement of screws should be close to the brim and directed parallel or toward the quadrilateral surface. Anterior column fractures often have a free brim fragment that should be reduced and fixed before reduction and fixation of the anterior column fragment.

4. Transverse fractures—The techniques for reducing transverse fractures are similar to those for reducing posterior column fractures. Often, a half-pin is used in the ischial tuberosity to help with rotational reduction. Fixation is performed with a combination of lag screws and a buttress plate. Although most transverse fractures are treated through the Kocher-Langenbeck approach, those with greater displacement of the anterior column than the posterior column or those with a high anterior column fracture line (i.e., through the dome) and a low posterior column fracture are best approached through the ilioinguinal approach.

5. Associated transverse and posterior wall fractures—Associated transverse and posterior wall fractures are reduced and fixed as previously described. Occasionally, the posterior wall involves the entire retroacetabular surface, making the reduction quite difficult to assess. In these cases, as well as cases with significant displacement of the anterior column, those in which the fracture line passes through the dome, and those with a separate greater sciatic notch piece, the extended iliofemoral approach may be indicated. ***These fractures have the highest incidence of preoperative sciatic nerve palsy.***

6. T-shaped fractures—T-shaped fractures can often be reduced using the posterior Kocher-Langenbeck approach. If the anterior column cannot be reduced, the surgeon first fixes the posterior column; the patient is then turned over for an ilioinguinal approach and the anterior column is reduced and fixed. Alternatively, an extended iliofemoral approach can be preformed for transtectal displaced T-type fractures.

7. Associated anterior wall or column and posterior hemitransverse fractures—Associated anterior wall or column and posterior hemitransverse fractures are usually reduced and fixed through the ilioinguinal approach. The posterior column is usually minimally displaced or nondisplaced and can be reduced with a laterally directed force on the posteroinferior quadrilateral surface.

Rarely, the posterior column requires reduction and fixation (after the anterior column has been reduced and fixed) through a separate Kocher-Langenbeck approach.

8. Both-column fractures—Both-column fractures usually can be reduced and fixed through an ilioinguinal approach. The fractures that enter the sacroiliac joint have associated marginal impactions, or have complex posterior column fractures (i.e., segmental, displaced posterior wall fractures; associated greater sciatic notch fragments; or significant displacement) and are better reduced and fixed through an extended iliofemoral approach. Alternatively, reduction of the anterior column may be performed first with internal fixation through an ilioinguinal approach (with care taken not to block later reduction of the posterior column). This is followed by a posterior approach. Reduction is obtained with a combination of clamps and forceps. At the time of injury, the two columns often rotate out as the head pushes in through the acetabulum like the opening of a saloon door. Therefore, the reduction is performed by rotating the columns back, like closing a saloon door.

9. Postoperative care—Postoperative care involves toe-touch weightbearing ambulation training as soon as possible. At 8 weeks, physical therapy is initiated with exercises, range of motion, and weightbearing-as-tolerated ambulation training. Assistive ambulation devices are used until strength has improved enough to prevent a limp.

VI. Complications—The most common complications include wound infections, iatrogenic nerve palsy, heterotopic bone formation, posttraumatic arthritis, and thromboembolic complications. Furthermore, a closed degloving injury over the greater trochanter containing hematoma and liquified fat between the subcutaneous tissue and deep fascia (Morel-Lavallee lesion) can occur. These lesions can lead to infection in up to 30% of cases and therefore need to be drained and debrided before or at surgery to decrease the risk of infection.

A. Posttraumatic Arthritis—Assuming the fracture is classified correctly and the proper approach is chosen, accuracy of the reduction is the most important factor in the clinical outcome and in preventing post traumatic arthritis.

B. Wound Infections—Bloody discharge may occur for 1 to 2 days after surgery and clear drainage may continue for up to 10 days. If drainage either increases or changes to a cloudy discharge, immediate incision and debridement of possible infection or hematoma is indicated. Patients with extraarticular infections may ultimately have a good functional result; deep or intraarticular infections are usually associated with a poor outcome.

C. Iatrogenic Nerve Palsy—Iatrogenic nerve palsy is the result of vigorous or prolonged retraction of the sciatic nerve, usually involving the peroneal division. Keeping the knee flexed to at least 60 with the hip extended during the posterior approach decreases the tautness of the sciatic nerve. In some centers, somatosensory-evoked potentials or motor-evoked potentials are monitored during surgery to watch for changes in amplitude or latency to prevent iatrogenic injury. The role of monitoring in acute acetabular surgery has not been established. Postoperative footdrop may resolve for up to 3 years after surgery, and tendon transfer procedures should not be contemplated until this time.

D. Heterotopic Bone Formation—Heterotopic bone formation is usually painless. It is most common after the extended iliofemoral approach and least common after the ilioinguinal approach. Proven risk factors for heterotopic bone formation include T-shaped fractures, associated head or chest trauma, and male patients. Indomethacin, 25 mg three times a day for 8 weeks, decreases the incidence of heterotopic ossification. Postoperative radiation (700 cGy, one-time dose), as well as the combination of the two modalities, has also been shown to be effective. Debriding necrotic muscle and reducing the amount of soft-tissue stripping off of the lateral aspect of the innominate bone can help reduce the risk of heterotopic bone formation. The correlation of heterotopic bone formation and range of motion is important because patients with apparent complete bone bridging on the AP X-ray film may have more than 110° of hip flexion. The 45° oblique views and CT scanning may be helpful for assessing the severity of heterotopic bone formation and should be used if excision is indicated (hip flexion <90° or a fixed rotational malalignment). When possible, surgery for removal of heterotopic bone should be delayed for 6 to 12 months until the heterotopic bone has matured. A bone scan can be ordered to determine the activity of the bone.

E. Deep Vein Thrombosis—Deep venous thrombosis and pulmonary embolism can occur. Although controversial, the author uses pneumatic compression boots from the time of admission until the patient is fully ambulatory after surgery. Once the drains are removed, pharmacologic prophylaxis (low–molecular-weight heparin) is also started. Contraindications to pharmacologic prophylaxis are splenic rupture and a severe head injury. In these cases and those with established deep vein thrombosis, a Greenfield filter is indicated before surgery.

SUGGESTED READINGS

Classic Articles

Fassler PR, Swiontkowski MF, Kilroy AW, et al. Injury of the sciatic nerve associated with acetabular fracture. *J Bone Joint Surg.* 1993;75A:1157–1166.

Hak DJ, Olson SA, Matta JM. Diagnosis and management of closed internal degloving injuries associated with pelvic and acetabular fractures: the Morel-Lavallee lesion. *J Trauma.* 1997;42:1046–1051.

Judet R, Judet J, Letournel E. Fractures of the acetabulum: classification and surgical approaches for open reduction. *J Bone Joint Surg.* 1964;46A:1615–1638.

Letournel E. *Fractures of the Acetabulum.* 2nd ed. New York, NY: Springer-Verlag; 1993.

Matta JM, Anderson L, Epstein H, et al. Fractures of the acetabulum: a retrospective analysis. *Clin Orthop.* 1986;205:220–240.

Matta JM. Fractures of the acetabulum: reduction accuracy and clinical results of fractures operated within three weeks of injury. *J Bone Joint Surg.* 1996;78A:1632–1645.

Matta JM, Mehne D, Roffi R. Fractures of the acetabulum: early results of a prospective study. *Clin Orthop.* 1986;205:241–250.

Matta JM. Operative indications and choice of surgical approach for fractures of the acetabulum. *Tech Orthop.* 1986;1:13–22.

Matta JM. Operative treatment of acetabular fractures through the ilioinguinal approach: a ten year perspective. *Clin Orthop.* 1994;305:10–19.

Matta JM, Letournel E, Browner B. Surgical management of acetabular fractures. *Instr Course Lect.* 1986;35:382–397.

Moed BR, McMichael JC. Outcomes of posterior wall fractures of the acetabulum. *J Bone Joint Surg Am.* 1989;89(6):1170–1176.

Olson SA, Matta JM. The computerized tomography subchondral arc: a new method of assessing acetabular articular continuity after fracture (a preliminary report). *J Orthop Trauma.* 1993;7:402–413.

Thomas KA, Vrahas MS, Noble JW Jr, et al. Evaluation of hip stability after simulated transverse acetabular fractures. *Clin Orthop Relat Res.* 1997;340:244–256.

Recent Articles

Griffin DB, Beaulé, Matta JM. Safety and efficacy of the extended iliofemoral approach in the treatment of complex fractures of the acetabulum. *J Bone Joint Surg.* 2005;87B(10):1391–1396.

Qureshi AA, Archdeacon MT, Jenkins MA, et al. Infrapectineal plating for acetabular fractures: a technical adjunct to internal fixation. *J Orthop Trauma.* 2004;18(3):175–178.

Olson SA, Kadrmas MW, Hernandez JD, et al. Augmentation of posterior wall acetabular fracture fixation using calcium-phosphate cement: a biomechanical analysis. *J Orthop Trauma.* 2007;21(9):608–616.

Textbook

Letournel E. *Fractures of the Acetabulum.* 2nd ed. New York, NY: Springer-Verlag; 1993.

CHAPTER 17

Hip Dislocations and Fractures of the Femoral Head

Steven C. Lochow and Steven A. Olson

I. Introduction—Hip dislocations and fracture-dislocations occur across all age groups and represent a spectrum of injuries that can result when abnormal load is placed on the hip. ***The position of the femur when the force is applied determines the pattern of injury.*** The force can be dissipated by any combination of femur fracture, intertrochanteric fracture, femoral neck fracture, hip dislocation, acetabular fracture, femoral head fracture, and pelvic fracture. Hip dislocations and femoral head fractures are considered together because a fracture of the femoral head cannot occur without subluxation or dislocation of the hip and the treatment rationale for both is similar.

II. Hip Dislocations
   A. Overview—Dislocations of the hip usually result from moderate to severe trauma. The majority (42% to 84%) occur as the result of a motor-vehicle accident. The remainder are associated with falls from a height, sports injuries, and industrial accidents. Posterior dislocations occur much more commonly than anterior dislocations (89% to 92%). Thirty percent of patients with a hip dislocation do not have an acetabular fracture, and most dislocations without fractures are posterior (approximately 80%). Dislocations with acetabular or femoral fractures are almost always posterior (approximately 90%). Historically, the assumed mechanism for posterior dislocation was dashboard impact. However, newer reports have shown that many of these injuries occur in the right hip, and the mechanism of such injuries is now believed to be related to the driver pressing on the brake with the right foot with the hip held in flexion, adduction, and internal rotation. Anterior dislocations often have an associated femoral head fracture and/or impaction. Hip dislocations have the potential for significant

long-term disability. Early literature showed poor results with frequent early arthritis and avascular necrosis (AVN). These early reports predated modern imaging modalities and current understanding of the vascularity of the femoral head. It is hoped that by incorporating recent advances, the results of the treatment of patients with these injuries can be improved.
   1. Historical overview—The modern phase in the management of dislocations of the hip dates from Henry Jacob Bigelow's publication in 1869. The clinical presentations and reduction maneuvers described are the same as those used today. In the 1950s, Thompson and Epstein's classification system and Stewart and Milford's classification system were devised. Trueta's description of the vascularity of the femoral head was also published in this time period. It was not until the advent of computed tomography (CT) in the 1970s that the treatment of hip dislocations evolved to its present state.
   B. Evaluation—The patient must be examined completely for associated injuries, particularly when the patient is unable to cooperate. Any injury to the pelvis, femur, or knee should raise suspicion of an injury to the hip. ***The position of the leg is often an indicator of hip dislocation, but this sign may be absent if there is a concomitant ipsilateral femoral neck or shaft fracture***.
   1. Clinical examination
      • Observation—Injuries to the soft tissues near the femur can localize the point of impact. Since dashboard injuries can cause hip dislocations, the physician should look for bruising about the knee. The resting position of the leg often indicates a dislocation. ***With a posterior dislocation, the leg is shortened and is held in flexion, adduction,***

and internal rotation. However, often with an irreducible posterior dislocation, the leg may rest in a neutral position. With an anterior dislocation, the leg is held in external rotation, abduction, and mild flexion or extension. The amount of flexion/extension depends on whether the dislocation is superior (pubic) or inferior (obturator).

- Palpation—A feeling of fullness in the soft tissues in the direction of displacement of the femoral head may be palpable.
- Neurovascular examination—*Sciatic nerve injuries* occur in 8% to 19% of posterior dislocations, mandating documentation of neural function at presentation. The *peroneal distribution* of the sciatic nerve is involved more often and usually more severely affected than the tibial distribution.

2. Radiographic evaluation—*Plain films should always be obtained to look for associated fractures before any reduction attempt*. A CT scan should be obtained, if time permits, before irreducible dislocations are taken to the operating room (OR) and after all reductions.

   - Plain films—An initial screening anteroposterior (AP) pelvis radiograph is required to evaluate for a suspected dislocation. When evaluating the plain films, the clinician should first look for associated injuries, paying particular attention to the femoral neck, femoral shaft, and acetabulum. The clinician should then carefully compare the congruency of the hip joints. *The head of an anteriorly dislocated hip appears larger on plain radiographs than the contralateral normal hip; a posteriorly dislocated hip appears smaller* (Fig. 17-1). If a dislocation is suspected, films of the entire femur, including the knee joint, are needed. These films should be carefully evaluated to rule out ipsilateral fractures, in particular nondisplaced fractures of the femoral head, the femoral neck, or the acetabulum. Anteromedial femoral head fractures are most common and will be demonstrated by Judet oblique radiographs. Postreduction plain films in at least two planes (AP and lateral or AP and Judet obliques) must be obtained to evaluate joint congruency and to look for the presence of associated fractures (Fig. 17-2). A postreduction CT is still required because small interposed fragments may be missed on plain films.

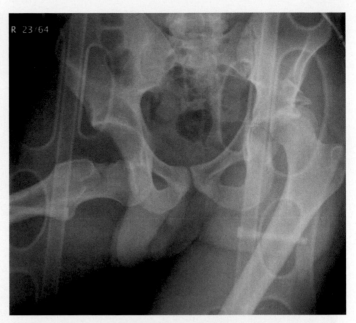

FIGURE 17-1 AP Radiograph demonstrates typical appearance of an anterior hip dislocation on the patient's right and a posterior fracture-dislocation on the left.

- CT—A CT scan of the hip should be obtained after reduction to assess the congruency of the hip joint. This assessment is best done by looking for lateral subluxation in the more proximal cuts that show the hip joint and by comparing the joint space in the more distal cuts of the affected hip to that of the uninjured hip. The postreduction CT scan is also the best means for checking for free osteochondral fragments within the joint (Fig. 17-3). Small foveal fragments may be left, but interposed fragments need to be addressed. If a hip cannot be closed reduced, and if time permits, an emergent preoperative CT scan is recommended to determine whether there are fragments within the joint that will necessitate an open reduction. After open reduction, even if a prereduction CT scan was obtained, a postreduction CT scan is advisable if there is any question regarding the concentricity of the reduction.
- Magnetic resonance imaging (MRI)—MRI can be useful for assessing the hip that has been reduced and has been found to be incongruent but without interposed tissue on CT scan. The MR image is better at evaluating the labrum, the muscles, and the capsule that may be incarcerated within the joint. The role of MRI in the assessment of early AVN, bone bruises, and chondral

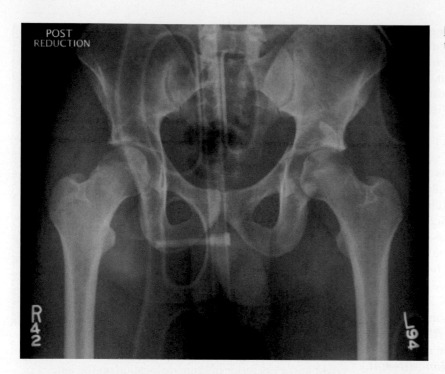

FIGURE 17-2 Postreduction radiograph of the patient shown in Figure 17-1.

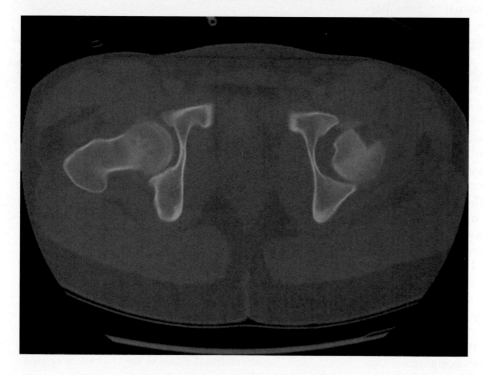

FIGURE 17-3 Axial CT scan demonstrates an incarcerated femoral head fragment.

injuries after hip dislocations has yet to be established. MRI may also show damage to the obturator externus muscle, which may represent injury to the medial circumflex femoral artery and possibly an increased risk of avascular necrosis.

C. Classification (Tables 17-1 to 17-4)—A classification system should help guide treatment and have prognostic value. The two modern classification systems (Comprehensive system and Brumback et al. system) guide clinicians more in terms of treatment than prognosis. The two historical systems (Thompson and Epstein system and Stewart and Milford system) were introduced before the advent of CT. If there is an associated fracture requiring treatment, the prognosis of the injury is usually determined by the quality of the reduction of the associated fracture. The prognosis of

TABLE 17-1

Thompson and Epstein's Classification of Posterior Hip Dislocations

Type	Description
I	With or without minor fracture of the acetabulum
II	With a large, single fracture off the posterior acetabular rim
III	With comminuted fractures of the acetabular rim (with or without a major fragment)
IV	With fracture of the acetabular rim and floor
V	With fracture of the femoral head

Source: From Thompson VP, Epstein HC. Traumatic dislocation of the hip: a survey of two hundred and four cases covering a period of twenty-one years. *J Bone Joint Surg.* 1951;33A: 746–778, with permission.

TABLE 17-2

Stewart and Milford's Classification of Hip Dislocations

Type	Description
I	No acetabular fracture or only a minor chip
II	Posterior rim fracture that is stable after reduction
III	Posterior rim fracture with hip instability after reduction
IV	Dislocation accompanied by fracture of the femoral head or neck

Source: From Stewart M, Milford LW. Fracture-dislocation of the hip: an endresult study. *J Bone Joint Surg.* 1954;36A:315–342, with permission.

TABLE 17-3

Comprehensive Classification of Hip Dislocations

Type	Description
I	No significant associated fractures: no clinical instability after concentric reduction
II	Irreducible dislocation without significant femoral head or acetabular fractures (reduction must be attempted under general anesthesia)
III	Unstable hip after reduction or incarcerated fragments of cartilage, labrum or bone
IV	Associated acetabular fracture requiring reconstruction to restore hip stability and joint congruity
V	Associated femoral head or femoral neck injury (fractures or impaction)

Source: From Levin PE. In: Browner BD, Jupiter JB, Levine AM, et al, eds. *Skeletal Trauma: Fractures, Dislocations, Ligamentous Injuries.* Vol 2. 2nd ed. Philadelphia, PA: WB Saunders; 1998, with permission.

TABLE 17-4

Brumback et al's Classification of Hip Dislocations

Type	Description
1	Posterior hip dislocation with femoral head fracture involving the inferomedial, non-weightbearing portion of the femoral head
1A	With minimum or no fracture of the acetabular rim and stable hip joint after reduction
1B	With significant acetabular fracture and hip joint instability
2	Posterior hip dislocation with femoral head fracture involving the superomedial weigh-bearing portion of the femoral head
2A	With minimum or no fracture of the acetabular rim and stable hip joint after reduction
2B	With significant acetabular fracture and hip joint instability
3	Dislocation of the hip (unspecified direction) with associated femoral neck fracture
3A	Without fracture of the femoral head
3B	With fracture of the femoral head
4	Anterior dislocation of the hip with fracture of the femoral head
4A	Indentation type; depression of the superolateral weight bearing surface of the femoral head
4B	Transchondral type; osteocartilaginous shear fracture of the weightbearing surface of the femoral head
5	Central fracture-dislocation of the hip with fracture of the femoral head

Source: From Brumback RJ, Kenzora JE, Levitt LE, et al. *Proceedings of the Hip Society 1986.* St. Louis, MO: Mosby; 1987, with permission.

a pure dislocation is determined by the incidence of AVN and chondral injuries, both of which are difficult to determine in the immediate postreduction period.

1. Thompson and Epstein (1951)—The classification system of Thompson and Epstein is based on the severity of the acetabular and/or femoral head fracture (Table 17-1).
2. Stewart and Milford (1954)—The classification system of Stewart and Milford is based on the stability of the hip after reduction and the condition of the femoral head (Table 17-2).
3. Comprehensive classification—The Comprehensive classification system is based on the reducibility of the hip, the presence of interposed fragments, the stability of the reduced hip, and associated fractures (Table 17-3).

4. Brumback et al.—The classification of Brumback et al. is based on the direction of dislocation and associated fractures (Table 17-4).

D. Associated Injuries—Associated injuries fall into two categories: those associated with the dislocation and those associated with the precipitating trauma. Additional organ-system injuries occur in 95% of patients with a traumatic hip dislocation secondary to a motor vehicle crash; 33% of patients have other orthopaedic injuries, 15% have abdominal injuries, 24% have closed-head injuries, 21% have thoracic injuries, and 21% have craniofacial injuries.

1. Injuries associated with the dislocation—The injury to the hip is determined by the vector of the traumatic load, the rate of load transmission, the point of load transmission, and the position of the leg at the time of impact. A centrally directed force on an abducted leg fractures the pelvis, the acetabulum, the femur, or a combination thereof. As the force is directed more posteriorly and the leg moves into adduction and flexion, a posterior fracture-dislocation is created; with more adduction, a pure dislocation occurs. A posterior impact or a force on an abducted and extended leg creates an anterior dislocation. As the rate of load transmission decreases, the pelvis can rotate, and pure dislocations become more likely. Conversely, when the rate of load transmission is rapid, the pelvis cannot rotate and a fracture of the acetabulum or the femoral head is more likely. *The incidence of femoral head fractures is higher with anterior dislocations* because the strong anterior ligaments do not easily allow for subluxation of the hip. The anterior wall of the acetabulum is substantial and resists fracturing more than the posterior wall, so the femoral head becomes the weak link and is fractured by the shear force.

   • Local bony injuries
   (a) Acetabular fractures—One study reported that 70% of patients with hip dislocations had an associated acetabular fracture. Fracture of the posterior wall is most common, but as force is directed more medially, any fracture pattern is possible.
   (b) Femoral head fractures—Femoral head fractures are covered in more detail later in this chapter but can include impactions as well as fractures. *Most femoral head fractures (90%) are seen with posterior dislocations since posterior dislocations are so much more common than anterior dislocations. However, a higher percentage of anterior dislocations have an associated femoral head fracture (68%) as compared to posterior dislocations (7%).*
   (c) Femoral neck fractures—Femoral neck fractures are uncommon in patients with hip dislocation. *Prereduction films need to be carefully assessed for displaced and nondisplaced fractures along the femoral neck.*
   (d) Femoral shaft fractures—Femoral shaft fractures are uncommon in patients with hip dislocation. These fractures make leg position no longer predictive of dislocation, and the leg cannot be used as a lever arm during reduction maneuvers.
   (e) Patellar fractures and knee dislocations—Patellar fractures and knee dislocations highlight the importance of X-ray films of the joint above and below the injury. If knee pathology is identified and the mechanism of injury is a motor-vehicle accident, there is a high incidence of ipsilateral hip injuries.

   • Soft tissue injuries
   (a) Blood supply to the femoral head—*Multiple sources supply blood to the femoral head. However, the medial femoral circumflex artery (MFCA) is the essential vessel.* This vessel anastomoses with a branch of the inferior gluteal vessel at the inferior border of the piriformis and then pierces the capsule deep to the piriformis insertion to run within the synovial reflection to enter the head at the superolateral articular margin (Fig. 17-4). The MFCA vascularizes areas not supplied by other vessels and can supply the entire femoral head. Injury to this vessel by avulsion, transection, thrombosis, or spasm leads to AVN. Posterior dislocations put this vessel at risk, whereas anterior dislocation relaxes the vessel, thus explaining the *2% to 17% rate of AVN with posterior dislocations* and the rare incidence with anterior dislocations. Additionally, the MCFA may arise from either the common femoral or more often from the profundus femoral artery. When the MCFA arises from the common femoral artery, a posterior dislocation causes a greater decrease in blood flow to the femoral head. This is theorized to

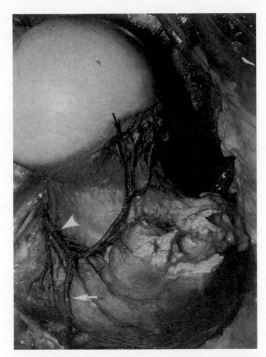

FIGURE 17-4 Posterosuperior view of the proximal femur. Note the medial femoral circumflex artery (*white arrowhead*), the lateral trochanteric vessel (*white arrow*), and the insertion of the terminal branches into the femoral head (*black arrow*). (Reprinted with permission from Gautier E, Ganz K, Krügel N, et al. Anatomy of the medial femoral circumflex artery and its surgical implications. *J Bone Joint Surg Br.* 2000;82(5):679–683.)

contribute to the variability in AVN rates after dislocation.

(b) Sciatic nerve injuries—***Reported rates of sciatic nerve injury range from 7% to 27%***. The incidence is approximately 5% in children. These occur exclusively with posterior dislocations, with the highest rate being seen in posterior fracture-dislocations as would be expected from the direction of the displaced posterior wall fragments. ***The peroneal distribution of the sciatic nerve is more frequently involved than the tibial distribution for unknown reasons***, although the posterior portion of the peroneal branch has been implicated because it would be stretched more. The mechanism of injury is proposed to be direct blunt trauma, stretching of the nerve around the posteriorly displaced head, or both. The sciatic nerve variant where the peroneal division branches through the piriformis muscle may place the nerve at increased risk as it is tethered by the piriformis. At least partial sciatic nerve recovery occurs in 60% to 70% of patients, with no clear correlation with injury or treatment.

(c) Ligamentum teres injuries—The ligamentum teres is torn during a dislocation. It can tear mid-substance, or more commonly, it can avulse a small piece of bone from the fovea. If the avulsed piece of bone is interposed between the articular surfaces after reduction, it needs to be removed. However, if it remains in the fovea and does not impinge on the head, it may be left.

(d) Acetabular labrum injuries—The acetabular labrum can be avulsed from the bony acetabular rim on either the side of or the opposite side from the dislocation and can become interposed during reduction. ***Labral injury can be a source of symptoms even after a successful reduction***.

(e) Joint capsule injuries—The joint capsule will be injured during all dislocations. When the femoral head has button-holed through the capsule, reduction can be diificult. The capsule may also become interposed during reduction.

(f) Muscle injuries—The short external rotators are frequently torn during posterior dislocations and may become interposed during reduction. The gluteus medius may be partially avulsed from its femoral insertions during obturator dislocations.

(g) Arterial injuries—Pulses should be evaluated during the physical examination because the femoral artery can be compressed during anterior dislocations.

2. Injuries associated with the trauma—It is important to establish the mechanism of injury to give insight into possible associated injuries.
   - Load transmission—The involved limb must be carefully examined from the point of impact all the way to the hip. Foot, ankle, leg, knee, and thigh injuries have all been reported. If the impact was posterior, the pelvis and lumbar spine should be evaluated.
   - Distant injuries—Dislocation of the hip is frequently the result of high-energy trauma, and 85% of patients have more than one injury (so the entire patient must be evaluated). These patients have often sustained a deceleration injury, and damage to the chest cavity or abdomen can occur. Seat belt injuries can also occur.

E. Treatment—The treatment of associated fractures is covered in detail in the chapters covering the specific injuries. Treatment is mentioned here only if it is altered by the presence of the hip dislocation. The treatment of hip dislocations follows a stepwise process that is outlined in Figure 17-5. These injuries represent an orthopaedic emergency requiring prompt reduction of the hip to protect the femoral head blood supply from further compromise. Additionally, urgent reduction minimizes further stretching of the sciatic nerve. The length of time to relocation has a direct influence on the severity of associated nerve injuries. The incidence of major sciatic nerve injuries was higher in patients transferred with the hip still dislocated, and in patients with a nerve injury who had a significantly longer time to reduction. A dislocation of the hip is an emergency of even greater urgency than an open fracture. *The rates of AVN and early arthritis are increased if the hip is left dislocated for more than 6 hours*.

1. Treatment of associated injuries—After the entire patient is thoroughly evaluated, injuries that are life threatening or need to be addressed are treated before reduction of the hip. A femoral shaft fracture needs to be temporized, and a femoral neck fracture needs to be stabilized before a hip reduction can be attempted. When open reduction is required, fractures of the proximal femur should be stabilized before hip reduction, whereas fractures of the acetabulum can be treated after hip joint reduction.

2. Closed reduction—*Except in cases with associated femoral neck fractures, a closed reduction should be attempted on all hip dislocations*. An associated femoral head fracture and/or a small posterior wall rim avulsion may indicate an associated labral avulsion which can become a mechanical block during closed reduction. A reduced hip with fragments in the joint is safer to the vascularity than a

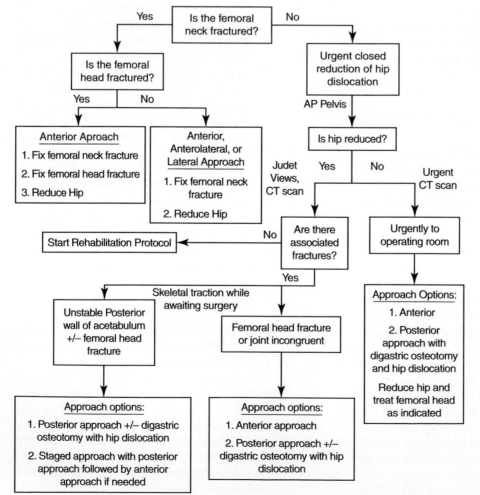

FIGURE 17-5 Algorithm for treatment of a hip dislocation.

dislocated hip. Ideally, only one attempt at reduction is required, so variables such as patient sedation, patient position, the experience of the reducer, and the amount of assistance should be maximized in favor of a successful reduction. Reduction maneuvers in the emergency department should be limited to one attempt. Iatrogenic fractures of the femoral neck have been reported after forceful attempts at reduction. The two described techniques for posterior hip dislocation reduction have not changed from the time of Bigelow.

- Techniques for posterior dislocations
  (a) Allis and Bigelow techniques (Fig. 17-6)— The patient is supine. Countertraction is applied to the ipsilateral anterior

superior iliac spine (ASIS). The leg is held with the knee flexed. Inline traction is applied, and the leg is slowly flexed, internally rotated, and adducted. Relaxing the anterior ligaments sometimes requires that the hip be flexed beyond 90° and the knee be pointed in the direction of the contralateral hip. With maximal traction the leg is gently rocked in internal and external rotation. Reduction of the hip is not subtle and is easily palpable and occasionally audible. The reduced hip is stabilized by external rotation, extension, and abduction. *A slow progression of the traction force is more effective than an abrupt tug*.

A   B

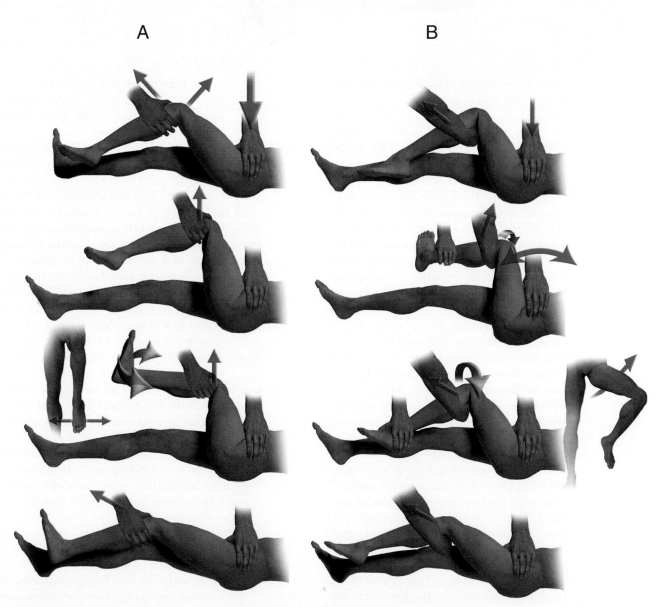

FIGURE 17-6 Reduction maneuvers for posterior dislocation of the hip. **A.** Allis. **B.** Bigelow.

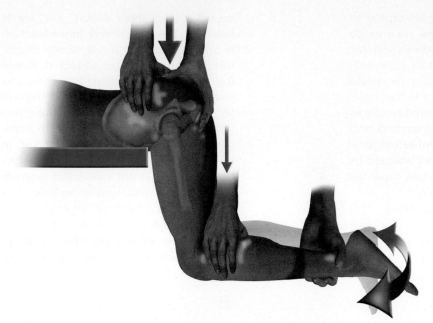

FIGURE 17-7 Stimson gravity-reduction technique for posterior dislocation of the hip.

General anesthesia is preferred, but conscious sedation is acceptable.

(b) Stimson technique (Fig. 17-7)—The patient is placed in the prone position with the hips flexed 90° off of the edge of the stretcher. The ipsilateral knee is bent 90°, and force is applied to the back of the proximal calf. The reduction maneuvers are the same as those used in the supine technique. The prone technique is contraindicated in the patient with multiple trauma but can be used for an isolated injury when full sedation is unavailable because it may be easier for the patient to relax the leg under the influence of gravity.

- Techniques for anterior dislocations

(a) Anterior dislocations are harder to reduce than posterior dislocations. If one or two attempts with optimal sedation are unsuccessful, the patient should be taken to the OR. The method of reduction differs from that previously described (for posterior dislocation) in that the position of the leg is reversed. With the leg in external rotation, abduction, and flexion, inline traction is applied. The leg is rocked in internal and external rotation to walk the head over the anterior acetabular rim. A lateralizing force on the proximal femur may assist with the reduction. This can be done by direct pressure over the femoral head

in the inguinal region or if in the operating room a Schanz pin in the proximal femur. The anterior capsule is usually the block to reduction.

3. Assessment of stability—The traditional teaching has been to clinically assess the stability of the hip joint immediately after reduction of the joint. This has come into question with the ability of CT to predict stability if there is a large posterior acetabular fracture. Subtle instabilities may be difficult to detect clinically. If the reduced hip is grossly unstable, skeletal traction should be placed. If the reduced hip remains located, the postreduction CT scan can be evaluated to determine if the hip will be definitely unstable (i.e., >50% posterior wall involvement). In cases in which stability cannot be predicted by CT (i.e., <50% posterior wall involvement), the evaluation for stability should be performed in the OR with the patient fully relaxed and with fluoroscopy to detect small degrees of subluxation.

- Posterior stability—The hip is flexed to 90°, and while it is held in neutral rotation and neutral abduction, a posteriorly directed force is applied to the leg. If the hip subluxes, it is unstable.
- Anterior stability—The hip is abducted, flexed, and externally rotated. If gravity can dislocate the hip, it is unstable.
- Hip instability—If the hip is unstable, the bony injury producing the instability needs

to be fixed by open reduction and internal fixation. The bony acetabulum covers approximately 40% of the femoral head, and the labrum extends the coverage to just over 50%. If there is no fracture, instability is unlikely.

4. Assessment of congruency—All reductions should have immediate postreduction films. If the hip is not reduced, another reduction is performed, preferably in the OR. If the hip is reduced, a CT scan is obtained to assess the congruency and look for fragments. *The joint space on the involved hip should be identical to that on the uninvolved hip*. A posteriorly dislocated hip may need a support under the greater trochanter to keep gravity from laterally subluxing the hip. If the hip is not congruent, the cause must be identified. If no bony cause is seen on CT, MRI may be performed to identify any soft tissue that has been interposed. Removal of the interposed tissue is mandatory. The operative approach is dictated by the location of the interposed tissue and its site of origin. There has been recent success with the use of hip arthroscopy to remove these fragments. The patient with interposed fragments or tissues in the hip joint should be placed in skeletal traction while waiting for operative removal/fixation.

5. Open reduction—Inability to obtain a closed reduction is usually the result of inadequate relaxation/paralysis, blockage by the hip capsule and/or short external rotators, or a femoral fracture that makes control of the hip difficult. Failure to obtain a closed reduction is an indication for an urgent and immediate open reduction. During an open procedure, it is paramount to protect the vascularity. Hips that cannot be reduced closed, hips with associated fractures that are unstable after reduction, and hips that are not congruent after reduction all need open treatment. If the dislocation, the instability, or the interposed fragment is posterior, a posterior approach should be chosen. However, in the rare case of an irreducible posterior dislocation with a femoral neck and/or femoral head fracture an anterior approach can be used. If the dislocation, the instability, or the interposed fragment is anterior, an anterior approach should be chosen. Choice of approach is covered in more detail under the femoral head fracture section. The surgical approaches are covered in detail in Chapter 16 and are only summarized in the next section.

6. Postreduction management—Weightbearing status is dictated by associated fractures if any are present. In a pure dislocation, weightbearing is as tolerated with crutches until leg control has been regained. *Early weightbearing does not predispose to the development of AVN* as previously contended. Appropriate hip precautions are recommended for 6 weeks following dislocation.

F. Relevant Anatomy and Surgical Techniques—The hip joint is a ball-and-socket configuration. The joint is highly constrained by soft tissues, including the stout fibrocartilaginous labrum, the transverse acetabular ligament, and the joint capsule. In a typical posterior dislocation without fracture, the posterior capsule is avulsed from its attachment to the labrum and the femoral head extrudes through the superior gemellus muscle or passes through the interval between the piriformis and the obturator internus. Complete coverage of the anatomy about the hip and of all the useful surgical approaches is beyond the scope of this chapter (see Chapter 16). Salient anatomic features and the three most common surgical approaches are highlighted.

1. Anatomy—The primary landmarks are the sciatic nerve, the location of the MFCA, and the structure of the labrum and capsule.
   - Sciatic nerve—The sciatic nerve divides into two branches (the peroneal and the tibial) within the pelvis. These exit the greater sciatic notch in a common sheath. A total of 85% of the time, the entire nerve exits inferiorly to the piriformis, and 15% of the time, a portion of the nerve may pass through or superior to the piriformis. The nerve then runs superficial to the short external rotators (the gemelli and the obturator internus) and lateral to the ischial tuberosity.
   - Blood supply to the femoral head—The blood supply to the femoral head has already been mentioned. It can be damaged at the time of injury. It can also be injured during anterior or posterior approaches to the hip. The MFCA is at risk at several locations along its course. The vessel enters the surgical field along the inferior border of the obturator externus. It then runs superiorly along the insertion of the short external rotators, approximately 1 cm from their insertion onto the intertrochanteric ridge (Fig. 17-8). It anastamoses with the branch of the inferior

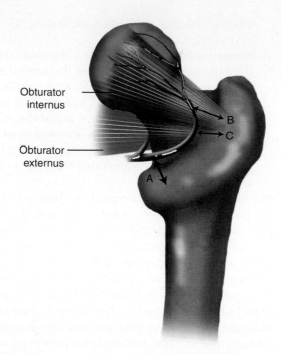

Obturator internus

Obturator externus

FIGURE 17-8 Anatomic location of the MFCA along the posterior neck of the femur. The vessel passes posterior to the obturator externus and anterior to the short external rotators, including the obturator internus. *A,* Proximity to the lesser trochanter; *B* and *C,* proximity to the muscular insertions.

gluteal artery that runs along the inferior border of the piriformis. The vessel distal to the anastamosis runs deep to the piriformis and perforates the capsule at the level of the piriformis insertion. The vessel then runs in the synovial reflection (this vessel has several different names depending on the author, and it is described here not by name but by location intentionally) up the lateral border of the neck to insert just distal to the articular margin (see Fig. 17-4). Injuries to the MFCA are most likely to occur when taking down the short external rotators, when opening the capsule, or when placing a retractor around the lateral femoral neck.

- Labrum—The labrum attaches to the bony acetabular rim, except inferiorly, where it attaches to the transverse acetabular ligament. The inner surface of the labrum is flush with the cartilage, and on its outer surface, there is a recess between it and the capsule. The labrum extends the coverage of the acetabulum to slightly over 50% but does not participate in the static load transmission across the hip. The deep fibers are circular and very strong, so the labrum does

not usually tear but is instead avulsed from its acetabular attachment. When labral injuries are encountered during open reduction, it is unclear as to whether repair or resection is appropriate.

- Capsule—The capsule is composed of two layers. The layers are not separable but do serve distinct functions. The ***inner fibers*** are longitudinal and run from the acetabulum parallel to the femoral neck to insert on the proximal femur, and they limit lateral subluxation. The ***outer fibers*** run obliquely in three identifiable groups: the two anterior bands and the posterior band. The anterior bands (the Y-shaped Bigelow's ligament) are more substantial; these are the iliofemoral ligament and the pubofemoral ligament. The posterior ligament is the ischiofemoral ligament. These outer fibers limit flexion and extension. The capsule is also strengthened by the reflected head of the rectus anteriorly and by the gluteus minimus superiorly.

2. Surgical approach—The surgical approach chosen depends on the location of the injury being addressed. A Kocher-Langenbeck approach is used for posterior exposure. Anterior exposure can be gained through a true anterior, an anterolateral, or a direct lateral approach.

- Posterior (Kocher-Langenbeck) Approach— Most of the salient points have been reviewed. The sciatic nerve must be protected, and only blunt retractors should be used. Protection of the MFCA requires that the dissection not go distally through the obturator externus because the vessel runs along its inferior border. If the short external rotators must be taken down, it should be done 1.5 to 2 cm away from their insertion. If the capsule is to be incised, it should be done from inside the joint along the acetabular rim under direct vision so as to not injure the vessel or the labrum. A retractor should never be placed along the lateral border of the neck, as is frequently done during total hip arthroplasty, because it can damage the artery running within the synovial reflexion.

- Anterolateral (Watson-Jones, Hardinge, Dall, or Trochanteric Slide) Approach—Because of the laterally placed skin incision, the anterolateral approach works well if access to both the anterior and posterior aspects of the hip is required, for example with an associated intertrochanteric fracture or femoral neck fracture. The trochanteric slide is a more extensive dissection, but it allows for surgical dislocation of the hip and full access to the acetabulum and the femoral head. This can also be accomplished through a posterior approach with a digastric trochanteric osteotomy as will be discussed later. The opening of the capsule should be performed as previously stated, and again, no retractors should be placed along the lateral femoral neck. Branches of the lateral femoral circumflex vessel are encountered along the anteromedial neck and may be sacrificed.

- Anterior (Smith-Petersen) approach—The anterior approach is advocated in anterior dislocations or dislocations with anterior femoral head fractures because the more medial dissection plane allows for easier placement of compression screws into the fracture fragment. Comparatively less dissection occurs with this approach. In the interval between the tensor laterally and the sartorius medially, the lateral femoral cutaneous nerve should be protected. This can be done by locating the nerve at the level of the **superficial circumflex iliac artery**, which penetrates the fascia just anterior to the nerve, or by staying within the fascia of the tensor. In the deeper dissection, the vessel overlying the rectus femoris is the **ascending branch of the lateral femoral circumflex artery**, which may be sacrificed.

G. Complications of Injury—Complications may be either local or systemic. The systemic complications are more often a result of the overall trauma than of the dislocation. The local complications include sciatic nerve injuries, AVN, arthritis, and recurrent dislocations.

1. Sciatic nerve injury—Sciatic nerve injury occurs in 7% to 27% of posterior hip dislocations. It is more common in fracture-dislocations than in pure dislocations. As previously mentioned, the prognosis for recovery is variable. **Nerve injury is not an indication for open reduction**. Electromyography at 3 months can be used to determine prognosis but usually does not change the management, which is to wait 18 to 24 months and then address the residual deficiency. Patients who lack ankle dorsiflexion should receive an ankle-foot orthosis early to avoid equinus contractures. No surgery to address the disability should be undertaken for at least 1 year.

2. **AVN**—AVN is reported to occur in 2% to 17% of cases of posterior dislocation of the hip (AVN is much rarer after anterior dislocation). These series do not report the possible differences in rates between surgical and nonsurgical cases or between pure dislocations and those with associated injuries. The rates of AVN increase if the hip is left dislocated for longer than 6 to 12 hours. This suggests that most injuries to the vessel are not avulsions or transections but are compressions, kinks, spasms, or a combination thereof. One report showed that the rate of AVN increased from 4.8% with a reduction within 6 hours to 52.9% after greater than 6 hours. Recent investigators suggest that the present rates of traumatic AVN may be on the lower end of the reported spectrum and that the higher rates previously reported may reflect damage to the vascularity during open procedures. If done carefully, open reduction should not increase the rate of AVN.

3. Arthritis—Arthritis is the common final pathway for all injuries to the articular surface. Damage to the cartilage can occur via many means. The progression to arthritis depends on the extent of the injury to the mechanical and biochemical properties of the articular cartilage. Likewise, fracture malunions and nonunions may be major contributors to long-range disability in patients with fracture-dislocations. Anterior dislocations are typically more prone to developing arthritis secondary to higher rates of impaction injuries.

- Third-body wear—Interposed bone (from the femoral head or the acetabulum), cartilage (labrum or articular surface), or soft tissue (muscle, tendon, or capsule) generates third-body wear within the hip and leads to early arthritis.
- Direct pressure—If the instantaneous load on the cartilage exceeds a certain threshold, direct chondral death can occur. This can occur at the time of impact or as the dislocated femoral head presses against the ilium.
- Shearing—As the hip dislocates, it is scraped along the acetabular rim and can shear off a portion of the articular cartilage.
- Nutritional deficiencies—The articular cartilage receives its nutrition from the synovial fluid, and it is not bathed in synovial fluid when in a dislocated position.

4. Recurrent dislocations—Recurrent dislocations are very rare. Most are posterior. Causes may include a combination of femoral version, acetabular version, soft-tissue impingement, labral avulsion, and capsular laxity. Treatment is directed toward the structures found responsible.

5. Heterotopic ossification—Heterotopic ossification in the soft tissues surrounding the hip joint may occur with and without open treatment. This may or may not have an affect on range of motion.

6. Persistent pain—Excluding the factors mentioned previously, the most common causes of continued pain after dislocation are labral injuries, ununited acetabular rim avulsion fractures, and dynamic instability. All cause intermittent symptoms and occasional clicking or catching. The diagnoses of labral injuries and avulsion fractures can be made with a positive impingement test, which correlates with the appropriate MR findings. Treatment should be tailored to the pathologic condition found. Arthroscopy has been advocated for many of these lesions.

H. Complications of Treatment
1. Infection—The infection rate is 3% to 5% for the surgical approaches described. Because of the capsular injury, if a deep infection occurs, a septic joint must be assumed and appropriately treated.

2. Sciatic nerve injury—The rate of injury as a result of the treatment of dislocations is unknown, but the rate with the Kocher-Langenbeck approach for acetabular fractures is 11% (range 2% to 17%). The nerve may become entrapped in heterotopic ossification and present as a delayed sciatic neurapraxia.

3. AVN—The rate of AVN resulting from the treatment of hip dislocations is unknown, but the higher rates from earlier series may be partially attributed to delays in reduction and to intraoperative damage to the MFCA.

4. Thromboembolism—Patients with hip dislocation generally require prophylaxis.

I. Outcomes—The outcomes of pure dislocations largely depends on the development of AVN, arthritis, and heterotopic ossification. Reported series show a range of good or excellent results from 48% to 95%. The outcome of a hip dislocation with an associated fracture is often determined by the outcome of the fracture. ***The most important prognostic factor in dislocations of the hip is the time to reduction (<6 to 12 hours) to avoid ongoing damage to the blood supply to the femoral head.*** One report indicated 88% good or excellent functional outcomes in hip dislocations reduced within 6 hours. For hips reduced greater than 6 hours, only 42% had good or excellent results. The second most important factor is to ensure that there is absolute congruency of the reduced joint to avoid ongoing damage to the articular cartilage.

III. Femoral Head Fractures
A. Overview—Femoral head fractures always occur as the result of hip dislocation or subluxation. Pertinent information about anatomy, presentation, evaluation, and management was presented in the previous section on hip dislocations. A total of 82% to 92% of hip dislocations are posterior and 4% to 18% are associated with femoral head fractures. Between 68% and 77% of anterior hip dislocations have an associated femoral head fracture. Despite this high incidence, only 10% of femoral head fractures result from anterior dislocation because of the preponderance of posterior dislocation. The two types of femoral head injuries are shear or cleavage injuries, which can occur with anterior or posterior dislocations, and impaction or crush injuries, which usually occur with anterior dislocations. The location, comminution, and displacement patterns are related to the position of the hip and the load applied to the hip during the traumatic event. The position of the leg at time of impact determines whether the hip dislocates with or without osseous injury. If the hip is flex and adducted, it is likely to dislocate without osseous injury. If the hip is extended and abducted, the axial force is directed more into the hip joint and results in a femoral head or acetabular fracture. With posterior dislocation, femoral head fractures typically involve the anteromedial aspect of the head. Impaction of the intact cancellous surface may occur as the dislocated hip rests on the retroacetabular surface. For anterior dislocations, the fracture is typically an infrafoveal impaction.

B. Evaluation—The evaluation is the same as that outlined in the section on hip dislocation.

C. Classification—There are two classifications systems for femoral head fractures. The Pipkin classification (Table 17-5 and Fig. 17-9), published in 1957, is an elaboration of the Thompson and Epstein Type V posterior hip dislocation. It includes associated injuries and provides prognostic information. The Pipkin classification system is the most commonly used system. Type I fractures are infrafoveal and are characterized by disruption of the ligamentum teres. Type II fractures are suprafoveal and are characterized by maintenance of the ligamentum teres to the fracture fragment. Type III fractures represent any head fracture with an associated femoral neck fracture. Type IV fractures represent any head fracture with an associated acetabular fracture. Brumback et al. introduced a classification system (see Table 17-4) in 1987 that included anterior and posterior fracture-dislocations. No large

TABLE 17-5

Pipkin's Classification of Posterior Hip Dislocations Associated with Femoral Head Fractures

Type	Description
I	Hip dislocation with fracture of the femoral head caudad to the fovea capitis femoris
II	Hip dislocation with fracture of the femoral head cephalad to the fovea capitis femoris
III	Type I or II injury associated with fracture of the femoral neck
IV	Type I or II injury associated with fracture of the acetabular rim

Source: From Pipkin G. Treatment of grade IV fracture-dislocation of the hip: a review. *J Bone Joint Surg.* 1957;39A:1027–1042, with permission.

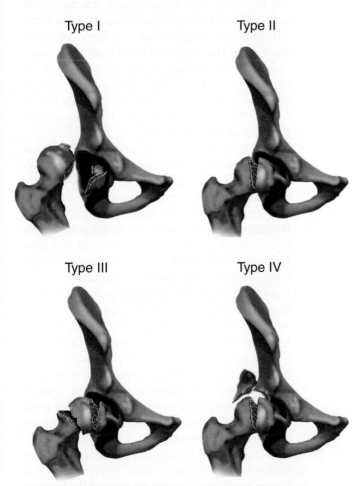

Type I Type II

Type III Type IV

<u>FIGURE 17-9</u> Pipkin's classification of posterior hip dislocations associated with femoral head fractures. Type I is a fracture fragment below the ligamentum teres. Type II is a fracture fragment including the ligamentum teres. Type III is either a type I or II injury with an associated femoral neck fracture. Type IV is either a type I or II injury with an associated acetabular fracture.

series has yet been published using this newer system. Impaction fractures of the femoral head do not have a classification system but do occur.

D. Anatomy—In addition to the musculature and osseous structure of the hip, the capsule and ligament teres are restraints to dislocation. The ligamentum teres represents a strong attachment between the acetabulum (cotyloid fossa) and the femoral head (fovea centralis). During a dislocation, the ligamentum may be torn or may remain attached to the femoral head fragment if the fracture exits cephalad to the fovea centralis (Pipkin II). Additionally, the ligamentum teres contains an arterial branch from the obturator artery and supplies 10% to 15% of the femoral head blood supply.

E. Associated Injuries—Associated injuries include damage to the sciatic nerve, the femoral neck, the acetabulum, the knee, and the femoral shaft. The acetabular labrum may also be injured. An avulsion of the labrum from the posterior acetabular rim may prevent a closed reduction in a posterior dislocation.

F. Treatment—Most femoral head fractures will require operative treatment. When the femoral head is fractured or dislocated, the femoral neck needs to be carefully evaluated for an injury. If the femoral neck is uninjured, a hip dislocation should be emergently reduced irrespective of the presence of a femoral head fracture. If closed reduction fails or if there is a femoral neck injury, open reduction is indicated. If a preoperative CT scan can be obtained with less than an hour's delay, it is helpful in elucidating loose bodies, soft tissue interposition, and impaction injuries and in selecting the appropriate surgical approach. After a reduction has been confirmed by plain films, a postreduction CT scan is required to assess the adequacy of the reduction of the hip joint and of the fracture fragments. Oblique Judet radiographs of the pelvis can also help elucidate the head fracture.

1. Pipkin type I—Closed treatment can be considered for isolated and small infrafoveal fractures. Closed management consists of protected weight bearing with appropriate hip precautions. If the fragment impinges the labrum or the acetabular cartilage and has more than a 1 mm step-off, the fragment should be excised if it is small or should be fixed if it is large. The displacement of the piece is typically caudal and anterior. Malunited inferomedial femoral head fractures may block hip motion. Large infrafoveal head fractures contribute to hip instability. For Type I fractures,

either an anterior or posterior approach may be used. The posterior approach may be used for small fragment excision but is less desirable for fragment fixation. The details of the approaches are in the following section on Type II fractures.

2. Pipkin type II—Suprafoveal fractures involve the weightbearing dome and the quality of the reduction is paramount. Minor incongruities are not tolerated by the hip joint. These injuries are treated with open reduction and internal fixation if not anatomically reduced. The choice of approach is somewhat controversial. The Smith-Peterson approach (anterior) is the most commonly advocated approach and can be performed supine on a radiolucent table or a traction table designed for acetabular surgery (Fig. 17-10). The fracture location is most commonly anteromedial, and this approach optimizes fracture reduction while preserving the posterior blood supply. The fracture fragment can often be visualized without redislocation. A surgical dislocation may be necessary for fracture visualization/ fixation as the fracture is more cephalad. Effort should be made to retain any soft-tissue attachment to the head fragment. The anteromedial position of the fragment makes visualization and fixation very difficult through a posterior approach.

For an irreducible posterior dislocation with a femoral head fracture, a Kocher-Langenbeck approach may be used. As mentioned previously, the femoral head may be buttonholed through the posterior capsule or through the short external rotators. These structures are difficult to access through an anterior approach. After making the standard posterior approach and releasing the short external rotators 1 to 2 cm from their insertion (the quadratus femoris must not be taken down to preserve the blood supply to the femoral head), the hip can often be dislocated through the traumatic capsulotomy for femoral head visualization and fragment excision/fixation. The capsulotomy may be extended along the rim of the acetabulum to increase visualization if necessary. Following the Kocher-Langenbeck approach, an additional anterior approach may be needed for fragment fixation. An alternative approach is to use a digastric trochanteric osteotomy with an anterior dislocation through a posterior Kocher-Langenbeck approach. With either approach, the femoral head blood supply must be preserved. Fairly unique to these injuries is the fixation of the fracture through the articular surface. Countersunk standard screws or variable-pitch headless screws may be used. The screws are typically of small diameter. The ligamentum teres may be transected to assist with open reduction. The ligamentum teres is often debrided to prevent interposition after reduction. With any approach, the capsule should be repaired and suture anchors may be used if necessary.

3. Pipkin type III—A Pipkin type III injury is the least common injury. Closed reduction of the hip dislocation is contraindicated. All patients should undergo surgical evaluation via an anterolateral (Watson-Jones) or anterior approach (Smith-Peterson) that allows access to both the anterior and posterior aspects of the hip joint. The femoral neck fracture must be stabilized before reduction of the hip dislocation. If the head fragment is large, often reduction of the neck and head fragments must occur simultaneously. If the patient is physiologically older and the reduced femoral head does not bleed from a 2-mm drill hole in the head, a hemiarthroplasty or a total hip arthroplasty may be considered.

4. Pipkin type IV—The type and location of the acetabular fracture dictates the surgical approach for the acetabulum. The acetabular exposure must not be compromised. The concomitant femoral head fracture can be treated through a separate anterior approach (Smith-Peterson) if necessary. However, often a posterior Kocher-Langenbeck approach will allow visualization of the posterior acetabulum, and then a digastric trochanteric osteotomy with anterior surgical dislocation can be done to access the femoral head. The femoral head fracture should either be fixed or excised to allow for early hip motion. Hip stability should be carefully considered especially after fragment excision. If possible, impaction injuries to either the acetabulum or the femoral head should be elevated and stabilized during the operative procedure.

G. Rehabilitation—The patient should undergo aggressive ROM exercises after open fixation of a Pipkin fracture. Toe-touch weight bearing is typically used for the first 8 weeks and then progressed to weight bearing as tolerated.

H. Surgical Techniques—The surgical approaches have been described. The following details the technique of using a digastric trochanteric osteotomy for dislocation and exposure of the

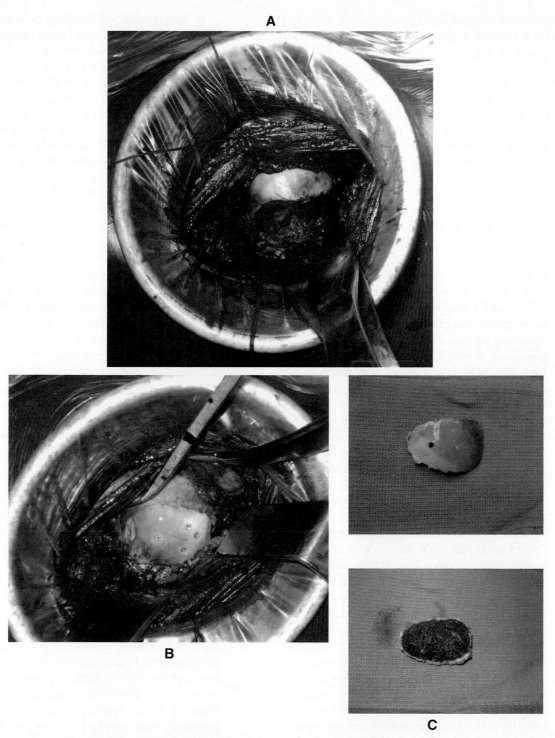

FIGURE 17-10 **A, B.** Intraoperative pictures demonstrating an anterior Smith-Peterson approach with hip dislocation. Large Pipkin type II injury is shown. **C.** The fragment was fixed with three headless screws.

femoral head and acetabulum. A standard incision for a Kocher-Langenbeck approach is made. The fascia lata is split in line with the skin. The posterior border of the gluteus medius is located, and the leg may be internally rotated to make this easier. An osteotomy is made with an oscillating saw just medial to tip of the

greater trochanter but lateral to the insertion of the short external rotators. The osteotomy extends distally to the posterior border of the vastus lateralis ridge. The osteotomized fragment is then rotated 90° and retracted anteriorly. The hip is then flexed and externally rotated. The plane between the piriformis and the gluteus minimus is located, and the minimus is reflected off the posterior, posterosuperior and anterior capsule. A Z-type capsulotomy is then made along the long axis of the femoral neck. The hip can then be dislocated with further flexion and external rotation and placed in a sterile bag on the opposite side of the table. By manipulation of the leg, a full view of the femoral head and acetabulum can be obtained. If needed, the short external rotators can be released 2 cm from their insertion to gain access to the posterior acetabulum.

I. Complications—The complications are a result of both the injury and the surgical treatment. The main complications are posttraumatic arthritis, heterotopic ossification, sciatic nerve palsy, and avascular necrosis.

1. AVN—AVN is reported at rates of 0% to 24%. AVN can be caused by injury to the MFCA and its terminal branches as a result of the dislocation or by injury to the interosseous blood supply as a result of the femoral head fracture. The incidence of AVN correlates with the length of time that the hip remains dislocated. When the large series are combined, the literature shows posterior dislocations to have a 13% incidence of AVN, which increases to 18% if there is an associated femoral head fracture. One study showed the Kocher-Langenbeck approach resulted in a 3.2-fold increase in osteonecrosis when compared to an anterior approach. Surgical incision of an intact ligamentum teres does not appear to increase the rate of avascular necrosis.

2. Sciatic nerve palsy—The sciatic nerve is at risk for palsy during posterior dislocations. The incidence of sciatic nerve injury is 7% to 27% for femoral head fractures. Motor loss that persists for longer than 3 months after hip fracture-dislocation has a poor prognosis.

3. Heterotopic ossification—The incidence of formation of heterotopic ossification is 2% to 54% in femoral head fractures. The extent of the heterotopic ossification increases with the severity of the bone and soft tissue trauma and the surgical approach chosen. There is a higher rate of heterotopic ossification with the Smith-Petersen approach than with the Watson-Jones approach, and both have a higher risk than the Kocher-Langenbeck approach. However, functionally significant ectopic bone formation rarely occurs. This may be minimized by sharp dissection. Additionally, the formation of heterotopic ossification increases in polytraumatized and brain injured patients.

4. Fracture malreduction and nonunion—The goal is to achieve less than 1 mm of articular step-off, but this is often difficult to obtain because of initial fracture comminution. If the fragment is not in the weightbearing dome, fragment excision can be considered. The anterior approach has shown to allow better fracture reduction. Fixation failure occurs most commonly with osteonecrosis or nonunion.

5. Hip joint malreduction—A malreduction is an absolute indication for repeat open reduction.

6. Degenerative arthritis—Posttraumatic arthritis occurs in 0% to 72% of femoral head fractures. Up to 50% of patients with Pipkin type II or IV posterior fracture-dislocations and most patients with Pipkin type III injuries develop degenerative arthritis. Fracture comminution and peripheral impaction increase the risk of posttraumatic arthritis.

J. Outcomes—The comparison of treatments is difficult because of the lack of a standardized evaluation system and the varying severities of these injuries. Present knowledge about results of treatment comes from retrospective series with small numbers and varying injuries with varying approaches. Few studies with long-term outcomes have been reported for hip dislocations with femoral head fractures. Follow-up studies of 2 to 5 years have shown fair or poor results in 57%. Good or excellent outcomes have only been reported in 40% to 70% of all patients. Ideally, similar injuries that have had different treatments would be compared, but because of the rarity of these injuries, this has not been possible. The reports over the last 40 years span the advent of CT and the use of different interventions but consistently show that up to 50% of patients with Pipkin type II or IV injuries and most patients with Pipkin type III injuries develop degenerative arthritis. Direct comparison between anterior and posterior surgical approaches for Pipkin I and II fractures showed the anterior approach was associated with less blood loss, shorter operating room time, and better visualization and fixation. The anterior approach was also associated with more functionally significant heterotopic ossification. Most current literature supports the idea that an anatomic reduction gives the best chance for good long-term results and treatment should focus on restoring the normal joint anatomy.

SUGGESTED READINGS

Classic Articles

Shim SS. Circulatory and vascular changes in the hip following traumatic hip dislocation. *Clin Orthop.* 1979;140:255–261.

Stewart M, Milford LW. Fracture-dislocation of the hip: an end-result study. *J Bone Joint Surg.* 1954;36A:315–342.

Thompson VP, Epstein HC. Traumatic dislocation of the hip: a survey of two hundred and four cases covering a period of twenty-one years. *J Bone Joint Surg.* 1951;33A:746–778.

Trueta J, Harrison MHM. The normal vascular anatomy of the femoral head in adult man. *J Bone Joint Surg.* 1953;35B:442–461.

Recent Articles

Baird RA, Schobert WE, Pais MJ, et al. Radiographic identification of loose bodies in the traumatized hip joint. *Radiology.* 1982;145:661–665.

Brumback RI, Kenzora JE, Levirt LE, et al. Fractures of the femoral head. In: *Proceedings of the 1986 Hip Society.* St Louis, MO: Mosby; 1987.

Dreinhofer KE, Schwarzkopf SR, Haas NP, et al. Isolated traumatic dislocation of the hip: long-term results in 50 patients. *J Bone Joint Surg.* 1994;76B:6–12.

Gardner MJ, Suk M, Helfet DL, et al. Surgical dislocation of the hip for fractures of the femoral head. *J Orthop Trauma.* 2005;19:334–342.

Ganz R, Gill TJ, Gautier K, et al. Surgical dislocation of the adult hip. *J Bone Joint Surg Br.* 2001;83-B:1119–1124.

Henle P, Kloen P, Sibenrock KA. Femoral head injuries: which treatment strategy can be recommended? *Injury.* 2007;38:478–488.

Hougaard K, Lindequist S, Nielsen LB. Computerised tomography after posterior dislocation of the hip. *J Bone Joint Surg.* 1987;69B:556–557.

Hougaard K, Thomsen PB. Traumatic posterior fracture-dislocation of the hip with fracture of the femoral head or neck, or both. *J Bone Joint Surg.* 1988;70A:233–239.

Olson SA, Matta JM. The computerised tomography subchondral arc: a new method of assessing acetabular articular continuity after fracture—A preliminary report. *J Orthop Trauma.* 1993;7:402–413.

Yang RS, Tsuany YH, Hang YS, et al. Traumatic dislocation of the hip. *Clin Orthop.* 1991;265:218–227.

Review Article

Tornetta P 3rd, Mustatari H. Hip dislocation: current treatment regimens. *J Am Acad Orthop Surg.* 1997;5:27–36.

Textbooks

Geller JA, Reilly MC. Hip dislocations and femoral head fractures. In: Stannard JP, Schmidt AH, Kregor PJ, eds. *Surgical Treatment of Orthopaedic Trauma.* New York, NY: Thieme; 2007.

Goulet JA, Levin PE. Hip dislocations. In: Browner BD, Jupiter JB, Levine AM, et al, eds. *Skeletal Trauma.* Vol 2. 3rd ed. Philadelphia, PA: WE Saunders; 2003.

Koval KJ, Cantu RV. Hip trauma. In: Fischgrund JS, ed. *Orthopaedic Knowkdge Update 9: Home Study Syllabus.* Rosemont, IL: American Academy of Orthopaedic Surgeons; 2008.

Nork, SE, Cannada LK. Hip dislocations and femoral head and neck fractures. In: Baumgaertner MR, Tornetta P, eds. *Orthopaedic Knowledge Update Trauma 3.* Rosemont, IL: American Academy of Orthopaedic Surgeons; 2005.

Tornetta P. Hip dislocations and fractures of the femoral head. In: Bucholz RW, Heckman JD, Court-Brown C, eds. *Rockwood and Green's Fractures in Adults.* Vol 2. 6th ed., Philadelphia, PA: Lippincott-Raven.

CHAPTER **18**

Fractures and Dislocations of the Shoulder Girdle

Gregory N. Drake and T. Bradley Edwards

I. Fractures of the Scapula
   A. Overview
      1. Function of the scapula—The scapula plays an important role in the mechanics of the shoulder girdle. It has 18 muscular attachments, which link the axial skeleton to the appendicular skeleton. Dyskinesis can lead to painful upper extremity use and if not treated, can be chronic in nature. The scapula is important for rotator cuff function, which is translated to upper extremity motion. It has several articulations, including the scapulothoracic, acromioclavicular, and glenohumeral joints.
      2. Frequency of injury—Fractures to the scapula are rare and account for 0.5% to 1.0% of all fractures and 3% to 5% of shoulder girdle injuries.
      3. Biomechanics—Shoulder elevation is composed of glenohumeral motion (120°) and scapulothoracic motion (60°). The scapula is the foundation for all complex upper extremity motions with its multiple muscle attachments. It acts as a fulcrum for the deltoid while allowing the rotator cuff muscles to keep the humeral head centered in the glenoid during abduction. The coracoid maintains vertical stability through soft-tissue attachments with the clavicle and muscles of the chest and arm. The acromioclavicular joint allows for horizontal and vertical stability.
   B. Mechanism of Injury
      1. Injury may occur from a direct blow to the scapula or with force acting through the humerus. As a general rule, scapular injuries require high-energy trauma and when seen should raise suspicion for other associated injuries including **rib fractures, hemo/pneumothorax, pulmonary contusion**, brachial plexus injury, cervical spine fracture, clavicle fracture, and arterial injury.
   C. Imaging
      1. Orthogonal—High-quality orthogonal views are the most helpful when evaluating scapular fractures. The AP scapula and transscapular Y view are the most helpful.
      2. Computed tomography (CT) scans—CT scans, particularly with three-dimensional reconstructions, may aid in diagnosis, and help with preoperative planning of periarticular and articular fractures.
      3. Stryker view—If a coracoid fracture is suspected, a 45° cephalic tilt view (Stryker view) is useful. If soft-tissue injury is diagnosed, an MRI may be useful.
   D. Classification (Fig. 18-1)
      1. Mayo
         • Type I—Involvement of the anteroinferior glenoid; the injury may be associated with complete dislocation or subluxation of the humeral head. The scapular body is intact.
         • Type II—Involvement of the superior third to half of the glenoid; the superior fragment

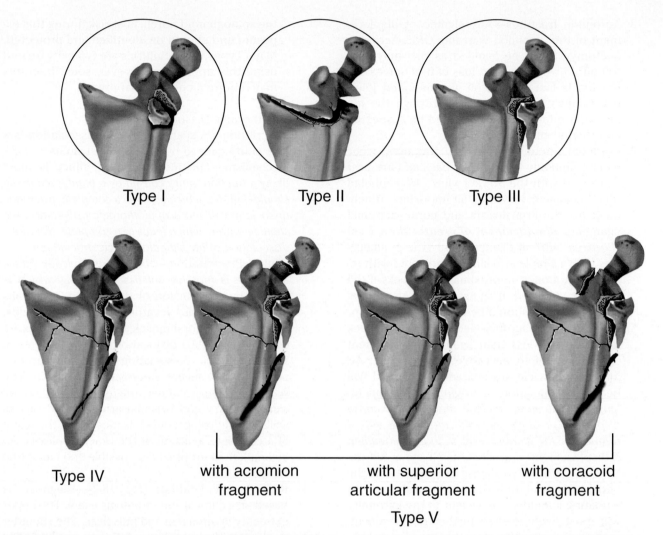

Type I　　　　Type II　　　　Type III

Type IV　　　　with acromion fragment　　　　with superior articular fragment　　　　with coracoid fragment

Type V

FIGURE 18-1　Mayo's modification of the Ideberg classification of intraarticular fractures of the glenoid distinguishes five types. The figure shows Types I through IV and three variants of Type V. Type V is a Type IV pattern plus an additional coracoid, acromion, or free superior articular fragment.

contains the intact coracoid. The scapular body is intact.
- Type III—Involvement of the inferior or inferoposterior glenoid; the injury includes the lateral scapular border. The scapular body is intact.
- Type IV—Involvement of the inferior glenoid with extension into the scapular body.
- Type V—Type IV with the addition of a coracoid, acromion, or free superior articular fragment.

E. Treatment
　1. Types
　　- Nonoperative—Indications include *scapular body fractures and periarticular/articular fractures with only minimal displacement*. These will generally heal well without complications.
　　- Surgical—Indications include *displaced glenoid fossa fractures and fracture-dislocations, glenoid neck fractures with displacement, coracoid and acromion fractures with displacement, and ipsilateral fractures of the clavicle and glenoid neck or a fracture of the glenoid neck associated with disruption of the soft tissues attaching the clavicle to the scapula*.

　2. Scapular body fractures—Although scapulothoracic motion is important in preservation of normal motion, *scapular body fractures do well with nonsurgical management*. Almost all of these fractures heal due to the abundant blood supply and musculature covering the surface of the scapula. If dyskinesis exists, it typically responds to therapy. If the fracture extends into the scapular spine and displacement is greater than 5 mm, open reduction and internal fixation (ORIF) is recommended. Be aware that these are *typically high-energy injuries and are associated with a high incidence of life-threatening injuries, including scapulothoracic dissociation*.

3. Acromion fractures—Any significant displacement of the acromion warrants ORIF. Acromionectomy should be avoided as this may lead to deltoid weakness and loss of function as the tension is lost across the glenohumeral joint. If the injury was transmitted through the humerus, a rotator cuff tear should be suspected and treated simultaneously.

4. Coracoid fractures—Coracoid fractures occur most commonly through the base and are best visualized with the Stryker view (45° cephalad tilt). Because it serves as an important attachment for the arm flexors and coracoacromial ligaments, ***displacement of greater than 1 cm requires ORIF***. If displacement is less, analgesics with a simple arm sling is indicated with return to motion at approximately 6 weeks if the pain has subsided. If an associated AC separation exists, this should be fixed in conjunction.

5. Glenoid neck fractures—Isolated glenoid neck fractures with less than 1 cm of displacement can be treated conservatively. Because the AC joint and clavicle are spared, the glenoid will heal in the position of original displacement. *Surgical indications include more than 1 cm of displacement of the glenoid, more than 40° of rotation of the glenoid, and a floating shoulder.* If displacement of greater than 1 cm is left untreated, abductor weakness can persist, and the patient may end up with pseudoparalysis. With a floating shoulder, the weight of the extremity will most likely lead to further displacement; therefore, surgical treatment is recommended.

6. Glenoid fossa fractures—*Glenoid fossa fractures require ORIF if greater than 25% of the anterior glenoid surface is fractured, if more than one-third of the posterior glenoid surface is fractured, if any subluxation of the humeral head exists, or if there is more than 5 mm displacement of the articular surface (in any of these instances are treated non-operatively,* a poor outcome is likely). Good to excellent results with surgical intervention are obtained in 80% of cases. Poor outcomes are related to iatrogenic nerve palsies. The goal of surgery is anatomic restoration of the articular surface.

F. Surgical Approaches
1. Anterior deltopectoral approach—This approach is used for Mayo Types I and II injuries.
2. Posterior Judet approach—This approach uses the internervous plane between the infraspinatus and the teres minor. The deltoid is released from the posterior acromion and retracted laterally giving a view of the posterior glenoid and lateral scapula. A posterior arthrotomy may be made to inspect the joint. The suprascapular nerve branch to the infraspinatus, which exits

the spinoglenoid notch, is at risk during this exposure and should be identified and protected. Mayo Types III to V injuries are typically treated using this approach; however, some fractures may require a combined approach.

II. Scapulothoracic Dissociation
A. Description—A scapulothoracic dissociation is a rare entity caused by high-energy trauma.
B. Mechanism—The mechanism of injury is most likely *a traction injury caused by a blunt force to the shoulder girdle, which leads to a complete, traumatic dissociation of the scapulothoracic articulation the shoulder girdle, which leads to a complete, traumatic dissociation of the scapulothoracic articulation.*
C. Clinical Presentation—*The skin is typically intact, and there is massive soft-tissue swelling,* which is caused by an avulsion of the deltoid, pectoralis minor, rhomboids, levator scapulae, trapezius, and latissimus dorsi muscles, as well as a fracture of the clavicle, AC dislocation, or SC dislocation. Scapulothoracic dissociation is typically accompanied by a severe neurovascular insult. The *subclavian artery and vein are usually torn,* and the axillary artery and brachial artery are at risk as well. The neurologic deficit is most often the result of a complete avulsion of the brachial plexus. An incomplete neuropraxia is possible and cannot be excluded.
D. Radiographic Findings (Fig. 18-2)—Diagnosis is based on a clinical and radiologic exam. The upper extremity is often flail and pulseless. The shoulder girdle exhibits massive soft-tissue swelling. The chest X-ray will show lateral displacement (measured as more than 50%) of the affected scapula. *The measurement may be performed as the distance from the sternal notch to the glenoid fossa or more commonly from the inferior angle of the scapula to the midline.* Close scrutiny of the chest X-ray must be performed to ensure that the image it is not rotated. Often there will be an associated clavicle fracture, AC dislocation, or SC dislocation.
E. Treatment—***Initial resuscitation should be followed by an emergent angiography if a pulseless extremity is diagnosed***. Rapid evaluation by a vascular surgeon is necessary and emergent surgical repair is required in the unstable patient. Following vascular repair, the clavicle and AC/SC joints should be surgically stabilized. Exploration of the brachial plexus, and cervical myelography should be done to determine the prognosis of the upper extremity. ***If a complete avulsion of the brachial plexus is found, a primary above-elbow amputation with early prosthetic fitting should be considered,*** as functional recovery is unlikely. Partial injuries have a fair prognosis and

Left   Right

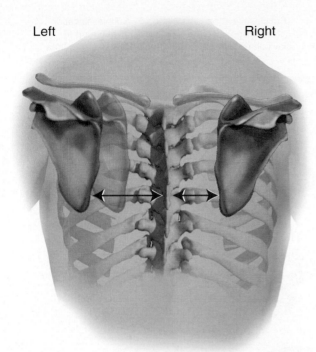

FIGURE 18-2 Scapulothoracic dissociation demonstrating lateral displacement (of at least 50%) on the injured left side as compared with the normal right side.

musculotendinous transfers may be performed at a later time.

III. Fractures of the Clavicle

A. Anatomy—The clavicle is the first bone to ossify (intramembranous ossification) in the fifth week of development and the last to fuse (medially). It is an S-shaped structure, which changes from a prismatic shape medially to a flattened shape laterally. It is anchored to the scapula via the AC and CC ligaments and to the trunk via the SC ligaments.

B. Function—The clavicle acts as a strut and is responsible for bracing the shoulder against motions, which would otherwise cause it to collapse. It also permits optimal muscle–tendon unit length to allow the thoracohumeral muscles to maintain optimal working distance. The clavicle acts to suspend the scapula both dynamically with an upward force from the trapezius through the CC ligaments and with a static force via the SC ligaments. It also affords protection for the closely related neurovascular structures. ***Biomechanically, the clavicle rotates 50° on its axis when the arm is elevated to 180°.***

C. Mechanism of Injury—Approximately 87% of clavicle fractures occur as a result of a fall onto the shoulder. Another 6% fracture secondary to a direct blow, and the remainder occur via indirect injury with force being transmitted up the humerus.

D. Classification (Fig. 18-3)—Allman described the initial classification; however, it was modified by Neer, Rockwood, and later Craig. The Craig classification combines the Allman and Neer types, providing more descriptive and functional information.

1. Group I (80% of all clavicule fractures)—Fracture of the middle third

2. Group II (12% to 15% of all clavicule fractures)—Fracture of the distal third
   - Type I—Minimal displacement (interligamentous)
   - Type II—Displaced secondary to a fracture line medial to the CC ligaments
     (a) Conoid and trapezoid attached (fracture medial to CC ligaments)
     (b) Conoid torn, trapezoid attached (fracture between the CC ligaments)
   - Type III—Fractures of the articular surface
   - Type IV—Periosteal sleeve fracture (children)
   - Type V—Comminuted with ligaments attached neither proximally nor distally, but to an inferior comminuted fragment

3. Group III (5% to 8% of all clavicule fractures)—Fractures of the proximal third
   - Type I—Minimal displacement
   - Type II—Displaced (ligaments ruptured)
   - Type III—Intraarticular
   - Type IV—Epiphyseal separation (children and young adults)
   - Type V—Comminuted

E. Diagnosis

1. Clinical examination—A thorough physical exam should be performed, as an injury to the brachial plexus and/or subclavian artery or vein may be present. Pneumothorax occurs in 3% of clavicle fractures.

2. Radiographic evaluation
   - Plain X-ray—An apical oblique view is helpful in the acute setting. This is done by placing a bump under the contralateral scapula, so the injured side will lie flat against the cassette. Angle the beam, 20° cephalad, will isolate the image away from the thoracic cage. To view an internally fixed clavicle, the abduction-lordotic view is helpful. To obtain this, have the patient abduct the arm 135° and angle the beam 25° cephalad.
   - Serendipity view and CT—A serendipity view and CT scan should be obtained if a SC injury is suspected. This will help determine if there is posterior displacement of the medial clavicle that threatens neurovascular structures.

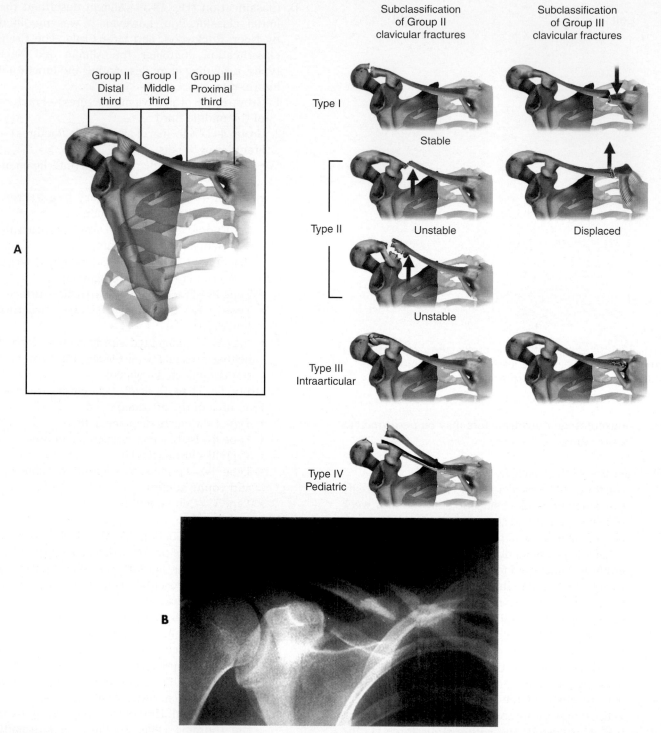

FIGURE 18-3 **A.** Classification of clavicular fractures with a detailed description of fractures of the distal third and the proximal third. **B.** Radiograph of a displaced fracture of the middle third of the clavicle.

F. Treatment
  1. Adults
    • Medial third fractures—Medial third fractures are generally treated nonoperatively. If there is posterior displacement with potential or apparent compromise

of neurovascular structures, surgery is recommended.
    • Middle third fractures—Middle third fractures are most commonly treated in a sling or figure of eight immobilization. Although the rate of fracture healing is quite high with

nonoperative treatment, several authors have suggested that the nonunion rate is much higher than previously thought.

(a) Factors leading to nonunion
- Advancing age
- Female gender
- Absence of cortical contact between the fracture ends
- Comminution

(b) Surgical indication—*A relative indication for surgery includes any clavicle fracture with greater than or equal to 20 mm of shortening.* These have a 91% nonunion rate, and consideration for ORIF must be given. Factors affecting absolute versus relative indications for surgery are as follows:
- Absolute indications for operative treatment
  1. Shortening of greater or equal to 20 mm
  2. Open injury
  3. Impending skin disruption with an irreducible fracture
  4. Vascular or progressive neurologic loss
  5. Scapulothoracic dissociation
- Relative indications for operative treatment
  1. Displacement greater than 20 mm
  2. Neurologic disorder
  3. Parkinson's disease
  4. Seizure disorder
  5. Head injury
  6. Multitrauma
  7. Floating shoulder
  8. Bilateral fractures
  9. Cosmesis
- Distal third fractures—Most distal third fractures heal well with nonoperative care. However, Type II fracture treatment is controversial. The nonunion rate for this type of fracture is quite high; however, the majority of them are asymptomatic without functional limitations. Therefore, *current literature suggests nonoperative management for type II distal third fractures, unless there is displacement greater than 20 mm.* Type III fractures are generally treated nonoperatively, and if chronic pain develops, the distal clavicle can be excised. Type IV fractures in children can generally be treated nonoperatively; however, if posterior or inferior displacement exists, surgery should be considered.

2. Infants—The clavicle has a high incidence of fracture at birth. A sling and swath for 2 weeks is adequate for healing and remodeling occurs over time.

3. Children (2 to 12 years)—Immobilization for 3 weeks or until the patient is pain free with motion is usually sufficient for healing.

4. Adolescents (13 to 16 years)—Treatment is similar to adult's with 4 to 6 weeks of immobilization.

G. Complications
1. Nonunion—Nonunion occurs in 0.9% to 5% of all fractures. It is most common in the middle third. ***Nonunions that show callus formation may respond to a bone stimulator; however, symptomatic atrophic nonunions require ORIF with autogenous bone graft.*** Asymptomatic nonunions are common and do not require treatment.
2. Malunion
3. Neurovascular insult—If problem persists after fracture healing, an osteotomy and ORIF may be required.

IV. AC Joint Injuries
A. Anatomy (Fig. 18-4)—The acromioclavicular (AC) joint is a diarthrodial joint with a fibrocartilaginous disk that varies in shape and size. It has a thin capsule that is stabilized by superior, inferior, anterior, and posterior ligaments. ***The most robust ligament is the superior AC ligament, which is primarily responsible for horizontal AC joint stability. Vertical stability is provided by the CC ligaments***, which also act as the primary support through which the scapula is suspended by the clavicle. Normal AC joints are 0.5 to 6 mm in width. Anything greater than 6 mm is considered abnormal. ***The normal CC distance is 1.1 cm to 1.3 cm***

B. Mechanism of Injury—Classically, the AC joint is injured by a direct blow to the acromion with the humerus in adduction. The magnitude of the blow will determine the severity of injury. Because of the inherent stability of the SC joint, the force is transmitted laterally, and the AC ligaments, CA ligament, and possibly the deltotrapezial fascia can be injured. An indirect injury can occur as well; however, this is much less common. Rugby and hockey players frequently sustain this injury.

C. Classification (Fig. 18-5)
1. Type I—Sprain of the AC ligament only.
2. Type II—AC ligaments and the joint capsule are disrupted. CC ligaments are intact. There is less than or equal to 50% vertical subluxation of the clavicle. The CC interval is only slightly increased.
3. Type III—The AC ligaments, joint capsule, and CC ligaments are disrupted. There is an AC joint dislocation with the clavicle displaced

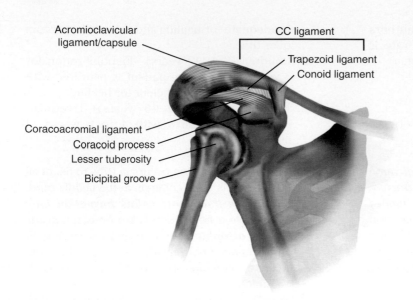

Acromioclavicular
ligament/capsule

CC ligament

Trapezoid ligament
Conoid ligament

Coracoacromial ligament
Coracoid process
Lesser tuberosity
Bicipital groove

FIGURE 18-4 Normal anatomy of the AC joint.

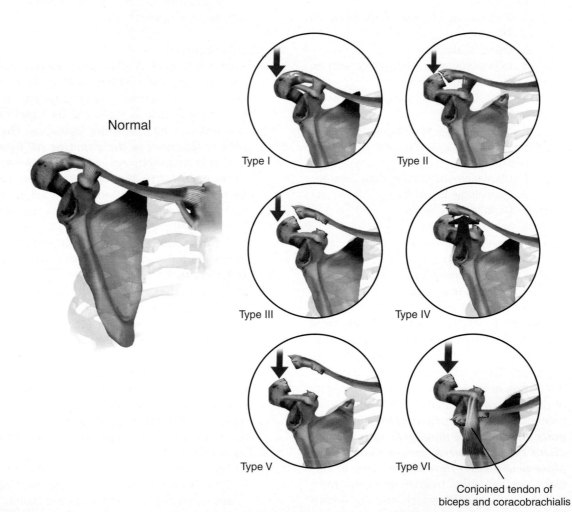

Normal

Type I

Type II

Type III

Type IV

Type V

Type VI

Conjoined tendon of
biceps and coracobrachialis

FIGURE 18-5 AC joint injury classification. Type 1, AC ligament sprain, AC and CC ligaments intact. Type II, AC ligament disrupted, CC ligament intact (usually sprained). Type III, AC and CC ligaments disrupted. Type IV, AC and CC ligaments disrupted, the distal (lateral) clavicle is displaced posteriorly through the trapezius muscle. Type V, AC and CC ligaments disrupted, attachments of the deltoid and trapezius muscles on the clavicle are disrupted, the clavicle is displaced superiorly. Type VI, AC and CC ligaments disrupted, the clavicle is displaced inferiorly (subcoracoid).

superiorly and there is complete loss of contact between the acromion and the clavicle. The CC interval is increased from 25% to 100%.

4. Type IV—The AC ligaments, joint capsule, and the CC ligaments are disrupted. There is an AC joint dislocation with the clavicle displaced posteriorly into the trapezius.

5. Type V—The AC ligaments, joint capsule, and the CC ligaments are disrupted. There is an AC joint dislocation with superior elevation of the clavicle in relation to the acromion (100% to 300% of normal). There is complete detachment of the deltoid and trapezius from the distal clavicle.

6. Type VI—The AC ligaments, joint capsule, and the CC ligaments are disrupted. There is an AC joint dislocation with the clavicle displaced inferior to the acromion and the coracoid process.

D. Diagnosis
1. Clinical examination—Clinical diagnosis with prominence, pain, and soft-tissue swelling over the distal clavicle
2. Radiographic evaluation—An AP view and Zanca view (15° cephalic tilt) are recommended to evaluate for joint displacement and intra-articular fractures. An axillary view is mandatory to determine AP displacement. Stress radiographs are no longer routinely used.

E. Treatment
1. Based on type
   • Types I and II—Nonoperative care with cryotherapy and analgesics. Sling for comfort and early range of motion (ROM). Return to sports when pain free.
   • Type III—Controversial. If professional baseball pitcher or heavy laborer, surgery may be the best option. All others should be treated nonoperatively with return to activities within 4 to 6 weeks. Most authors report excellent results, whether repair is early or late; therefore, a trial of nonoperative care may be in the patient's best interest.
   • Types IV, V, and VI—Surgical repair with reconstruction of the CC ligaments.
2. Surgical options
   • Dynamic muscle transfer—The tip of the coracoid is transferred to the undersurface of the clavicle along with the coracobrachialis and the short head of the biceps. The rate of nonunion is high, and this procedure has generally fallen out of favor.
   • Primary AC joint fixation—Bioabsorbable materials are now being used more often, as a second operation does not need to be performed to remove hardware. Smooth tip K-wires are not recommended as migration may occur.
   • Primary CC ligament fixation—Bosworth was the first to describe transfixing the clavicle to the coracoid. There have been problems with pull out, thus the repair should be augmented by reconstructing the CC ligaments.
   • Excision of the distal clavicle—Weaver and Dunn presented this type of repair, and currently, variations of this technique are the most widely used method to reconstruct the AC joint. The CA ligament is often transferred to the undersurface of the clavicle and the repair is protected with a loop of tissue from the clavicle to the coracoid.

V. SC Joint Injuries
A. Incidence—SC joint dislocations are rare and account for only 3% of all shoulder girdle injuries. Anterior dislocations are more common due to the strong posterior SC ligaments. The majority are caused by motor vehicle accidents and contact sports.
B. Anatomy—The SC joint is a diarthrodial joint, which has the least amount of osseous stability of all the major joints in the body. ***The medial clavicular epiphysis is the last to fuse at 23 to 25 years of age***. Strong ligaments may cause a fracture through the physis, which may be misdiagnosed as a dislocation.
   1. Ligaments
      • Intra-articular disk ligament—Dense, fibrous structure that acts as a check-rein against medial displacement
      • Costoclavicular ligament—Provides stability of the joint during rotation and elevation of the clavicle
      • Interclavicular ligament—Aids in suspending the shoulder
      • Capsular ligament—Covers the anterosuperior and posterior portions of the SC joint
C. Biomechanics—The SC joint is able to move in all planes. It has approximately 35° of motion superior, anterior, and posterior, and is able to rotate about the clavicle's long axis 45° to 50°.
D. Mechanism of Injury—A high-energy mechanism is needed for a SC joint dislocation to occur. A direct or indirect force may be the cause. Anterior dislocations are more common because the posterior capsular ligaments are stronger.
E. Diagnosis
   1. Clinical examination—Pain and soft-tissue swelling at the SC joint. The patient may present carrying the injured extremity in the contralateral arm. The patient may have trouble in breathing, a choking sensation, or difficulty in swallowing.

2. Radiologic examination—AP and lateral X-rays are difficult to interpret. Therefore, other views are used to evaluate the SC joint.
   - Hobbs view—90° cephalocaudal view that is taken with the patient leaning over the table so the anterior and lower rib cage is against the table.
   - Serendipity view (Fig. 18-6)—40° cephalic tilt view of both SC joints and the medial clavicles. If the medial clavicle is dislocated anteriorly, the clavicle will appear to be displaced superiorly when compared with a horizontal line drawn from the normal clavicle. If the medial clavicle is dislocated posteriorly, the clavicle will appear displaced below the horizontal line.
   - CT (Fig. 18-7)—CT is the best study to evaluate the SC joints. This can distinguish between fractures and dislocations, and both joints can be visualized at the same time for comparison.

F. Treatment
   1. Traumatic injuries
      - Mild sprain (Type I injury)—The ligaments are intact and the joint is stable. Treatment is with cryotherapy and a sling for comfort with early ROM.
      - Moderate sprain (Type II injury)—The capsular, intra-articular disk, and costoclavicular ligaments are partially disrupted with subluxation of the joints—reduce by drawing the shoulders backward; sling and swath to prevent motion of the arm. Protect for 4 to 6 weeks with gradual return to motion.
      - Severe dislocation (Type III injury)
        (a) Anterior SC dislocation—If the patient presents within 7 to 10 days after injury, an attempt at reduction can be performed. These are typically unstable and will dislocate again. If the reduction stays in place, immobilization should be maintained for at least 6 weeks. *Operative management of irreducible anterior dislocations is not recommended*.
        (b) Acute posterior dislocation—*If the patient presents within 7 to 10 days of injury, an attempt at closed reduction is advised*. Initially, a thorough exam should be performed to rule out pulmonary or vascular problems and if necessary a thoracic surgeon should be present during reduction should a complication occur. If the reduction is successful, the SC joint is typically stable.

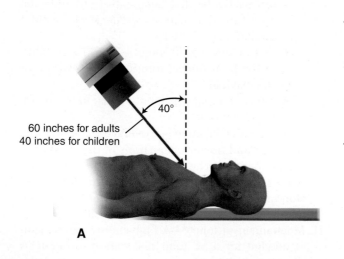

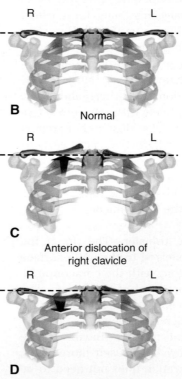

FIGURE 18-6
A. Positioning for the serendipity view for evaluation of the SC joints. B to D. Interpretation of the serendipity view. L, left; R, right. **B.** Normally, both clavicles are in the same plane. **C.** In a patient with an anterior dislocation of the medial end of the clavicle (anterior SC dislocation), the clavicle appears to be displaced superiorly. **D.** In a posterior SC dislocation, the clavicle appears to be displaced inferiorly.

60 inches for adults
40 inches for children

40°

A

R   L

B   Normal

R   L

C   Anterior dislocation of right clavicle

R   L

D   Posterior dislocation of right clavicle

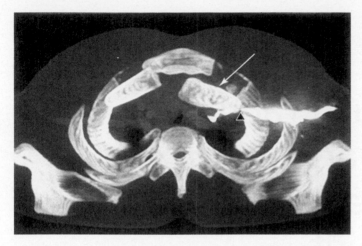

FIGURE 18-7 CT scan showing a posterior SC dislocation (*arrow*) with compression of the subclavian artery (*arrowhead*). (From Brinker MR, Miller MD. *Fundamentals of Orthopaedics*. Philadelphia, PA: WB Saunders; 1999. Courtesy Fondren Orthopedic Group LLP, Texas Orthopedic Hospital, Houston.)

(c) Chronic posterior SC dislocation—*If closed reduction fails or a chronic posterior dislocation presents, an operative procedure should be performed, because most adult patients cannot tolerate compression of the mediastinum. A thoracic surgeon should be part of the surgical team as the risk of fatal complications is high.* The operation can be aimed at stabilizing the SC joint or performing a medial clavicle resection with stabilization to the first rib. *Never attempt a fixation of the SC joint with metallic pins, Steinmann pins, Kirschner wires, threaded pins with bent ends, or Hagie pins, as all are associated with migration and serious complications.*

SUGGESTED READINGS

Classic Articles

Boyer MI, Axelrod TS. Atrophic nonunion of the clavicle, treatment by compression plate, lag-screw fixation and bone graft. *J Bone Joint Surg Br.* 1997;79-B:301–303.

Brinker MR, Bartz RL, Reardon PR, Reardon MJ. A method for Open Reduction and Internal Fixation of the Unstable Posterior Sternoclavicular Joint Dislocation. *J orthop Trauma.* 1997;11:378-381

Deafenbaugh MK, Dugdale TW, Staeheli JW, et al. Nonoperative treatment of Neer type II distal clavicle fractures: a prospective study. *Contemp Orthop.* 1990;20:405–413.

Ebraheim NA, An HS, Jackson WT, et al. Scapulothoracic dissociation. *J Bone Joint Surg Am.* 1988;70:428–432.

Froimson AI. Fracture of the coracoid process of the scapula. *J Bone Joint Surg Am.* 1978;60:710–711.

Herscovici D, Fiennes AGT, Allgower M, et al. The floating shoulder: ipsilateral clavicle and scapular neck fractures. *J Bone Joint Surg.* 1992;74B:362–366.

Hill JM, McGuire MH, Crosby LA. Closed treatment of displaced middle-third fractures of the clavicle gives poor results. 1997;79B(4):537–539.

Lansen E, Bjerg-Mielson A, Christensen P. Conservative or surgical treatment of acromioclavicular dislocation: a prospective, controlled randomized study. *J Bone Joint Surg.* 1986;68A:552–555.

Leung KS, Lam TP. Open reduction and internal fixation of ipsilateral fractures of the scapular neck and clavicle. *J Bone Joint Surg.* 1993;75A:1015–1018.

Mayo KA, Benirschke SK, Mast JW. Displaced fractures of the glenoid fossa. *Clin Orthop.* 1998;347:122–130.

Nuber GW, Bowen MK. Acromioclavicular joint injuries and distal clavicle fractures. *J Am Acad Orthop Surg.* 1997;5:11–18.

Rockwood CA. Reconstruction of chronic and complete dislocations of the acromio-clavicular joint. *Clin Orthop.* 1998;347:138–149.

Simpson NS, Jupiter JB. Clavicular nonunion and malunion: evaluation and surgical management. *J Am Acad Orthop Surg.* 1996;4:1–8.

Recent Articles

Herscovici D. Scapula fractures: To fix or not to fix? *J Orthop Trauma.* 2006;20(3):227–229.

Robinson CM, Cairns DA. Primary nonoperative treatment of displaced lateral fractures of the clavicle. *J Bone Joint Surg Am.* 2004;86:778–782.

Robinson CM, Court-Brown CM, McQueen MM, et al. Estimating the risk of nonunion following nonoperative treatment of a clavicular fracture. *J Bone Joint Surg Am.* 2004;86:1359–1365.

Review Article

Wirth MA, Rockwood CA. Acute and chronic traumatic injuries of the sternoclavicular joint. *J Am Acad Orthop Surg.* 1996;4:268–278.

Textbooks

DeLee JC, Drez D. *DeLee & Drez's Orthopedic Sports Medicine Principles and Practice.* 2nd ed. Philadelphia, PA: WB Saunders.

Rockwood CA, Matsen FA, Wirth MA, et al, eds. *The Shoulder.* 3rd ed. Philadelphia, PA: WB Saunders.

CHAPTER 19

Proximal Humerus Fractures and Dislocations and Traumatic Soft-Tissue Injuries of the Glenohumeral Joint

Jerry S. Sher and Philip R. Lozman

I. Proximal Humerus Fractures

A. Overview—Fractures of the proximal humerus are classified according to the patterns of displacement of the four major segments. These include the humeral head, the greater and lesser tuberosities, and the humeral shaft. A proximal humerus fracture is considered displaced if any major segment is displaced more than 1.0 cm or angulated greater than 45°. As described by Neer, this classification system is based on anteroposterior and lateral radiographs. Recently, the use of three right-angle trauma series radiographs has improved the accuracy in diagnosing fracture displacement. Computed tomography (CT) can be helpful in preoperative planning by delineating the degree of displacement and rotation of the fracture fragments, especially with fractures that involve the tuberosities and humeral head.

Proximal humerus fractures comprise 4% to 5% of all fractures. In younger patients, these fractures are commonly associated with violent trauma, whereas in older patients, minor trauma and decreased bone mineral density lead to the majority of proximal humerus fractures.

The proximity of the neurovascular bundle to the glenohumeral joint makes it subject to injury with proximal humeral fractures, and necessitates a thorough neurovascular examination. ***The finding of a palpable distal pulse does not eliminate the possibility of a vascular injury due to the rich collateral circulation of the proximal humerus***.

The majority of proximal humerus fractures are minimally displaced and can be treated with immobilization and early range of motion. Displaced fractures are optimally treated by closed or open reduction to restore anatomic alignment. In some cases, prosthetic replacement is the treatment of choice based on the disruption of the blood supply to the humeral head.

B. Physical Examination

1. Shoulder—The shoulder must be well visualized. Gowns are used to expose the entire shoulder for women, while men can be undressed from the waist up.

2. Cervical spine—The cervical spine should be examined prior to the shoulder, and radiographs obtained if there is any concern of concomitant injury.

3. Neurovascular examination—The neurovascular evaluation of the extremity is essential and can usually be obtained in a fractured extremity with gentle motion and isometric contraction. The presence of sensibility in the axillary distribution (lateral arm) is not a reliable test of the integrity of axillary motor function. Neurovascular injuries occur in 5% to 30% of complex proximal humerus fractures.

C. Imaging

1. Radiographs

• Trauma series (Fig. 19-1)—Three right angle views of the shoulder are essential to determine the relationship of the four major segments of the shoulder in space. These views are taken in the sagittal, coronal, and axial ***planes of the scapula***, rather than the body.

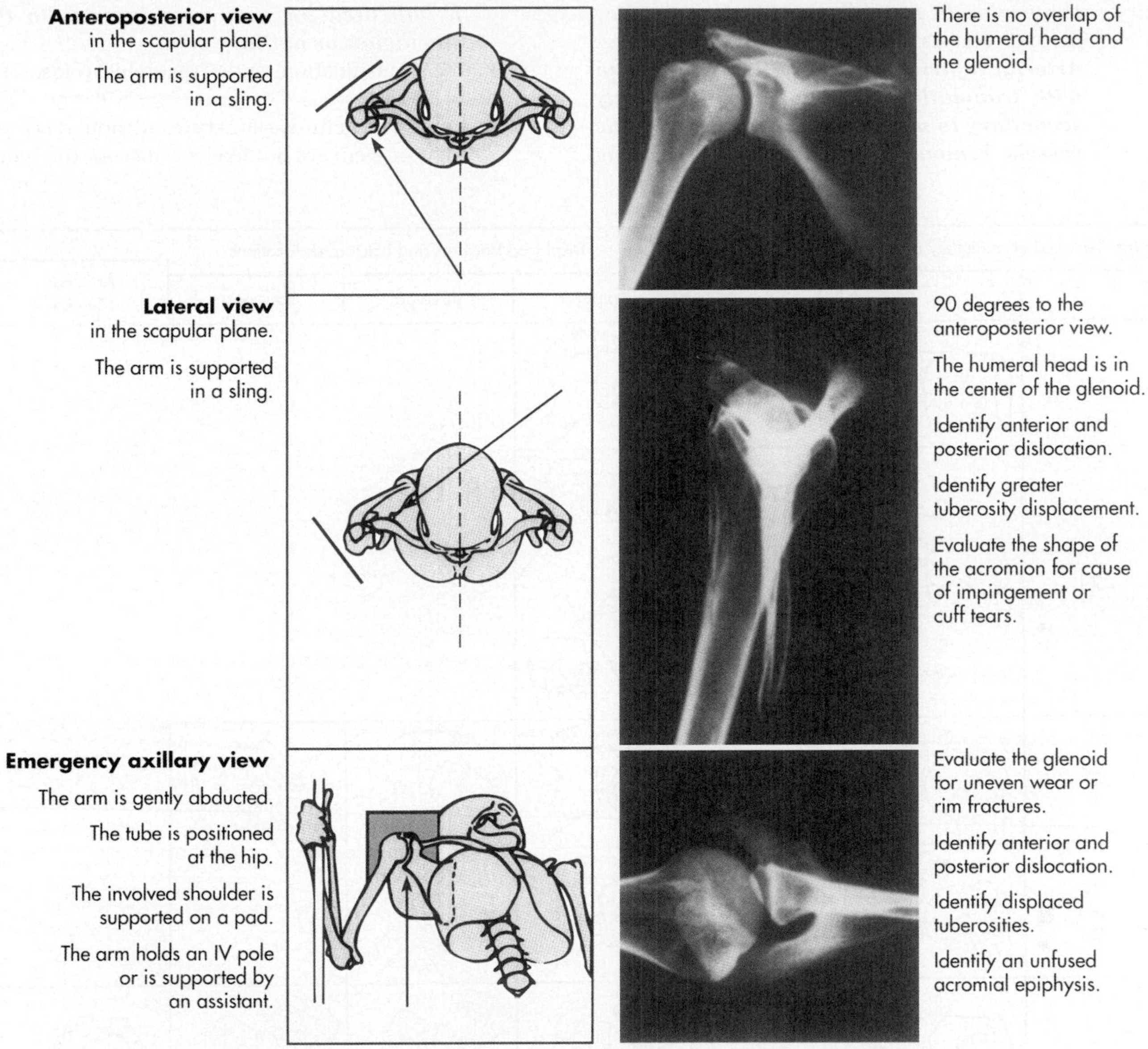

Anteroposterior view
in the scapular plane.

The arm is supported
in a sling.

There is no overlap of
the humeral head and
the glenoid.

Lateral view
in the scapular plane.

The arm is supported
in a sling.

90 degrees to the
anteroposterior view.

The humeral head is in
the center of the glenoid.

Identify anterior and
posterior dislocation.

Identify greater
tuberosity displacement.

Evaluate the shape of
the acromion for cause
of impingement or
cuff tears.

Emergency axillary view

The arm is gently abducted.

The tube is positioned
at the hip.

The involved shoulder is
supported on a pad.

The arm holds an IV pole
or is supported by
an assistant.

Evaluate the glenoid
for uneven wear or
rim fractures.

Identify anterior and
posterior dislocation.

Identify displaced
tuberosities.

Identify an unfused
acromial epiphysis.

FIGURE 19-1 Trauma series views of the shoulder (From Norris TR. In: Chapman MW, Madison M, eds. *Operative Orthopaedics*. Philadelphia, PA: JB Lippincott; 1988, with permission.)

- Rotational anteroposterior (AP) views—Supplement to the trauma series, these views reveal the greater tuberosity in external rotation and humeral head impression fractures with internal rotation.
2. CT scanning
   - Low-dose CT scanning—Low-dose CT provides extremely accurate imaging to evaluate complex proximal humeral fractures, and in some cases can change the treatment plan as contemplated, based on the initial radiographs.
   - Three-dimensional CT scanning—3D CT is now available in many institutions using the standard data obtained from the initial scan.

These images allow depiction of the relationship of the fractures in any direction.
3. MRI scanning—MRI is used in the determination of soft-tissue injuries involving the rotator cuff and the neurovascular structures around the shoulder. MRI also allows early assessment of osteonecrosis following trauma, which may not be evident on plain films for a number of years.
4. Arteriography and venography—Arteriography and venography are required when a vascular injury is suspected, as the finding of a distal pulse does not rule out an arterial injury. The ***circumflex vessels connect with***

the profunda brachii through the ascending deltoid vessels and feed the distal arteries. *Arterial injuries are more likely to be seen with traumatic dislocations in the elderly secondary to noncompliant, atherosclerotic vessels. Venous duplex ultrasound scanning*

in indicated for suspected injuries to the subclavian or axillary vein.

D. Injury Classification and Treatment (Figs. 19-2 and 19-3)

1. One-part fractures—Fractures without displacement of 1 cm are not likely to disrupt the blood

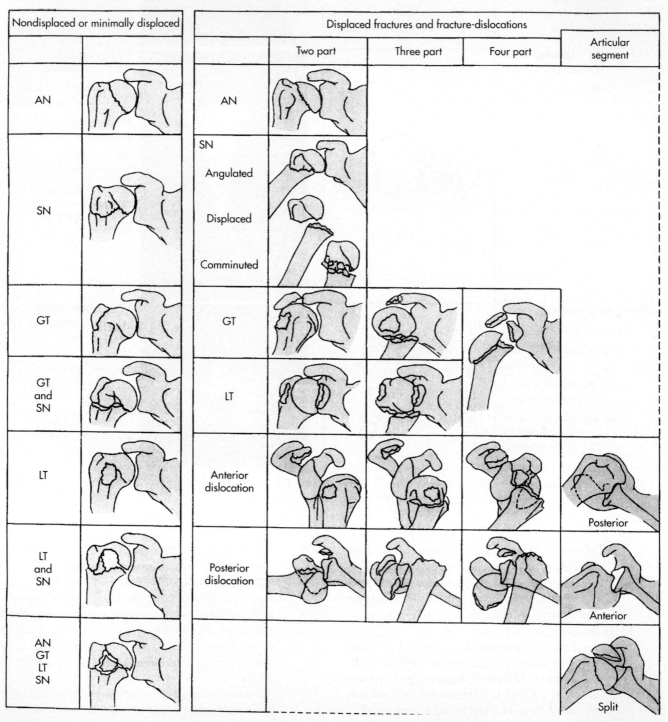

FIGURE 19-2 Four-part classification of proximal humerus fractures and fracture-dislocations. *AN,* Anatomic neck; *GT,* greater tuberosity; *LT,* lesser tuberosity; *SN,* surgical neck. (Redrawn from Browner BD, Jupiter JB, Levine AM, et al., eds. *Skeletal Trauma: Fractures, Dislocations, Ligamentous Injuries.* Vol 2, 2nd ed. Philadelphia, PA: WB Saunders; 1998, with permission.)

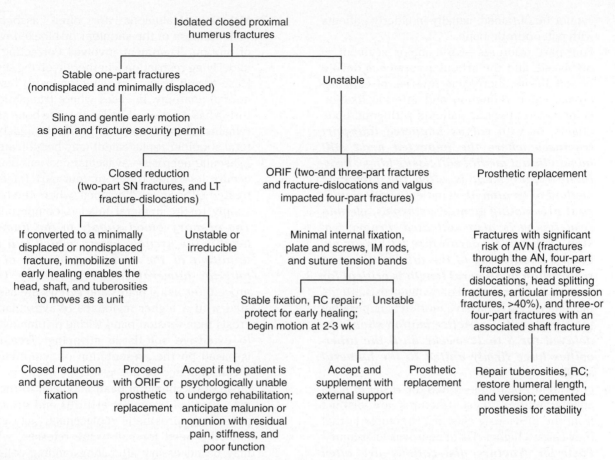

FIGURE 19-3   Algorithm for isolated closed proximal humerus fractures. *AN, Anatomic neck;* AVN, *avascular necrosis;* IM, *intramedullary;* LT, lesser tuberosity; *ORIF, open reduction with internal fixation;* RC, rotator cuff; *SN,* surgical neck. (Reprinted with permission from Browner BD, Jupiter JB, Levine AM, et al., eds. *Skeletal Trauma: Fractures, Dislocations, Ligamentous Injuries.* Vol 2, 2nd ed. Philadelphia, PA: WB Saunders; 1998.)

supply to the humeral head and are referred to as minimally displaced. The surrounding soft tissues (periosteum, capsule, and rotator cuff) tend to hold the fragments together and allow near anatomic healing. These fractures are optimally treated by immobilization and early functional exercises to avoid stiffness. ***Functional outcome improves if physical therapy is initiated within 2 weeks of the injury.***

2. Two-part fractures—Isolated two-part fractures involving the tuberosities are rare, and usually occur as a consequence of a glenohumeral dislocation.

    • Two-part lesser tuberosity fractures—Usually associated with ***posterior glenohumeral dislocation***. Axillary radiographs and CT scanning are useful in confirming the diagnosis. Displaced fragments require open reduction and internal fixation.

    • Two-part greater tuberosity fractures—May accompany an ***anterior glenohumeral***

dislocation and are associated with longitudinal tears of the rotator cuff. ***Surgical treatment is indicated for fractures with more than 0.5 cm of displacement or 45° of rotation***, with repair of the rotator cuff.

    • Two-part surgical neck fractures—Classified as impacted and stable or displaced and unstable. Treatment for displaced fractures includes open reduction and internal fixation versus percutaneous pin fixation.

3. Three-part fractures—Include displacement of three segments including the humeral head, the shaft, and one tuberosity. Closed reduction is difficult to obtain due to the unopposed muscle pull on the remaining tuberosity. Axillary radiographs allow best visualization of the rotation of the articular surface of the humeral head. Open reduction and internal fixation using tension band wiring which incorporates the rotator cuff tendon provides good fixation. Prosthetic replacement is indicated when secure fixation

cannot be obtained, usually in elderly patients with osteoporotic bone.

4. Four-part fractures—Each major segment is displaced, and the articular surface is devoid of soft tissue, increasing the risk of osteonecrosis. Open reduction and internal fixation is indicated in young patients with good bone quality, or with *valgus impacted four-part fractures where the impacted head still has an intact medial soft-tissue hinge. Prosthetic replacement is often the preferred method of treatment*. In patients *with significant preexisting glenoid arthrosis, glenoid resurfacing is also indicated. Proper tension of the cuff musculature with near anatomic positioning of the tuberosities and restoration of humeral length is critical for functional recovery*. Following prosthetic replacement, early passive motion is imperative to prevent stiffness. *Active motion should be delayed for 8 to 12 weeks until the tuberosities have firmly united to the humeral shaft.*

5. Fracture-dislocations—Often the result of high-energy injuries, these fractures are distinct from the previously classified fractures in that they carry a higher risk of neurovascular injury. *Posterior fracture dislocations are often missed* due to poor radiographic evaluation, thus necessitating the three view trauma series in all shoulder injuries.

6. Head-splitting fractures—*Head-splitting fractures are most commonly treated with hemiarthroplasty;* however, if large fragments and good bone quality are present, open reduction and internal fixation can be attempted. Articular impression fractures are commonly associated with chronic dislocations, and stability usually depends upon the percentage of articular surface defect. Defects less than 20% tend to be stable after immobilization, whereas defects up to 40% or more may require soft-tissue transfers or hemiarthroplasty.

E. Complications

1. Nonunion—A number of factors can lead to nonunion of proximal humerus fractures including inadequate fixation or immobilization, traction at the fracture site, soft-tissue interposition, and osteonecrosis. *Nonunion most commonly occurs in patients with two-part surgical neck fractures.* Treatment is aimed at anatomic reduction and stable fixation of the fracture fragments as described for acute fractures. When this goal cannot be met, prosthetic replacement is the treatment of choice.

2. Malunion—Malunions are often associated with stiffness of the shoulder or blocked range of motion. Treatment involves correcting the underlying restriction whether involving the release of soft tissues or osteotomies to restore normal anatomy. In cases where traumatic arthritis has developed, or inadequate bone stock remains after correction, hemiarthroplasty or total shoulder replacement may be indicated.

3. Avascular necrosis—Avascular necrosis usually occurs following three- or four-part fractures treated either closed or open, where the blood supply to the humeral head is compromised. *The primary blood supply to the humeral head is the arcuate artery, which is a continuation of the ascending branch of the anterior humeral circumflex artery.* Open procedures using plates and screws are associated with a higher incidence of avascular necrosis than tension band wiring or pinning due to extensive soft-tissue stripping. Treatment is based on the presentation of symptoms as a consequence of the avascular necrosis. Collapse of the humeral head may lead to the development of traumatic arthritis and disabling pain. Early prosthetic replacement may eliminate the need for soft-tissue releases, which may be necessary after longstanding collapse of the humeral head.

4. Neurologic injury—*The musculocutaneous nerve is at risk of injury from proximal humerus fractures, dislocations, or excessive traction of the conjoint tendon during open reduction and internal fixation*. Symptoms can present as numbness and tingling along the anterolateral aspect of the forearm, which is supplied by *the terminal branch of the musculocutaneous nerve, the lateral antebrachial cutaneous nerve*.

5. Arthrodesis—Indications include a young patient with nonfunctioning shoulder musculature, prior deep infection, loss of articular cartilage, and severe pain refractory to conservative treatment. The shoulder should be positioned in such a way that the arm rests comfortably without winging of the scapula and the hand can be used functionally: *20° of flexion, 30° of abduction and 40° of internal rotation is the optimal position for a shoulder arthrodesis.*

II. Acute Dislocations of the Shoulder (Glenohumeral Joint)

A. Overview—Approximately 30% of the humeral head articulates with the glenoid at any given arm position (angle). The minimally constrained design of the glenohumeral joint affords it a wide arc of motion at the expense of inherent instability of the shoulder. Unlike the hip joint, the osseous structures of the glenohumeral joint contribute only a small portion to the joint's overall stability. Rather, *the surrounding soft tissues, which include the rotator cuff, glenoid labrum, and glenohumeral capsular ligaments, are of paramount importance in maintaining stability of the articulation.*

B. Evaluation

1. Mechanism of injury—Patients with acute dislocations commonly note an episode of significant trauma. In the case of anterior dislocations, force applied to an abducted and externally rotated arm is usually involved. Such injuries can occur after a fall or motor-vehicle accident, or during contact sports. Posterior dislocations typically involve significant trauma and also can occur secondary to falls, car accidents, or seizure disorders.

2. Presentation

   • Anterior dislocations—Patients with anterior dislocations typically manifest a loss of the normal deltoid contour. Palpation of the shoulder demonstrates prominence of the acromion process laterally and posteriorly, and a prominent humeral head can often be felt anteriorly. *The arm is often maintained in a partial externally rotated and abducted position.*

   • Posterior dislocations—Posterior dislocations are not as common and represent approximately 5% of dislocations of the shoulder. Clinical deformities are not as evident, but can include prominence of the humeral head posteriorly and of the coracoid process anteriorly. There may be a mild loss of the normal deltoid contour with notable flattening anteriorly. *The arm is typically held in an adducted and internally rotated position.* Patients typically experience a loss of arm external rotation as the humeral head is wedged against the posterior aspect of the glenoid.

   • Posterior subluxation—*Recurrent posterior subluxation can occur after an initial posterior directed force on the humeral head relative to the glenoid in the elevated arm such as a baseball player sliding into base. It can also be a sequela after a primary posterior dislocation. Clinical findings typically include a posterior prominence during midranges of forward*

arm elevation that disappears with a palpable clunk during terminal elevation and abduction.

3. Physical examination—The evaluation of patients with acute dislocations should include a thorough neurovascular examination both before and after any attempts at closed reduction. Injuries to the axillary nerve and artery occur infrequently, but they should be noted. Few patients have an expanding subdeltoid hematoma, indicating an underlying vascular injury. *Palpable distal pulses may be present despite an injury to the axillary artery because of the abundant collateral circulation surrounding the shoulder.*

4. Radiographic evaluation—Standard radiographs should be obtained to confirm the direction of the dislocation and evaluate the shoulder for associated fractures and any possible obstructions to reduction. An AP view in the plane of the scapula, an axillary view, and the scapular lateral (Y) view can aid in the detection of glenoid rim fractures, articular impression fractures of the humeral head, and fractures of the tuberosities. A standard AP radiograph alone may not be sufficient for detecting posterior dislocations because the displacement typically occurs at a right angle to the plane of the film. On a normal AP radiograph, the humeral head typically fills the glenoid fossa. *A vacant glenoid sign* refers to a partial vacancy of the glenoid fossa, and *a positive rim sign* refers to a space between the anterior glenoid rim and humeral head of greater than 6 mm. These signs suggest a posterior dislocation as viewed on the AP film. *The axillary radiograph remains the single most important X-ray film in assessing the presence and direction of a glenohumeral dislocation.*

5. Classification (Table 19-1)—Glenohumeral instability has commonly been categorized into one of two groups: traumatic unidirectional and atraumatic multidirectional. However, instability can also be considered as a continuum with these categories at the extremes and varying forms in between. For example, an athlete with global glenohumeral ligamentous laxity may develop symptoms after a traumatic event and manifest findings consistent with both traumatic and atraumatic forms of instability. When glenohumeral instability is described, the timing, frequency, degree, direction, and volition should all be considered.

TABLE 19-1

Classification of Glenohumeral Instability

Description	Group
Timing	Acute vs. chronic
Frequency	Recurrent vs. isolated event
Degree	Subluxation vs. dislocation
Direction	Unidirectional vs. bidirectional vs. multidirectional
Volition	Involuntary vs. voluntary vs. positional

C. Associated Injuries
1. Axillary nerve palsy—The axillary nerve is vulnerable to injury as it courses along the anteroinferior aspect of the glenohumeral joint. The nerve may be subject to excessive compression and traction with luxation of the humeral head. The incidence of axillary nerve injuries after acute dislocation has been reported to range from 5% to 33%. Age, degree of trauma at the time of injury, and duration of the dislocation all appear to have an impact on both the incidence and prognosis of nerve injury. In addition, proximal humerus fractures, blunt trauma, and gunshot injuries all have been associated with axillary nerve palsy. *EMG studies are indicated and can document the status of recovery 3 months after injury when physical examination reveals persistent absence of deltoid muscle function.*
2. Vascular injury—Vascular injury is more commonly seen in elderly patients after acute dislocations. Stiffer, less pliable vessels predispose these patients to such injuries, which can involve the axillary artery or vein or branches of the axillary artery, including the subscapular, thoracoacromial, and circumflex arteries. Vessel damage may occur at the time of injury or during reduction. A loss or decrease in the radial pulse may not always be present because of the abundant collateral circulation. An expanding subdeltoid hematoma may be evident, and arteriography should be performed if the diagnosis is suspected.
3. Glenoid rim fracture—Displaced fractures involving more than 20% of the glenoid rim decrease the effective surface area of glenoid articulation and can predispose patients to recurrent instability. *The anterior band of the inferior glenohumeral ligament inserts onto the glenoid labrum at the anteroinferior aspect of the glenoid rim. An avulsion*

fracture of this ligament will result in a bony Bankart lesion and occurs less frequently than an isolated soft tissue avulsion of the anteroinferior labrum from the glenoid rim (Bankart lesion). Malunion of such fractures also disrupts the concavity of the already shallow glenoid fossa, further compromising joint stability. Surgical treatment with anatomic reduction and fixation of the fractured fragments is recommended (Fig. 19-4).
4. Rotator cuff tear—Rotator cuff tears occur in 14% to 63% of patients after acute anterior or inferior dislocations. *The incidence increases in older persons and has been reported in 63% of patients over 50 years of age. Patients should be reevaluated 7 to 10 days after the initial injury to look for associated soft-tissue injuries.* By 10 days the acute symptoms will have subsided to some degree and may allow for better evaluation of the rotator cuff. Typically, patients are unable to sufficiently elevate the arm in the post-injury period. There may be

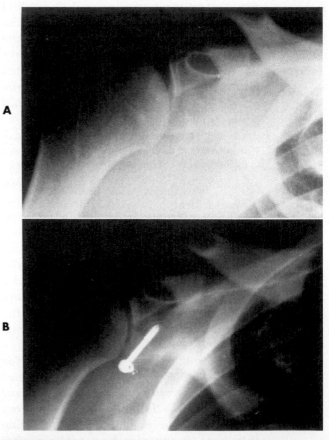

A

B

FIGURE 19-4 Preoperative **(A)** and postoperative **(B)** AP radiographs of a patient with a fracture of the anteroinferior glenoid rim associated with a traumatic anterior glenohumeral dislocation.

weakness in external rotation. The supraspinatus is commonly torn with variable degrees of infraspinatus involvement. Patients with recurrent anterior instability generally have disruption of the subscapularis tendon. ***An MRI is the study of choice when a rotator cuff tear is suspected.*** Satisfactory treatment can be achieved with primary repair of the tendon without reconstruction of the capsulolabral complex. ***The "lift-off test" described by Gerber can be performed to assess the functional integrity of the subscapularis.*** The arm is placed behind the back and the patient is asked to lift the hand from his back through further internal rotation of the arm. Inability to maintain the arm in this lifted position is a positive test suggestive of a subscapularis tendon tear (Fig. 19-5).

- Tensile failure—Traumatic lesions of the rotator cuff may also occur secondary to occult underlying instability. Such findings are more commonly seen in throwing athletes. It has been suggested that the rotator cuff lesions are the result of a continuum progressing from instability to subluxation, impingement, and tension overload of the cuff with resultant tearing. Articular surface partial-thickness tearing of the supraspinatus or

subscapularis is commonly seen. Repeated mechanical stress causes failure of the glenohumeral static restraints and places increased demands on the dynamic stabilizers. The rotator cuff is subject to injury through both repetitive tensile loading and secondary impingement mechanisms.

5. Tuberosity fractures—Fractures of the greater tuberosity may occur in association with anterior dislocations. Although tearing of the rotator cuff is not typically seen with posterior dislocations, avulsion fractures of the lesser tuberosity may occur. ***Recurrent instability is rare after these injuries, and ranges from 1% to 4%.*** Fracture-dislocations of the shoulder are generally more stable after healing compared with simple dislocations. In a simple shoulder dislocation, all of the energy of the injury is used to tear the capsular and ligamentous structures. In a fracture-dislocation, some of the energy is dissipated by the bone (tuberosity fracture), so the ligamentous component of the injury is less, and therefore there are fewer long-term problems with shoulder instability.

D. Treatment and Treatment Rationale

1. Initial management—Initial treatment of an acute glenohumeral dislocation should follow a complete physical and radiographic evaluation, including assessment of the patient's neurovascular status before and after reduction. Closed reduction should be performed in a relaxed and sedated patient. Intravenous sedation with a narcotic agent and benzodiazepine is routinely used in an emergency department setting before reduction. Inadequate sedation can lead to a traumatic reduction, inciting further injury to an already-compromised joint. Various reduction techniques have been described and include traction-counter traction methods, the modified Stimson maneuver (application of weight to the flexed arm in the prone patient [anterior dislocation]), and digital reduction of the humeral head within the axilla during applied traction on the partially abducted and externally rotated arm (Milch technique). The decision to proceed with surgical or nonsurgical management should include consideration of the patient's age, activity level, type of injury, number of prior dislocations, chronicity of the injury, and anticipated demands after treatment. Many of these injuries can be effectively treated with nonoperative measures. ***Patients with traumatic anterior subluxation events may describe a sensation of the shoulder "popping out***

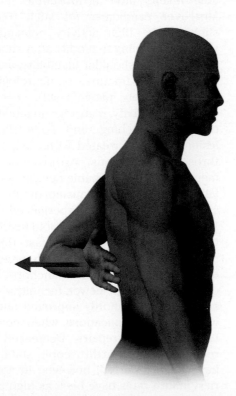

FIGURE 19-5 Lift-off test demonstrated clinically. Inability to maintain the arm in the lifted position is a positive test suggestive of a subscapularis tendon tear.

and then back into place." MRI studies may not always demonstrate a labrum tear or Hill-Sachs lesion. Initial treatment should include a short period of rest and immobilization followed by a physical therapy rehabilitation program. Patients with recurrent dislocations, dislocations associated with displaced tuberosity or glenoid rim fractures, irreducible dislocations by closed means, chronic dislocations, and young patients with acute primary anterior dislocations can be considered candidates for surgical treatment.

2. Nonoperative management—Nonoperative treatment typically includes a period of immobilization followed by a progressive rehabilitation program. Prolonged immobilization does not decrease recurrence rates in anterior instability and may contribute to joint stiffness, especially in older patients. However, recent data suggests that a short period of immobilization of up to 3 weeks with the arm in external rotation for first time anterior dislocations may result in lower recurrence rates as arm position in external rotation can effect better coaptation of a torn anteroinferior labrum against the glenoid neck. A progressive rehabilitation program beginning with range of motion exercises should be initiated as soon as possible. End arcs of abduction and external rotation should be avoided initially in anterior dislocators to afford adequate soft-tissue healing while minimizing the chance of contracture. Subsequent therapeutic measures include rotator cuff and periscapular muscle strengthening in an attempt to restore dynamic stability. *Initial treatment for patients with multidirectional instability should consist of physical therapy to include scapular stabilization and rotator cuff strengthening exercises.* Posterior dislocations should be initially immobilized in a neutral rotation arm sling after successful closed reduction. If the joint is unstable, then immobilization in an orthosis in 10° to 20° of abduction, external rotation, and extension is recommended for approximately 6 weeks to allow for adequate soft-tissue healing. *Placement of the extremity in internal rotation should be avoided for the first 4 to 6 weeks.* A supervised physiotherapy program is then initiated to regain shoulder motion and strength and to restore function. *Patients, especially the elderly, who have had a chronic posterior dislocation for several months or years and who demonstrate functional use of the extremity with minimal symptoms* can often be successfully treated with observant management.

3. Operative management
   • Open treatment—Techniques for both acute primary anterior dislocations and recurrent anterior instability demonstrate consistently good results, with recurrence rates under 5%. Direct repair of any Bankart lesions and capsulorrhaphy are carried out depending on the surgical findings. Displaced tuberosity fractures are also addressed and internally fixed with screws or sutures as needed.
   • Arthroscopic treatment—Arthroscopic stabilization techniques for acute, traumatic, first-time anterior dislocations in young patients have been performed with satisfactory results in experienced hands. *In patients who sustain an acute anterior dislocation that requires a manual reduction, a Perthes-Bankart lesion (avulsion of the anterior capsulolabral complex rather than an isolated labrum detachment [Bankart]) will be observed in 80% to 95% of patients.* Patients under 25 years of age with acute Bankart lesions, hemarthrosis, good soft-tissue quality, and a lack of undue capsular stretching obtain favorable results after arthroscopic methods. Moreover, candidates for such treatment should have high activity demands that they are unwilling to modify after treatment, have no prior shoulder instability, and have no associated fractures or neurologic injuries. Conversely, patients with generalized ligamentous laxity, recurrent instability with capsular stretching, and large Hill-Sachs lesions are best treated with open (not arthroscopic) methods. Arthroscopic treatment using bioabsorbable devices for direct labral repair and/or capsulorrhaphy yields successful results in experienced hands. While arthroscopic transglenoid fixation has been commonly used in the past, this technique has been supplanted more recently by direct repair using suture anchors. Recent data suggests that newer techniques using suture anchors affords improved outcomes with fewer complications when compared to transglenoid repairs. Decreased recurrence rates after arthroscopic stabilization have been reported; however, in some series, failure rates have been as high as 40%. Therefore, proper patient selection and sufficient experience with arthroscopic techniques necessitates good functional results.

Complications associated with transglenoid fixation include articular cartilage and suprascapular nerve injuries. The suprascapular nerve is vulnerable as it traverses the spinoglenoid notch. At this level, the nerve has already innervated the supraspinatus muscle and begins to branch, supplying the infraspinatus muscle. *An improperly directed transglenoid pin (too horizontal) can impale the nerve causing partial or complete denervation of the infraspinatus muscle.*

E. Anatomic Considerations and Surgical Techniques
1. Introduction—Numerous properties contribute to the stability of the glenohumeral joint. Abnormalities in any of these structures or properties may predispose a patient to an instability event or may be the consequence of a traumatic episode. No one essential lesion is associated with all instability patterns. Therefore, a broad approach with consideration of osseous, labral, and capsular injuries should be used. Rotator cuff and neural function must also be evaluated.
2. Osseous factors (Fig. 19-6)—The glenoid articulates with approximately 25% to 30% of the humeral head at any given arm position. Gross and radiographic inspection of a normal joint suggests an apparently flat glenoid and a larger, convex humeral head. However, the radius of curvature of the glenoid closely approximates that of the humeral head (*conformity*), and the differences observed represent a mismatch in the surface areas of the two articular surfaces (*constraint*). *Thus, the minimally constrained architecture affords the glenohumeral joint a wide arc of motion at the expense of inherent stability.*
3. Negative intraarticular pressure—A slightly negative intraarticular pressure is present in the glenohumeral joint. Moreover, the joint is

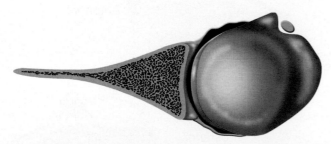

FIGURE 19-6   The bony glenoid is relatively flat; the articular cartilage is thinner in the center and thicker at the periphery. The articular cartilage of the humeral head is thicker in the center and thinner in the periphery.

a sealed compartment with a limited volume, and distraction of the joint increases its negative pressure, resisting further displacement. This concept is analogous to pulling on the plunger of a plugged syringe. It is generally accepted that the negative-pressure effect provides restraint at low loads or at rest, since the forces generated in the shoulder with muscle activity far exceed those provided by this property. *The negative-pressure effect acts to limit inferior translation in the adducted arm at rest.*

4. Glenoid labrum (Fig. 19-7)—The glenoid labrum is a fibrous ring that encompasses the glenoid and serves as an anchor point for the glenohumeral ligaments and biceps tendon. *It extends the load bearing area of the glenoid and increases its depth as much as 50%.* An intact superior labrum stabilizes the shoulder by increasing its ability to withstand external rotation forces by an additional 32%. *Tears of the superior labrum anterior and posterior (SLAP lesions) increases the strain on the inferior glenohumeral ligament by greater than 100%.*

5. Glenohumeral ligaments (Fig. 19-8)—The glenohumeral ligaments have been described as areas of thickening within the joint capsule. They act as static restraints to excessive translation and rotation at the extremes of motion. Much of their function has been learned through biomechanical testing and selective sectioning in anatomic specimens.

   • Superior glenohumeral and coracohumeral ligaments—The superior glenohumeral and coracohumeral ligaments lie within the rotator interval, which is bordered by the superior aspect of the subscapularis and the anterior aspect of the supraspinatus. The superior glenohumeral ligament is variable in size and course. These structures act as a static restraint to excessive inferior translation in the adducted arm. Other potential functions include limitation of external rotation in the adducted arm and restraint against excessive posterior translation in the flexed, adducted, and internally rotated arm.

   • Middle glenohumeral ligament—The middle glenohumeral ligament is part of the anterior capsule and typically courses past the intraarticular portion of the subscapularis tendon at an acute angle. It may be absent in up to 30% of individuals and can demonstrate a sheet-like or cord type of morphology. It functions as a primary restraint against

FIGURE 19-7 The inferior glenoid labrum can be thought of as a wedge (chock) preventing a wheel (the humeral head) from rolling downhill.

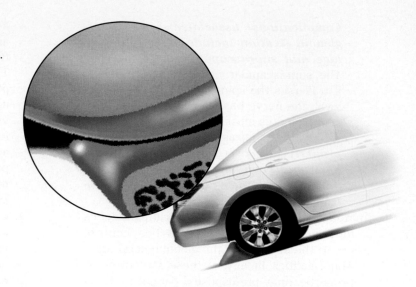

anterior instability of the partially abducted arm and a secondary restraint to inferior instability in the adducted arm.

• Inferior glenohumeral ligament complex— The inferior glenohumeral ligament complex consists of an anterior band, posterior band, and an interposed axillary pouch. This complex lies at the inferior aspect of the glenohumeral joint and remains lax in the adducted arm. In the abducted arm, the complex becomes taut and supports the humeral head in a hammock-type fashion in which the axillary pouch cradles the humeral head directly inferiorly and the anterior and posterior bands provide stability against excessive anterior and posterior humeral translations, respectively. ***The anterior band of the***

inferior glenohumeral ligament is the primary stabilizer against anterior instability in the abducted and externally rotated arm (see Fig. 19-8).

6. Rotator Cuff—The rotator cuff is made up of four muscles that act through coordinated and synchronous action to provide dynamic stability to the glenohumeral joint. The muscles' close proximity to the center of rotation of the joint makes them well suited to maintain a stable glenohumeral fulcrum during active motion of the arm. Dynamic stability is achieved through direct joint compression in addition to asymmetric contraction and "steering" of the humeral head into the glenoid during active arm movement. Compression is achieved by the perpendicular vector pull of the humeral

FIGURE 19-8 Glenohumeral ligaments in the abducted arm. Note the reciprocal tightening of the inferior glenohumeral ligament complex (both the posterior band of the inferior glenohumeral ligament and the anterior band of the inferior glenohumeral ligament tighten) and the relative loosening of the superior and middle glenohumeral ligaments.

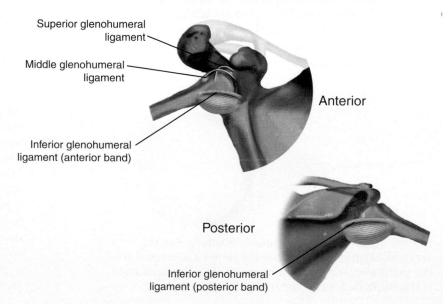

head into the glenoid, which minimizes tendencies toward joint subluxation. The infraspinatus and the smaller teres minor muscles are the primary external rotators of the humerus. The supraspinatus and subscapularis muscles contribute to arm abduction and internal rotation, respectively.

7. Anatomic course of the axillary nerve—The proximity of the axillary nerve to the glenohumeral capsule predisposes the nerve to injury through both traumatic and iatrogenic mechanisms. Open shoulder operations that require anterior capsulotomy can result in inadvertent injury to the nerve if care is not taken to identify its location and protect it during dissection. Posterior approaches to the shoulder, which are utilized infrequently, may also result in nerve injury if dissection is mistakenly carried out in the interval between the teres minor and major.

The axillary nerve takes a circuitous path before innervating the deltoid and teres minor muscles. It arises from the posterior cord of the brachial plexus and courses across the inferolateral border of the subscapularis approximately 3 to 5 mm medial to the musculotendinous junction. It passes inferior to the glenohumeral axillary recess and along with the posterior humeral circumflex artery, exits the quadrangular space, where it divides into two branches. The posterior branch splits and innervates the teres minor and posterior deltoid before terminating as the superior lateral cutaneous nerve. The anterior branch winds around the humerus and innervates the remaining deltoid muscle. It becomes subfascial and intramuscular at a point between the anterior and middle heads of the deltoid.

8. Bankart reconstruction—The Bankart repair can be performed through an inferior axillary incision. The deltopectoral interval is developed and the cephalic vein mobilized. The subscapularis tendon is divided medial to its insertion on the lesser tuberosity and is dissected from the underlying capsule. Care is taken to preserve the anterior humeral circumflex vessels at the junction of the upper two-thirds and lower one-third of the subscapularis. The capsular incision can be laterally based adjacent to the humeral head or medially based at the glenoid margin. On exposure of the joint, transosseous repair of labral detachments can be accomplished, and glenoid rim fractures, if present, can be reduced and internally fixed. Capsulorrhaphy or capsular shift is also carried out in cases in which redundancy of the capsule is noted.

9. Capsular reconstruction—Avulsion of the glenohumeral ligaments and joint capsule from their humeral insertion can lead to recurrent instability. This injury is found less frequently than Bankart lesions and was reported in 7% of patients undergoing surgery for recurrent instability. Patients tended to be older, on average, than those with instability for other causes. *Diagnosis can be made by MRI, and open repair of the lateral joint capsule disruption has been successful in preventing recurrent symptoms.*

F. Complications of the Injury
1. Recurrence—*Age at the time of the initial dislocation appears to be the most important determinant in predicting the likelihood of recurrence.* Reports on the frequency of recurrence fall within a variable range. *First-time dislocators under the age of 20 demonstrate the highest recurrence rate, with frequencies ranging up to 95%.* Patients 20 to 25 years of age have demonstrated recurrence rates of 28% to 75%. Patients older than 25 have recurrence rates less than 50%, and persons over the age of 40 demonstrate recurrence rates less than 10%. *However, a rotator cuff tear is the most common cause of recurrent instability following first time dislocations in patients over 40 years of age.* While the incidence of recurrence does not seem to be affected by the type and duration of immobilization after the initial dislocation, some recent data suggests that there may be a role for short-term immobilization of the arm in external rotation for first time anterior dislocators (this position may better reduce a torn anteroinferior labrum to the glenoid neck).

2. Arthrofibrosis—Arthrofibrosis is more likely to develop in patients over 30 years of age. Inadequate rehabilitation, poor patient compliance, and the degree of trauma at the time of injury are all factors predisposing to joint stiffness.

III. Other Traumatic Soft-Tissue Injuries of the Shoulder
A. Rotator Cuff Tears—*Acute rotator cuff tears can occur after a fall directly onto the shoulder or outstretched upper extremity*, sudden extreme hyperextension or hyperabduction, lifting a heavy object, or catching a heavy falling object. Subsequent swelling and ecchymosis in the upper arm can often develop. In younger patients, a small avulsion fracture of the greater tuberosity may be present as the insertion of the

supraspinatus to the greater tuberosity is robust and typically less prone to failure than the osseous greater tuberosity itself. ***Patients typically develop acute pain and a precipitous loss of function with either difficulty or an inability to elevate the arm.*** Those patients demonstrating significant loss of function are best treated with surgical repair of the rotator cuff. ***Initial postoperative management in the immediate postoperative period includes passive forward elevation and external rotation within a safe zone determined at surgery.*** Early active range of motion or resistive exercises increases the risk of failure of the tendon repair.

Patients with chronic massive rotator cuff tears may have pain with variability in observed shoulder function. Those with long-standing tears may demonstrate functional use of the arm with sufficient compensatory action of the remaining intact rotator cuff and surrounding musculature. If there is significant extension of a supraspinatus tear into the posterior rotator cuff (infrasplnatus) or concomitant tearing of the subscapularis anteriorly, then considerable loss of shoulder strength and function can be anticipated. Cephalad migration of the humeral head relative to the glenoid may ensue. In these patients, the coracoacromial ligament acts as a static secondary restraint to further cephalad and anterior migration of the humeral head. ***If attempts at surgical repair are undertaken and the rotator cuff is found to be irreparable, then in addition to debridement, the coracoacromial ligament should be preserved. Moreover, patients with shoulder pain, irreparable rotator cuff tears, cephalad migration of the humeral head and glenohumeral arthritis are best treated with a humeral head arthroplasty.***

Arthroscopic techniques for repair of large rotator cuff tears include single or double row repairs with the use of suture anchors and attempts at restoration of the anatomic footprint of the torn tendon onto the greater tuberosity of the humerus. After carrying out soft-tissue releases, as in open techniques, initial side-to-side closure of large L-shaped or U-shaped tears (margin convergence) is recommended. ***Margin convergence decreases the size of the overall tendon defect and also decreases the stress in the rotator cuff at the free margin and greater tuberosity interface.***

B. Tears of the Superior Glenoid Labrum—Tears of the superior labrum can occur after a direct fall onto the involved extremity resulting in either traction or compression forces to the glenohumeral joint. Repetitive stress such as pitching can also progressively toggle the superior labrum from the glenoid neck (like extracting a root from the ground by repetitively pulling it from side to side rather than straight up). The superior labrum serves as the anchor for the long head of the biceps tendon that in turn is attached to the superior glenoid neck. Several types of superior labrum tears have been described that range from isolated tears of the superior labrum to those also involving the anterior and posterior labrum and/or capsule with associated instability (Fig. 19-9). ***T2 weighted MRI findings may show increased signal between the superior labrum and glenoid neck.***

C. Tears of the Pectoralis Major Tendon—Tears of the pectoralis major tendon are relatively uncommon and can occur after a fall that causes excessive eccentric contraction of the muscle. Use of anabolic steroids can predispose patients to tendon rupture and this possibility should be considered. Typical findings in acute cases include deformity of the anterior axillary fold, weakness in internal rotation and adduction and ecchymosis of the upper arm. ***The treatment of choice in young patients is open exploration and surgical repair.*** Tears occurring within the pectoralis muscle or at the myotendinous junction are best treated nonsurgically and the diagnosis can be confirmed by MRI.

D. Dislocation of the Long Head of the Biceps Tendon—The biceps tendon is supported within the bicipital groove by the medial aspect of the subscapularis tendon, the transverse ligament and coracohumeral ligament-superior glenohumeral ligament pulley. ***Medial dislocation of the tendon can occur with an injury to these supporting structures that lie in the region of the rotator interval. Patients with a rupture of the subscapularis tendon and dislocation of the long head of the biceps are best treated with primary repair of the subscapularis and tenodesis of the biceps.***

E. Latissimus Dorsi Injury—Tears of the latissimus dorsi tendon have been reported as a cause of pain in the thrower's shoulder. The mechanism of injury involves an eccentric overload during the follow-through phase of throwing. ***Tenderness along the posterior axillary fold and pain and weakness with resisted extension of the shoulder can be found on physical examination in patients with complete tears of the latissimus dorsi tendon.*** Current treatment recommendations are nonoperative and include a short period of rest, followed by physical therapy.

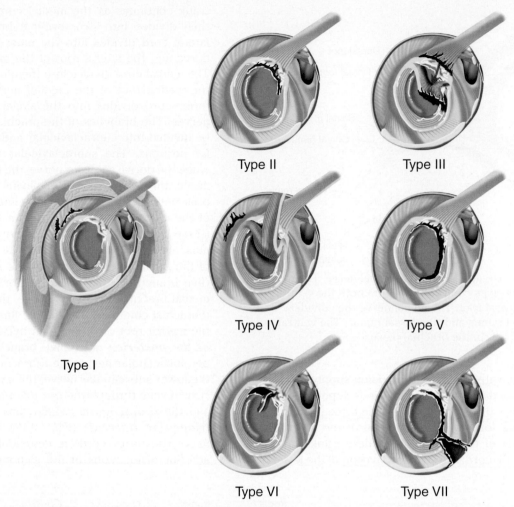

Type II   Type III

Type IV   Type V

Type I

Type VI   Type VII

FIGURE 19-9 Types of Superior Glenoid Labrum Tears. **Type I**. Lesion is characterized by fraying or degeneration of the superior labrum and a normal biceps tendon. **Type II**. Notable for detachment of the superior labrum and biceps anchor from the superior rim of the glenoid. **Type III**. There is a bucket handle tear of the superior labrum with an intact biceps anchor. **Type IV**. There is a bucket handle tear of the superior labrum with tearing of the biceps tendon. **Type V**. There is a type II detachment that also extends into the anterior labrum. **Type VI**. There is a type II detachment with a parrot beak or flap tear of the labrum. **Type VII**. There is a type II detachment with extension into the middle glenohumeral ligament.

F. Biceps Brachii Transection—***Transection of the biceps brachii muscle has been reported and can occur as a result of a cord wrapped around the upper arm***. A posterior subcutaneous hematoma can be found on physical examination and confirmed on MRI. Patients should be evaluated for concurrent neurovascular injury.

IV. Brachial Plexus Injuries
A. Overview—Trauma to the brachial plexus involves a spectrum of injuries that varies in both the extent and degree of neurologic compromise. Less severe injuries may result in isolated sensory abnormalities. Higher-energy mechanisms can produce significant motor deficits and loss of functional use of the arm. An understanding

of brachial plexus anatomy aids in the clinical evaluation of these lesions and allows the development of appropriate treatment strategies.
B. Anatomy (Figs. 19-10 and 19-11)—This complex of nerves extends from the cervical spine into the axilla, supplying motor, sensory, and sympathetic nerve fibers to the upper limb. The brachial plexus is formed by the ventral rami (Fig. 19-10) of nerves from C5 to T1, which lie between the scalenus anterior and medius muscles. The ventral rami from C5 and C6 unite to form the upper trunk of the brachial plexus. The ventral ramus of C7 continues as the middle trunk, and the ventral rami of C8 and T1 form the lower trunk of the brachial plexus. Each of the trunks divides into anterior and posterior divisions behind the

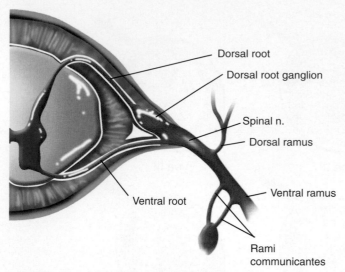

FIGURE 19-10 Organization of the spinal nerve. The spinal nerve receives contributions from both the ventral root and the dorsal root. The spinal nerve then divides into the ventral ramus and the dorsal ramus. The ventral rami of C5 to T1 form the brachial plexus.

clavicle, with the anterior division supplying the flexors and the posterior divisions supplying the extensors of the upper limb. The three posterior divisions form the posterior cord; the anterior divisions of the upper and middle trunks form the lateral cord; the anterior division of the lower

trunk continues as the medial cord. Each cord then divides into two terminal branches. The lateral cord divides into the musculocutaneous nerve and the lateral root of the median nerve. The medial cord divides into the ulnar nerve and the medial root of the median nerve. The posterior cord divides into the axillary and radial nerves. The branches of the brachial plexus can be divided into supraclavicular and infraclavicular portions. The supraclavicular branches include the dorsal scapular nerve, the long thoracic nerve, the nerve to the subclavius, and the suprascapular nerve. The infraclavicular branches of the cords include *those of the lateral cord* (three branches): the lateral pectoral nerve, the musculocutaneous nerve, and the lateral root of the median nerve; *those of the medial cord* (five branches): the medial pectoral nerve, the medial brachial cutaneous nerve, the medial antebrachial cutaneous nerve, the ulnar nerve, and the medial root of the median nerve; and *those of the posterior cord* (five branches): the upper subscapular nerve, the thoracodorsal nerve, the lower subscapular nerve, the *axillary nerve* (which runs through the *quadrangular space*), and the *radial nerve* (which runs through the *triangular interval*) (Fig. 19-12). The axillary nerve (posterior cord) is commonly injured in anterior dislocations of the glenohumeral joint.

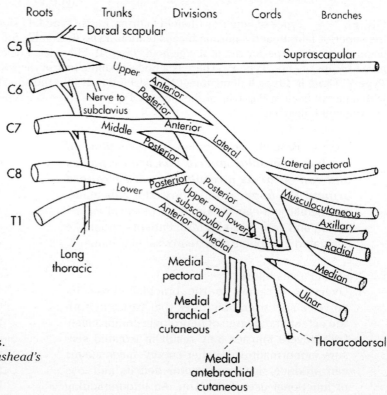

FIGURE 19-11 Organization of the brachial plexus. (Reprinted with permission from Jenkins DB. *Hollinshead's Functional Anatomy of the Limbs and Back*. 7th ed. Philadelphia, PA: WB Saunders; 1998.)

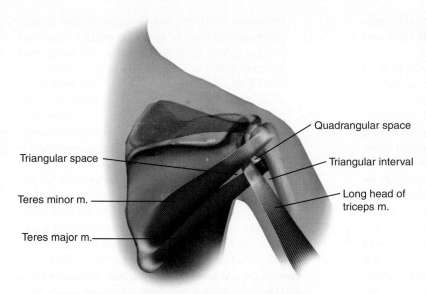

FIGURE 19-12 Important anatomic relationships. The ***quadrangular space*** is bordered by the teres minor (superiorly), the teres major (inferiorly), the long head of the triceps (medially), and the proximal humerus (laterally). The posterior humeral circumflex vessels and axillary nerve pass through this space. The ***triangular space*** is bordered by the teres minor (superiorly), the teres major (inferiorly), and the long head of the triceps (laterally). It contains the circumflex scapular vessels. The ***triangular interval***, bordered by the teres major (superiorly), the long head of the triceps (medially), and the humerus (laterally), allows visualization of the profunda brachii artery and radial nerve.

Severe stretch injuries to the lower portions of the brachial plexus (C8 and T1) can result in ***injury to preganglionic (proximal to the dorsal root ganglion) sympathetic fibers*** for head and neck innervation to the spinal nerves and stellate ganglion, resulting in ptosis, anhidrosis, and papillary dilation ***(Horner's syndrome). Penetrating wounds to the axilla resulting in interosseous wasting and hand weakness are likely secondary to injuries to the inferior trunk emanating from the C8 and T1 nerve roots and giving rise to the ulnar nerve.***

C. Evaluation

   1. Mechanism of injury—The majority of closed injuries occur as a result of inferior-directed traction applied to the superior aspect of the shoulder. The head and shoulder are forcefully separated, placing undue traction on the brachial plexus. Motorcycle accidents are one common mechanism for such injuries.

   2. Types of injuries
      - Root avulsion—A root avulsion represents a central nervous system injury and carries a poor prognosis. To date, there is no reliable method of restoring continuity and function of the nerve root to its avulsed portion of the spinal cord.
      - Supraclavicular peripheral nerve injuries— The injury occurs distal to the nerve root (commonly in the supraclavicular fossa). This category carries a more favorable prognosis compared with a nerve root avulsion. Because this represents a peripheral nervous system injury, surgical exploration and repair with possible nerve grafting

represents one option that may afford an improved outlook for functional recovery.

- Infraclavicular peripheral nerve injuries— The brachial plexus may be vulnerable to injury in its infraclavicular region by direct compression or pressure from fracture fragments or joint dislocations. The mechanism typically involves lower-energy events as compared with those seen in the supraclavicular cases. Accordingly, the injuries tend to be more confined and of a lesser degree of severity. They carry a relatively better prognosis than the supraclavicular injuries.

- Burners (stingers)—Burners or stingers represent a transient injury to the brachial plexus that typically occurs during contact sports. Sports such as American football and wrestling commonly give rise to this injury. The head and neck are characteristically impacted or moved to one side resulting in a stretch and/or compression to the brachial plexus. Sharp pain, radiating from the neck to hand, with burning, numbness, tingling, and weakness may occur. ***Unilateral arm symptoms are typical.*** The symptoms usually last for seconds to minutes in most patients and can persist for days in 5% to 10% of cases. Recurrent episodes may be associated with cervical spinal stenosis. Initial treatment includes removal from contact sports until symptoms have completely resolved. Persistent weakness, neck pain, bilateral symptoms, or recurrent episodes require further evaluation that may include radiographs, MRI, and neurologic testing.

Uncomplicated cases benefit from strengthening and conditioning of the cervical and shoulder musculature.

3. Physical examination—Careful evaluation of all upper-extremity muscle groups, including the shoulder, helps determine the location and extent of the injury. ***Physical examination may demonstrate a flail arm; however, the presence or absence of rhomboid (dorsal scapular nerve) and serratus anterior (long thoracic nerve) activity should be carefully noted.*** Absence of function of the rhomboids (major and minor) and the serratus anterior, in addition to absence of function of the rotator cuff and deltoid, suggests a nerve root avulsion (the long thoracic and dorsal scapular nerves arise from the proximal trunks of the plexus where the spinal nerves exit the intervertebral foramina). Presence of function of the rhomboids and the serratus anterior muscles suggests a more peripheral lesion distal to the innervation of these muscles.

4. Electrodiagnostic studies—Electromyography (EMG) and nerve conduction tests performed at least 1 month after the injury may help further delineate the extent and location of the plexus injury. A myelogram with a follow-up CT scan can also help determine the presence of a nerve root avulsion.

D. Prognosis

1. Root avulsions—Root avulsions of the upper trunk are fortunately rare and carry a bleak chance of spontaneous functional recovery. Surgical reconstruction of root avulsions is not possible, and fusion of the glenohumeral joint for the management of a flail arm is generally unsuccessful because of the loss of function of important scapular stabilizers.

2. Upper-trunk injuries—injuries involving the upper trunk commonly occur proximal to the suprascapular nerve origin. Loss of function of the supraspinatus and posterior rotator cuff as well as the deltoid muscle can be expected with a resultant loss in the ability to elevate the arm. Moreover, treatment of injuries of the upper trunk fare better with regard to return of elbow flexion than to restoration of functional shoulder activity. In general, the prognosis for adult brachial plexus injuries is not as promising as that typically described for birth palsies.

3. Guidelines—Consideration of some general guidelines can help categorize various injuries with respect to prognosis. The prognosis for distal injuries is more favorable than that for proximal injuries. The prognosis for incomplete motor loss is more favorable than that for complete motor loss, and the prognosis for a confined or focal injury is more favorable than that for a broader injury (the incidence of neuropraxia is higher in the more focal injuries). If there is no clinical or electrodiagnostic evidence of recovery within 9 months, the prognosis for significant improvement remains poor.

E. Treatment—Treatment strategies should be tailored to each patient based on specific clinical findings. Initial management should include functional splinting and physical therapy to minimize the potential for joint contractures while maintaining functional arcs of motion. If surgical management may benefit the patient, consideration can be given to nerve exploration and repair with possible grafting, muscle transfers, and arthrodesis. Operative treatment is best performed before 6 months following injury have elapsed. Beyond 6 months, irreversible changes in the muscles begin to occur, further decreasing the chance of significant functional recovery. Most patients with traction injuries undergoing nerve exploration require nerve grafting, since primary repair of the neural elements is typically not possible. Results after such procedures can be unpredictable and depend on the nature and extent of the injury. Multiple tendon transfers have been described in an attempt to restore elbow flexion and shoulder function. Such transfers offer a viable alternative to neural reconstructions, which have yielded unpredictable results in adult traumatic injuries. Transfers of the pectoralis major, trapezius, biceps, triceps, teres major, and latissimus dorsi have all been reported. Treatment should be tailored to an individual's specific clinical findings. Glenohumeral arthrodesis for a flail arm remains a viable treatment option in attempt to restore some degree of upper extremity function and minimize painful subluxation of the joint. Neural innervation of the scapular stabilizers (trapezius and serratus anterior) should be protected from injury if reasonable function is to be expected after surgery. ***Fusion of the glenohumeral joint should be in 30° of arm abduction, 20° of forward flexion, and 40° of internal rotation.*** In a healthy individual, the ratio of glenohumeral to scapulothoracic motion during elevation of the arm is approximately 2:1.

V. Long Thoracic Nerve Palsy

A. Overview—Injury to the long thoracic nerve results in paralysis of the serratus anterior muscle

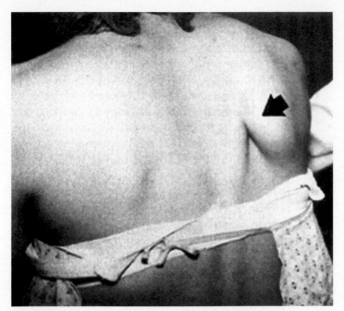

FIGURE 19-13 Clinical example of scapular winging (*arrow*) in a patient with along thoracic nerve palsy. (From Miller MD, Cooper DE, Warner JJP. *Review of Sports Medicine and Arthroscopy*. Philadelphia, PA: WB Saunders; 1996, with permission.)

and is clinically manifested by the presence of shoulder pain, scapular winging (Fig. 19-13), and difficulty in arm elevation. Causes are multiple and in addition to trauma include mechanical, toxic, and infectious etiologies. Up to 15% of cases are of unknown etiology. Nerve compression as a result of anterior scapular motion or traction associated with posterior scapular movement is felt to be responsible, in part, for injury to the relatively unprotected nerve at the inferior angle of the scapula in susceptible individuals.

B. Treatment—Although the majority of cases of isolated palsy of the long thoracic nerve resolve within 12 months, a few patients fail to improve with expectant management. Surgery can be considered in patients who continue to have symptoms refractory to conservative measures with no evidence of spontaneous recovery. Transfer of the pectoralis major tendon (extended with a fascia lata graft) to the inferior pole of the scapula has demonstrated consistently good results in most cases. Opinions differ as to the optimal time for operation after the initial neurologic insult; however, it is generally recommended that surgery be delayed for at least 6 to 12 months. Consideration should be given to the mechanism of injury, residual symptoms, functional deficit, physical demands, and electrodiagnostic

studies before operative management is contemplated. Nerve exploration and reconstruction might be considered as an alternate surgical option; however, poor accessibility of the long thoracic nerve, extended time involved between the injury and ultimate anticipated return of nerve function, and the uncertain return of serratus activity can add significant morbidity and likely exceed the potential pitfalls of pectoralis major transfer.

VI. Quadrangular Space Syndrome—Quadrangular space syndrome represents an uncommon entity; the diagnosis is often difficult to make and is also frequently overlooked.

A. Anatomy—The **quadrangular space** is bordered superiorly and inferiorly by the teres minor and major, respectively. The humeral shaft and the long head of the triceps make up the lateral and medial borders, respectively (see Fig. 19-12). Both the posterior humeral circumflex artery and axillary nerve travel through the quadrangular space, where they may be subject to abnormal compression.

B. Evaluation

1. Signs and symptoms—Symptoms of poorly localized shoulder pain, paresthesias not necessarily of a dermatomal distribution, and focal tenderness overlying the quadrilateral space characterize the disorder. Symptoms may be exacerbated with forward flexion or abduction and external rotation of the arm. Clinically, deltoid weakness or atrophy is not always present, since pain may precede any objective decrease in deltoid strength or mass. Furthermore, such findings can demonstrate considerable variability among individuals and are likely related to the degree and duration of nerve compression. Individuals between 22 and 35 years of age are typically afflicted, and symptoms may be mistaken for thoracic outlet syndrome or other shoulder disorders. This disorder has also been observed in throwing athletes with shoulder pain and paresthesia.

2. Diagnostic studies—Diagnostic studies may include electrodiagnostic tests, arteriograms, and MRI. The role of arteriography is not clearly established but can be of value in selected cases. Occlusion of the posterior humeral circumflex artery may be evident when the arm is abducted and externally rotated. Positive findings on arteriography provide indirect evidence of neuropathy as the axillary nerve exits the quadrangular space with the

posterior humeral circumflex artery. Electro-diagnostic studies are helpful in confirming the presence of axillary nerve compression when results are positive; however, a negative EMG does not preclude the diagnosis. A few patients have quadrangular space syndrome despite normal EMG findings. MRI, although expensive, can provide useful information, especially when the diagnosis is equivocal. MRI can help rule out alternate sources of shoulder pain and also may aid in revealing early deltoid atrophy, which is not otherwise discernable on clinical examination.

C. Treatment—Considering the infrequency of the diagnosis and the fact that many patients do not demonstrate sufficient symptoms to warrant neurolysis, only a few individuals ultimately require surgical intervention. Patients with clinical evidence of this syndrome in the absence of deltoid denervation or dysfunction may benefit from activity modification and stretching exercises alone. Those with symptoms refractory to conservative measures or manifestations of deltoid denervation and positive findings on EMG or arteriography should be considered as candidates for nerve decompression. Optimal timing of surgical decompression becomes difficult to outline in consideration of the variable stages of presentation and the indeterminate natural history of this disorder. However, nerve exploration before 6 months from the time of injury is generally preferred, since it may minimize the potential for irreversible changes within the deltoid muscle and axillary nerve. Surgical decompression of the axillary nerve can be adequately achieved through a posterior approach without detachment of the deltoid origin from the scapular spine. With the arm in abduction, the posterior border of the deltoid can be easily identified and gently retracted cephalad to expose the underlying quadrangular space. Care should be taken to avoid injury to the posterior humeral circumflex artery on exploration. Satisfactory results have been reported in the majority of patients after the use of an extensile surgical approach.

VII. Thoracic Outlet Syndrome
   A. Overview—Thoracic outlet syndrome is typically characterized by neurologic symptoms radiating along the upper extremity that can include pain, numbness, tingling, burning and weakness. Hand or arm swelling and aching along the neck or shoulder can also occur. Symptoms may be aggravated with arm elevation and occur as a result of compression of the neurovascular structures as they travel through a narrowed thoracic outlet. Venous compression occurs in 2% to 3% of cases and arterial compression occurs in 1% to 2% of cases. Contributing factors include obesity, poor posture, cervical muscular contracture, trauma, pregnancy or congenital factors (cervical rib). Possible sites of compression include: (a) the superior thoracic outlet secondary to the presence of a cervical rib; (b) *the scalene interval, formed by the scalene anterior and middle attachments onto the first rib (this can be a site of compression of the subclavian vein or surrounding neurovascular structures through scalene muscle hypertrophy in well-developed athletes)*; (c) the costoclavicular space, or interval between the first rib and the clavicle (this can be narrowed secondary to inferior depression of the clavicle by factors including hypertrophy of the subclavius muscle, clavicle fracture with callus formation, and muscular weakness resulting in drooping or downward depression of the upper extremity); and (d) the subcoracoid region (the final potential site for compression prior to the neurovascular structures entering the axilla).

   B. Evaluation—Diagnosis can be elusive as symptoms are often vague and physical signs are indistinct. Affected patients typically show signs of lower brachial plexus involvement involving C8 and T1. Symptoms include paresthesias along the medial aspect of the arm and hand and loss of fine motor hand dexterity. Provocative tests such as the Adson test (loss of radial pulse with the arm at the side and with extension and rotation of the head and neck to the involved side) and Wright hyperabduction test (loss of pulse with arm abduction to 90° and external rotation) require the reproduction of symptoms to be considered positive. Diagnostic studies may include cervical radiographs to evaluate the presence or absence of a cervical rib and MRI exams to evaluate the anatomy and course of the brachial plexus. Noninvasive vascular studies and angiography may also be of benefit to assess arterial and venous patency. Lastly, electrodiagnostic studies may aid in assessing nerve compression and help in establishing the diagnosis.

   C. Treatment—Treatment is directed at reducing compression at the thoracic outlet. Stretching exercises to minimize contractures at the thoracic outlet and cervical and shoulder strengthening aimed at improving posture can be helpful. Carrying heavy objects over the shoulder should be avoided to minimize further outlet compression. Surgery is indicated for refractory cases with significant pain that have failed conservative treatment and that demonstrate a discernible neurologic deficit or vascular compromise. Isolated first rib resection, anterior scalenotomy or both procedures combined have been performed with varied success and recurrence rates.

SUGGESTED READINGS

Classic Articles

Cofield RH, Briggs BT. Glenohumeral arthrodesis: operative and long-term functional results. *J Bone Joint Surg.* 1979;61A:668–677.

Colachis SC, Strohm BR, Brechner VL. Effects of axillary nerve block on muscle force in the upper extremity. *Arch Phys Med Rehabil.* 1969;50:647–654.

Dehne E, Hall RM. Active shoulder motion in complete deltoid paralysis. *J Bone Joint Surg.* 1959;41-A:745–748.

Gerber C, Schneeberger AG, Vinh TS. The arterial vascularization of the humeral head: an anatomical study. *J Bone Joint Surg.* 1990;72A:1486–1494.

Hawkins RJ, Neer CS. A functional analysis of shoulder fusions. *Clin Orthop.* 1987;223:65–76.

Howell SM, Galinat BJ, Renzi AJ, et al. Normal and Abnormal mechanics of the glenohumeral joint in the horizontal plane. *J Bone Joint Surg.* 1988;70-A:227–232.

Howell SM, Imobersteg AM, Seger D, et al. Clarification of the role of the supraspinatus muscle in shoulder function. *J Bone Joint Surg.* 1986;68A:398–404.

Itoh Y, Sasaki T, Ishiguro T, et al. Transfer of latissimus dorsi to replace a paralysed anterior deltoid. *J Bone Joint Surg.* 1987;69-B:647–651.

Kumar VP, Balasubramaniam P. The role of atmospheric pressure in stabilizing the shoulder. *J Bone Joint Surg.* 1985;67-B:719–721.

McLaughlin HL, Cavallaro WU. Primary anterior dislocation of the shoulder. *Am J Surg.* 1950;80:615–621.

Neer CS 2nd. Displaced proximal humerus fractures: II. Treatment of three- and four-part displacement. *J Bone Joint Surg.* 1970;52A:1090–1103.

Neviaser RJ, Neviaser TJ, Neviaser JS. Concurrent rupture of the rotator cuff and anterior dislocation of the shoulder in the older patient. *J Bone Joint Surg.* 1988;70A:1308–1311.

Poppen NK, Walker PS. Normal and abnormal motion of the shoulder. *J Bone Joint Surg.* 1976;58A: 195–201.

Poppen NK, Walker PS. Forces at the glenohumeral joint in abduction. *Clin Orthop.* 1978;135: 165–170.

Rowe CR. Prognosis in dislocations of the shoulder. *J Bone Joint Surg.* 1956;38-A:957–977.

Rowe CR. Re-evaluation of the position of the arm in arthrodesis of the shoulder in the adult. *J Bone Joint Surg.* 1974;56A:913.

Snyder SJ, Wuh HCK. Arthroscopic evaluation and treatment of the rotator cuff and superior labrum anterior posterior lesion. *Op Tech Orthop.* 1991;1:207–220.

Staples OS, Watkins AL. Full active abduction in traumatic paralysis of the deltoid. *J Bone Joint Surg.* 1943;25:85–89.

Turkel SJ, Panio MW, Marshall JL, et al. Stabilizing mechanisms preventing anterior dislocation of the glenohumeral joint. *J Bone Joint Surg.* 1981;63A:1208–1217.

Recent Articles

Arciero RA, Wheeler JH, Ryan JB, et al. Arthroscopic Bankart repair versus nonoperative treatment for acute, initial anterior shoulder dislocations. *Am J Sports Med.* 1994;22:589–594.

Bigliani LU, Dalsey RM, McCann PD, et al. An anatomical study of the suprascapular nerve. *Arthroscopy.* 1990;6:301–305.

Bigliani LU, Kurzweil PR, Schwartzbach CC, et al. Inferior capsular shift procedure for anterior-inferior shoulder instability in athletes. *Am J Sports Med.* 1994;22:578–584.

Boileau P, Villalba M, Hery JY. Risk factors for recurrence of shoulder instability after arthroscopic Bankart repair. *J Bone Joint Surg.* 2006;88A:1755–1763.

Bokor DJ, Conboy VB, Olson C. Anterior instability of the glenohumeral joint with humeral avulsion of the glenohumeral ligament. A review of 41 cases. *J Bone Joint Surg.* 1999;81B:93–96.

Burkhart SS. A stepwise approach to arthroscopic rotator cuff repair based on biomechanical principles. *Arthroscopy.* 2000;16:82–90.

Burkhead WZ, Scheinberg RR, Box G. Surgical anatomy of the axillary nerve. *J Shoulder Elbow Surg.* 1992;1:31–36.

DeBerardino TM, Arciero RA, Taylor DC, et al. Prospective evaluation of arthroscopic stabilization of acute, initial anterior shoulder dislocations in young athletes: two- to five year follow-up. *Am J Sports Med.* 2001;29:586–592.

Cooper DE, O'Brien SJ, Warren RF. Supporting layers of the glenohumeral joint. An antomic study. *Clin Orthop.* 1993;289:144–155.

Flatow EL, Cuomo F, Maday MG, et al. Open reduction and internal fixation of two-part displaced fractures of the greater tuberosity of the proximal part of the humerus. *J Bone Joint Surg.* 1991;73A:1213–1218.

Flatow EL, Raimundo RA, Kelkar R. Active and passive restraints against superior humeral translation: the contribution of the rotator cuff, the biceps tendon and the coracoacromial arch. *J Shoulder Elbow Surg.* 1996;6:172.

Francel TJ, Dellon AL, Campbell JN. Quadrilateral space syndrome: diagnosis and operative decompression technique. *Plastic Recon Surg.* 1991;87:911–916.

Friedman AH, Nunley JA, Urbaniak JR, et al. Repair of isolated axillary nerve lesions after infraclavicular brachial plexus injuries: case reports. *Neurosurgery.* 1990;27:403–407.

Gerber C, Sebesta A. Impingement of the deep surface of the subscapularis tendon and the reflection pulley on the anterosuperior glenoid rim: a preliminary report. *J Shoulder Elbow Surg.* 2000;9:483–490.

Gibb TD, Sidles JA, Harryman DT, et al. The effect of capsular venting on glenohumeral laxity. *Clin Orthop.* 1991;268:120–127.

Hanna CM, Glenny AB, Stanley SN, et al. Pectoralis major tears: comparison of surgical and conservative treatment. *Br J Sports Med.* 2001;35:202–206.

Harryman DT, Sidles JA, Harris SL, et al. The role of the rotator interval capsule in passive motion and stability of the shoulder. *J Bone and Joint Surg.* 1992;74A:53–66.

Harryman DT, Walker ED, Harris SL, et al. Residual motion and function after glenohumeral or scapulothoracic arthrodesis. *J Shoulder Elbow Surg.* 1993;2:275–285.

Hodgson SA, Mawson SJ, Stanley D. Rehabilitation after two-part fractures of the neck of the humerus. *J Bone Joint Surg.* 2003;85B:419–422.

Hovelius L, Augustini BG, Fredin H, et al. Primary anterior dislocation of the shoulder in young patients. A ten year prospective study. *J Bone Joint Surg.* 1996;78A:1677–1684.

Hovelius L, Olofsson A, Sandstrom B. Nonoperative treatment of primary anterior shoulder dislocation in patients forty years of age and younger. A prospective twenty-five year follow-up. *J Bone Joint Surg.* 2008;90A:945–952.

Iannotti JP, Gabriel JP, Schneck SL, et al. The normal glenohumeral relationships. An anatomical study of one hundred and forty shoulders. *J Bone Joint Surg.* 1992;74A:491–500.

Itoi E, Hatakeyama Y, Sato T, et al. Immobilization in external rotation after shoulder dislocation reduces the risk of recurrence. A randomized controlled trial. *J Bone Joint Surg.* 2007;89A:2124–2131.

Itoi E, Newman SR, Kuechle DK, et al. Dynamic anterior stabilisers of the shoulder with the arm in abduction. *J Bone Joint Surg.* 1994;76B:834–836.

Jakob RP, Miniaci A, Anson PS, et al. Four-part valgus impacted fractures of the proximal humerus. *J Bone Joint Surg.* 1991;73B:295–298.

Jakobsen BW, Johannsen HV, Suder P, et al. Primary repair versus conservative treatment of first-time traumatic anterior dislocation of the shoulder: a randomized study with 10-year follow-up. *Arthroscopy.* 2007;23:118–123.

Kauppila LI. The long thoracic nerve: possible mechanisms of injury based on autopsy study. *J Shoulder Elbow Surg.* 1993;2:244–248.

Killewich LA, Bedford GR, Black KW, et al. Diagnosis of deep venous thrombosis: a prospective study comparing duplex scanning to contrast venography. *Circulation.* 1989;79:810.

Kim SH, Ha KI, Cho YB, et al. Arthroscopic anterior stabilization of the shoulder: two to six year follow-up. *J Bone Joint Surg.* 2003;85A:1511–1518.

Kirley A, Werstine R, Ratjek A, et al. Prospective randomized clinical trial comparing the effectiveness of immediate arthroscopic stabilization versus immobilization and rehabilitation in first traumatic anterior dislocations of the shoulder: long-term evaluation. *Arthroscopy.* 2005;21:55–63.

Koval KJ, Gallagher MA, Marsicano JG, et al. Functional outcome after minimally displaced fractures of the proximal part of the humerus. *J Bone Joint Surg.* 1997;79:203–207.

Maffet MW, Gartsman GM, Moseley B. Superior labrum-biceps tendon complex lesions of the shoulder. *Am J Sports Med.* 1995;23:93–98.

McIlveen SJ, Duralde XA, D'Alessandro DF, et al. Isolated nerve injuries about the shoulder. *Clin Orthop.* 1994;306:54–63.

Neer CS, Satterlee CC, Dalsey RM, et al. The anatomy and potential effects of contracture of the coracohumeral ligament. *Clin Orthop.* 1992;280:182–185.

Neviaser RJ, Neviaser TJ. Recurrent instability of the shoulder after age 40. *J Shoulder Elbow Surg.* 1995;4:416–418.

Otis JC, Jiang CC, Wickiewicz TL, et al. Changes of the moment arms of the rotator cuff and deltoid muscles with abduction and rotation. *J Bone Joint Surg.* 1994;76A:667–676.

Post M. Pectoralis major transfer for winging of the scapula. *J Shoulder Elbow Surg.* 1995;4:1–9.

Resch H, Povacz P, Frohlich R, et al. Percutaneous fixation of three- and four-part fractures of the proximal humerus. *J Bone Joint Surg.* 1997;79B:295–300.

Richards RR, Beaton D, Hudson AR. Shoulder arthrodesis with plate fixation: functional outcome analysis. *J Shoulder Elbow Surg.* 1993;2:225–239.

Robinson CM, Page RS, Hill RM, et al. Primary hemiarthroplasty for treatment of proximal humeral fractures. *J Bone Joint Surg.* 2003;85A:1215–1223.

Rodosky MW, Harner CD, Fu FH. The role of the long head of the biceps muscle and superior glenoid labrum in anterior stability of the shoulder. *Am J Sports Med.* 1994;22:121–130.

Soslowski LJ, Flatow EL, Bigliani LU, et al. Articular geometry of the glenohumeral joint. *Clin Orthop.* 1992;285:182–190.

Taylor DC, Arciero RA. Pathologic changes associated with shoulder dislocations. Arthroscopic and physical examination findings in first-time traumatic anterior dislocations. *Am J Sports Med.* 1997;25:306–311.

Vastamaki M, Kauppila LI. Etiologic factors in isolated paralysis of the serratus anterior muscle: a report of 197 cases. *J Shoulder Elbow Surg.* 1993;2:240–243.

Walch G, Boileau P. Subluxations and dislocations of the tendon of the long head of the biceps. *J Shoulder Elbow Surg.* 1998;7:100–108.

WarnerJP, Micheli LJ, Arslanian LE, et al. Patterns of flexibility, laxity, and strength in normal shoulders and shoulders with instability and impingement. *Am J Sports Med.* 1990;18:366–375.

Warner JP. Frozen shoulder: diagnosis and management. *J Am Acad Orthop Surg.* 1997;5:130–140.

Zuckerman JD, Scott AJ, Gallagher MA. Hemiarthroplasty for cuff tear arthropathy. *J Shoulder Elbow Surg.* 2000;9:169–172.

Review Articles

Blom S, Dahlback LO. Nerve injuries in dislocations of the shoulder joint and fractures of the neck of the humerus. *Acta Chir Scand.* 1970;136:461–466.

Cahill BR, Palmer RE. Quadrilateral space syndrome. *J Hand Surg.* 1983;8-A:65–69.

Leffert RD. Brachial plexus injuries. *N Engl J Med.* 1974;291:1059–1067.

Narakas A. Surgical treatment of traction injuries of the brachial plexus. *Clin Orthop.* 1978;133:71–90.

Textbooks

Arciero RA, Deberardino TM. Acute and chronic dislocations of the shoulder. In: Norris TR, ed. *Orthopaedic Knowledge Update Shoulder and Elbow.* Rosemont, IL: American Academy of Orthopaedic Surgeons; 1997:67–76.

Jobe CM. Gross anatomy of the shoulder. In: Rockwood CA, Matsen FA, eds. *The Shoulder.* Philadelphia, PA: WB Saunders; 1990.

Kozin SH. Injuries of the brachial plexus. In: Iannotti JP, Williams GR, eds. *Disorders of the Shoulder: Diagnosis and Management.* Philadelphia, PA: Lipincott Williams & Wilkins; 1999.

Leffert RD. Neurological problems. In: Rockwood CA, Matsen FA, eds. *The Shoulder.* Philadelphia, PA: WB Saunders; 1990.

Matsen FA, Fu FH, Hawkins RJ, eds. *The Shoulder: A Balance of Mobility and Stability.* Rosemont, IL: American Academy of Orthopaedic Surgeons; 1993.

Matsen FA, Thomas SC, Rockwood CA. Glenohumeral instability. In: Rockwood CA, Matsen FA, eds. *The Shoulder.* Philadelphia, PA: WB Saunders; 1990.

Sher JS, Iannotti JP, Warner JP. Deltoid injuries. In: Warner JP, Iannotti JP, Gerber C, eds. *Complex and Revision Problems in Shoulder Surgery.* Philadelphia, PA: Lippincott Raven; 1997:399–413.

Sher JS, Iannotti JP, Williams GR. Shoulder reconstruction. In: *Orthopaedic Knowledge Update V.* Rosemont, IL: American Academy of Orthopaedic Surgeons; 1996:245–257.

Watson-Jones R. *Fractures and Joint Injuries.* In: Wilson JN, ed. Edinburgh, New York: Churchill Livingstone; 1976.

CHAPTER 20

Fractures of the Humeral Shaft

Robert Probe and Ian Whitney

I. Overview—Humeral shaft fractures represent approximately 3% of all fractures. Multiple treatment options are available and include both operative and nonoperative management. The majority of humeral shaft fractures may be treated via nonsurgical means with a high success rate. Most low-energy fractures may be amenable to closed treatment because of internal soft-tissue splinting and the biologic potential of the humerus. In high-energy fractures, soft-tissue disruption and extensive fracture comminution are frequently observed rendering closed treatment less predictable.

II. Anatomy
   A. Osteology—The humeral shaft can be defined as extending from the pectoralis major insertion proximally to the supracondylar ridge distally. The shaft of the humerus assumes a more triangular shape distally. The anterolateral surface of the humerus contains the deltoid tuberosity as well as the sulcus for the profunda brachii artery and the radial nerve. The spiral groove located on the posterior humeral shaft contains the radial nerve as it passes distally.
   B. Musculature—The humeral musculature is divided by medial and lateral intermuscular septa into anterior and posterior compartments. The triceps brachii muscle fills the posterior compartment. The anterior compartment contains the biceps brachii, the coracobrachialis, and the brachialis muscles. Deforming muscle forces often lead to predictable patterns of fracture displacement. *Fractures that occur between the pectoralis major insertion and the deltoid insertion display adduction of the proximal fragment and lateral displacement of the distal fragment. Humeral shaft fractures distal to the deltoid muscle insertion often result in abduction of the proximal fragment.*

C. Nerves
   1. Musculocutaneous nerve—*The musculocutaneous nerve pierces the coracobrachialis muscle 5 to 8 cm distal to the coracoid process* and then branches to supply the coracobrachialis, the biceps brachii, and the brachialis muscles. It continues distally and becomes the lateral antebrachial cutaneous nerve.
   2. Median nerve—The median nerve accompanies the brachial artery medial to the humeral shaft and crosses lateral to medial (in relation to the artery) in the distal arm. *It lies medial to the artery in the antecubital fossa.*
   3. Radial nerve—The radial nerve, formed from the posterior cord of the brachial plexus, spirals around the humerus in a medial to lateral direction. It supplies the triceps as well as innervation to the lateral portion of the brachialis muscle. It emerges through the intermuscular septum between the brachialis and the brachioradialis muscles.
   4. Ulnar nerve—The ulnar nerve travels down the arm medial to the brachial artery. It traverses behind the medial epicondyle of the humerus.
   D. Vasculature—The endosteal blood supply of the humeral shaft comes from branches of the brachial artery. Periosteal branches may arise from the brachial artery, the profunda brachii artery, and the posterior humeral circumflex artery. In addition, numerous small muscular branches contribute to the periosteal circulation.

III. Clinical Examination—The majority of patients with humeral shaft fractures have the common signs and symptoms of fracture, including swelling, pain, deformity, and crepitation. Motor-vehicle accidents, direct blows, and falls on the upper extremity are common mechanisms of injury. The humeral shaft also concentrates rotational force applied to the upper extremity and is subject to fracture under these loading conditions. A complete physical examination is performed before concentrating on the upper extremity.

A complete neurovascular examination of the entire upper extremity is performed. Because of the high incidence of injury, *the function of the radial nerve must be documented before any reduction maneuver or surgical intervention*. The joints above and below the humerus, as well as the ipsilateral wrist, are examined to exclude other injuries. The skin should be examined for abrasions, lacerations, contusions or a combination thereof. The compartments of the arm should be palpated to assess for the possibility of a compartment syndrome.

IV. Radiographic Evaluation—A complete radiographic evaluation is mandatory in the workup of a humeral shaft fracture. An anteroposterior radiograph and a lateral radiograph that includes both the elbow joint and the glenohumeral joint are essential. While obtaining radiographs, the examining physician should place the X-ray cassette in various positions about the upper extremity rather than manipulating the patient's fractured limb. Simple limb rotation does not provide orthogonal views of the proximal humeral shaft and results in an incomplete radiographic analysis. Pathologic fractures may require other imaging studies, before definitive treatment, to evaluate a neoplasm and exclude occult lesions.

A. Fracture Classification—There are numerous classification strategies for describing and reporting on humeral shaft fractures. Most fracture classification schemes are based on plain radiography and rely on fracture geometry. In practice, treatment for humeral shaft fractures frequently depends on other variables, including bone quality, concomitant injuries, soft-tissue injuries, or neurovascular insult. Simple fracture patterns include those of transverse, oblique, and spiral geometry. More complex patterns include segmental fractures, severely comminuted fractures, open fractures, and humeral shaft fractures with dislocation of either the shoulder or the elbow. *The Holstein-Lewis fracture is a spiral fracture in the distal third of the humeral shaft that typically presents with a lateral spike on the distal fragment. This pattern has been associated with a radial nerve injury because of proximity and tethering of the nerve adjacent to this lateral spike*. Open fractures should be evaluated according to the Gustilo and Anderson Classification. Moreover, pathologic conditions such as osteoporosis, metastatic or primary tumors, and other associated conditions are important in regards to fracture description.

V. Treatment

A. Closed Treatment—The majority of fractures of the humeral shaft are treated adequately via closed methods. The fracture character, the patient's age and occupation, and the presence of associated injuries all influence fracture management. Transverse and oblique humeral shaft fractures are commonly best treated closed. Options for closed treatment include hanging arm cast, shoulder spica cast, Velpeau dressing, coaptation splint, and a *functional brace*. Because of low cost, effectiveness and minimal complications, the use of a functional brace has become the preferred method of treatment. The ideal humeral shaft fracture amenable to a functional brace is the long oblique shaft fracture with soft-tissue stability provided by an intact medial and lateral intramuscular septum. A functional brace is generally applied to the humerus after 3 to 14 days of fracture splinting. Active elbow flexion and extension are required to assist fracture healing during bracing. This method has been reported to result in humeral shaft fracture healing in more than 90% of patients. Functional bracing has proven a reliable method of treatment for extraarticular supracondylar fractures but is less effective in the treatment of proximal humeral fractures because of the physical constraints of the axilla. The hanging arm cast is used less frequently because it requires that the patient stay erect the majority of the time. Additionally, frequent follow-up is mandatory to monitor for excessive fracture distraction. The Velpeau (or sling-and-swathe) dressing may be useful in children under the age of 8 years. The coaptation splint may be used before application of the functional fracture brace. In summary, whenever possible, closed treatment should be performed with the functional brace.

B. Operative Treatment—Despite the success of closed treatment, a number of relative indications for operative treatment exist. These are listed in Table 20-1. If surgical stabilization is chosen for one of these indications, a number of surgical options exist.

1. Plate osteosynthesis

    • Open reduction and plate osteosynthesis has proven a reliable method of achieving union in humeral shaft fractures. *Advantages of plate osteosynthesis include the ability to explore the radial nerve during fixation, minimal morbidity to the shoulder joint, low complication rates, early restoration of function, and the opportunity to apply direct reduction techniques to the fracture fragments*. Furthermore, bone defects

TABLE 20-1

Relative Indications for Operative Treatment of Humeral Shaft Fractures

Segmental fractures

Lower-extremity fractures that require arm use for mobilization

Open fractures

Vascular injury

Bilateral humeral shaft fractures

Floating elbow injury

Most pathologic fractures

Inability to obtain and maintain an acceptable closed reduction

Fractures associated with radial nerve palsy after a closed reduction

Large body habitus

Parkinson's disease

Ipsilateral brachial plexus lesion(s)

may be addressed with autologous bone graft, bone substitutes, or allograft in the rare cases when a biological adjunct is felt to be necessary to accomplish healing. Plate osteosynthesis may be equally successful with either absolute stability or relative stability. In cases without significant comminution, lag screw placement neutralized with a plate is the preferred technique. Alternatively, when lag screw placement is impractical, compression plating is acceptable. As the fracture pattern increases in complexity, bridge fixation should be considered. With this technique, length, alignment and rotation of the arm is restored with the plate secured to the proximal and distal segment to maintain this position. This technique may be applied through traditional open exposure or with a percutaneous technique.

- Dynamic compression plates—The AO group recommends a ***4.5-mm broad dynamic compression (DC or LC-DCP) plate with a minimum of six (preferably eight) cortices both proximal and distal to the humeral shaft fracture***. The rationale for broad DC use is that it allows multiplanar screw placement, increasing fixation strength. Humeral shafts with a smaller bone diameter may not accept a 4.5-mm broad plate and use of a 4.5-mm narrow or 3.5-mm plate is acceptable in these circumstances.

- Locked plating—Locked screws have dramatically expanded the utility of plating as a treatment of humeral shaft fractures. ***The opportunity to gain stable fixation in osteoporotic bone and in fractures with short metaphyseal segments has broadened the range of fractures amenable to plate fixation***. In both of these clinical situations, the locked relationship of the screw to the plate prevents screw toggle, which translates into improved longevity of fixation. Locking plates are most commonly used on the humerus with a "hybrid" construct. In this mode, conventional screws are placed first creating stability through traditional plate/bone friction generated by the compressing effect of the tightened screw. This stability is then maintained by the addition of a sufficient number of locking screws that are relatively protected from loosening. An alternative use of a locking plate is in the "internal–external fixator" mode. In this technique, the plate is not compressed to the bone but held off of the bone with locking screws. While this technique has the theoretical advantage of minimizing periosteal disruption, superior clinical results have not yet been documented. While locking plates have proven advantageous in osteoporotic bone, they do not offer benefit in cases of normal bone quality.

2. Intramedullary fixation
- Rigid intramedullary interlocking nails—Antegrade intramedullary nail fixation is applicable to proximal and middle third fractures. In the distal third, the flattening shape of the medullary canal precludes sufficient insertion depth and presents a contraindication. The advantages of intramedullary nails include limited exposure and the preserved fracture biology with indirect reduction. Static interlocking is generally recommended to enhance both rotational and axial stability. ***Complications associated with antegrade nailing of humeral shaft fractures include rotator cuff injury, shoulder pain, and proximal prominent hardware***. In an attempt to avoid these shoulder complications, retrograde nail placement has been utilized with a posterior starting point above the olecranon fossa. While avoiding shoulder complications this off axis starting point presents difficulty passing a nail and places a large stress riser in the supracondylar region. ***Pathologic fractures present***

a relative indication for intramedullary stabilization as this stabilizes longer sections of bone that are at risk for future oncologic weakening. Patients with concomitant lower-extremity injuries that are expected to require crutch assistance have traditionally been treated with intramedullary fixation. It has been presumed that this affords fixation better suited to weight bearing activity. However, recent clinical series have also supported plate fixation in these situations. Intramedullary reaming in humeral shaft fractures remains a controversial topic. The soft-tissues, exposed by fracture displacement, should never be subjected to revolving reamers because of the potential for radial nerve injury. Open nailing decreases the risk of neurovascular injury but also decreases the benefit of indirect reduction and limited exposure.

- Flexible intramedullary nail fixation—Flexible intramedullary nails may be useful in both adult and pediatric humeral shaft fractures. Many surgeons prefer the lower morbidity and simpler techniques associated with these flexible implants. Flexible intramedullary devices may be inserted in an anterograde or retrograde fashion. When utilized, multiple nails are recommended for rotational control. Complications with flexible nails include implant migration, nonunion and rotational instability.

3. External fixation—Open fractures, infected nonunions, burn patients, and cases with segmental bone loss may be best stabilized with an external fixator. *External fixation pins should be inserted in a controlled fashion under direct vision to guard against neurovascular injury.* In Gustilo Type III open fractures, external fixation is an excellent option. However, Type I and Type II open fractures may be stabilized using plate osteosynthesis or an intramedullary nail. The external fixator is usually placed as a temporizing device during soft-tissue healing and before functional bracing or definitive fixation. External fixation is generally not recommended as the definitive fracture management in the humeral shaft.

C. Surgical Approaches
  1. Posterior approach to the humeral shaft (Fig. 20-1)—The posterior approach uses the

FIGURE 20-1 Posterior approach to the humeral shaft.

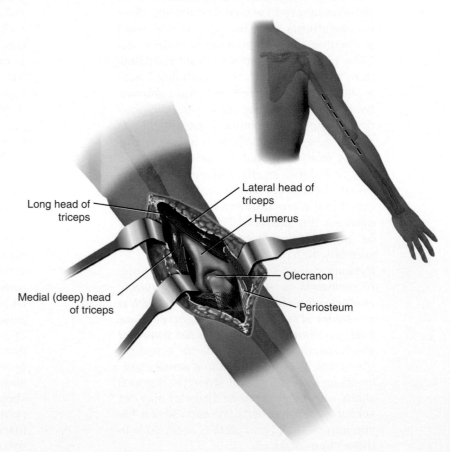

Long head of triceps

Lateral head of triceps

Humerus

Medial (deep) head of triceps

Olecranon

Periosteum

interval between the long and lateral heads of the triceps muscle. The deep (medial) head is subsequently divided, and the humeral shaft is exposed. Dangers associated with this approach include damage to the radial nerve and damage to the profunda brachii artery. These two important structures must be identified and protected. In addition, care should be taken not to injure the ulnar nerve or the lateral brachial cutaneous nerve.

2. Anterolateral approach to the humeral shaft (Fig. 20-2)—In the anterolateral approach, the humeral shaft is exposed by developing the plane between the deltoid muscle and the pectoralis major muscle proximally and through the brachialis muscle distally. Dangers associated with this approach include the musculocutaneous nerve and the radial nerve as it enters the anterior compartment distally.

3. Posterolateral approach to the humeral shaft (Fig. 20-3)—This approach essentially follows the lateral intermuscular septum and allows humeral exposure from the lateral condyle to the proximal crossing of the axillary nerve. In addition to this being an extensile exposure, its major advantage is the ability to explore the radial nerve in both the posterior and anterior compartments.

VI. Complications—Complications that may occur while treating humeral shaft fractures include osteomyelitis, malunion, delayed union or nonunion, vascular injury, and radial nerve injury.

A. Osteomyelitis—Osteomyelitis of the humerus is rare but may accompany open fractures or operative treatment. The diagnosis may be difficult unless gross signs of infection are present. Open fractures and immune suppression place a patient at risk. Irrigation and debridement and the administration of organism-specific antibiotics with or without hardware removal remain the cornerstone of treatment. Nuclear medicine studies, including a combined indium-111-labeled leukocyte and technetium-99m methylene diphosphonate scintography, may be useful during the diagnostic workup for infection. The placement of antibiotic-impregnated polymethylmethacrylate may be required to eliminate an infection. In the event that sequestrum removal is necessary, the arm is able to preserve function with resection of up to 3 cm of bone making acute shortening a viable option for limb reconstruction.

B. Malunion—A large amount of angular and rotational deformity may be tolerated in the humerus before it limits function of the upper limb. Generally, ***up to 20° to 30° of angular deformity and 15° of rotational malalignment are***

FIGURE 20-2 Anterolateral approach to the humeral shaft.

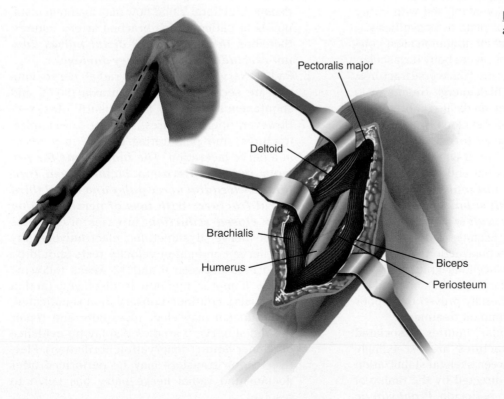

Pectoralis major

Deltoid

Brachialis

Humerus

Biceps

Periosteum

FIGURE 20-3 Posterolateral approach to the humeral shaft allows for extensile exposure and visualization of the radial nerve in both the posterior and anterior compartments of the arm.

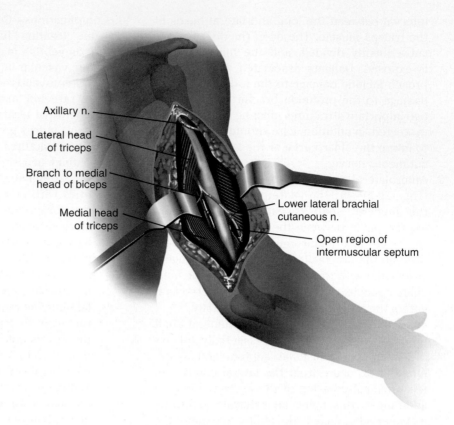

Axillary n.

Lateral head of triceps

Branch to medial head of biceps

Medial head of triceps

Lower lateral brachial cutaneous n.

Open region of intermuscular septum

considered acceptable. Surgical correction of a malunion frequently requires a corrective osteotomy, which may be stabilized with either an intramedullary nail or plate osteosynthesis.

C. Nonunion—A humeral shaft nonunion most commonly occurs in cases of severe bony devascularization, segmental fractures, transverse fractures, poor fracture fixation, high-energy trauma or in patients with significant medical comorbidities. Humeral shaft nonunion develops in only 2% to 5% of fractures. The keys to management are reduction of the fracture fragments, assuring adequate biologic potential and stable fixation. *Open reduction with internal fixation using a 4.5-mm DC plate with supplemental cancellous autogenous bone graft is the treatment of choice for nonunion*. Segmental defects likely require an advanced reconstruction with vascularized fibular graft, cancellous graft, or acute shortening. Intramedullary fixation alone and exchange nailing have generally proven to be poor choices for humeral nonunion treatment.

D. Vascular Injury—Vascular injuries associated with humeral shaft fractures are exceedingly rare. Prioritization between skeletal stabilization and vascular repair is directed by the timing of injury and residual limb perfusion. *Prophylactic*

fasciotomies should be considered because of the risk of reperfusion compartment syndrome. Collateral blood flow may maintain distal pulses in patients with brachial artery injuries; therefore, *the presence of distal pulses does not preclude brachial artery damage*.

E. Radial Nerve Injury—Most radial nerve injuries are secondary to neurapraxia (90%), and spontaneous recovery is frequently observed. However, open fractures, Holstein-Lewis spiral fractures, and penetrating trauma may result in a nerve laceration. *The indications for primary nerve exploration include open fractures with radial nerve palsy and distal third spiral fractures with loss of nerve function after closed reduction*. In cases of complete radial nerve dysfunction, electromyography and nerve conduction velocity tests should be performed between 6 and 12 weeks following injury. If motor function is displayed (action potentials), continued observation is indicated. The clinician may elect to explore and repair the radial nerve if studies display no evidence of reinnervation (denervation fibrillation). Elective tendon transfers may be performed after documented radial nerve palsy has failed to resolve.

SUGGESTED READINGS

Classic Articles

Healy WL, White GM, Mick CA, et al. Nonunion of the humeral shaft. *Clin Orthop.* 1987;219: 206–213.

Holstein A, Lewis GB. Fractures of the humerus with radial-nerve paralysis. *J Bone Joint Surg.* 1963;45A:1382–1388.

Ingman AM, Waters DA. Locked intramedullary nailing of humeral shaft fractures: implant design, surgical technique, and clinical results. *J Bone Joint Surg.* 1994;76B:23–29.

Sarmiento A, Kinman PB, Calvin EG, et al: Functional bracing of fractures of the humeral shaft. *J Bone Joint Surg.* 1977;59A:59–601.

Recent Articles

Gosler MW, Testroote M, Morrenhof JW, et al. Surgical versus non-surgical interventions for treating humeral shaft fractures in adults. *Cochrane Database Syst Rev.* 2012;1:CD008832.

Heineman DJ, Bhandari M, Poolman RW. Plate fixation or intramedullary fixation of humeral shaft fractures—an update. *Acta Orthop.* 2012.

Kurup H, Hossain M, Andrew JG. Dynamic compression plating versus locked intramedullary nailing for humeral shaft fractures in adults. *Cochrane Database Syst Rev.* 2011;(6):CD005959.

Shin SJ, Sohn HS, Do NH. Minimally invasive plate osteosynthesis of humeral shaft fractures: a technique to aid fracture reduction and minimize complications. *J Orthop Trauma.* 2012.

Textbook

Zagorski JB, Zych GA, Latta LL, et al. Modern concepts in functional fracture bracing: the upper limb. *Instr Course Lect.* 1987;36:377–401.

CHAPTER 21

Fractures and Dislocations of the Elbow

O. Alton Barron and Damien Davis

I. Overview—The elbow provides the critical linkage as the shoulder moves the hand through space. The normal elbow has an average extension to flexion arc of 0° to 145°. Normal pronation and supination are approximately 80° and 85°, respectively. Functional arcs fall within these limits, with activities of daily living requiring 50° each of pronation and supination and a 100° arc of extension to flexion between 30° and 130°. Less than 130° of elbow flexion diminishes the ability to feed and groom oneself. Fractures and dislocations of the elbow should be evident on routine anteroposterior (AP), lateral, and oblique radiographs. The radiocapitellar view provides an additional and clearer view of this joint. Information from these plain radiographs is almost always sufficient for the surgeon to decide between operative and nonoperative treatment. Once a decision is made to pursue operative treatment, plain radiographs with gentle traction applied to the arm after anesthesia may further clarify fracture anatomy, especially in the case of distal humerus fractures. Computed tomography (CT) is indicated to assess the articular surfaces when the decision to pursue operative treatment on the basis of articular displacement is equivocal after plain radiographs. It is also more ideal to assess fragment size and configuration prior to surgery.

II. Distal Humerus Fractures (Fig. 21-1)
  A. Anatomy—The distal humerus consists of an obliquely oriented articular surface comprised of the spool-like trochlea and the hemispheric capitellum, each supported by a condylar column. The olecranon fossa lies between these columns proximal to the articular surface. Its sometimes paper-thin floor is the confluence between the anterior and posterior cortices of the distal humerus and contributes little osseous support. The longitudinal axis of the spool-shaped trochlea is internally rotated 3° to 8° with respect to the humerus and inclines laterally 5° to 8°, thereby creating the valgus carrying angle of the extended elbow. In the male, the mean carrying angle is 11° to 14°, and in the female, it is 13° to 16°. The roughly hemispheric capitellum is centered 1 to 1.5 cm anterior to the central axis of the humeral shaft. The humerocapitellar angle in the adult is 30°. The medial column diverges at an angle of 45° with the humeral shaft, whereas the lateral column diverges 20° to 25°. The medial epicondyle, forming the distal extent of the medial column, lies just posterior to the rotational axis of the trochlea. Thus a cam effect is created, with different portions of the medial collateral ligament (MCL) becoming taut at different angles of flexion. Conceptualizing distal humerus fractures as involving one or both columns simplifies accurate identification and management. Isolated capitellar fractures are discussed separately.
  B. One-Column Fractures—These fractures involve part or all of the trochlea. Milch and Jupiter have classified these, depending on how much of the trochlea remains with the involved column. High-columnar fractures involve the majority of the trochlea, and the radius and ulna are displaced with the fractured column. Low-columnar fractures involve a smaller portion of the trochlea, and the radius and ulna remain with the intact humeral column and shaft. For fractures displaced more than 2 mm, anatomic reduction with stable internal fixation allows for early motion and yields consistently better results than closed management. For nondisplaced fractures, the position of immobilization should *relax* the musculature originating from that column (i.e., pronation for medial column fractures, supination for lateral column fractures). Rigid fixation of high columnar fractures with plates provides improved rigidity over screws alone; low

Lateral epicondyle fracture
Surgical approach—Lateral
Treatment—ORIF
Type of hardware—Screw, suture anchors

Columnar, intraarticular fracture
Surgical approach—Olecranon osteotomy
Treatment—ORIF, ulnar nerve transposition
Type of hardware—Plates and screws

Radial head/neck fracture
Surgical approach—Kocher, Kaplan,
              Pankovich
Treatment—ORIF vs. excision
Type of hardware—T-plate, screws,
              prosthesis

Medial epicondyle fracture
Surgical approach—Medial
Treatment—ORIF
Type of hardware—Screw, suture anchor

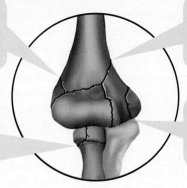

Capitellum fracture
Surgical approach—Lateral
Treatment—ORIF vs. excision
Type of hardware—PA lag or headless screw

Supracondylar fracture
Surgical approach—Olecranon osteotomy
Treatment—ORIF with or without ulnar
              nerve transposition
Type of hardware—Plates and screws

Coronoid fracture
Surgical approach—Injury/fixation
              dependent
Treatment—ORIF if indicated
Type of hardware—Lag screw, anchor,
              suture

Olecranon tip fracture
Surgical approach—Posterior
Treatment—Excision
Type of hardware—None

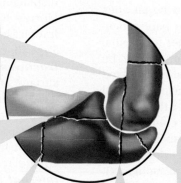

Monteggia injury
Surgical approach—Posterior
Treatment—ORIF
Type of hardware—Compression plate

Olecranon fracture
Surgical approach—Posterior
Treatment—ORIF
Type of hardware—Tension band wire

FIGURE 21-1 Treatment of elbow fractures. Although there may be alternative treatments of equal merit, this is the standard information at this time. *ORIF,* Open reduction with internal fixation; *PA,* Posteroanterior.

columnar fractures without comminution may be adequately stabilized with screws. In either case, the articular reduction must be anatomic. This can be achieved through indirect reduction at times, but may require an olecranon osteotomy in certain cases. For lateral column fractures where the lateral trochlea is fractured off with the capitellum, a chevron olecranon osteotomy can be levered open on a medial (ulnar) soft-tissue hinge. This provides for adequate articular visualization and anatomic restoration while leaving the medial structures (i.e., the ulnar nerve and MCL) undisturbed. This also simplifies reduction and fixation of the osteotomy.

C. Two-Column Fractures—Fractures involving both columns are either intra-articular or extra-articular. While common in children, extra-articular columnar fractures (i.e., supracondylar fractures) are

rare in adults (except perhaps in osteoporotic older individuals). Fixation in the presence of closed physes is similar to that used in intraarticular fractures. In adults, efforts must be made to achieve anatomic reductions and *rigid* internal fixation, despite the allure of percutaneous pin fixation. Shear forces are too great, and postoperative fracture displacement occurs too often with limited fixation. Intra-articular bicolumnar fractures frequently result from high-energy trauma and may be extensively comminuted. Common fracture patterns include the T, Y, H, and the laterally or medially inclined "lambda" fractures. The high risk for stiffness and loss of motion after such fractures is best minimized by stable fixation and early motion. If sufficient stability to permit early range of motion (ROM) cannot be achieved, then anatomic restoration of the articular surface should take precedence. Joint contractures in the presence of healed, congruent articular surfaces can be effectively treated with a soft-tissue release. Two-column distal humerus fractures are best approached posteriorly. Given the relatively high incidence of ulnar neuropathy associated with these injuries (early and late), some recommend anterior transposition of the ulnar nerve at the time of fracture fixation. This can be easily performed from the posterior approach.

An olecranon osteotomy, most reliably and inexpensively stabilized with a tension band wiring technique, affords access to the entire articular surface. The osteotomy should be an apex distal osteotomy centered over the bare articular area of the trochlear notch. Larger fragments, whether columnar or intraarticular, should be stabilized first. The columns are most rigidly fixed with plates along their posterior aspects. Dual plating along the columns is stronger than Y plating or other constructs. The lateral column, with its gently curved posterior aspect, usually accommodates 3.5-mm dynamic compression plates (stronger torsional forces and bending moments). The more malleable 3.5-mm reconstruction plates are better for more distal fractures requiring plate bends with smaller radii of curvature. The use of two plates along the lateral column (one posterior, one lateral) has also been described. The contour of the medial epicondyle usually requires a reconstruction plate posteriorly or a one-third tubular plate along its medial ridge. Alternatively, "prebent" plates are available and can be used in a similar fashion. The trochlea, which is usually fractured in the sagittal plane, is best stabilized with screws along its axis; these may be passed through the various plates for added stability. Since the articular cartilage of the trochlea covers 270° of its surface, fixation of articular fragments is best accomplished with headless compression screws or lag screws countersunk below the subchondral bone. Provisional pin fixation and patience, with accurate contouring of plates, greatly facilitate stable fixation. Even prebent plates often require some additional bending to conform to each patient's unique anatomy.

Total elbow arthroplasty (TEA) has been used to treat primarily elderly, low-demand osteoporotic patients with comminuted bicolumnar fractures not amenable to open reduction and internal fixation. Such elbow fractures in patients with pre-existing degenerative conditions of the elbow, such as rheumatoid arthritis, are also candidates for primary TEA. It is important not to perform an olecranon osteotomy if TEA is necessary, as this can result in inadequate fixation of the ulnar prosthesis. In higher-demand elbows, however, the surgeon should strive for optimal fracture fixation and bone healing (even if a later contracture release becomes necessary). Postoperative care should include active motion as soon as it is appropriate, depending on the fixation achieved (immediately if at all possible).

III. Capitellum Fractures (Fig. 21-1)—Fractures of the capitellum are rare. The usual configuration is a shear fracture in the coronal plane with superior displacement of the articular surface. Bryan and Morrey have classified these as Type I, complete fractures; Type II, osteochondral fractures; and Type III, comminuted fractures (Table 21-1). *Type I fractures* consist of the hemisphere of the articular surface and the underlying cancellous bone (typically referred to as the Hahn-Steinthal fracture). Occasionally, Type I fractures may be amenable to closed reduction if attempted early. However, it is difficult to achieve and subsequently maintain adequate reduction. *When required and possible, internal fixation is best accomplished with lag screws from posterior to anterior into the posterior portion of the lateral condyle.* A lateral approach with subperiosteal release of the common extensor origin is used to expose the capitellum and posterior aspect of the distal lateral column. *Type II fractures* are less common and consist of an osteochondral shell of the anterior capitellar cartilage (i.e., the Kocher-Lorenz fracture). Occasionally, these fractures are amenable to fixation with headless anterior-to-posterior compression screws if there is enough cancellous subchondral bone for stable fixation. *Highly comminuted (Type III) and osteochondral fractures may not be amenable to stable internal fixation. Excision of fragments is then recommended as long as the integrity of the radioulnar interosseous ligament and MCL has been confirmed.* In the presence of longitudinal radioulnar instability, excision of the capitellum is analgous to excision of a nonrepairable radial head. In either case, proximal radial migration leads to positive ulnar variance and ulnocarpal impaction. Although avascular necrosis (AVN) of the fragment is rare, delayed excision of a necrotic fragment is appropriate. Excision of capitellar fragments, whether performed initially or delayed, may lead to elbow stiffness. Arthroscopic excision results in improved motion compared with open excision.

IV. Elbow Dislocation (Fig. 21-2)

A. Anatomy—Dislocation of the elbow joint in the adult population has an annual incidence of

TABLE 21-1

Important Elbow Injury Classifications

Type	Description	Treatment or Age Group
Radial head fractures		
Mason Classification		
I	Nondisplaced	Nonoperative
II	Displaced	ORIF vs. excision
III	Comminuted	Excision with or without replacement
IV	Associated with elbow dislocation	Replacement based on stability
Hotchkiss Classification		
I	Marginal fracture or minimally displaced with no motion block	Nonoperative
II	>2-mm displacement and amenable to fixation	ORIF
III	Comminuted fracture not amenable to fixation	Excision with or without replacement
Coronoid fractures		
Regan and Morrey Classification		
I	Tip avulsion	None
II	<50%, MCL insertion intact	Usually non-operative
III	≥50%, MCL disrupted	ORIF
Monteggia Lesions		
Bado Classification		
I	Anterior dislocation of the radial head	Children to young adults
II	Posterior dislocation of the radial head	Elderly
III	Lateral dislocation of the radial head	Children
IV	With a radial shaft fracture	Adults
Capitellum fractures		
Bryan and Morrey Classification		
I	Complete fracture	Closed reduction vs. ORIF
II	Osteochondral (shear) fracture	Excision
III	Comminuted fracture	Excision

ORIF, Open reduction with internal fixation.

13 per 100,000 people. That is about the same incidence as proximal interphalangeal joint dislocations, but less than shoulder dislocations at 17 per 100,000. The osseous anatomy of the elbow is inherently stable and contributes the majority of resistance to varus and valgus forces. The column model (Greek temple) of elbow stability depicts the humerus as spanning the articular surfaces of the radial head and the coronoid process of the ulna. Valgus forces are resisted primarily at the radiocapitellar joint (the lateral column), whereas varus forces are resisted primarily at the ulnohumeral joint (the medial column). The ulnohumeral articulation provides 55% of the resistance to varus with the elbow extended and 75% of the resistence with the elbow flexed 90°. The radiocapitellar joint, though transmitting up to 60% of the axial force from the hand to the humerus, contributes only 30% of the resistance to valgus force at the elbow. In cases of ligament disruption, the osseous columns contribute more of the resistance to varus and valgus loads. The anterior band of the MCL originates from the anterior portion of the medial epicondyle (the center of the ulnohumeral motion axis) and inserts onto the medial base of the coronoid. The lateral,

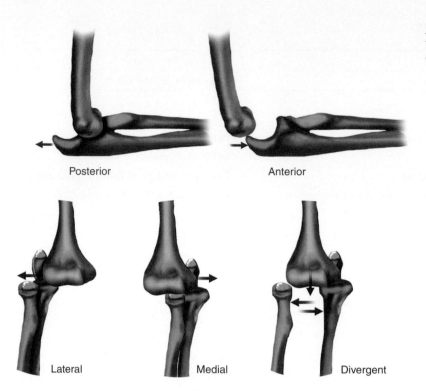

FIGURE 21-2 Elbow dislocations. Note that the classification is based on the direction of displacement of the forearm bones.

Posterior   Anterior

Lateral   Medial   Divergent

or radial, collateral ligament (LCL) originates from the lateral epicondyle of the humerus at the axis of ulnohumeral motion and inserts into the annular ligament and into the proximal ulna just lateral to the lesser sigmoid notch (Fig. 21-3). Classically, the anterior band of the MCL is considered the primary stabilizer of the ulnohumeral joint, but the role of the LCL, especially the ulnar portion, has been clearly delineated. The MCL contributes 70% of the resistance to valgus loads in the intact elbow. The anterior capsule also provides some resistance to both valgus and varus stress, primarily with the elbow in extension. Clinically, the MCL may provide adequate stability against valgus force even in the case of radial head resection. Biomechanical studies of the LCL, however, suggest that stability to varus force depends on both an intact LCL and a competent coronoid process (>50% intact). The lateral ulnar collateral ligament (LUCL) cradles the radial head and prevents its posterior subluxation along with preventing lateral opening of the ulnohumeral joint. Such instability is termed posterolateral rotatory instability (PLRI). Injuries to the LCL complex have been created biomechanically with application of a supination, hyperextension load. Testing of elbow stability with the forearm in pronation to tighten the LCL has been suggested; testing in supination may lead to confusion between PLRI and MCL laxity if a

"clunk" is felt during valgus testing. The collateral ligaments usually fail in their midsubstance, although avulsion fractures, especially laterally, may occur, usually in adults. An attenuated MCL has been associated with valgus instability but not with recurrent dislocation, whereas an incompetent LUCL has been associated with subluxation and recurrent dislocation. An incompetent LUCL leading to PLRI can frequently be detected by the pivot shift test. A supination valgus moment is applied to the flexed elbow with the patient supine. The subluxation is felt as the elbow is extended and a reduction clunk is felt as the elbow is flexed again. The flexor-pronator group and the extensor group of muscles serve as secondary dynamic stabilizers of the elbow joint, as do the triceps, brachialis, and biceps muscles. These muscles span the elbow joint, resisting applied moments, and increasing joint reactive forces (thereby increasing the osseous stability). Grossly unstable elbow dislocations are often associated with rupture of these dynamic stabilizers as well as the static ligamentous restraints.

B. Evaluation and Treatment—Despite the inherently stable osseous configuration of the joint, dislocations of the elbow represent 20% of all dislocations. The injury occurs most often in young people as a result of relatively high-energy trauma but can nevertheless occur after a seemingly minor fall onto an outstretched hand. ***Some***

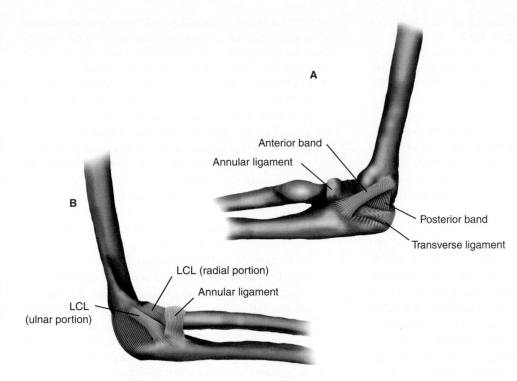

FIGURE 21-3 Elbow joint. **A.** Medial collateral ligament with its important anterior band. **B.** Lateral collateral ligament (LCL).

A

Anterior band
Annular ligament
Posterior band
Transverse ligament

B

LCL (radial portion)
Annular ligament
LCL (ulnar portion)

90% of elbow dislocations are posterior. Anterior, medial, or lateral dislocations are rare; divergent dislocations (radius and ulna displaced in different directions with disruption of the proximal radioulnar joint) are extremely rare. As the ulnohumeral joint dislocates, the radial head and coronoid are sometimes fractured (in up to 10% and 18%, respectively, of all elbow dislocations); more rarely the olecranon tip is fractured. At surgical exploration, over 90% of elbow dislocations demonstrate osteochondral fractures that may be attributed to the initial trauma or to subsequent overzealous reduction maneuvers. The humeral epicondyles may fracture as well, representing avulsion of the collateral ligaments. These fragments, along with injured soft tissue, can become incarcerated within the joint, necessitating operative intervention. True lateral and AP X-rays are required to confirm a congruent reduction. A CT scan is also informative as to the exact location of the fragment and more subtle impaction and shear fractures, especially those involving the medial coronoid. An incongruent reduction is an indication for surgical exploration with open reduction.

1. Reduction—Reduction under appropriate sedation that provides sufficient muscle relaxation should be followed by an examination of joint stability and ROM. This allows the examiner to gauge the extent of injury to various stabilizers as well as the limits of motion

appropriate for early rehabilitation. ***Blocked motion usually indicates an incarcerated osteochondral fragment.*** Stability to varus and valgus stress should be tested in 30° of flexion and full pronation. ***The simple elbow dislocation stable beyond 45° of flexion should generally be splinted in 90° of flexion and neutral pronation/supination. Pronation tightens the LCL and may be used to improve postreduction stability.*** However, certain patients, especially younger athletes, may enjoy a more rapid recovery of function if open repair of critical ligaments and muscle tendon units is performed acutely.

2. Repair of ruptured ligaments—***Repair of ruptured ligaments in an elbow that is stable past 45° of extension does not improve results. If, however, the elbow requires immobilization in extreme flexion, then the LCL and/or MCL should be repaired.*** The flexor/pronator and extensor origins are generally ruptured in these cases and should be reattached to the humerus at the time of ligament repair. If the elbow remains unstable even after ligament repair (rare but more common when associated with unstable fractures), the surgeon should consider a dynamic external fixator. Devices now available allow for control of varus and valgus, flexion and extension, and joint distraction. Still the trend continues to be toward anatomic repairs and reconstruction

of critical stabilizers such that the need for dynamic fixators is minimized.

3. Associated fractures—The treatment of associated fractures (radial head, capitellum, coronoid process, and olecranon) is discussed in each of those sections.

4. Active motion—*Active* motion should be instituted 5 to 10 days after an elbow dislocation to minimize stiffness and heterotopic ossification. Early *passive* motion may lead to redislocation and heterotopic ossification. Patient apprehension is overcome by having the patient lie supine with the injured arm held above the chest (i.e., with the shoulder in 90° of forward elevation). From this position, active extension of the elbow against gravity is allowed. This position is most advantageous in that if the patient loses control of the arm, it will fall into elbow flexion, a position of greater stability. This can decrease patient apprehension of redislocation and facilitate rehabilitation. Dynamic extension splints should be considered if extension is not improving by 5 weeks following the injury.

C. Associated Injuries—Neurovascular injury is fairly rare in association with elbow dislocation. The ulnar nerve is most commonly involved because of excessive traction during posterior dislocations. The median nerve, the second most commonly injured, may become entrapped after reduction, emphasizing the importance of prereduction and postreduction neurovascular examinations. Brachial artery disruptions are rare and are usually associated with open injuries. Doppler evaluation or arterial imaging is recommended in cases of asymmetric pulses or other signs of arterial compromise. Examination of distal pulses may be unreliable because of collateral circulation around the elbow. Since elbow dislocations frequently result from a force applied to the outstretched hand, other injuries resulting from this mechanism may occur and should be sought radiographically and clinically. Carpal fractures and dislocations, distal radius fractures, and injuries to the interosseous membrane of the forearm have been reported.

V. Olecranon Fractures (Fig. 21-1)—Intra-articular fractures of the olecranon most commonly result from a direct blow to the posterior elbow sustained during a fall. The less common extra-articular (avulsion) fractures are usually smaller fragments. These most often occur via indirect trauma (e.g., an eccentric triceps contraction against a fixed forearm as in a fall onto an outstretched hand). True lateral radiographs of the elbow are required to accurately assess these injuries. Articular impaction fractures of the trochlear notch or fracture extension into the coronoid process may occur and must be identified.

A. Undisplaced Fractures—Colton classified an "undisplaced" olecranon fracture as having less than 2 mm of displacement, being stable with elbow flexion to 90°, and allowing active extension of the elbow. Careful follow-up of such fractures treated nonoperatively is needed to detect subsequent fracture displacement.

B. Displaced Fractures—Displaced olecranon fractures should be treated operatively except when the patient cannot tolerate any surgery. Displaced noncomminuted fractures are generally amenable to treatment with a tension band wiring construct, with the pins best placed into the anterior cortex of the ulnar shaft to minimize the risk of pin migration. However, great care must be exercised to avoid injury to the anterior interosseous neurovascular bundle, which lies adjacent to the anterior proximal ulna. The tension wire should be passed deep to the triceps tendon to rest against the cortex of the olecranon while maintaining an awareness of the nearby ulnar nerve within the cubital tunnel. Tension band wiring may be insufficient for complex olecranon fractures associated with comminution, instability, or substantial extension into the coronoid process. *The most common complication associated with tension band wiring of the olecranon is prominence of the Kirschner wires at the insertion site into the olecranon.* This irritates the triceps tendon, necessitating hardware removal. Avulsion fractures may sometimes be fixed with a heavy nonabsorbable suture. *Comminuted fractures of the olecranon may require plate fixation if the proximal piece is large enough to accommodate two or three screws,* or excision if the fragments cannot be reconstructed. A plate placed laterally (when possible) minimizes the risk of painful and/or prominent hardware because the medial and posterior aspects of the olecranon are frequently used to rest the arm or to bear weight. In the rare cases requiring excision, advancement of the triceps mechanism into cancellous bone of the ulnar shaft results in adequate function in older individuals. The literature suggests that excision of as much as two-thirds of the olecranon has yielded good results in very low-demand elbows. However, resection of 25% of the olecranon process reduces the resistance to valgus load by 50%. Thus, excision is contraindicated in the presence of anterior soft-tissue damage, when the fracture involves the coronoid process, or in younger, active patients. After excision, the triceps should be advanced so that the tendon is congruent with the articular surface of the trochlear notch. Immediate or early motion after stable internal fixation of olecranon fractures engenders the best results. After excision, the repair of the triceps to the proximal ulna should be protected as necessary. Intraoperative assessment of the stability of this repair should be used to guide postoperative rehabilitation.

VI. Proximal Ulna Fractures—Olecranon fractures that extend into the coronoid are better regarded as proximal ulna fractures, since they represent a more complex injury to the elbow and require different fixation techniques. Comminution is frequent. These fractures are termed trans-olecranon fracture-dislocations of the elbow and occur when a high-energy direct posteroanterior blow is applied to the dorsal aspect of the forearm with the elbow in mid-flexion. This results in an olecranon fracture and an anterior dislocation of the forearm with respect to the distal humerus. A transolecranon fracture-dislocation is often misdiagnosed as an anterior Monteggia lesion. **The transolecranon fracture-dislocation is different from a Bado I Monteggia lesion, because in the former, there is loss of stability in the ulnohumeral joint but the radioulnar relationship is preserved via an intact annular ligament.** Recognition of these injuries as fracture-dislocations facilitates an appropriate approach to restoring elbow stability. ***In cases of transolecranon fracture-dislocation of the elbow, anatomic restoration of the olecranon is critical to restore osseous resistance to anterior translation of the forearm. Simple transverse or oblique fractures may be treated via tension-band wiring or other fixation based on sound biomechanical principles.*** If the trochlear notch is comminuted, the ulnar fracture is generally amenable to plate fixation, since the olecranon fragment is usually of sufficient size to allow for rigid fixation with two or three cancellous screws. Restoration of the articular surface of the trochlear notch (with bone graft as necessary), including fixation of the coronoid process (which restores the integrity of the MCL), may then allow for early motion.

A. Monteggia Fractures (Fig. 21-4)—Monteggia fractures represent only 1% to 2% of forearm fractures. **Disruption of the annular ligament with dislocation of the proximal radioulnar joint, combined with an associated fracture of the proximal ulna, distinguishes the Monteggia lesion from fracture-dislocations of the elbow.** The radial head may be displaced anteriorly (Bado Type I), posteriorly (Bado Type II), or laterally (Bado Type III). Injuries with an associated

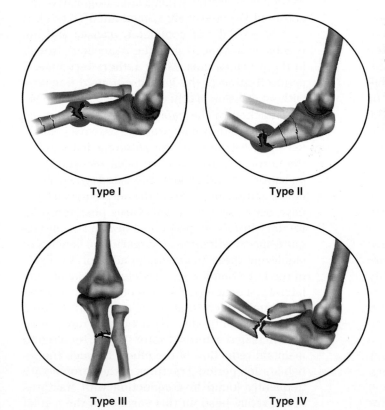

Type I   **Type II**

Type III   **Type IV**

FIGURE 21-4 Classification of Monteggia injuries (Bado). **Type I.** Anterior angulation of the ulnar fracture and anterior dislocation of the radial head. **Type II.** posterior angulation of the ulnar fracture and posterior dislocation of the radial head. **Type III.** fracture of the proximal ulna metaphysis and lateral dislocation of the radial head. **Type IV.** anterior dislocation of the radial head and fracture of both the radius and ulna.

fracture of the radial shaft have been designated as Bado Type IV (see Table 21-1). Associated ulnar fractures are generally distal to the coronoid process but may involve the trochlear notch. Dislocation of the radial head, especially posteriorly or laterally, may include disruption of the LCL, possibly leading to late instability of the elbow if unrecognized. ***Posterior interosseous nerve (PIN) palsy is most commonly seen in Bado Type I (anterior) fractures and may occur in a delayed fashion if the radial head is not promptly reduced.*** Appropriate management of these injuries is predicated on anatomic reduction and fixation of the ulna fracture. If stable anatomic fixation of the ulna with reduction of the proximal radioulnar joint is achieved, early motion should be instituted to minimize stiffness. Proximal radioulnar instability is rare in this setting, and annular ligament reconstruction is unnecessary. Ulnohumeral stability should be tested during surgery to detect possible injury to the LCL; repair of the LCL should be performed in the presence of any lateral instability. ***Malreduction of the ulna fracture can lead to persistent radial head subluxation, valgus instability, and post-traumatic arthrosis. Other, less common causes of persistent radial head subluxation include interposition of soft-tissue in the joint and lateral ligamentous injuries.***

B. Coronoid Fractures (Figs. 21-1 and 21-5)—Coronoid fractures are classified according to the percentage of the coronoid that is fractured (see Table 21-1). Fractures of the tip of the coronoid (Regan and Morrey Type I) do not cause instability and do not require treatment unless one or more fragments become incarcerated within the joint. The anterior capsule inserts 6.4 mm distal to the tip of the coronoid process. Therefore, Type I injuries do not signify capsular avulsion but may be a sign of previous elbow instability (i.e., an elbow dislocation or subluxation that spontaneously reduced). Fractures involving more than the tip but less than half the height of the coronoid signify a capsular avulsion injury (Regan and Morrey Type II). These Type II injuries are not frequently associated with elbow instability and can usually be treated nonoperatively. However, some Type II injuries of the coronoid may result in posterior subluxation of the elbow when tested in more than 45° of elbow extension; these fractures should be stabilized with screws, heavy sutures through drill holes, or suture anchors. Fractures involving 50% or more of the coronoid (Regan and Morrey Type III) compromise elbow

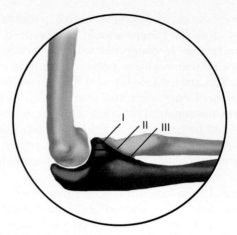

FIGURE 21-5   Coronoid fracture classification (Regan and Morrey). Note that Type I and Type II fractures involve less than 50% of the coronoid and are usually amenable to nonoperative treatment, whereas Type III fractures involve 50% of more of the coronoid and usually require operative stabilization.

stability by disrupting the osseous integrity of the ulnohumeral articulation, by disrupting the anterior capsule, and by rendering the MCL incompetent. They are associated with instability to anterior, valgus, and varus forces (even in the case of an intact LCL and radial head) as well as elbow extension. Therefore, Type III coronoid fractures should be repaired. Although fracture fixation is preferred, when a large fragment of the coronoid is extensively comminuted (rarely), it may be partially or completely excised and the brachialis advanced into the cancellous trough in the proximal ulna. Many authors recommend suture fixation of the largest coronoid fragment without excision of other small fragments if these are attached to the capsule. In this case, these smaller fragments may promote osseous healing. Recently, fractures of the anteromedial facet of the coronoid process have been recognized as an important and underappreciated type of coronoid fracture. Fractures of the anteromedial facet have been associated with varus posteromedial rotatory instability-pattern elbow injuries and require special attention at surgery. The benefits of stabilizing these fragments in addition to repair of the LCL complex are now clearly evident. Collateral ligament repair should be performed when a coronoid fracture is associated with residual elbow instability after reduction. In rare cases, an articulated external fixator may be required to maintain reduction of the elbow through the rehabilitation period. Fractures of the coronoid are frequently found in conjunction with fractures of the radial head. In this case, both the medial and lateral columns of the elbow are disrupted. ***When these fractures are associated with elbow dislocation (the "unhappy triad" of the elbow), recurrent instability and posttraumatic arthrosis often result. In this setting, smaller fractures of the coronoid may require fixation to provide additional stability.***

VII. Radial Head Fractures (Figs. 21-1 and 21-6)—Radial head fractures are generally created by the axial load sustained during a fall on an outstretched arm and are often associated with other injuries sustained by this mechanism (e.g., wrist). The PIN lies in close proximity and may also be injured. Careful evaluation of neurovascular status and motion is necessary, with the latter often difficult due to the fracture hemarthrosis. Intra-articular injection of local anesthetic through the posterolateral "soft spot" and subsequent aspiration of the hemarthrosis provides dramatic joint decompression with pain reduction, and greatly improved motion. In this manner, joint crepitus and loose fracture fragments can be identified. The forearm and wrist should be evaluated both clinically and radiographically for possible radioulnar dissociation (i.e., the Essex-Lopresti lesion). Posteroanterior radiographs in neutral forearm rotation of both wrists should be used to assess ulnar variance and possible distal radioulnar joint widening.

A. Classification and Treatment (Table 21-1)—Mason classified these injuries according to the degree of displacement or comminution of the radial head. ***Type I fractures are nondisplaced and may not be seen on radiographs. A posterior fat-pad sign is pathologic and should warrant further radiographs, including a radial head-capitellar view.*** Mason Type II fractures involve less than 30% of the articular surface but have more than 2 mm of fracture displacement. Mason Type III fractures involve comminution of the entire radial head. Controversy

exists with regard to the treatment of the Mason Type II injury (displaced fractures), and this system does little to guide treatment. Hotchkiss has classified these injuries more practically as those not requiring operative treatment (Type I), those requiring either open reduction with internal fixation (ORIF) or excision (Type II), and those that are too comminuted to be amenable to ORIF and should be excised (Type III). In the case of excision, the intact MCL provides adequate resistance to valgus force. Isolated radial head fractures should be reduced and stabilized if possible and excised if not. Elderly patients with low-demand elbows may lower the threshold for excision, but the current trend is towards ORIF whenever feasible. Any suspicion of valgus instability should lead the surgeon to seriously consider prosthetic radial head replacement rather than simple excision. ***Complications following excision of the radial head include muscle weakness, wrist pain, valgus elbow instability, heterotopic ossification, and arthritis. Displacement of fragments more than 2 mm increases the risk of arthrosis and is an indication for ORIF. Failure to achieve functional ROM after administration of a local anesthetic block is an indication for operative treatment as well.*** Impacted radial neck fractures are generally stable and amenable to treatment with early motion. Angulated fractures of the radial neck with an intact radial head are more frequently encountered in children but when encountered in adults, may require operative treatment, especially if angulated more than 30°. For comminution leading to shortening or displacement, fixation with appropriate hardware is advisable.

Radial head fractures associated with elbow dislocation (10% of all radial head fractures) are more difficult to treat. Excision after dislocation has been associated with high rates

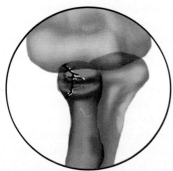

Type I

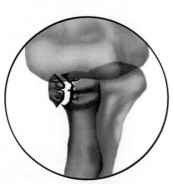

Type II

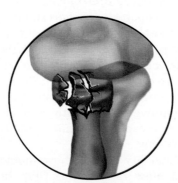

Type III

FIGURE 21-6 Mason classification of radial head fractures. (Type IV [radial head fracture with an elbow dislocation] fracture is not shown.)

of degenerative arthrosis and recurrent dislocation. Inadequate restoration of radial length (with either ORIF or replacement) alters the tension of the healing soft tissues. The restoration and maintenance of appropriate radial length may be more difficult in cases of interosseous membrane/ligament disruption (Essex-Lopresti lesion). More than 1 cm of shortening of the radial shaft indicates disruption of the interosseous membrane. Open treatment with internal fixation or prosthetic replacement with a metallic implant in this setting is critical to avoid the late sequelae of the Essex-Lopresti lesion.

Approaches to the radial head include the Kocher (between the anconeus and the extensor carpi ulnaris), the Kaplan (between the extensor carpi radialis brevis and the extensor digitorum communis, with pronation to protect the PIN), and the Pankovich (between the ulna and the supinator, from posterior).

When the radial neck is intact, headless self-compressing screws can secure radial head fragments to the remaining head and neck while being countersunk below the articular cartilage. In cases of radial neck comminution, mini-fragment plates can be placed more easily through the Kaplan approach. The point directly opposite the radial notch when the radius is halfway between maximal pronation and supination indicates the center of the "safe zone" for the placement of plates. Articular fragments should be supported with bone graft as necessary. AVN and nonunion may complicate highly comminuted fractures. Fixation of the radial head should be adequate enough to allow for a period of ligamentous healing. Excision of the radial head in the case of nonunion or AVN may be safely performed after the ligamentous integrity of the elbow is restored. *In cases of elbow dislocation and an unreconstructable radial head, excision of the radial head followed by prosthetic replacement is appropriate.* Silastic replacement does not restore valgus stability but yields better short-term results than simple excision. *However, silastic implants have been associated with synovitis and wear debris, and are rarely indicated.* Metallic implants restore more stability to valgus and have been shown to improve results, with more recent designs better recapitulating native radial head and neck anatomy.

Intraoperative stability of the elbow should be demonstrated after radial head ORIF or replacement and repair of the LCL, and lateral soft tissue restraints to the humeral epicondyle (with suture through bone tunnels or suture anchors). If instability is demonstrated, repair of the MCL and the medial soft tissues should follow. An external fixator is rarely required, but should be used if the elbow remains unstable after repair or reconstruction of the medial soft tissues.

VIII. Complications of Elbow Injuries
  A. Neurovascular Injury—Isolated or combined injuries to the median, ulnar, radial, and posterior and anterior interosseous nerves, and the brachial artery may occur as a result of the initial trauma or very infrequently, may have an iatrogenic origin. *The PIN is located adjacent to the radial neck, placing it at risk for a traction injury with dislocation of the proximal radius, as seen with Monteggia injuries.* The PIN is also the most at risk from iatrogenic injury, specifically during plating of radial neck fractures. Ulnar neuropathy is commonly seen after elbow trauma. Acutely, the ulnar nerve is at risk for traction neuropathy or from shards of bone. Late compressive neuropathy occurs within the cubital tunnel as the scar tissue matures. Controversy still exists regarding prophylactic ulnar nerve transposition during open reduction and internal fixation of distal humerus fractures. The nerve should be transposed subcutaneously if any hardware places it at risk.

As in other musculoskeletal injuries, the likelihood of neurovascular insult is tied to the mechanism of injury and the amount of energy imparted to the tissues. The ulnar, radial, and posterior interosseous nerves usually sustain neurapraxic and occasionally axonotmetic injuries as a result of direct blunt trauma or the cavitary effects of low-velocity gun shot wounds. Although the median and anterior interosseous nerves also commonly sustain such injuries, these two nerves along with the brachial artery and its branches are more susceptible to macroscopic injury as a result of their anterior midline location. The shards of bone dispersed from the distal humerus and proximal ulna in higher-energy injuries can impale these structures, especially in posterior fracture-dislocations and Monteggia lesions. Since these latter fractures usually require operative treatment, this allows for intraoperative inspection and surgical repair as indicated. Other specifics of neurovascular injuries are discussed in the sections on the specific fractures.

B. Posttraumatic Stiffness—Loss of motion is a common sequela of elbow injuries. Simple elbow dislocations frequently result in loss of the terminal 15° of extension. Loss of motion is more common after complex elbow dislocations (i.e., those with associated fractures). Extension seldom improves more than 6 months after injury. Arthrofibrosis, particularly involving the anterior joint capsule, is frequent unless early motion is instituted.

If 6 months have passed since the injury or motion gains have reached a plateau, *and* the elbow lacks extension beyond 35° or flexion beyond 100°, then operative release should be considered. Good results have been reported with open (i.e., medial, lateral, or combined approaches) and arthroscopic releases. In cases of stiffness after minimal trauma (e.g., isolated radial head fractures), arthroscopic release affords good results. The MCL and LCL should be preserved during open release. Symptomatic instability has been reported after lateral release when the LCL is injured.

The release of a posttraumatic contracture in the setting of malunion or nonunion is considerably more difficult, and poor results are common. Restoration of osseous anatomic structures in the acute setting with immobilization to achieve union should therefore take precedence over early motion in cases of tenuous fixation.

C. Heterotopic Ossification—Heterotopic ossification about the elbow involves, in order of frequency, the posterolateral joint, the anterior joint (or musculature), and the collateral ligaments. The risk of heterotopic ossification after injury to the elbow is similar for elbows treated operatively and nonoperatively. Increasing severity of the injury, delayed reduction of a dislocation, forced passive motion, central nervous system injury, repeat surgery during the first few weeks of treatment, and burns all have been associated with an increased risk for heterotopic ossification. Early motion, nonsteroidal anti-inflammatory agents (efficacy documented in the hip but not the elbow), and postoperative radiation (up to 1,000 cGy but with an increased risk of radiation-associated neuritis at the elbow as a result of the subcutaneous position of the nerves) decrease the incidence of heterotopic ossification. *Radiographic maturation of heterotopic bone (cortical and trabecular patterns) is the best predictor of an acceptable risk of recurrence after excision in the absence of risk factors. Early excision yields satisfactory results compared with the more*

standard, late excision. Serum alkaline phosphatase levels, total serum protein levels, and bone scans are less accurate and do not need to be monitored. Surgical excision is reserved for cases of functional impairment.

IX. Summary—Elbow fractures and dislocations occur in the context of a unique articulation with complex biomechanics. A full understanding of the osseous and ligamentous anatomy of the elbow is necessary for effectively evaluating and treating elbow trauma. More recent efforts at anatomic reduction and stable internal fixation of fractures with repair of soft-tissue stabilizers are proving superior to nonoperative or limited surgical techniques. Residual elbow stiffness is a frequent sequela to these injuries regardless of treatment and often must be addressed with additional surgical procedures.

SUGGESTED READINGS

Classic Articles

Bado JL. The Monteggia lesion. *Clin Orthop.* 1967;50:1971–1986.

Cobb TK, Morrey BF. Total elbow arthroplasty as primary treatment for distal humerus fractures in elderly patients. *J Bone Joint Surg Am.* 1997;79:826–832.

Dushuttle RP, Coyle MP, Zawadsky JP, et al. Fractures of the capitellum. *J Trauma.* 1985;25:317–321.

Fyfe IS, Mossad MM, Holdsworth BJ. Methods of fixation of olecranon fractures: an experimental mechanical study. *J Bone Joint Surg Br.* 1985;67:367–372.

Garland DE, Hanscom DA, Keenan MA, et al. Resection of heterotopic ossification in the adult with head trauma. *J Bone Joint Surg Am.* 1985;67:1261–1269.

Grantham SA, Norris TR, Bush DC. Isolated fracture of the humeral capitellum. *Clin Orthop.* 1981;161:262–269.

Hume MC, Wiss DA. Olecranon fractures: a clinical and radiographic comparison of tension-band wiring and plate fixation. *Clin Orthop.* 1992;285:229–235.

Jessing P. Monteggia lesions and their complicating nerve damage. *Acta Orthop Scand.* 1975;46:601–609.

Josefsson PO, Johnell O, GEntz CF. Long-term sequelae of simple dislocation of the elbow. *J Bone Joint Surg Am.* 1984;66:927–930.

Jupiter JB, Leibovic SJ, Ribbans W, et al. The posterior Monteggia lesion. *Trauma.* 1991;5:395–402.

King GJ, Lammens PN, Milne AD, et al. Plate fixation of comminuted olecranon fractures: an in vitro biomechanical study. *J Shoulder Elbow Surg.* 1996;5:437–441.

Macko D, Szabo RM. Complications of tension-band wiring of olecranon fractures. *J Bone Joint Surg Am.* 1985;67:1396–1401.

McKee MD, Jupiter JB, Bamberger HB. Coronal shear fractures of the distal end of the humerus. *J Bone Joint Surg Am.* 1996;78:48–54.

Moor TJ. Functional outcome following surgical excision of heterotopic ossification in patients with traumatic brain injury. *J Orthop Trauma.* 1993;7:11–14.

O'Driscoll SW, Morrey BF, Korinek S, et al. Elbow subluxation and dislocation: a spectrum of instability. *Clin Orthop.* 1992;280:186–197.

Peters CL, Scott SM. Compartment syndrome in the forearm following fractures of the radial head or neck in children. *J Bone Joint Surg Am.* 1995;77:1070–1074.

Stein F, Grabias SL, Deffer PA. Nerve injuries complicating Monteggia lesions. *J Bone Joint Surg Am.* 1971;53:1432–1436.

Recent Articles

Agarwal A. Type IV Monteggia fracture in a child. *Can J Surg.* 2008;51(2):E44–E45.

Bae DS, Kadiyala RK, Waters PM. Acute compartment syndrome in children: contemporary diagnosis, treatment and outcome. *J Pediatr Orthop.* 2001;21:680–688.

Chalidis B, Papadopoulos P, Sachinis N, et al. One-stage shoulder and elbow arthroplasty after ipsilateral fractures of the proximal and distal humerus. *J. Orthop Trauma.* 2008;22(4):282–285.

Clare DJ, Corley FG, Wirth MA. Ipsilateral combination Monteggia and Galeazzi injuries in an adult patient: a case report. *J Orthop Trauma.* 2002;16(2):130–134.

Deuel CR, Wolinsky P, Shepherd E, et al. The use of hinged external fixation to provide additional stabilization for fractures of the distal humerus. *J Orthop Trauma.* 2007;21(5):323–329.

Doornberg JN, de Jong IM, Lindenhovius AL, et al. The anteromedial facet of the coronoid process of the ulna. *J Shoulder Elbow Surg.* 2007;16(5):667–670.

Duckworth AD, Kulijdian A, McKee MD, et al. Residual subluxation of the elbow after dislocation or fracture-dislocation: treatment with active elbow exercises and avoidance of varus stress. *J Shoulder Elbow Surg.* 2008;17(2):276–280.

Duckworth AD, Ring D, Kulijdian A, et al. Unstable elbow dislocations. *J Shoulder Elbow Surg.* 2008;17(2):281–286.

Dunning CE, Zarzour ZD, Patterson SD, et al. Muscle forces and pronation stabilize the lateral ligament deficient elbow. *Clin Orthop.* 2001;388:118–124.

Egol KA, Immerman I, Paksima N, et al. Fracture-dislocation of the elbow functional outcome following treatment with a standardized protocol. *Bull NYU Hosp Jt Dis.* 2007;65(4):263–270.

Esser RD, Davis S, Taavao T. Fractures of the radial head treated by internal fixation: late results in 26 cases. *J Orthop Trauma.* 9:318–323.

Forthman C, Henket M, Ring DC. Elbow dislocation with intra-articular fracture: the results of operative treatment without repair of the medial collateral ligament. *J Hand Surg Am.* 2007;32(8):1200–1209.

Frankle MA, Herscovici D Jr, DiPasquale TG, et al. A comparison of open reduction and internal fixation and primary total elbow arthroplasty in the treatment of intra-articular distal humerus fractures in women older than 65. *J Orthop Trauma.* 2003;17:473–480.

Furry KL, Clinkscales CM. Comminuted fractures of the radial head: arthroplasty versus internal fixation. *Clin Orthop.* 1998;353:40–52.

Judet T, Marmorat JL, Mullins MM. Effective treatment of fracture-dislocations of the olecranon requires a stable trochlear notch. *Clin Orthop Relat Res.* 2005;(435):276–277.

Kälicke T, Muhr G, Franger TM. Dislocation of the elbow with fractures of the coronoid process and radial head. *Arch Orthop Trauma Surg.* 2007;127(10):925–931.

Konrad GG, Kundel K, Kreuz PC, et al. Monteggia fractures in adults: long-term results and prognostic factors. *J Bone Joint Surg Br.* 2007;89(3):354–360.

Lindenhovius AL, Felsch Q, Doornberg JN, et al. Open reduction and internal fixation compared with excision for unstable displaced fractures of the radial head. *J Hand Surg Am.* 2007;32(5):630–636.

Maeda H, Yoshida K, Doi R, et al. Combined Monteggia and Galeazzi fractures in a child: a case report and review of the literature. *J Orthop Trauma.* 2003;17(2):128–131.

Mehdian H, McKee M. Management of proximal and distal humerus fractures. *Orthop Clin North Am.* 2000;31:115–127.

Moushine E, Akiki A, Castagna A, et al. Transolecranon anterior fracture dislocation. *J Shoulder Elbow Surg.* 2007;16(3):352–357.

Nalbantoglu U, Kocaoglu B, Gereli A, et al. Open reduction and internal fixation of Mason type III radial head fractures with and without an associated elbow dislocation. *J Hand Surg Am.* 2007;32(10):1560–1568.

Obremskey WT, Bhandari M, Dirschl DR, et al. Internal fixation versus arthroplasty of comminuted fractures of the distal humerus. *J Orthop Trauma.* 2003;17:463–465.

Papandrea RF, Morrey BF, O'Driscoll SW. Reconstruction for persistent instability of the elbow after coronoid fracture-dislocation. *J Shoulder Elbow Surg.* 2007;16(1):68–77.

Pugh DM, Wild LM, Schemitsch EH, et al. Standard surgical protocol to treat elbow dislocations with radial head and coronoid fractures. *J Bone Joint Surg Am.* 2004;86:1122–1130.

Ring D, Hannouche D, Jupiter JB. Surgical treatment of persistent dislocation or subluxation of the ulnohumeral joint after fracture-dislocation of the elbow. *J Hand Surg [Am].* 2004;29(3):470–480.

Ring D, Jupiter J, Gulotta L. Articular fractures of the distal part of the humerus. *J Bone Joint Surg Am.* 2003;85:232–238.

Ring D, Jupiter JB, Sanders RW, et al. Transolecranon fracture-dislocation of the elbow. *J Orthop Trauma.* 1997;11:545–550.

Ring D, Jupiter JB, Simpson NS. Monteggia fractures in adults. *J Bone Joint Surg Am.* 1998;80:1733–1744.

Ring D, Jupiter JB, Zilberfarb J. Posterior dislocation of the elbow with fractures of the radial head and coronoid. *J Bone Joint Surg Am.* 2002;84-A(4):547–551.

Ring D, Jupiter JB. Fracture-dislocation of the elbow. *J Bone Joint Surg Am.* 1998;80:566–580.

Ring D, Quintero J, Jupiter JB. Open reduction and internal fixation of fractures of the radial head. *J Bone Joint Surg Am.* 2002;84:1811–1815.

Ring D, Tavakolian J, Kloen P, et al. Loss of alignment after surgical treatment of posterior Monteggia fractures: salvage with dorsal contoured plating. *J Hand Surg Am.* 2004;29(4):694–702.

Schneeberger AG, Sadowski MM, Jacob HA. Coronoid process and radial head as posterolateral rotatory stabilizers of the elbow. *J Bone Joint Surg [Am].* 2004:86-A(5):975–982.

Strauss EJ, Tejwani NC, Preston CF, et al. The posterior Monteggia lesion with associated ulnohumeral instability. *J Bone Joint Surg Br.* 2006;88(1):84–89.

Van Riet RP, Morrey BF. Documentation of associated injuries occurring with radial head fracture. *Clin Orthop Relat Res.* 2008;466(1):130–134.

Villanueva P, Osorio F, Commessatti M, et al. Tension-band wiring for olecranon fractures: analysis of risk factors for failure. *J Shoulder Elbow Surg.* 2006;15(3):351–356.

Review Articles

Boyer MI, Galatz LM, Borelli J Jr, et al. Intra-articular fractures of the upper extremity: new concepts in surgical management. *Instr Course Lect.* 2003;52:591–605.

Cohen MS, Hastings H 2nd. Acute elbow dislocations: evaluation and management. *J Am Acad Orthop Surg.* 1998;6:15–23.

Hotchkiss RN. Displaced fractures of the radial head: Internal fixation or excision? *J Am Acad Orthop Surg.* 1997;5:1–10.

Textbooks

Jupiter JB, Kellam JF. Diaphyseal fractures of the forearm. In: Broward B, Jupiter J, Levine A, et al, eds. *Skeletal Trauma*. 2nd ed. Philadelphia, PA: WB Saunders; 1992:1421–1454.

Kellam JF, Fischer TJ, Tornetta P 3rd, et al, eds. *Orthopedic Knowledge Update: Trauma 2*. Rosemont, IL: American Academy of Orthopaedic Surgeons; 2000.

Morrey BF. Radial head fracture. In: Morrey BF, ed. *The elbow and Its Disorders*. 3rd ed. Philadelphia, PA: WB Saunders; 2000.

CHAPTER 22

Forearm Injuries

Lisa K. Cannada

I. Forearm fractures are a common injury often occurring from a fall or a direct blow. Twenty six percent of fractures involving both bones of the forearm occur in children younger than 15 years of age.

   The treatment for these injuries depends on a number of factors. These include the patient's age, bone quality, physiologic health, specific injury pattern, associated injuries, and physical demands. There are four main types of forearm fractures: (a) an isolated fracture of the radius or ulna, (b) fracture of the radius with a distal radial ulnar joint (DRUJ) dislocation (Galeazzi fracture), (c) fracture of the ulna with a radial head dislocation (Monteggia fracture), and (d) a both bone forearm fracture of the radius and ulna. The treatment of most fractures of the forearm, except some isolated ulnar shaft fractures, is operative.

II. Anatomy—The forearm is complex with two mobile parallel bones, which essentially function as a joint with a proximal and distal radioulnar joint (DRUJ). There are several muscles that originate in the forearm and insert on the hand and provide hand function. Thus, it is of paramount importance following a forearm fractures to restore rotation of the forearm, range of motion of the wrist and elbow, and grip strength.

A. Bones
   1. Radius—Proximally the radius has a radial notch for articulation with the ulna, and distally there is a notch for articulation as well. There is a tuberosity in the proximal portion of the radius for insertion of the biceps. The radius has a bow, which must be restored during fracture treatment. Every 5° loss of radial bow results in a 15° loss of pronation and supination. After open reduction internal fixation (ORIF) of a both bone forearm fracture, the recovery of grip strength and forearm motion correlates with restoration of the normal radial bow.
   2. Ulna
B. Interosseous Membrane—The interosseous membrane is between the two bones and is very important in assisting with forearm function as well. The interosseous membrane is of key importance for forearm stability. The interosseous membrane can be considered as proximal, middle, and distal thirds with the middle third being the strongest and most significant contributor to longitudinal stability of the forearm.
C. Muscles
   1. Volar
      • The mobile wad consists of the brachioradialis, the extensor carpi radialis longus (ECRL) and the extensor carpi radialis brevis (ECRB) The radial nerve provides innervation.
      • The flexor pronator group is arranged in three layers. The median and ulnar nerves provide innervation.
      (a) The superficial layer—The superficial layer has four muscles arising from the medial humeral epicondyle spanning out across the forearm. It is easy to remember these in their orientation if you place your hand at the medial epicondyle with the palm on the anterior surface of the forearm. The thumb represents a pronator teres. The index finger represents the flex carpi radialis, the middle finger represents the palmaris longus (which is absent in approximately 10% of the population), and the ring finger represents the flexor carpi ulnaris.
      (b) The middle layer is the flexor digitorum superficialis.

(c) The deep layer is the flexor digitorum profundus, flexor pollicus longus, and pronator quadratus.

2. Dorsal
   • Superficial—The superficial extensor muscles fan out from the lateral epicondyle of the humerus. From the ulnar side to the radial side, they are the:
     (a) anconeus
     (b) extensor carpi ulnaris
     (c) extensor digiti minimi
     (d) extensor digitorum communis
   • Deep
     (a) The abductor pollicis longus, extensor pollicis longus and extensor pollicis brevis provide motor function to the thumb and cross the forearm from the ulnar to the radial side in an oblique manner.
     (b) The remaining deep muscles are the supinator and the extensor indicis.

D. Nerves
   1. Radial nerve
      • The radial nerve has a superficial sensory branch along the lateral aspect of the forearm. It runs under the brachioradialis muscle.
      • The anterior branch of the radial nerve supplies the mobile wad muscles (brachioradialis, ECRL, ECRB).
      • The deep branch is the posterior interosseous nerve (PIN) (Fig. 22-1). The PIN passes between the two heads of the supinator and emerges distally over the origin of the abductor pollicis longus lying along the interosseous membrane. In 25% of patients, the PIN is directly on bone near the biceps tuberosity.
     (a) To protect the nerve, do not place retractors on the posterior surface of the proximal radius.
     (b) ***With proximal exposure of the forearm, supinate the forearm to protect the nerve***.

   2. Median nerve—The median nerve enters the forearm and antecubital fossa region and splits the pronator teres running between the flexor digitorum superficialis and the flexor digitorum profundus.

   3. Ulnar nerve—The ulnar nerve travels under the flexor carpi ulnaris and lies on the flexor digitorum profundus in the forearm. The ulnar artery lies on the radial side of the nerve.

E. Arteries—The radial and ulnar arteries are branches of the brachial artery.
   1. Radial artery—Proximally, the radial artery lies just medial to the biceps tendon and angles across the arm lying on the supinator, the pronator teres and the origin of the flexor pollicis longus. The radial artery is palpable on the distal anterior radius.
   2. Ulnar artery—The ulnar artery runs between the flexor digitorum profundus and superficialis;

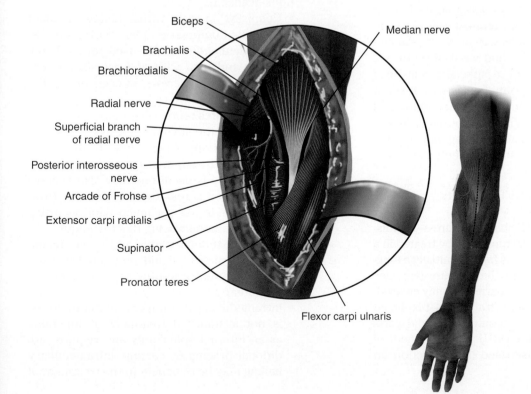

Biceps
Brachialis
Brachioradialis
Radial nerve
Superficial branch of radial nerve
Posterior interosseous nerve
Arcade of Frohse
Extensor carpi radialis
Supinator
Pronator teres
Median nerve
Flexor carpi ulnaris

FIGURE 22-1 Course of the posterior interosseous nerve in the proximal forearm.

distally, it runs between the flexor carpi ulnaris and the flexor digitorum superficialis.

III. Surgical Approaches
   A. Volar (Henry) Approach—This extensile approach uses an internervous plane between the radial nerve and the median nerve. The muscular interval is between the brachioradialis and the pronator teres/flexor carpal radialis.
   B. Dorsal (Thompson) Approach—The internervous plane is between the radial nerve and the PIN. The dorsal approach of Thompson utilizes the interval between the extensor carpal radialis brevis and the extensor digitorum communis/extensor pollicis longus.
   C. Approach to the Ulna—The ulnar is approached between the extensor carpi ulnaris and the flexor carpi ulnaris right along the bone. The internervous plane is between the PIN and the ulnar nerve.
   D. Cross-Sectional Anatomy of the Forearm (Fig. 22-2).

IV. Physical Evaluation—The patient with a forearm fracture often has obvious signs and symptoms of a fracture, with deformity and crepitus. The physical examination should include the elbow and wrist. Close evaluation of the soft tissue is necessary to assess for any evidence of open fracture, soft-tissue injury, and injury of the median, radial, and ulnar nerves. It is also important to evaluate the patient for compartment syndrome (discussed later in this chapter).

V. Radiographic Evaluation—Radiographic evaluation of the forearm includes an anteroposterior (AP) and lateral view of the forearm as well as AP, lateral and oblique views of the elbow and wrist. If there is a fracture of the radial head, a special radial head radiographic view may be obtained as well. It is not necessary to include computer tomography and magnetic resonance imaging for routine forearm fractures. Magnetic resonance imaging may provide further information regarding ligamentous disruption and joint involvement.

VI. Specific Injury Patterns and Treatments
   A. Radial Shaft Fractures
      1. Nondisplaced radial shaft fractures—Nondisplaced radial shaft fractures may be treated in a cast until the fractures is healed. Initially a long-arm cast is used until the fracture becomes "sticky" and then a short-arm cast may be used.
      2. Displaced radial shaft fractures—Displaced radial shaft fractures require ORIF and careful assessment of the DRUJ. The treatment of DRUJ injuries is discussed in the section on Galeazzi fractures.
   B. Ulnar Shaft Fractures—Isolated ulna fractures often occur as the result of an altercation with the ulna broken when the forearm is used in self-defense. These injuries are therefore commonly known as a nightstick fracture.
      1. The recommended treatment for an isolated ulnar fracture that is stable is functional bracing. The key here is that the central third of the interosseous membrane remains intact.
      2. Ulnar shaft fractures that are displaced with more than 10° of angulation or more than 50% fracture displacement require ORIF.
   C. Both-Bone Forearm Fractures
      1. Pediatric—Closed reduction and splinting followed by casting is an acceptable treatment method in the pediatric population. In children younger than age 9, up to15° of angulation and 45° of malrotation is acceptable. In children older than age 9, up to 10° of angulation and 30° of malrotation is acceptable. In children with forearm fractures, *there have been case reports of scarring or tendinous entrapment.* Close physical examination is the key to diagnosis.
      2. Adult—For the adult population, casting does not allow for maintenance of reduction and thus is not an accepted form of treatment. The treatment of choice for an adult both bone forearm fracture is ORIF with plate and screw fixation. Currently there are several plate options available.
         • Compression plate with a Limited Contact Dynamic Compression plate (LCDC)—LCDC is recommended to be used for both the radius and ulna with at least six cortices purchased with screws on each side of the fracture.
         • Locking plates represent a newer type of fixation. With the advent of locked plates, certain indications have evolved—*the main one being osteoporotic bone.* If a combination plate is used, one may also achieve compression across the fracture site. However, there is not yet much data regarding clinical outcomes using this technique.
         • One-third tubular plates and pelvic reconstruction plates fail and should not be used for diaphyseal fractures in both bones of the forearm.
         • Intramedullary fixation of forearm fractures is not a standard treatment. It functions as an internal splint only and requires additional bracing or casting. Intramedullary nailing may be of benefit in the treatment of

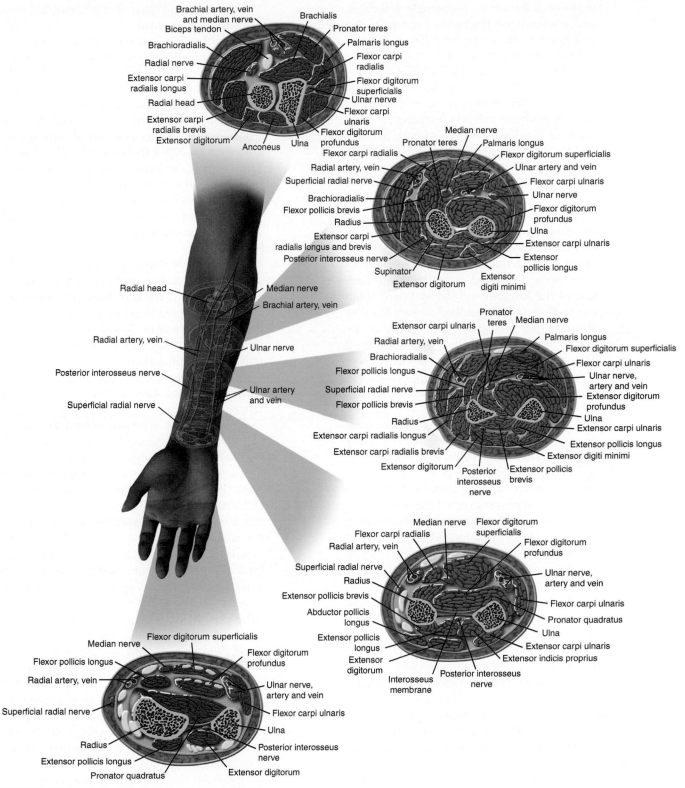

FIGURE 22-2 Cross-sectional anatomy of the forearm.

segmental fractures, pathologic fractures, and comminuted fractures, especially due to a gunshot injury. Intramedullary fixation is best used for fractures of the diaphysis and should not be used for injuries near the proximal or distal end of the bone. Intramedullary nail fixation is more commonly used in pediatric forearm fractures.

- External fixation—The use of external fixation for forearm fractures is generally not indicated. There is significant risk of injury to neurovascular structures in addition to pin site complications. External fixation should typically be reserved for extremely unstable patients or those with significant open contaminated injuries.

- Other techniques—Various techniques have been described regarding plate fixation of the forearm and the standard treatments have been described above. Another strategy that has gained popularity is the use of longer plates (such as those used with a bridge plating technique) with fewer screws. Two recent studies support the use of long plates with screws capturing only four cortices on either side of the fracture with two cortices being close to the fracture on each end and two being further away from the fracture. Long-term results of this technique are pending.

3. Bone grafting in both-bone forearm fractures— Bone graft is necessary only if there is no cortical contact. Previously it was recommended that bone grafting be completed at the time of fixation if comminution exceeded one third of the bone's diameter. However, there was a review of 319 diaphyseal forearm fractures with variable comminution which were treated with open reduction and internal fixation without bone grafting (although significant comminution was present in <5% of the cases). Those fractures which had significant comminution had a prolonged time to union but still managed to heal.

D. Monteggia Fracture Dislocations
1. Classification—The classification system most commonly used is the Bado classification which describes the direction of the dislocation of the radial head. This type of fracture does not reduce with closed reduction techniques.
- An anterior dislocation is a Type I
- A posterior dislocation is a Type II
- A lateral dislocation is a Type III
- A Type IV injury involves anterior dislocation of the radial head with fracture of both

the radius and ulna in the proximal one-third of the forearm.
2. Treatment—The standard of care is ORIF of the ulna. With restoration of the ulnar anatomy, the radial head often reduces with closed methods. If the radial head does not reduce through closed methods, then open reduction is indicated, as there may be soft-tissue interposition. ***Associated injuries include up to 20% incidence of a PIN injury. The correct technique for a comminuted proximal ulnar fracture is a posterior plate that acts as a tension band.*** The plate should not be applied medially, as it will not resist the compressive forces.

E. Galeazzi Fracture
1. Description—A Galeazzi fracture is a radial shaft fracture in conjunction with disruption of the DRUJ. The fracture most commonly occurs in the distal third at the metaphyseal/diaphyseal junction. Closed reduction is not an acceptable treatment option because of the multiple muscle attachments and deforming forces. The deforming forces include the pronator quadratus, brachioradialis, thumb extensors and the weight of the hand (gravity).
2. Treatment—This fracture is also known as a "fracture of necessity" because the injury necessitates ORIF with plate and screw fixation and reduction of the distal radialulnar joint. It is very important to evaluate the DRUJ after plating of the radius. The joint often is reduced in a supinated position where it should be casted for 6 weeks. A Muenster cast is an excellent cast to be used for this type of injury as it allows elbow flexion and extension but discourages pronation and supination. If the DRUJ cannot be maintained with closed methods, percutaneous reduction and pinning should be performed. ***The most common reason for inability to obtain a closed reduction is interposition of the extensor carpi ulnaris in the DRUJ.*** The location of the radial shaft fracture may give some clue as to whether the distal radial joint is unstable. In a recent study, the DRUJ was unstable in 55% of patients when a radial shaft fracture occurred less than the 7.5 cm from the mid-articular surface of the radius. If the radial fracture was more than 7.5 cm from the mid articular surface of the radius, the DRUJ was unstable in only 6% of patients.

F. Floating Elbow/The Polytraumatized Patient—A floating elbow injury occurs if the radius or ulnar or both are fractured along with the humerus; ORIF is the treatment of choice. In the pediatric population, there is a significant increased risk of compartment syndrome with a floating elbow injury.

In the polytraumatized patient, operative intervention should be considered early in order to permit mobilization.

VII. Complications of Forearm Injuries
   A. Compartment Syndrome
      1. Overview—Compartment syndrome is a rare complication in patients with forearm fractures but should not to be missed. The incidence is low, under 3%. However, there is a higher incidence with proximal ulna fractures caused by high-energy trauma. *Compartment syndrome can also occur with gunshot wounds to the forearm without fracture.*
      2. Etiology
         • High-energy comminuted fractures
         • Significantly displaced fractures
         • Severe soft injuries
         • Crush injuries
         • Vascular injuries
         • Tight closure of the fascial compartments after surgery
         • Prolonged tissue compression
         • Casting which is too tight
         • Patient physiology (anti-coagulation medication)
      2. Clinical Evaluation—A high index of suspicion for compartment syndrome is warranted in the patient with progressive forearm pain. The pain is characteristically out of proportion to the patient's injuries. The arm may be tense and swollen. Passive stretch of the muscles in the involved compartment causes significant discomfort. The deepest muscles are affected first and are abnormal earliest in the physical examination, thus the flexor digitorum profundus and flexor pollicis longus are commonly affected first as they are the deepest muscles. The next muscles affected are the flexor digitorum superficialis and pronator teres. The patient may present with a compartment syndrome or it may develop over time so close monitoring is essential.
      3. Treatment—The immediate treatment is urgent fasciotomy. Most often, it is the volar compartment in the forearm that develops compartment syndrome. It is important to completely release the volar compartment including the carpal tunnel. The additional forearm compartments are the dorsal compartment and the mobile wad compartment.

   B. Infection—The surgical infection rate in forearm fractures is generally low, anywhere from 0.8% to 7%. With open fractures, the rate may increase up to 20%. The treatment is irrigation and debridement and intravenous antibiotics, which are culture specific. Whenever possible, hardware should be retained until fracture healing occurs.

   C. Fracture Nonunion—The rate of nonunion of forearm fractures is 12% or more, depending upon many factors. An increased risk of nonunion is seen in open fracture, severely comminuted fractures, segmental fractures, fractures with bone loss, cases of plate fixation mismatch, and those treated with an intramedullary nail. The most common treatment of a fracture nonunion of the forearm is autogenous bone graft. It is important that the bone graft be laid just about the nonunion site after it is taken down and not across the interosseous membrane as that increases the risk of synostosis.

   D. Nerve Injuries—Nerve injuries are more related to the complications in the soft-tissue stresses due to excessive swelling or iatrogenic due to retraction of the soft tissues during surgical exposure. Injury to the median nerve with a diaphyseal fracture has been reported but is uncommon. The most common risk during surgical exposure of the middle and distal thirds of the forearm is the superficial radial nerve. The PIN is at risk during exposure of the proximal forearm. The clinical presentation of specific muscles lost in the various nerve injuries is shown in Table 22-1 and Figures 22-3 through 22-6.

   E. Functional Outcome—*Recovery of grip strength and forearm motion following ORIF correlates best with restoration of the radial bow* (long-term outcomes have not yet been well documented). McKee evaluated patients with both bone forearm fractures treated with open reduction and internal fixation at an average of 5.4 years following surgery; compared to the uninjured arm, the injured arms had approximately a 30% decrease in forearm pronation and supination. There was also a significant decrease in wrist flexion (16%), wrist extension (37%) and grip strength (25%). These deficits were found despite the patients being several years out from their injury.

   F. Synostosis—Synostosis is more common in patients with head injuries, burns, genetic predisposition to soft-tissue injury or if bone fragments or bone graft is in the area of the interosseous membrane. The likelihood of radial-ulnar synostosis

TABLE 22-1

Nerve Injuries

Injured Nerve	Clinical Presentation	Specific Muscle Lost
Radial nerve (see Fig. 22-3)		
High	Wrist-drop deformity	EDC
		EPL
		APL
		ECRB
		ECRL
		BR
Low	Wrist-drop deformity	EDC
		EPL
		APL
Ulnar nerve[a]		
High	Ulnar clawhand deformity (intrinsic-minus deformity) (see Fig. 22-4)	Adductor pollicis
		Interossei
		FDP (to the ring and small fingers)
		FCU
		Lumbricals (to the ring and small fingers)
Low	Severe ulnar clawhand deformity	Adductor pollicis
		Interossei
		Lumbricals (to the ring and small fingers)
Median nerve		
High	Ape-hand deformity (see Fig. 22-5)	PT
		FCR
		FDP (to the index and long fingers)
		FPL
		APB
		Lumbricals (to the index and long fingers)
Low	Thenar wasting (see Fig. 22-5)	APB
		Lumbricals (to the index and long fingers)

[a]*Note:* A low-ulnar nerve injury paradoxically results in a worse deformity than a high-ulnar injury because in a low-ulnar nerve injury, the FDP to the ring and small fingers retains innervation and results in an even worse clawing deformity. *EDC,* Extensor digitorum communis; *EPL,* Extensor pollicis longus; *APL,* Abductor pollicis longus; *ECRB,* Extensor carpi radialis brevis; *ECRL,* Extensor carpi radialis longus; *BR,* Brachioradialis; *FDP,* Flexor digitorum profundus; *FCU,* Flexor carpi ulnaris, *PT,* Pronator teres; *FCR,* Flexor carpi radialis; *FPL,* Flexor pollicis longus; *APB,* Abductor pollicis brevis.
Source: From Brinker MR, Miller MD. *Fundamentals of Orthopaedics.* Philadelphia, PA: WB Saunders; 1999, with permission.

is increased with high-energy fractures with extensive comminution or when there is violation of the interosseous membrane with screws or the surgical approach. This can lead to loss of pronation and supination. Compared with heterotopic ossification around other joints, the treatment in the forearm is early excision. Excellent results have been reported with resection of a forearm synostosis within 4 months of injury and then utilizing a protocol postoperatively including radiation or Indomethacin. Occurrence of a forearm synostosis in the proximal one-third in general leads to more disability and less favorable results.

G. Refracture after Plate Removal—This may occur with the use of large plates, removal of the plate too early in the postoperative period and

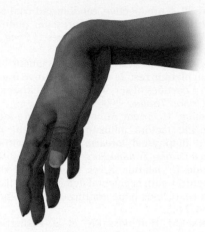

FIGURE 22-3 Wrist-drop deformity of a radial nerve injury.

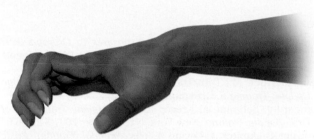

FIGURE 22-4 Clawhand (intrinsic-minus) deformity. Loss of intrinsic muscle function (usually from ulnar [and median] nerve injury) and overpull of the extrinsic extensors on the metacarpophalangeal joints lead to extension at the metacarpophalangeal joints and flexion at the interphalangeal joints.

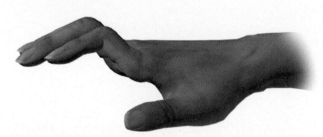

FIGURE 22-5 Ape-hand deformity (median nerve injury) associated with thenar wasting. Note the hyperextension of the metacarpophalangeal joints and the inability to flex or oppose the thumb.

failure to protect the forearm after the plate is removed. ***The incidence of refracture after hardware removal using large fragment plates approaches 20%.*** The patients often refracture through the large screw holes. It is important to not remove the plate until the fracture is healed and bone remodeling is observed on radiographs. The patient should be limited to

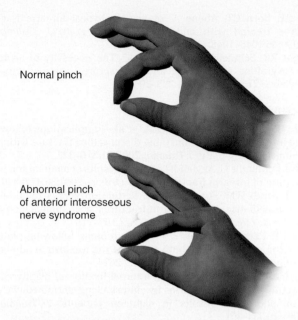

Normal pinch

Abnormal pinch of anterior interosseous nerve syndrome

FIGURE 22-6 Deficit of the anterior interosseous nerve is manifested by loss of active flexion of the index distal interphalangeal and thumb interphalangeal joints, giving a characteristic abnormal pinch.

decreased physical activities for 8 to 12 weeks following plate removal.

SUGGESTED READINGS

Classic Articles

Bado JL, Springfield T. The Monteggia lesion. *Clin Orthp Rel Res.* 1967;50:71–86.

Chapman MW, Gordon JE, Zissimos AG. Compression plate fixation of acute fractures of the diaphysis of the radius and ulna. *J Bone Joint Surg Am.* 1989;71:156–169.

Chung KC, Spilson SV. The frequency and epidemiology of hand and forearm fractures in the United States. *J Hand Surg Am.* 2001;26(5):908–915.

Deluca PA, Lindsey RW, Ruwe PA. Refracture of bones of the forearm after removal of compression plates. *J Bone Joint Surg Am.* 1988;70:1372–1376.

Jupiter JB, Ring D. Operative treatment of post-traumatic proximal radioulnar synostosis. *J Bone Joint Surg Am.* 1998;80:248–257.

Moed BR, Fakhouri AJ. Compartment syndrome after low velocity gunshot wounds to the forearm. *J Ortho Trauma.* 1991;5:134–137.

Sarmiento A, Latta LL, Zych G. et al. Isolated ulnar shaft fractures treated with functional braces. *J Orthop Trauma.* 1998;12:420–423.

Schemitsch EH, Richards RR. The effect of malunion on functional outcome after plate fixation of fractures of both bones of the forearm in adults. *J Bone Joint Surg Am.* 1992 74:1068–1078.

Tarr RR, Garfinkel AI, Sarmiento A. The effects of angular and rotational deformity on both bones of the forearm. *J Bone Joint Surg Am.* 1984;66:65–70.

Wei SY, Born CT, Abene A, et al. Diaphyseal forearm fractures treated with and without bone graft. *J Trauma.* 1999;46:1045–1048.

Wright RR, Schmeling GJ, Schwab JP. The necessity of acute bone grafting in diaphyseal forearm fractures: a retrospective review. *J Trauma.* 1977;11:288–294.

Recent Articles

Arora R, Lutz M, Hennerbichler A, et al. Complications following internal fixation of unstable distal radius fracture with a palmar locking-plate. *J Trauma.* 2007;21:316–322.

Crow BD, Mundis G, Anglen JO. Clinical results of minimal screw fixation of forearm fractures. *Am J Orthop.* 2007;36:477–480.

Do TT, Strub WM, Foad SL, et al. Reduction versus remodeling in pediatric distal forearm fractures: a preliminary cost analysis. *J Pediatr Orthop B.* 2003;12:109–115.

Droll KP, Perma P, Potter J, et al. Outcomes following plate fixation of fractures of both bones of the forearm in adults. *J Bone Joint Surg Am.* 2007;89:2619–2624.

Gao H, Luo CF, Zhang CQ, et al. Internal fixation of diaphyseal fractures of the forearm by interlocking intramedullary nail: short-term results in eighteen patients. *J Trauma.* 2005;19:384–391.

Ghobrial TF, Egleseder WA, Bleckner SA. Proximal ulna shaft fractures and associated compartment syndromes. *Am J Orthop.* 2001;30:703–707.

Goldfarb CA, Ricci WM, Tull F, et al. Functional outcome after fracture of both bones of the forearm. *J Bone Joint Surg Br.* 2005;87:374–379.

Haas N, Hauke C, Schutz M, et al. Treatment of diaphyseal fractures of the forearm using the Point Contact Fixator (PC-Fix): results of 387 fractures of a prospective multicentric study (PC-Fix II). *Injury.* 2001;32(suppl 2):B51062.

Larson AN, Rizzo M. Locking plate technology and its applications in upper extremity fracture care. *Hand Clin.* 2007;23:269–278.

Leung F, Chow SP. A prospective, randomized trial comparing the limited contact dynamic compression plate with the pint contact fixator for forearm fractures. *J Bone Joint Surg Am.* 2003;85:2343–2348.

Lindvall EM, Sagi HC. Selective screw placement in foararm compression plating: results of 75 consecutive fractures stabilized with 4 cortices of screw fixation on either side of the fracture. *J Orthop Trauma.* 2006;20:157–162.

Mikek M, Vidmar G, Tonin M, et al. Fracture-related and Implant-specific factors influencing treatment results of comminuted diaphyseal forearm fractures without bone grafting. *Arch Orthop Trauma Surgery.* 2004;124:393–400.

Ring D, Allende C, Jafarnia K, et al. Ununited diaphyseal forearm fractures with segmental defects: plate fixation and autogenous cancellous bone grafting. *J Bone Joint Surg Am.* 2004;86:2440–2445.

Ring D, Waters PM, Hotchkiss RN, et al. Pediatric floating elbow. *Pediatr Orthop.* 2001;21:456–459.

Solomon HB, Zadnik M, Egleseder WA. A review of outcomes in 18 patients with floating elbow. *J Orthop Trauma.* 2003;17:563–570.

Textbooks

Hoppenfeld S, deBoer P. *Surgical Exposures in Orthopaedics: The Anatomic Approach.* 3rd ed. Philadelphia, PA: Lippincott Williams & Wilkins; 2003:141–172.

Baumgaertner M, Tornetta P, eds. *Orthopaedic Knowledge Update: Trauma 3.* Rosemont, IL: AAOS; 2005:199–220.

Stannard J, Schmidt A, Kregor P, eds. *Surgical Treatment of Orthopaedic Trauma.* New York, NY: Thieme; 2007:340–363.

Browner B, Jupiter J, Levine A, eds. *Skeletal Trauma: Basic Science, Management, and Reconstruction.* Vol 2, 3rd ed. Philadelphia, PA: Saunders; 2003:1363–1403.

CHAPTER 23

Fractures and Dislocations of the Wrist

R. Jay French

I. Fractures of the Distal Radius
  A. Overview—Fractures of the distal radius are the most common fractures of the upper extremity, representing 17% of all fractures treated each year. Although they are seen most frequently among older women (ages 60 to 70), young adults make up a significant portion of cases. *For those patients older than 60 years of age, almost 70% will have significant osteoporosis of the hip or spine.* High-energy injuries resulting in complex fracture patterns have led to the development of newer treatment modalities. *Residual articular incongruity greater than 2 mm leads to post-traumatic arthritis in most, if not all, patients.* As a result, traditional methods of nonoperative treatment of high-energy injuries have been abandoned in favor of surgical techniques that restore articular anatomic structures.
  B. Mechanism of Injury—Approximately 90% of all distal-radius fractures are caused by *compressive loading* on the dorsiflexed wrist. *The degree of comminution is proportional to the energy transferred to the bone, with high-energy injuries causing more comminution and increasingly complex fracture patterns*.
  C. Anatomy
    1. Bony anatomy
      • Distal radius—The distal radius is composed of three concave articular surfaces: scaphoid fossa, lunate fossa, and sigmoid notch (Fig. 23-1).
      • Articulation between the distal radius and the ulna—The articulation between the distal radius and the ulna occurs at the sigmoid notch, forming the distal radioulnar joint (DRUJ) and allowing forearm rotation.
      • Triangular fibrocartilage complex (TFCC)—The TFCC has multiple attachments to the ulna and carpus and may be injured in combination with a distal radius fracture (see later section on the DRUJ).
      • Biomechanics—The radius normally carries 80% of the axial load across the wrist. This percentage may change after fracture if there is radial shortening or dorsal tilt of the radial articular surface. *As fracture deformity increases, greater loads are shifted to the ulnar side of the wrist.* A dorsal tilt of 30° results in 50% load transmission to the ulna.
      • Wrist range of motion—Normal ranges of motion of the wrist joint are as follows: dorsiflexion, up to 80°; palmar flexion, up to 85°; radial deviation, up to 25°; ulnar deviation, up to 35°; and pronation/supination, up to 90°. These ranges often decrease after injury as a result of fracture deformity, prolonged immobilization, or both.
    2. Ligamentous anatomy—The extrinsic ligaments of the wrist stabilize the carpus to the distal radius and ulna. The intrinsic ligaments of the wrist link the individual carpal bones and are discussed later in this chapter.
      • Volar ligaments—*The volar extrinsic ligaments are stronger and clinically more important.* They include the radioscaphocapitate (RSC), long radiolunate (LRL), short radiolunate (SRL), ulnolunate (UL), and ulnotriquetral (UT) ligaments (Fig. 23-2). The radioscapholunate ligament (ligament of Testut) is now believed to be a neurovascular pedicle and does not provide ligamentous support.
      • Dorsal ligaments—The dorsal extrinsic ligaments are less well defined and include the dorsal radiocarpal (DRC) and dorsal intercarpal (DIC) ligaments (Fig. 23-3). *Because they are less well defined, they are not very effective at restoring palmar tilt during fracture reduction (by ligamentotaxis).*

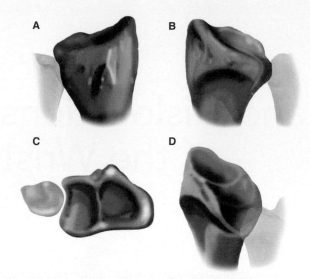

FIGURE 23-1 Distal radius. **A.** Dorsal view of Lister's tubercle. **B.** Palmar view of the scaphoid and lunate fossae distally as well as the sigmoid notch ulnarly. Vascular foramina can be noted on the palmar and dorsal aspects of the distal radius. **C.** End-on view of the distal radius and radioulnar joint showing the scaphoid fossa, lunate fossa, and ulnar head resting in the sigmoid notch. **D.** Sigmoid notch from the ulnar aspect.

- Triangular fibrocartilage (TFC)—The TFC attaches to the carpus through the volar UT and UL ligaments (see Fig. 23-2). The TFC with its accompanying attachments is called the TFCC.
3. Radiographic   measurements   (Fig.   23-4)— Radiographic measurements are important in assessing fracture reduction and residual deformity.

- Radial inclination—The normal range is 15° to 30°; the average is 23° (posteroanterior [PA] view).
- Radial length—The normal range is 11 to 12 mm; the average is 12 mm (PA view).
- Volar tilt—The normal range is up to 20°; the average is 11° (lateral view).

D. Classification of Fractures
1. Common eponyms—Although eponyms are imprecise, they continue to be used by orthopaedists to describe distal radius fractures.
- Colles' fracture (Colles, 1814)—Colles' fracture is typically extra-articular with dorsal comminution, dorsal displacement, and radial shortening (Fig. 23-5).
- Smith's fracture (Smith, 1847)—Smith's fracture is a "reverse Colles' fracture" with volar displacement. There are three types: Types I, II, and III (Fig. 23-6).
- Barton's   fracture   (Barton,   1838)—Barton's fracture is an intra-articular fracture (a fracture-dislocation of the wrist). ***These fractures can be volar or dorsal and are usually unstable*** (see Fig. 23-6). (A Smith Type II fracture is the same as a volar Barton's fracture.)
- Chauffeur's   fracture   (Edwards,   1910)—A Chauffeur's fracture is an intra-articular fracture of the radial styloid. ***It may be associated with disruption of the scapholunate ligament*** (Fig. 23-7).
- Die-Punch (Lunate Load) fracture (Rutherford, 1891; Scheck, 1962)—A die-punch fracture is

FIGURE 23-2 Volar extrinsic ligaments of the wrist.

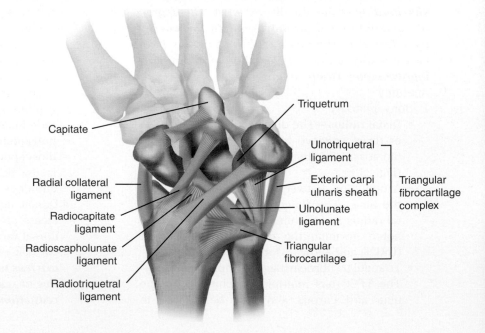

Capitate

Radial collateral ligament

Radiocapitate ligament

Radioscapholunate ligament

Radiotriquetral ligament

Triquetrum

Ulnotriquetral ligament

Exterior carpi ulnaris sheath

Ulnolunate ligament

Triangular fibrocartilage

Triangular fibrocartilage complex

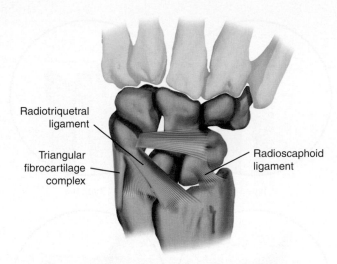

Radiotriquetral ligament

Triangular fibrocartilage complex

Radioscaphoid ligament

FIGURE 23-3 Dorsal extrinsic ligaments of the wrist.

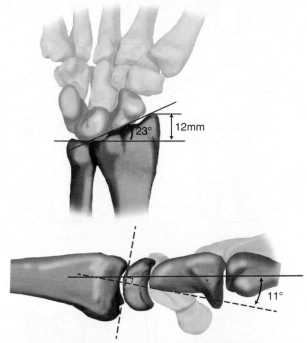

FIGURE 23-4 Radiographic measurements important in assessing fracture reduction and residual deformity: *radial inclination* (shown here as a normal 23°), *radial length* (shown here as a normal 12 mm), and *volar tilt* (shown here as a normal 11°).

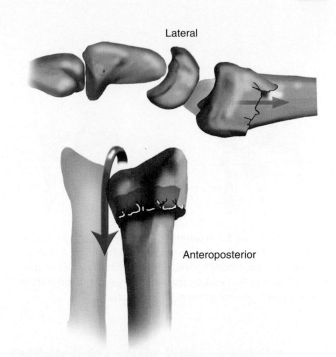

Lateral

Anteroposterior

FIGURE 23-5 Typical deformity seen in a Colles' fracture, showing dorsal comminution and displacement with shortening of the radius relative to the ulna.

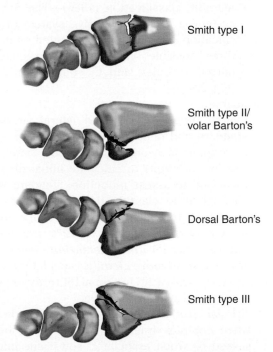

Smith type I

Smith type II/ volar Barton's

Dorsal Barton's

Smith type III

FIGURE 23-6 Thomas' classification of Smith's fractures. **Type I.** extra-articular fracture with volar tilt and displacement of the distal fragment. **Type II.** intra-articular fracture with volar and proximal displacement of the distal fragment along with the carpus (the same as a volar Barton's fracture). A dorsal Barton's fracture is illustrated for comparison, showing the dorsal and proximal displacement of the carpus and distal fragment on the radial shaft. **Type III.** extra-articular fracture with volar displacement of the distal fragment and carpus. (In Type III, the fracture line is more oblique than in Type I.)

an intra-articular depression fracture of the lunate fossa of the distal radius (Fig. 23-7).

2. Modern classification systems—Modern classification systems are treatment-oriented and more specific.
   • Frykman classification (1937)—Frykman Types I to VIII are classified according to fracture pattern (Fig. 23-8).

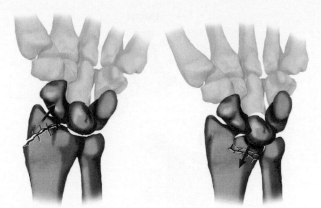

FIGURE 23-7 *Left*, Chauffeur's fracture with the carpus displaced ulnarly by the radial styloid fracture. *Right*, Lunate load (die-punch) fracture with depression of the lunate fossa of the radius that allows proximal migration of the lunate and/or proximal carpal row.

- Melone's classification (1984)—Melone's Types I to V are determined by the orientation of the four main intra-articular fragments (Fig. 23-9).
- AO/ASIF classification (1986)—The AO/ASIF system is a comprehensive system of classification. Fractures are classified as one of three possible types: A, extra-articular; B, partial articular; and C, complete articular (Fig. 23-10).

E. Evaluation
   1. Plain radiographs—PA and lateral views are standard and demonstrate most fractures. Radiographic measurements can be made (see previous section) to calculate initial displacement and to assess reduction. Standard views also facilitate classification of fractures and choice of treatment. ***Oblique views detect occult carpal fractures (12% incidence), whereas the PA ulnar-deviation view shows the scaphoid more clearly.*** Facet lateral views are taken with a 20° proximal tilt to give a better view of the articular surface.
   2. Special studies—Special studies are helpful when complex fracture patterns must be assessed or when associated soft-tissue injuries are suspected.
      - Computed tomography (CT)—The 1- to 2-mm sections in the sagittal plane are ***most effective in demonstrating articular depression (die-punch) fractures. Axial views are best for evaluating the distal radioulnar joint and should include the opposite, uninjured wrist for comparison.*** Three-dimensional reconstructions provide anatomic images and can be useful in surgical planning.

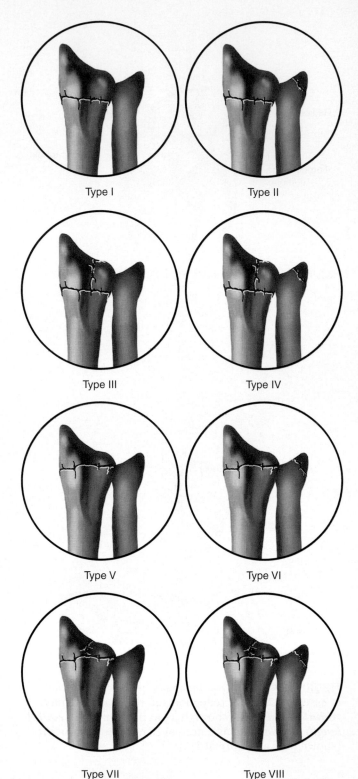

Type I   Type II

Type III   Type IV

Type V   Type VI

Type VII   Type VIII

FIGURE 23-8 Frykman classification of distal radius fractures. Types I, III, V, and VII do not have an associated fracture of the ulnar styloid. Fractures III through VII are intra-articular fractures. (Types III and IV involve the radiocarpal joint, Types V and VI involve the radioulnar joint, and Types VII and VIII involve both the radiocarpal and the radioulnar joints.) Higher-classification fractures have a worse prognosis.

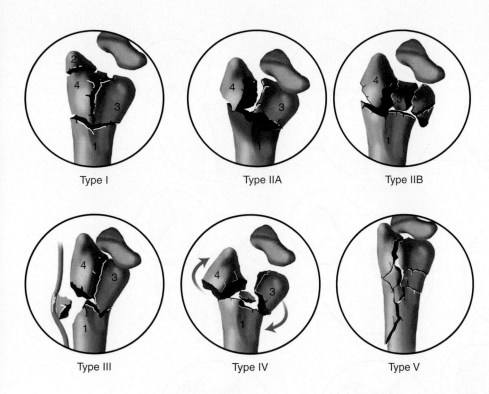

FIGURE 23-9 Melone's classification of subtypes of four-part intra-articular fractures.

Type I

Type IIA

Type IIB

Type III

Type IV

Type V

- Magnetic resonance imaging (MRI)—MRI should be reserved for suspected soft-tissue injuries (TFCC or scapholunate ligament tears).
- Radionuclide bone imaging—Radionuclide bone imaging may have a role in the detection of occult fractures or the evaluation of reflex sympathetic dystrophy (RSD) as a late complication.

F. Associated Soft-Tissue Injuries—Associated soft-tissue injuries are common in high-energy fractures.
1. Open fracture—Management should include emergent irrigation and debridement, administration of intravenous antibiotics, and early fracture stabilization (external fixation). Wound coverage may require skin grafting or local flap.
2. Median nerve injury—Median nerve injury, usually a neurapraxic injury, commonly improves after fracture reduction. If there is no improvement after 48 hours of observation, exploration and carpal tunnel release are indicated.
3. TFCC injury—TFCC injury has been documented in up to 50% of cases of distal radius fractures when there is an associated ulnar styloid fracture. It often causes late ulnar-sided wrist pain. When the ulnar styloid fracture occurs at the base and is displaced, DRUJ instability is likely present and should be treated.
4. Carpal ligament injury—A complete tear of the scapholunate ligament (most common) can lead

to scapholunate instability and if untreated, carpal collapse and posttraumatic arthritis.
5. Tendon injury—Acute tendon laceration is rare but may be seen in fractures with gross displacement. *Attritional rupture of the extensor pollicis longus (EPL) tendon may be a late sequela* (see later section).
6. Arterial injury—A rare but serious complication, arterial injury (radial or ulnar artery) requires emergent evaluation and repair.
7. Compartment syndrome—Compartment syndrome is seen in approximately 1% of distal radius fractures. The cardinal signs of *pain (with passive finger motion), paralysis, and paresthesia* should alert the treating physician to this condition. Appropriate fasciotomy of the involved compartments (volar forearm is the most common) is mandatory and most successful when performed early.

G. Treatment
1. Principles
- Assessment of stability—*The stability of the fracture is the most important point to consider when determining treatment. Hallmarks of an unstable fracture include articular depression greater than 2 mm, radial shortening greater than 5 mm, and dorsal tilt greater than 20°. Metaphyseal comminution involving both the volar and dorsal cortices is also indicative of an unstable fracture pattern.* In general, a stable fracture can be treated

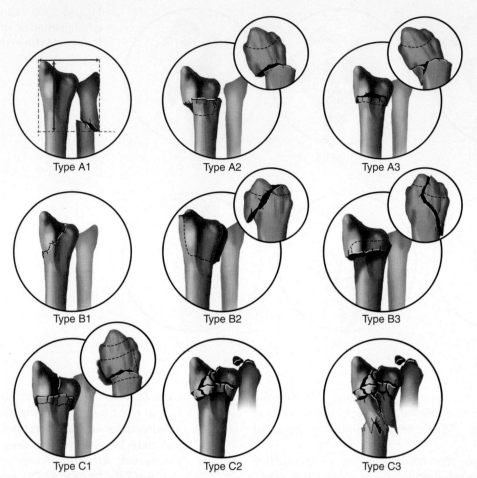

FIGURE 23-10 AO/ASIF classification of distal radius fractures based on the ABC system. The subgroups are not shown. Type A is an extra-articular metaphyseal fracture. The junction of the metaphysis and diaphysis is identified by the "square" or "T" method (the greatest width on the frontal plane of the distal forearm; illustrated on A1). Type A1 is an isolated fracture of the distal ulna. Type A2 is a simple distal radius fracture. Type A3 is a radius fracture with metaphyseal impaction. Type B is an intra-articular rim fracture (preserving the continuity of the epiphysis and metaphysis). Type B1 is a fracture of the radial styloid. Type B2 is a dorsal rim fracture (dorsal Barton's). Type B3 is a volar rim fracture (volar Barton's is the same as a Smith Type II). Type C is a complex intra-articular fracture (disrupting the continuity of the epiphysis and metaphysis). Type C1 is a metaphyeal fracture with radiocarpal joint congruity preserved. Type C2 has articular displacement. Type C3 has diaphyseal–metaphyseal involvement. Injury of the distal radioulnar joint is possible in any of these fractures.

by closed reduction and plaster immobilization, whereas an unstable fracture requires some form of internal or external fixation. ***Certain fracture patterns are known to be unstable by nature, and as a result, should almost always be treated surgically. These include displaced articular margin fractures: Barton's and Chauffeur's fractures (AO Types B1 to B3).*** DRUJ stability also needs to be assessed on injury radiographs. Widening of the DRUJ or ulnar styloid fracture displacement is indicative of instability.

- Assessment of reduction—Recent studies have highlighted the importance of achieving and maintaining a near anatomic reduction when treating distal radius fractures in younger patients. Guidelines for an acceptable reduction are (in order of importance) ***articular step-off less than 2 mm, radial shortening less than 5 mm, and dorsal tilt less than 10°.*** Failure to achieve and maintain an adequate reduction results in predictable sequelae and potential long-term disability.

2. Methods of reduction
   - Closed reduction—Closed reduction relies on ***ligamentotaxis*** to restore alignment and correct fracture deformity. Traction/countertraction is used and can be combined

with varying degrees of palmar flexion, ulnar deviation, and pronation of the distal fragment. Volar tilt cannot be reliably restored by longitudinal traction alone because of the nature of the radiocarpal ligaments *(the volar ligaments tighten first)*. Alternatively, palmar displacement of the carpus improves volar tilt by using the dorsal periosteal hinge (Fig. 23-11). However, this maneuver requires an intact volar cortical strut without comminution. Postreduction radiographs should be carefully inspected to identify any residual articular step-off or fragment depression (die-punch type).

- Open reduction—Open reduction is indicated when closed reduction has failed to achieve an acceptable result. Articular depression and die-punch fractures often require open reduction through a limited dorsal approach and manual elevation of fragments. Other surgical approaches are recommended for different fracture patterns.

  (a) Limited dorsal approach (proximal to Lister's tubercle)—The limited dorsal approach is indicated for a simple depressed fragment that can be elevated under fluoroscopic control. Fixation is achieved with percutaneous K-wires (oblique or transverse) and may be supplemented with bone graft.

  (b) Formal dorsal approach (through the third dorsal compartment and combined with a dorsal arthrotomy)—The formal dorsal approach is indicated for complex joint involvement requiring direct visualization of the articular surface. Fixation is achieved with either K-wires or a dorsal plate. Several low-profile plates have been developed for this specific application. Bone graft or bone graft substitute is usually necessary to support the elevated fragments. SL ligament injuries can also be repaired using the dorsal approach.

  (c) Standard volar approach *(the interval is between the flexor carpi radialis tendon and the radial artery)*—The standard volar approach is indicated for volarly displaced articular margin (Barton's) fractures. Fixation is usually achieved with a T-plate. This approach is now commonly used to fix dorsally

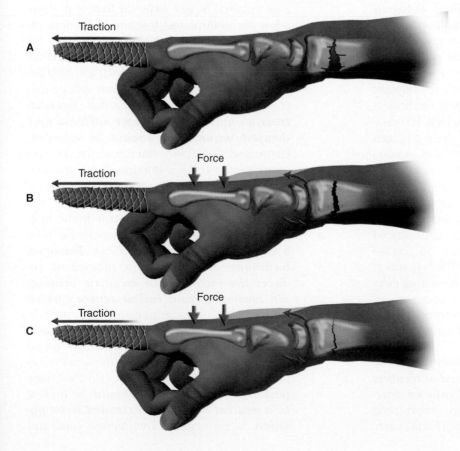

A. Traction

B. Traction Force

C. Traction Force

FIGURE 23-11 In a dorsally displaced distal radius fracture, reduction can be obtained by two distinct and separate forms of ligamentotaxis. **A.** The ligamentotaxis obtained by forces of longitudinal traction restores skeletal length, but the distal fragment remains dorsally tilted. **B** and **C.** A palmar translating force (applied by the physician) attempts to sublux the midcarpal joint, creating a force that is transmitted through the proximal carpal row via capsular ligaments to the distal radial fragment, *tilting its articular surface palmarly*.

displaced fractures as well. Fixed angle locking plates can be employed to support these fractures.

(d) Extensile volar approach (the interval is between the ulnar artery and nerve and the carpal canal)—The extensile volar approach is indicated for treatment of complex articular fractures involving the DRUJ and lunate fossa. ***This approach also allows for carpal tunnel release.***

(e) Dorsal radial approach (the interval is between the first and second dorsal compartments)—The dorsal radial approach is indicated for displaced radial styloid fractures. Fixation is achieved with pins or screws.

(f) Combined volar and dorsal approach—The combined volar and dorsal approach is indicated only in the most severe high-energy fractures with both volar and dorsal articular fragmentation.

- Bone grafting—The use of bone graft or bone graft substitute is indicated when there has been significant depression of the radial articular surface. After elevation of the fragments, bone graft is used to fill the metaphyseal defect. This technique prevents late collapse and may allow for earlier mobilization of the radiocarpal joint. Cancellous autograft (iliac crest) has been used traditionally but may be replaced by allograft or graft substitute in certain cases. Bone graft can be used with either pin or plate fixation as long as adequate bone stock is available for implant purchase. In addition to allograft cancellous chips (*osteoconductive* effect), new formulations are now marketed with demineralized bone matrix (DBM) which may have *osteoinductive* properties. Graft substitutes are produced from a variety of ceramics including calcium sulfate, calcium phosphate, hydroxyapatite and silicone dioxide (bioactive glass). More recent products have been produced using recombinant technology to create bone morphogenic proteins (BMPs), which have the ability to induce bone forming cells (*osteogenic* potential).

3. Methods of stabilization—Stabilization techniques can be used alone or in combination as dictated by the fracture type.
   - Plaster cast or splint—***A plaster cast or splint is the traditional method of treating nondisplaced and stable displaced fractures after closed reduction.*** Sugar tong splints and long-arm and short-arm casts

have been recommended in different combinations, depending on the fracture type and amount of displacement. Regardless of the specific choice, serial radiographs (at 1- to 2-week intervals) are necessary to check for subsequent displacement. ***Fractures that displace in plaster are by definition unstable and should be treated by other means.***

- Pins and plaster—Pins and plaster has become less popular with the advent of external fixation frames. Complication rates may be as high as 50%.

- Percutaneous pin fixation—***Percutaneous pin fixation is indicated for unstable extra-articular fractures after successful closed reduction.*** Certain intra-articular fractures may also be amenable to this treatment, particularly those without significant comminution. Various techniques of pinning have been described and are often combined with external fixation. They include radial styloid pinning, combination radial styloid and dorsal pinning (usually crossed), and intrafocal (Kapandji) pinning placed through the fracture site.

- External fixation—Once the treatment of choice for unstable, comminuted distal radius fractures, external fixation has become less popular with the advent of locking fixed angle plates. Newer external fixator designs allow for multiplanar fracture reduction, including palmar translation, which can be used to restore volar tilt. External fixation frames are often combined with pin fixation to improve fracture stability and reduce distraction forces across the carpus. ***Overdistraction may lead to finger stiffness and delayed union, and should be avoided.*** Depressed articular fractures usually require limited open reduction, bone grafting, and supplemental pin fixation in addition to external fixation (Fig. 23-12). When this combination is used, the fixator frame may be removed earlier (4 to 6 weeks vs. 6 to 8 weeks), reducing wrist stiffness. ***The open technique of fixator pin placement reduces the incidence of eccentric drilling, pin loosening, and radial sensory nerve injury.*** Additional complications may include pin tract infection, pin breakage, and complex regional pain syndrome. Median nerve compression can occur when the wrist is immobilized in extreme flexion (Cotton-Loder position), so ***the fixator should be locked in a neutral or slightly extended wrist position.*** In rare cases of combined volar and

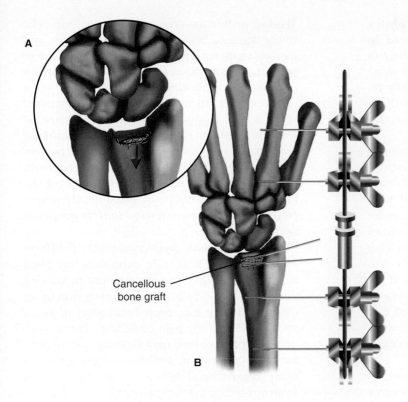

Cancellous bone graft

FIGURE 23-12 **A.** Depressed fracture of the distal radius with a portion of the lunate fossa of the radius dorsally and proximally displaced. **B.** Treatment of the fracture with application of an external fixation device, carpal distraction, elevation of the depressed fragment and fixation with two K-wires, and cancellous bone grafting of the bony defect left behind by elevation of the depressed fracture fragment.

dorsal articular involvement, the external fixator must be applied in combination with open reduction with internal fixation (ORIF) of the articular fragments. The plate is usually applied volarly (as a preliminary step) and is followed by dorsal fragment reduction using ligamentotaxis.

- Internal fixation—ORIF has become more popular since the development of *volar locking plates.* These plates utilize fixed angle screws or pegs to support the intact subchondral bone of the distal radius. Even in cases of severe comminution the locked screws prevent collapse and hold the fragments out to length. The plate is usually applied to the volar aspect of the bone where it is well tolerated and tendon problems are minimized. Elevation of depressed articular fragments and bone grafting can be performed through the fracture site by pronating the proximal fragment. Use of these plates has allowed earlier wrist motion and produced better results when compared to external fixation. Although most distal radius fractures are amendable to volar plating, certain fractures will still require a dorsal or radial approach.

(a) Radial styloid fractures (Chauffeur's, AO Type B1)—When displaced, radial styloid fractures must be reduced anatomically through a dorsal radial approach.

Percutaneous pins or lag screws may be used for fracture fixation.

(b) Articular margin fractures (Barton's, AO Types B2 and B3)—An AO T-plate is applied either volarly or dorsally depending on the direction of fracture displacement. *These fractures are inherently unstable and require buttress plate fixation across the oblique fracture line.*

(c) Complex articular fractures (AO types C1 to C3)—Often, complex articular fractures cannot be reduced by other means, necessitating ORIF. The surgical approach is dictated by fracture location. For volar articular fragments, an extensile volar approach, followed by buttress plate fixation, is recommended. Of particular concern is the volar ulnar fragment of the distal radius, which may be difficult to reduce and fix through a standard volar approach. Failure to stabilize this fragment may lead to persistent volar collapse. *This type of lunate facet fracture should be approached through an extended carpal tunnel incision.* Dorsal fragmentation requires a formal arthrotomy and fixation with a low-profile plate specifically designed for this location. *Dorsally applied plates still carry a higher risk of tenosynovitis than volar plates and many (30% to 50%) will need to be removed after fracture healing is complete.* These fractures are the most challenging to treat and occasionally require combinations of internal and external fixation and combined volar and dorsal approaches.

- Arthroscopic evaluation and treatment—Techniques of wrist arthroscopy have recently been applied to the treatment of distal radius fractures. Indications have not fully evolved, but several points can be made. Arthroscopy provides an excellent view of the distal radial articular surface; during reduction maneuvers, the joint surface can be visualized directly, avoiding residual articular step-off. Associated carpal ligament and TFCC tears can be easily identified and treated. Arthroscopic evaluation is not without risk, which may include fluid extravasation and neurovascular injury.

- Treatment of ulnar styloid fractures—Treatment of these associated fractures has traditionally received little attention. *However, in cases of ulnar styloid base fractures, particularly if widely displaced, instability of the DRUJ will be present.* In these cases, ORIF of the styloid fracture is recommended either by tension band wiring or by mini-screw fixation. Because of its attachments to the ulnar styloid, fracture fixation will generally stabilize the TFCC.

H. Late Complications—For acute complications, see earlier section on associated soft-tissue injuries.

   1. Malunion—***Extra-articular malunion*** usually involves dorsal tilt and loss of radial length. These deformities in turn lead to ***ulnocarpal impingement, DRUJ incongruity, and midcarpal instability.*** Chronic symptoms can include pain, weakness, and loss of motion. Functional limitations can be disabling, especially in younger patients. ***Corrective surgery is indicated in these cases and involves radial opening wedge (triplanar) osteotomy with corticocancellous bone graft. Intra-articular malunion*** is even more serious, with an early onset of ***radiocarpal arthritis in 90% of wrists with more than 2 mm of articular step-off.*** Surgical treatment usually involves a salvage-type procedure such as arthrodesis or arthroplasty.

   2. Nonunion—Nonunion is a rare complication that has occasionally been reported as a result of overdistraction by external fixation.

   3. Tendon problems—Tendon problems are relatively common after distal radius fracture and include tendon adhesion, tendinitis (from a dorsal plate), and tendon rupture. ***The EPL tendon is most often involved*** and may rupture as a result of mechanical attrition within a narrowed third dorsal compartment. ***The incidence of tendon rupture is greater in nondisplaced fractures, suggesting that stripped periosteum, as in the case of a displaced fracture, protects the EPL tendon.*** Direct repair of the EPL tendon is usually not possible; therefore, ***treatment involves extensor indicis proprius tendon transfer.***

   4. Complex regional pain syndrome (CRPS)—Also known as RSD, this condition has been reported after distal radius fracture in varying percentages (2% to 20%). Overdistraction by an external fixator has been implicated in some studies. Disabling pain, swelling, finger stiffness, and osteopenia may develop and require long-term treatment. Avoidance of this problem by aggressive hand therapy, edema control, and fixator removal (as early as possible) helps prevent permanent sequelae. When present, CRPS should be treated by a combination of therapy, medications, and stellate ganglion blockade.

I. Rehabilitation—Postfracture rehabilitation should begin early, with finger range of motion exercises starting as soon as the cast or fixator is applied. Overdistraction of the fixator may limit tendon excursion and should be avoided. Similarly, a cast that impedes finger motion may lead to permanent stiffness. After cast or fixator removal, exercises may be advanced as the patient tolerates. Removable splints are helpful in allowing intermittent wrist motion while still protecting a healing fracture. Some patients may require a more formal program supervised by an occupational or physical therapist. Plate fixation may improve wrist function by allowing earlier range of motion.

II. Fractures of the Carpal Bones
   A. Fractures of the Scaphoid
      1. Overview—***Scaphoid fractures are the most common carpal fracture*** and are typically seen in young men. Radial deviation and wrist dorsiflexion greater than 90° may lead to scaphoid fracture during a fall on the outstretched hand. ***Fractures of the scaphoid waist are most frequent.*** Early evaluation and appropriate treatment are important in avoiding nonunion, avascular necrosis (AVN), and late carpal collapse.
      2. Anatomy—***The proximal pole of the scaphoid is completely intra-articular (with no***

capsular attachments) and receives all of its blood supply from distal (volar and dorsal) branches of the radial artery (Fig. 23-13). Fractures of the proximal pole depend on intraosseous arterial flow and heal more slowly than distal fractures. They also have a higher risk of nonunion and AVN.

3. Evaluation—*"Snuffbox tenderness"* is a classic sign and should alert the physician to the possibility of scaphoid fracture. The diagnosis is confirmed radiographically with standard PA, lateral, and oblique views of the wrist. A PA view with ulnar deviation *(scaphoid view)* shows the scaphoid in profile and should be ordered when the appearance of the initial radiographs is equivocal. Associated ligamentous injuries must be ruled out by careful radiographic assessment or arthrography. When no fracture is seen initially, the wrist should be splinted for 1 to 2 weeks, and another X-ray study should be performed after fracture resorption has occurred. Occult fractures may be detected in this manner or through the use of bone isotope scanning or MRI. *CT scanning has proved useful in the assessment of established nonunions with carpal collapse.*

4. Classification systems—Most systems highlight the importance of fracture location in regard to treatment and risk of late complications. Waist fractures are most common (65%), followed by proximal pole (25%) and distal pole (10%) fractures.
   • Russe system—The Russe system divides scaphoid fractures into transverse, horizontal, oblique, and vertical oblique patterns. *Vertical oblique fractures are considered unstable.*
   • Herbert system—The Herbert system is more comprehensive and also includes delayed union and nonunion (Fig. 23-14).

5. Treatment—Treatment is determined by location and degree of displacement.
   • Nondisplaced fractures—Nondisplaced fractures are usually stable and can be treated by closed methods. The use of a short-arm thumb spica cast is standard and usually results in healing within 6 to 12 weeks. *Proximal pole fractures heal more slowly* (12 to 24 weeks). Long-arm cast immobilization (for the initial 6 weeks) has been recommended for proximal pole fractures and waist fractures with a vertical oblique pattern.
   • Displaced fractures—*Fractures with more than 1 mm of displacement or any angulation are considered unstable and require operative treatment.* ORIF is usually performed through a volar (Russe) approach between the flexor carpi radialis tendon and the radial artery. *The volar blood supply is compromised in this approach, but is not as crucial as the dorsal arterial branch, which feeds 80% of the scaphoid.* Reduction of the fracture should be anatomic and fixation achieved with either K-wires or screws. The Herbert screw is headless, multipitched (to provide fracture compression), and well suited for this purpose. Newer versions include cannulated and tapered screw designs. When rigid fixation is achieved, immediate range of motion is possible. If there is significant comminution, however, K-wires may be indicated either with or without supplemental bone graft. When K-wires are used, a short period of immobilization (2 to 3 weeks) is recommended.
   • Special considerations—In cases of displaced proximal pole fractures, a dorsal approach is required. This is carried out through the third dorsal compartment using careful technique

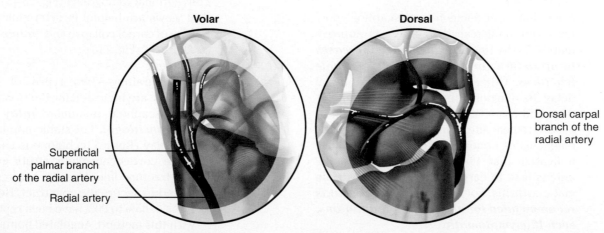

Volar   **Dorsal**

Superficial palmar branch of the radial artery

Radial artery

Dorsal carpal branch of the radial artery

<u>FIGURE 23-13</u>   Blood supply of the scaphoid.

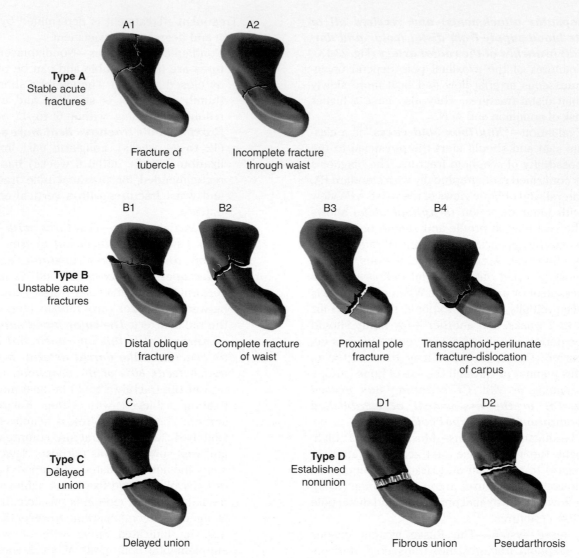

Type A
Stable acute
fractures

Fracture of
tubercle

Incomplete fracture
through waist

Type B
Unstable acute
fractures

Distal oblique
fracture

Complete fracture
of waist

Proximal pole
fracture

Transscaphoid-perilunate
fracture-dislocation
of carpus

Type C
Delayed
union

Delayed union

Type D
Established
nonunion

Fibrous union

Pseudarthrosis

FIGURE 23-14   Classification system of Herbert for scaphoid fractures, delayed unions, and nonunions.

to preserve the dorsal arterial branches. Fixation is with K-wires or screws.

6. Complications
   - Nonunion—The incidence of scaphoid nonunion for undisplaced fractures is approximately 5% to 10%. *The incidence increases to up to 90% for displaced proximal pole fractures.* Other risk factors include initial delay in diagnosis, inadequate immobilization, and associated ligamentous instability. Failure to heal after 6 months establishes the diagnosis of nonunion. Recent studies have indicated that virtually all unstable nonunions lead to carpal collapse and posttraumatic arthritis. For this reason, *treatment is recommended for all scaphoid nonunions, even if asymptomatic.*

   (a) Radiographic assessment—Thin-cut (1- to 2-mm) CT scans show more detail than conventional tomograms (Fig. 23-15). Sagittal views are helpful in determining the degree of carpal collapse and *"humpback deformity"* (Fig. 23-16).

   (b) Treatment
      - Bone grafting—Two types of bone grafting are indicated for the treatment of a scaphoid nonunion: *inlay and interpositional.* For stable nonunions the inlay (Russe) technique is used to place corticocancellous struts across the fracture line. Usually, K-wires are added to secure the construct. Healing rates of 85% to 90% have been reported with this method. Angulated nonunions

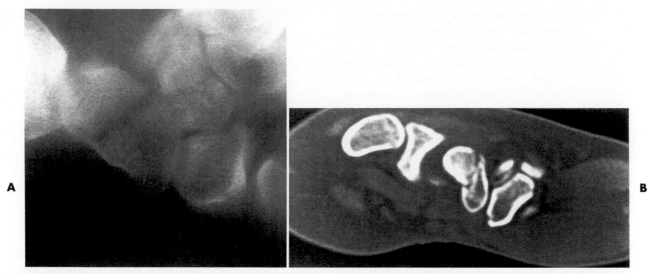

FIGURE 23-15   **A.** Lateral polytome showing an obvious fracture line across the waist of the scaphoid. **B.** CT scan showing the scaphoid waist fracture, with angulation. (From Browner BD, Jupiter JB, Levine AM, et al, eds. *Skeletal Trauma: Fractures, Dislocations, Ligamentous Injuries.* 2nd ed. Philadelphia, PA: WB Saunders; 1998, with permission.)

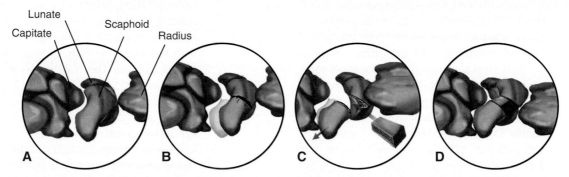

FIGURE 23-16   Correction of dorsal intercalary segment instability and humpback deformity. **A.** Normal alignment. **B.** Fractured humpback scaphoid with a dorsiflexed lunate. **C.** Opening wedge in the scaphoid showing placement of the interpositional graft. **D.** Grafted scaphoid with correction of the instability and deformity.

with a dorsal humpback deformity require interpositional grafting (see Fig. 23-16). Fernandez has described the use of a trapezoidal iliac crest graft to correct the angulation and carpal collapse pattern. Fixation is achieved with screws or K-wires. In both types of grafting procedures, a volar approach is used, and care is taken to preserve the vascularity of the fragments.

- Salvage procedures—Salvage procedures are indicated when nonunion has led to carpal collapse and secondary degenerative changes. Proximal row carpectomy, intercarpal arthrodesis, or radiocarpal arthrodesis is recommended in patients with chronic wrist pain and stiffness. Radial styloidectomy and scaphoid interposition arthroplasty may be combined with other procedures or performed independently in the younger patient with less severe symptoms. Silicone implants have been used in the past but are now avoided because of silicone synovitis. Newer techniques include the use of collagen grafts (tendon or fascia), allografts, or titanium spacers.

- Proximal pole excision—When a small proximal fragment is not amenable to bone grafting, proximal pole excision and fascial hemiarthroplasty are recommended.

- Electric stimulation—Pulsed electromagnetic field stimulation has been investigated as a noninvasive treatment for scaphoid nonunion. Although controversial, there appears to be some benefit (shorter healing time) when electrical stimulation is combined with bone grafting procedures.

- Malunion—Malunion of the scaphoid may occur when a displaced or angulated fracture is allowed to heal without anatomic reduction. In most cases, there is apex dorsal angulation resulting in a fixed humpback deformity. A *dorsal intercalated segmental instability (DISI)* pattern of carpal collapse ensues, resulting in pain, loss of motion, and decreased grip strength (see Fig. 23-16). Treatment in a young patient includes osteotomy, volar wedge bone graft, and internal fixation. Once degenerative arthritis has begun, treatment is limited to a salvage procedure such as proximal row carpectomy, intercarpal arthrodesis, or complete wrist fusion.

- Posttraumatic arthritis—As previously noted, articular degeneration can occur when the normal carpal kinematics are disturbed. Scaphoid nonunion and malunion result in abnormal stress across the radiocarpal joint, leading to predictable patterns of carpal arthritis. Scaphoid nonunion advanced collapse is analogous to scapholunate advanced collapse (SLAC) and describes a pattern of posttraumatic arthritis (see section on carpal dislocations and instability patterns). Salvage procedures are indicated for the painful wrist with scaphoid nonunion or advanced collapse.

- AVN
  - (a) Incidence—*The incidence of AVN of the scaphoid depends on the location of the fracture, with those of the proximal one fifth leading to osteonecrosis in 90% to 100% of cases.* Fractures of the scaphoid waist have an AVN incidence of 30% to 50%. The reason for this phenomenon is that the tenuous blood supply that enters the scaphoid distally is disrupted during fracture (see Fig. 23-13). *The displacement of fragments more than 1 mm increases the chance of AVN by 50%.*
  - (b) Evaluation—The diagnosis of AVN can often be made with plain films when there is evidence of a relatively radiodense proximal scaphoid fragment. *MRI is the most sensitive and specific test and is indicated when the appearance of radiographs is equivocal.* T1-weighted MR

images usually show a decreased signal corresponding to a loss of marrow elements. Surgical biopsy with the absence of punctate bleeding bone is the most definitive test for AVN.

  - (c) Treatment—When AVN occurs in a nondisplaced fracture or after operative fixation of a displaced fracture, revascularization can occur by creeping substitution. This process is slow and may take longer than 1 year to complete. *In the majority of cases, AVN is associated with scaphoid nonunion.* When AVN and nonunion occur together, the treatment is more difficult, and the results less encouraging. Usually bone grafting (inlay or interpositional) is combined with internal fixation. Healing rates vary between 50% and 90% depending on the vascularity of the proximal fragment as evidenced by punctate bleeding. Other treatments include vascularized bone grafting, proximal pole excision, and pulsed electromagnetic field stimulation. When vascularized bone grafting is used for proximal pole AVN, a dorsal pedicle is elevated from the 1,2 intracompartmental supraretinacular artery (1,2 ICSRA). Volarly, a pedicle from the pronator quadratus and underlying bone can be used for more distal AVN and nonunions. Salvage procedures are again indicated once the degenerative process has progressed.

- Carpal instability—Carpal instability may persist after scaphoid fracture as a result of concurrent ligament disruption. Usually this occurs as a result of a perilunate injury (discussed later in this chapter). These injuries need to be identified early and repaired surgically.

B. Isolated Carpal Fractures (Excluding Scaphoid)—Fractures of the carpal bones are often associated with dislocation patterns referred to as *greater arc injuries* (Fig. 21-17). In these cases, the carpal fracture represents an avulsion injury indicative of a more serious carpal dislocation. The treating physician must be aware of these injuries and suspect ligamentous involvement when an isolated fracture is seen on radiographs. These combined fracture-dislocations are discussed further in the section on carpal dislocations and instability patterns.

1. Fractures of the lunate—Isolated fractures of the lunate are rare and must be distinguished from Kienböck's disease (see later section). *Volar pole fractures are most common and*

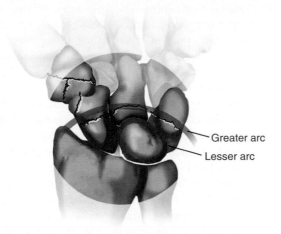

Greater arc
Lesser arc

FIGURE 23-17 Johnson described the "vulnerable zone of the carpus," the shaded area of the carpus in which most of his experimentally produced injuries occurred. Greater arc injuries occurred through bone, and lesser arc injuries were purely ligamentous. Many possible combinations and variants of these "pure" injury patterns can be seen clinically.

may require ORIF if displaced. Marginal chip fractures are treated nonoperatively.

2. Fractures of the triquetrum—Fractures of the triquetrum most commonly occur as impaction fractures of the proximal pole. During forced dorsiflexion and ulnar deviation, the ulnar styloid may shear off a small fragment termed a *chisel.* Chisel fractures may be treated closed, whereas displaced body fractures require ORIF.

3. Fractures of the capitate—Capitate fractures may occur in combination with scaphoid fractures *(scaphocapitate syndrome)* during extreme dorsiflexion of the wrist. This represents a serious injury in which the proximal pole of the capitate may rotate out of position by up to 180°. Because the fragments remain colinear, the diagnosis is difficult and may be missed. Treatment includes ORIF of both the scaphoid and capitate fractures. The complications of nonunion and AVN may occur as a result of the disrupted blood supply to the proximal capitate.

4. Fractures of the hamate—Fractures of the hamate can be divided into hook (hamular process) fractures and body fractures. Hooks of hamate fractures are caused by a direct blow to the hand and are often seen in baseball players or golfers. The diagnosis may be missed initially and may lead to chronic symptoms and nonunion. Occasionally, these fractures may affect the flexor tendons to the ring or small finger causing tendinitis or tendon rupture.

When symptomatic, the fragment should be excised. Carpal tunnel views or a CT scan demonstrates the acute fracture or nonunion. Fractures of the hamate body are often associated with dislocation of the fourth and fifth metacarpal bases. These injuries require open reduction and pinning of the fracture as well as the involved carpometacarpal joints.

5. Fractures of the trapezium—Fractures of the trapezial ridge are analogous to hook of hamate fractures and are treated similarly (by excision) if they progress to nonunion. As in other carpal fractures, displaced body fractures require ORIF, whereas nondisplaced fractures are treated closed.

6. Fractures of the trapezoid—Trapezoid fractures are rare as isolated injuries, but may occur with dislocation of the index metacarpal. Interpretation of routine radiographs is difficult, and tomography or CT scanning may be necessary to make the diagnosis. ORIF is indicated for fracture-dislocation of the metacarpal base. Nondisplaced body fractures are treated nonoperatively.

C. AVN of the Carpal Bones

1. Scaphoid—AVN of the scaphoid as a post-traumatic complication has been discussed previously. When osteonecrosis occurs without apparent trauma, the diagnosis is *Preiser's disease.* The etiology has been debated and may include steroid use, microtrauma, or a connective tissue disorder. Because of the rarity of this condition, formal treatment guidelines are not available. In general, all conservative measures should be exhausted before aggressive bone grafting or scaphoid excision is contemplated.

2. Capitate—Displaced fractures of the capitate can lead to AVN of the vulnerable proximal pole. This is analogous to AVN of the scaphoid. Treatment should be symptomatic unless degenerative changes progress and involve the midcarpal joint. Scaphocapitate arthrodesis or proximal pole excision has been recommended when nonoperative treatment fails.

3. Lunate—Osteonecrosis of the lunate, or *Kienböck's disease,* has been well described in the orthopaedic literature. Theories of causation vary and include both vascular and traumatic etiologies. The current consensus is that microtrauma may lead to AVN in a susceptible lunate. Predisposing factors include negative ulnar variance of the wrist and a one-vessel lunate vascular pattern. *Negative ulnar variance is thought to increase the load across the lunate.* Negative ulnar variance is found in

only 23% of normal individuals but in almost 80% of those with Kienböck's disease. ***The lunate vascularity pattern*** has also been implicated with a one-vessel lunate (20% of the population) at a higher risk than a two-vessel lunate (80% of the population).

- Diagnosis—The diagnosis of Kienböck's disease is made radiographically with the appearance of a sclerotic, fragmented, or collapsed lunate. The stages of the disease follow a predictable pattern of degeneration and are summarized in Table 23-1.
- Treatment (see Table 23-1)—Initial treatment is conservative, with splinting and rest helpful in 50% of cases. Surgical intervention in the early stages (I or II) involves joint-leveling procedures such as ulnar lengthening or radial shortening. Stage III is defined by lunate collapse and is treated with scaphotrapezial-trapezoid fusion, lunate excision arthroplasty, or combined procedures. After degenerative changes become extensive, stage IV treatment is limited to proximal row carpectomy or complete wrist fusion.

III. Carpal Dislocations and Instability Patterns
  A. Overview—The bony and ligamentous structures of the wrist together form a complex mechanism that allows for the transmission of force and a stable range of motion. When injury occurs, the delicate balance can be altered, resulting in loss of function and instability. The successful treatment of carpal injuries requires an understanding of the intricate anatomy and kinematics of the wrist joint.

TABLE 23-1

Stages of Kienböck's Disease

Stage	Radiography	Treatment
I	Sclerosis	Conservative/splinting
II	Fragmentation	Joint leveling (radial shortening or ulnar lengthening)
III	Collapse	Controversial (most treat like stage II ± scaphocapitate or triscaphe [STT] and capitohamate fusion)
IV	Radiocarpal and intercarpal DJD	Salvage (wrist fusion or proximal row carpectomy)

STT, Scaphotrapezial-trapezoid; *DJD*, degenerative joint disease.
Source: From Bruce JF. In: Miller MD, ed. *Review of Orthopaedics.* 2nd ed. Philadelphia, PA: WB Saunders; 1996, with permission.

B. General Concepts—The geometry of the seven carpal bones (excluding the pisiform, which is a sesamoid) has been described in terms of theoretic models. Of the various concepts, the row theory has been most popular and best explains carpal dynamics.
  1. Row theory—The row theory, the traditional model of the wrist, divides the carpal bones into proximal and distal rows separated by the midcarpal joint. The proximal row includes the scaphoid, lunate, and triquetrum, each held together by intrinsic interosseous ligaments. The distal row consists of the trapezium, trapezoid, capitate, and hamate, also connected by intrinsic ligaments. The midcarpal joint is spanned by the extrinsic ligaments and accounts for 50% to 60% of total wrist motion. Some motion occurs within the proximal row, but the distal row bones are relatively fixed. ***The scaphoid functions as a link between the two rows, integrating motion and providing stability.*** No tendinous attachments occur on the bones of the proximal row. Instead ***distal forces act on the proximal row as an intercalated segment.*** Their motions are guided by their unique bony anatomy and ligamentous support.
  2. Ligamentous anatomy—The ligaments of the wrist are divided into intrinsic and extrinsic structures.
     - Intrinsic ligaments—***The intrinsic ligaments of the wrist run between adjacent carpal bones within the same row. The most important of the intrinsic ligaments are the scapholunate and lunotriquetral interosseous ligaments.*** They are located on either side of the lunate and hold it in a balanced position. The scapholunate ligament is stronger dorsally, and the lunotriquetral ligament is stronger volarly.
     - Extrinsic ligaments—***The extrinsic ligaments of the wrist span carpal bones in different rows*** and attach to the distal radius and ulna. The volar extrinsic ligaments (see Fig. 23-2) are thicker and functionally more important than the dorsal extrinsic ligaments. These volar ligaments form a double V pattern (apex distal) with a weak area over the capitolunate joint known as the ***space of Poirier.*** The RSC (also called the radiocapitate) ligament spans both the radiocarpal and the midcarpal joints and is an important stabilizer of the scaphoid. ***The radioscapholunate ligament is mostly a mesentery of vessels and has little***

mechanical function. Dorsally, the extrinsic ligaments converge on the triquetrum in a Z configuration (see Fig. 23-3). The most important of these are the DRC ligament and the DIC ligament.

3. Kinematics—Carpal movements are complex and occur in three planes at both the radiocarpal and the midcarpal joints. A unique mechanism allows the proximal row to flex with radial deviation and extend with ulnar deviation. This normally occurs in a synchronous fashion but may be impaired in certain instability patterns (see later section).

C. Patterns of Injury—No single classification system can easily describe all the various carpal injuries. Specific patterns, however, are well known and can be used to guide treatment and predict outcomes.

1. Progressive perilunar disruption—Four stages have been described as a mechanism for sequential ligamentous failure: Stage I, scapholunate ligament tear *(scapholunate dissociation)*; Stage II, capitolunate ligament tear; Stage III, lunotriquetral ligament tear *(perilunate dislocation)*; and Stage IV, dorsal radiolunate ligament tear *(lunate dislocation).* This system explains how lunate dislocation can occur as the result of a perilunate injury.

2. Lesser arc and greater arc patterns (see Fig. 23-17)—Perilunar injury can involve ligamentous failure, carpal fracture, or a combination of both. When an injury is purely ligamentous, it is termed a *lesser arc pattern.* A *greater arc pattern,* on the other hand, involves a carpal fracture. The most common of these injuries is the *transcaphoid perilunate fracture-dislocation.* Various combinations of these two patterns can exist simultaneously.

3. Axial disruption patterns—Axial or longitudinal injuries have recently been classified according to their lines of cleavage through the carpus (Fig. 23-18). These rare injuries usually result from a blast or severe crush of the hand and wrist.

D. Patterns of Instability—Instability patterns may develop after an injury (see previous section) or may be nontraumatic in etiology (such as in rheumatoid arthritis). Commonly, a carpal injury may occur and go unnoticed until it progresses to a more severe and symptomatic form of instability (such as a scapholunate ligament tear progressing to advanced collapse). For this reason, there is considerable overlap between acute injury and chronic posttraumatic instability.

1. Dorsal and volar instability patterns
   • DISI—DISI refers to a pattern in which the scaphoid and lunate become disconnected or disassociated as the result of a scaphoid fracture or a scapholunate ligament tear. Because the lunate is separated from its scaphoid attachment, it rotates dorsally under the influence of the triquetrum (via the lunotriquetral ligament). Similarly, the scaphoid is unsupported and rotates (collapses) into flexion. This is also termed *rotatory subluxation of the scaphoid.* Radiographically, this pattern leads to an *increased scapholunate angle (>60°)* as measured on the lateral radiographic film (Fig. 23-19, *A*). The *normal scapholunate angle ranges from 30° to 60° (average, 47°).* In addition, the capitolunate angle (normal, up to 15°) and radiolunate angle (normal, up to 15°) are also increased. The PA view shows widening of the scapholunate interval (>3 mm) or evidence of a scaphoid fracture. Other findings include the *"cortical ring" sign* of the scaphoid and a triangular appearance of the lunate (Fig. 23-20). With time, the DISI pattern leads to proximal migration of the capitate as it subluxes dorsally over the rotated lunate. This results in degenerative wear and arthrosis. Eventually, SLAC occurs with its progressive arthritic changes.
   • Volar intercalated segmental instability (VISI)—VISI is much rarer than DISI and less well understood. In the VISI pattern, there is a disruption of the lunotriquetral ligament and probably also a disruption of the DRC ligaments. The net result is volar flexion of the lunate and a volar shift of the carpus. Lateral radiographs demonstrate a *decreased scapholunate angle (<30°)* as well as increased capitolunate and radiolunate angles (Fig. 23-19, *B*).

2. Dissociative and nondissociative and complex and adaptive instability patterns
   • Carpal instability dissociative (CID)—*Carpal instability dissociative* refers to intrinsic ligament disruptions that occur between carpal bones of the same row. Examples include scapholunate ligament tears causing scapholunate dissociation and lunotriquetral ligament tears causing lunotriquetral dissociation.
   • Carpal instability nondissociative (CIND)—*Carpal instability nondissociative* refers to extrinsic ligament disruptions that occur between carpal rows. *Midcarpal instability is an example* in which there is disruption

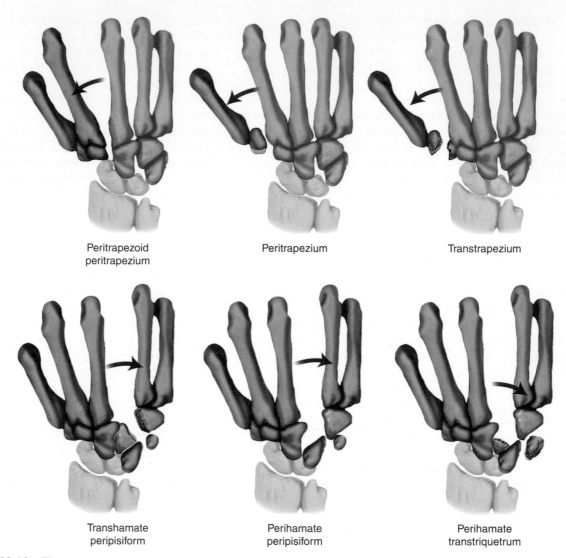

Peritrapezoid
peritrapezium

Peritrapezium

Transtrapezium

Transhamate
peripisiform

Perihamate
peripisiform

Perihamate
transtriquetrum

FIGURE 23-18   The most common patterns of axial (longitudinal) carpal instability.

(or laxity) of the extrinsic ligaments that connect the proximal and distal carpal rows. Because the appearance on radiographs is usually normal, the diagnosis must be made by physical examination or by the use of fluoroscopy.

• Carpal instability complex (CIC)—*Carpal instability complex* is a combination of both the dissociative and the nondissociative types and includes all types of perilunate dislocations.

• Carpal instability adaptive (CIA)—*Carpal instability adaptive* refers to carpal instability that develops as an adaptive response to some prior malalignment. The most common example is midcarpal instability caused by the dorsal articular tilting of a malunited distal radius fracture.

3. Static and dynamic instability patterns— Recently, the terms *static* and *dynamic* have been used to separate and classify instability patterns.

• Static instability—*Static instability* patterns are fixed and can be identified on plain radiographs. Examples include most DISI and VISI patterns with their characteristic angular measurements (see previous section).

• Dynamic instability—*Dynamic instability* refers to functional instability that is transient and intermittent. These abnormalities are not present on routine radiographs but can be identified with stress views (e.g., clenched-fist PA view showing **dynamic scapholunate instability**) or fluoroscopy (e.g., **midcarpal instability**). The history and physical examination are also important in diagnosing

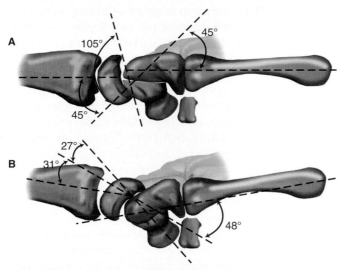

FIGURE 23-19 **A.** Dorsal intercalated segmental instability. The scapholunate angle is high (105°), the capitolunate angle is high (45°), and the radiolunate angle is high (45°). The intercalated segment is represented by the lunate. **B.** Volar intercalated segmental instability. The scapholunate angle is low (27°).

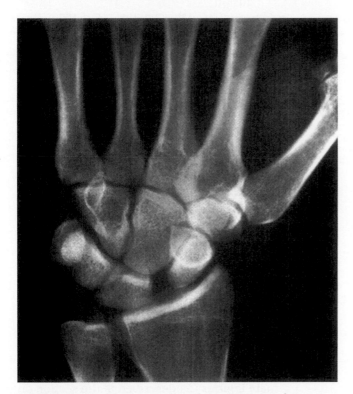

FIGURE 23-20 The key radiographic features of rotatory subluxation of the scaphoid (scapholunate dissociation) are seen on this anteroposterior view of the wrist: widening of the space between the scaphoid and lunate, a foreshortened appearance of the scaphoid, and the "cortical ring" shadow, which represents an axial projection of the abnormally oriented scaphoid. (From Green DP, ed. *Operative Hand Surgery*. 3rd ed. New York, NY: Churchill Livingstone; 1993, with permission.)

dynamic instability that may present as a painful "clunk" with radial and ulnar deviation of the wrist.

E. Evaluation—As previously noted, carpal injuries may be acute or chronic. In an acute situation, there is associated swelling and deformity, and the diagnosis may be obvious. Chronic injuries, however, may present with milder symptoms, and the diagnosis may be missed. Although acute and chronic instabilities may have similar radiographic appearances, their treatment and prognosis are very different.

1. Acute injury—With an acute wrist injury, the history and physical examination may be straightforward. The most common mechanism is a fall on the dorsiflexed wrist with associated ulnar deviation. For these injuries, a thorough examination is important to rule out neurovascular compromise or compartment syndrome of the hand. Plain radiographs (PA, lateral, and oblique views) show displacement of the carpus (e.g., perilunate dislocation) or malalignment (e.g., scapholunate dissociation, DISI). Rarely, stress views are needed to demonstrate an occult injury. A clenched-fist PA view may highlight subtle scapholunate dissociation.

2. Chronic injury—Additional studies are often needed in the evaluation of a chronic or subacute injury. Arthrography has been used extensively to diagnose tears of the scapholunate and lunotriquetral ligaments. Triple-injection techniques are important in evaluating the flow of dye between the radiocarpal, midcarpal, and DRUJs. When abnormal flow is present, a ligamentous tear is suspected. Unfortunately, arthrograms are helpful only in evaluating the intrinsic ligaments, so extrinsic ligament disruptions may be missed. Also, as many as 70% of asymptomatic wrists may have some abnormality noted on an arthrogram. MRI has become more popular in evaluating the wrist as techniques and image detail has improved. Cineradiography and fluoroscopy are indicated in the workup of dynamic instability. In many of these cases, all other test results are normal, but fluoroscopy demonstrates a midcarpal shift corresponding to a painful clunk on physical examination. ***Wrist arthroscopy now allows the most comprehensive and direct evaluation of the carpal ligaments***. The exact type and degree of ligament disruption can be identified and in some cases treated arthroscopically. Also, arthroscopy can provide information about

articular wear, chondral fractures, and synovial hypertrophy.

3. Special tests—A number of maneuvers have been developed to help diagnose specific patterns of instability. The ***Watson test*** is performed by applying dorsally directed thumb pressure over the volar scaphoid tubercle during radial and ulnar deviation of the wrist. A palpable clunk that often elicits pain is diagnostic of ***scapholunate dissociation.*** Another test is the ***ballottement or shuck test*** in which the triquetrum and lunate are shifted volarly and dorsally in an attempt to elicit any instability or pain. A positive ballottement test is indicative of ***lunotriquetral dissociation.*** Both of these tests should be performed on the opposite, uninvolved wrist as well as the injured wrist to rule out normal variants.

F. Treatment

1. Lesser arc injuries—Lesser arc injuries are purely ligamentous and may involve disruption of the intrinsic or extrinsic ligaments.

   • Scapholunate dissociation—***Tear of the scapholunate interosseous ligament leading to dissociation is the most common carpal injury.*** Early diagnosis and appropriate treatment are important in preventing midcarpal changes (DISI) and late collapse (SLAC arthrosis).

     (a) Acute treatment—Acute treatment consists of ORIF with ligament repair. The surgical approach is dorsal, between the third and fourth dorsal compartments. Reduction is achieved under direct visualization by manipulation of the scaphoid using thumb pressure (volarly) and K-wire joysticks to "derotate" the flexed scaphoid. Pins are used to hold the reduction and are usually passed from the scaphoid into the lunate and capitate. The ligament should be repaired back to bone (usually the scaphoid) with suture anchors or through drill holes. When sufficient ligament is not present, the repair is augmented with dorsal capsule used to stabilize and suspend the scaphoid ***(Blatt capsulodesis).*** Other types of ligament reconstructions have been described, most using tendon grafts or bone-ligament constructs. Postoperative regimens vary, but protected motion can be started after a period of immobilization. Pins are usually removed after 8 to 12 weeks.

     (b) Chronic treatment—Chronic scapholunate dissociation (>8 weeks old) without arthrosis is treated operatively with either a soft-tissue procedure or limited arthrodesis. After reduction of the scaphoid, ligament repair with capsular augmentation is performed. K-wires are again used to hold the reduction and are left in place for 8 to 12 weeks. In cases of insufficient soft tissue or irreducibility, limited arthrodesis is recommended. Different options include scaphotrapezial–trapezoid fusion, scapholunate fusion, or scaphocapitate fusion.

     (c) Treatment of SLAC with associated arthrosis—SLAC with arthrosis is treated with some type of salvage procedure. The most popular technique combines scaphoid excision with a midcarpal (four-corner) fusion. Other surgical options include proximal row carpectomy, wrist arthroplasty, and complete wrist fusion.

   • Lunotriquetral dissociation—Lunotriquetral dissociation results from disruption of the lunotriquetral ligament. Unlike scapholunate dissociation, lunotriquetral dissociation is rare and not very well understood. A staging system has been developed to guide treatment of these injuries. Stage I represents isolated tears of the lunotriquetral interosseous ligament without midcarpal (VISI) involvement. These injuries are treated nonoperatively with splinting, anti-inflammatory medications, and local injections. Stage II injuries have disruption of the lunotriquetral interosseous ligament and are associated with a dynamic VISI. Stage III injuries are more severe and are characterized by a static VISI collapse pattern. Treatment of Stage II and III injuries is controversial but may include soft-tissue reconstruction (using dorsal capsule or tendon graft) or limited arthrodesis (lunotriquetral or four-corner fusion).

   • Perilunate dislocation—Staging of perilunate injuries (as described in the section on progressive perilunar disruption) includes Stage I to IV, with Stage III representing ***perilunate dislocation*** and Stage IV representing ***lunate dislocation.*** These two injuries are closely related and are treated as one entity by most authors. For example, dorsal perilunate and volar lunate dislocations are considered together, and volar perilunate and dorsal lunate dislocations are grouped as one.

(a) Dorsal perilunate and volar lunate dislocation—***Dorsal perilunate and volar lunate dislocations are the most common types of perilunate injury.*** When they occur, there is complete disruption of all perilunar ligaments except the SRL ligament, which remains attached to the volar aspect of the lunate. The lunate may remain in its fossa (Stage III, perilunate dislocation) or be displaced volarly into the carpal canal (Stage IV, true lunate dislocation). These displacements may be seen on lateral radiographs as a continuum of the injury pattern (Fig. 23-21). Treatment consists of emergent closed reduction and splinting followed by definitive ORIF. Some patients may present with acute carpal tunnel syndrome caused by the displaced lunate. These cases require emergent carpal tunnel release and fixation. Although closed reduction and percutaneous pinning have been recommended by some authors, more reliable results can be achieved using open methods, usually through combined volar and dorsal approaches. The dorsal approach is between the third and fourth dorsal compartments, whereas the volar approach proceeds through the carpal canal. In a complete lunate dislocation, the lunate is found within the carpal canal and can be reduced with a small elevator. The "rent" through the volar capsule and ligaments should be repaired in both lunate and perilunate dislocations. Dorsally, the normal alignments of the scaphoid, lunate, and capitate are restored and the bones pinned in place using K-wires. Ligamentous repair dorsally is not as simple as the volar repair but should be attempted and augmented with capsule if necessary. Postoperative management is variable, but there is general consensus that the pins should remain in place for at least 8 weeks. Final range of motion is limited because of the extensive damage and may not reach 50% of normal in many cases. ***Late cases of perilunate dislocations (>8 weeks) may not be reparable and are usually treated by proximal row carpectomy.***

(b) Volar perilunate and dorsal lunate dislocations—Volar perilunate and dorsal lunate dislocations are much less common but are treated in a similar fashion. Again, combined volar and dorsal approaches are used to restore the normal anatomic relationships and allow for ligamentous repair.

2. Greater arc injuries—***Greater arc injuries are distinguished by an associated carpal fracture.*** Treatment is directed at restoring normal carpal alignments in addition to reducing and fixing the fractures. They may occur separately or in various combinations.

• Transscaphoid perilunate fracture-dislocation—***A transscaphoid perilunate fracture-dislocation combines fracture of the scaphoid with perilunar dislocation and is the most common greater arc pattern.*** The initial treatment is similar to that for lesser arc injuries, with emergent closed reduction and splinting performed to avoid neurovascular compromise. Definitive treatment should include ORIF of the scaphoid fracture, usually carried out through a volar (Russe) approach. The fracture is fixed with a screw or K-wires, and attention is then directed to the alignment of the lunate and capitate. If there is a VISI deformity as a result of lunotriquetral ligament disruption, a dorsal approach is added to reduce and pin the carpus. Of the two variations, volar and dorsal, volar dislocations are more severe and more likely to require two approaches. Postoperative care is the same as that for ligamentous injuries but with added complications because of the scaphoid fracture. These ***include nonunion and AVN of the scaphoid, both of which are more likely when there is an associated perilunar dislocation***.

• Transradial styloid perilunate fracture-dislocation—Treatment of transradial styloid perilunate fracture-dislocation includes ORIF of the radial styloid fracture in addition to reduction and pinning of the perilunar joints. When fracture comminution precludes adequate fixation, the fragments should be excised and the soft tissues reattached to bone. Failure to do this may result in residual instability of the radiocarpal joint.

• Scaphocapitate syndrome—As the name implies, scaphocapitate syndrome combines fracture of the capitate and perilunar dislocation either with or without a scaphoid fracture. Often, the proximal pole of the capitate rotates 90° to 180° and is seen on

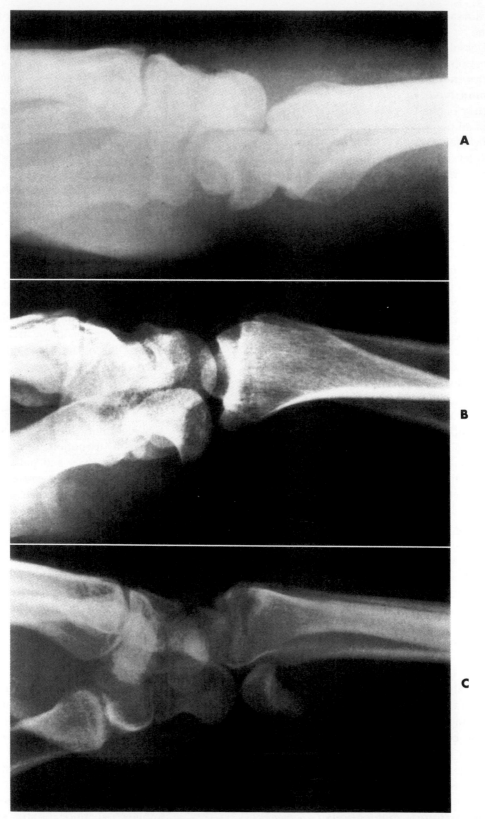

FIGURE 23-21   Carpal dislocations make up a spectrum of injury, and the initial lateral radiograph in a patient with a carpal dislocation may depict a configuration at any point in the spectrum. **A.** "Pure" dorsal perilunate dislocation. **B.** Intermediate stage. **C.** "Pure" volar lunate dislocation. (From Green DP, ed. *Operative Hand Surgery*. 3rd ed. New York, NY: Churchill Livingstone; 1993, with permission.)

anteroposterior radiographs as a squared-off fragment. ORIF is indicated for all fractures along with appropriate restoration of carpal alignment. AVN may occur in the proximal fragment of the capitate fracture.

- Transtriquetral perilunate fracture-dislocation—Transtriquetral perilunate fracture-dislocation occurs when the fracture line extends into the triquetrum, leaving its proximal pole attached to the lunate. Treatment and postoperative care are similar to those for the other greater arc injuries.

3. Axial disruption injuries—Axial disruption injuries are rare, usually caused by high-energy trauma to the hand and wrist. Disruption and dislocation occur along an axial plane perpendicular to the lines of perilunar injury. Different patterns have been described and classified according to their location (see Fig. 23-18). Axial radial disruptions involve the first and second metacarpals as well as the trapezium and trapezoid. Axial ulnar injuries usually result in a separation between the capitate and hamate and the third and fourth metacarpals. They are treated by ORIF through a dorsal approach. Many of these injuries are associated with extensive soft-tissue damage.

4. Midcarpal instability—Different types of midcarpal instability have recently been identified. These instability patterns are considered nondissociative because they involve the extrinsic ligaments (between carpal rows) and not the intrinsic ligaments (within a carpal row). Often, they develop insidiously over time and are seen in patients with generalized ligamentous laxity. Occasionally, they may result from a perilunar injury. Clinically, midcarpal instability may present with a painful clunk as the proximal and distal rows shift suddenly. Treatment of this problem is controversial but may include soft-tissue reconstructive procedures or ultimately, midcarpal arthrodesis.

IV. Injuries of the DRUJ
   A. Overview—Fractures, dislocations, and soft-tissue injuries of the DRUJ have received more attention recently as the importance of this joint has become evident. Failure to treat these injuries appropriately can lead to disabling pain, instability, or loss of motion. Treatment should include restoration of normal joint alignment and repair of the soft tissues that may lead to late instability. A thorough understanding of the anatomy of this joint is critical in the evaluation and treatment of these injuries.

   B. Anatomy—The DRUJ is a diarthrodial trochoid articulation between the concave sigmoid notch of the radius and the convex head or "seat" of the distal ulna (Fig. 23-22). Two-thirds of the distal ulna is covered by articular cartilage, but its nonarticular dorsal surface is grooved to accommodate the extensor carpi ulnaris (ECU) tendon (sixth dorsal compartment). Pronation and supination occur through an arc of 180°, of which approximately 30° is due to translational movement. Because the radius of curvature of the sigmoid notch is larger than that of the ulnar seat, *the radius slips volarly during full pronation and dorsally during full supination.* At these extremes of rotation, there is only 10% contact between the articular surfaces, and stability must be provided by the soft-tissue (ligamentous) restraints. *The most important of these ligamentous stabilizers is the TFCC. The TFCC is composed of the following structures (Fig. 23-23): TFC, ulnocarpal ligaments (including the UL, UT, and ulnocapitate ligaments), volar and dorsal radioulnar ligaments, meniscal homologue, sheath of the ECU tendon, and ulnar collateral ligament.*

   The TFC is at the heart of this complex and forms a *load-bearing component* that transmits compressive force between the carpus and ulna. *It attaches to the distal radius at the sigmoid notch and runs to the fovea at the base of the ulnar styloid.* The thickness of the TFC varies from 2 mm at its center to 5 mm at its periphery. Typically, there is an inverse relationship between ulnar variance and TFC thickness; ulna-negative wrists have a thicker TFC, and ulna-positive wrists have a thinner TFC. The vasculature of the TFC

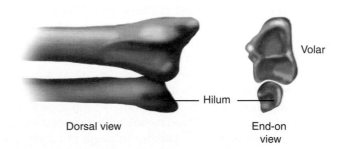

Volar

Hilum

Dorsal view   End-on view

FIGURE 23-22 Radioulnar articulation in neutral or zero rotation as viewed from the dorsum and from end on. Note that the arc of the notch circumscribes a circle of greater diameter than that of the ulnar head. (Illustration by Elizabeth Roselius. From Green DP, ed. *Operative Hand Surgery.* 4th ed. New York, NY: Churchill Livingstone; 1999, with permission.)

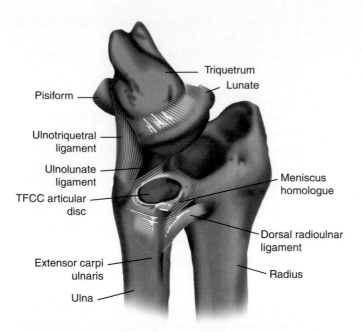

Pisiform

Triquetrum

Lunate

Ulnotriquetral ligament

Ulnolunate ligament

TFCC articular disc

Meniscus homologue

Extensor carpi ulnaris

Dorsal radioulnar ligament

Radius

Ulna

FIGURE 23-23 Anatomy of the ulnocarpal joint and the TFCC, including the pisiform, triquetrum, lunate, ulna, radius, TFCC-articular disc, meniscus homologue, extensor carpi ulnaris, dorsal radioulnar ligament, ulnotriquetral ligament, and ulnolunate ligament. The volar radioulnar ligament and ulnar collateral ligament are not shown.

is provided by volar and dorsal branches of the anterior interosseous artery, which perfuses the outer 20%; the central area remains avascular. The volar and dorsal radioulnar ligaments are intimately associated with the TFC and are the *primary stabilizers of the DRUJ*. These ligaments provide support during full pronation and supination. The ulnocarpal ligaments, of which the most important are the UL and UT, connect the TFC to the carpus and support the volar side of the joint. The ulnar collateral ligament runs from the fovea to the base of the fifth metacarpal and includes the vestigial meniscal homologue, which can vary in its presentation. When fully developed, the meniscus may include an ossicle known as a *lanula*, which is present in 4% of wrists. The major dorsal support of the TFCC is the ECU tendon sheath. It is composed of a fibroosseous tunnel separate from the extensor retinaculum. Although not included in the TFCC, the pronator quadratus muscle is thought to be an important dynamic stabilizer of the DRUJ. During pronation and supination, this muscle contracts to provide compressive force across the joint. *The fovea is described as the axis of rotation of the forearm*. It is located at the base of the ulnar styloid and forms the important attachment site for the volar and dorsal

radioulnar ligaments. *Fractures at the base of the ulnar styloid disrupt these attachments and result in DRUJ instability*. When displaced, these fractures require ORIF to prevent chronic instability.

C. Evaluation

1. Physical examination—Acute injuries of the DRUJ may occur as isolated events or may be associated with fractures of the wrist and forearm. Accordingly, the examination must include the elbow and forearm as well as the wrist. Swelling, tenderness, and limitation of motion may accompany these injuries and be associated with deformity. When the ulna is dislocated dorsally, there may be a prominence of the ulnar head. Conversely, a depression may be seen and felt when a volar ulna dislocation has occurred. Pronation and supination may be limited or completely blocked depending on the degree of injury. Chronic problems associated with the DRUJ may be more difficult to diagnose. In these cases, a careful examination of each structure is necessary. Palpation may elicit tenderness, and provocative maneuvers can identify instability of the DRUJ. Clicks or clunks are considered significant if they are associated with pain and if they are not found on the opposite, uninvolved wrist. The piano key sign refers to a prominent and unstable distal ulna. It is indicative of dorsal instability.

2. Diagnostic imaging

- Plain radiographs—Plain radiographs should include PA and lateral views of the wrist taken in neutral forearm rotation. The PA view should demonstrate both the radial and ulnar styloids and allow for the calculation of ulnar variance. *(Note that variance changes with forearm rotation.)* The PA view may show separation of the radius and ulna, indicating a dislocation of the joint. A true lateral view shows dislocation of the DRUJ and distinguishes between volar and dorsal displacement of the ulna. Radiographs of the forearm and elbow should also be included to check for radial shaft and radial head fractures.

- CT—CT scanning, especially with three-dimensional reconstruction, provides useful information about complex fracture patterns. Axial cuts can identify subtle joint disruptions and should include both wrists for comparison purposes.

- MRI—MRI has been used to identify soft-tissue injuries of the wrist, including ligament disruption and tears of the TFC. Areas of injury are usually represented by a low-intensity signal on T1-weighted images, whereas fluid around a tear appears bright on T2-weighted images. Newer machines with dedicated wrist coils have improved the accuracy of MRI to greater than 90%.

- Radionuclide bone imaging—Radionuclide bone imaging is an important tool in the evaluation of unexplained wrist pain. It is a sensitive test that can be used to detect occult fracture, infection, tumor, or CRPS.

- Arthrography—Arthrography has been used extensively in the evaluation of the DRUJ. Triple-injection techniques instill dye into the DRUJ as well as the radiocarpal and midcarpal joints. When combined with serial radiographs or fluoroscopy, the flow of dye can demonstrate ligamentous and TFC tears. A drawback of arthrography is the existence of asymptomatic "communicating defects," which may be demonstrated and confused with pathologic tears. Normal findings with DRUJ injection include the prestyloid recess and pisotriquetral joint communication.

3. Arthroscopy—The use of arthroscopy in the diagnosis and treatment of wrist pathology has grown tremendously. It is now considered the gold standard for evaluation of the TFC and the carpal ligaments. Arthroscopic evaluation has led to the development of a classification system for TFCC abnormalities (Table 23-2). Class 1 lesions are traumatic, whereas class 2 lesions are degenerative. Many of these problems can now be treated arthroscopically or be combined with minimally open techniques. Evaluation of the DRUJ itself is more difficult, but arthroscopy can provide diagnostic information about the articular cartilage of the joint.

D. Treatment—Problems of the DRUJ include isolated dislocations, combined fracture-dislocations, soft-tissue injuries, and chronic joint disorders. The treatment of each problem is different; therefore, each needs to be addressed separately.

1. Isolated dislocations of the DRUJ— Hyperpronation may lead to dorsal dislocation of the ulna (more common), whereas hypersupination may cause volar dislocation. As the injury occurs, there is sequential disruption of the radioulnar ligaments, the TFCC, and the capsule of the DRUJ. **Simple dislocations** are those that can be reduced closed and that are usually stable after reduction. Treatment consists of long-arm cast immobilization for 4 to 6 weeks in either **supination (for dorsal**

TABLE 23-2
TFCC Abnormalities
Class 1: Traumatic
A. Central perforation
B. Ulnar avulsion With distal ulnar fracture Without distal ulnar fracture
C. Distal avulsion
D. Radial avulsion With sigmoid notch fracture Without sigmoid notch fracture
Class 2: Degenerative (ulnocarpal abutment syndrome)
A. TFCC wear
B. TFCC wear + lunate and/or ulnar chondromalacia
C. TFCC perforation + lunate and/or ulnar chondromalacia
D. TFCC perforation + lunate and/or ulnar chondromalacia + lunotriquetral ligament perforation
E. TFCC perforation + lunate and/or ulnar chondromalacia + lunotriquetral ligament perforation + ulnocarpal arthritis

Source: From Buterbaugh GA. In: *American Society for Surgery of the Hand: Hand surgery Update.* Rosemont, IL: American Academy of Orthopaedic Surgeons; 1996, with permission.

dislocations) or pronation (for volar dislocations). Complex dislocations are characterized by irreducibility or instability after closed reduction. This is due to interposed soft tissue, usually the ECU tendon and sheath. These injuries must be treated open. A dorsal approach is used to free the trapped ECU tendon and reduce the DRUJ. Reduction is followed by repair of the TFC back to the ulna and pin fixation of the DRUJ. If an ulnar styloid fracture is present, it should be fixed with a K-wire, a tension band, or interosseous wiring. Postoperative management should include long-arm cast immobilization for 6 weeks, followed by pin removal and joint rehabilitation.

2. Fractures of the ulna with an associated DRUJ injury—Fractures of the ulnar styloid need to be evaluated in terms of DRUJ stability. Because of the TFCC attachments, **fractures at the styloid base (fovea) result in greater instability than those at the tip**. These injuries are usually seen in combination with displaced fractures of the distal radius. In this situation, the distal radius fracture needs to be reduced and stabilized first, followed by evaluation of the DRUJ. If the joint is unstable to manual

stress or with forearm rotation, ORIF of the ulnar styloid fracture should be considered. Alternatively, the ulnar styloid fracture can be reduced closed and the DRUJ stabilized by pin fixation or by inclusion into an external fixation frame. Fractures of the ulnar head may also result in instability of the DRUJ. These articular fractures, if displaced, need to be treated surgically to restore joint congruency and stability. In rare situations, a severely comminuted fracture of the ulnar head may require partial or complete excision.

3. Fractures of the distal radius with an associated DRUJ injury—Fracture of the distal radius with DRUJ injury is seen when the distal radius fracture line extends into the DRUJ or when there is an associated TFCC disruption or ulnar styloid fracture. In each of these cases, treatment of the DRUJ injury should not be ignored. Recent studies have shown a correlation between distal radius malunion and late ulnar-sided wrist pain. ***Fractures that heal with more than 25° of dorsal tilt or more than 5 mm of shortening cause DRUJ disruption and lead to decreased forearm rotation and ulnocarpal impaction.*** Similarly, fractures of the lunate fossa involving the sigmoid notch should be anatomically reduced to avoid intra-articular malunion and posttraumatic arthritis of the DRUJ. This can be carried out using limited open reduction and pin fixation or formal ORIF. Another problem is late instability due to TFCC rupture or ulnar styloid base fracture. As previously noted, these injuries need to be treated surgically (by ORIF) when the DRUJ is unstable. A classification system by Fernandez divides ulnar-sided injuries into Types A (stable), B (unstable), and C (potentially unstable) (Fig. 23-24). Type A injuries are treated closed, whereas Types B and C injuries usually require operative fixation.

4. Fractures of the radial shaft with an associated DRUJ injury—Also known as ***Galeazzi fractures***; fractures of the radial shaft with DRUJ injury account for 5% to 7% of all forearm fractures. Because of their association with DRUJ injuries, radial shaft fractures should always raise the suspicion of a more distal problem. Careful clinical and radiographic evaluation of the wrist may show subluxation or dislocation of the DRUJ. In general, a radial shaft fracture within 7.5 cm of the wrist joint is more likely to be associated with dislocation of the DRUJ. Treatment includes ORIF of the radial shaft fracture, followed by reduction and evaluation

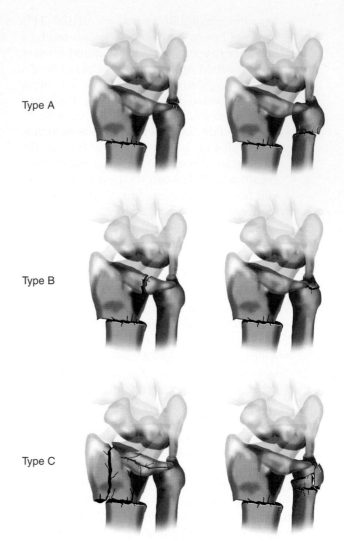

Type A

Type B

Type C

FIGURE 23-24 The classification of Fernandez allows ulnar-sided lesions to be categorized and incorporated as part of the overall treatment plan.

of the DRUJ. When a simple dislocation or subluxation is present, the DRUJ injury is treated closed and immobilized in either ***supination (for dorsal dislocations) or pronation (for volar dislocations)*** for 6 weeks. In rare cases of unstable simple dislocations, a transfixing pin is placed across the joint and removed after 6 weeks. Complex dislocations cannot be reduced closed and are treated by open reduction and repair of the TFCC back to the ulna. A pin is usually added to protect the repair and stabilize the DRUJ for 4 to 6 weeks.

5. Fractures of the radial head with an associated DRUJ injury—Known as the ***Essex-Lopresti injury,*** fractures of the radial head with DRUJ injury occur when an axial load is applied to the forearm, causing disruption of the DRUJ

and interosseous membrane and fracture of the radial head. Again, careful examination of the wrist should be performed in every patient with a radial head fracture. ***The significance of this injury is the destabilization of the entire radius.*** Failure to appreciate and treat this problem can lead to the late complications of instability, pain, and loss of forearm rotation. In addition, comminuted fractures of the radial head are at risk for proximal migration of the radius and should not be excised. ORIF is the preferred treatment and is combined with distal pin fixation of the radius and ulna. In the event that radial head excision is unavoidable, a silastic or titanium spacer should be implanted to prevent proximal radial migration. Because the interosseous membrane heals very slowly, these patients should be followed for at least 2 years. If removal of the spacer is planned, it should be delayed for the same amount of time.

6. Injuries of the TFC—Acute tears of the TFC may result from rotational forces acting on the wrist or from an axial load sustained during a fall. If there is no associated fracture or dislocation, initial treatment consists of splinting followed by gradual mobilization. If symptoms persist despite conservative management, further workup is indicated. Patients with painful clicking and evidence of a TFC tear on MRI or arthrogram may be candidates for arthroscopic treatment. Traumatic tears of the TFC have been classified into four subgroups based on their anatomic location (see Table 23-2). Class 1A lesions are central tears of the articular disc and when symptomatic, are usually treated by arthroscopic debridement. Because they occur in the avascular central region, they are not amenable to repair. Class 1B injuries are associated with DRUJ dislocation and represent complete tears from the fovea or fracture of the styloid base. Management of these tears usually includes suture repair of the TFC (using suture anchors or drill holes) or ORIF of the ulnar styloid fracture. Class 1C tears are located distally and include disruption of the UL ligament, the UT ligament, or both. Class 1D lesions represent avulsions of the TFC from its radial attachment at the sigmoid notch. These injuries are often associated with a distal radius fracture of the lunate fossa and require anatomic reduction and fixation. The treatment of many of these tears remains controversial. Most can be treated either using arthroscopic or open repair. Regardless of the method chosen, immobilization is usually necessary for 6 to 8 weeks to allow healing of the repaired structures.

E. Complications
1. Late instability—Chronic instability may be seen after injury of the DRUJ and its stabilizing structures. In cases of mild subluxation, reattachment of the TFC to the ulna can be accomplished with suture repair through drill holes or by use of suture anchors. If a styloid nonunion is present, it can be reduced and fixed to the ulna with a K-wire, screw, or tension band wire. For small nonunions, excision of the fragment and repair of the soft tissues are recommended. In cases of gross instability, TFC repair may be augmented with a tendon graft reconstruction. Various procedures are available for reconstructing the radioulnar or ulnocarpal ligaments depending on the site of instability.

2. Posttraumatic arthritis—Posttraumatic arthritis may result from intra-articular malunion of the DRUJ or chronic instability. Initial treatment is conservative with long-arm splinting (prevents forearm rotation), oral anti-inflammatory medications, and local corticosteroid injections. Many patients respond to these treatments. Patients for whom conservative care fails are candidates for operative treatment. Surgical options include distal ulnar resection (Darrach procedure), hemiresection arthroplasty, and distal radioulnar fusion. Of these procedures, hemiresection arthroplasty of the ulna has become the most popular. It has evolved from the more radical Darrach procedure into a technique that preserves the TFC and limits bone excision to the joint margins only. A free tendon graft is used as an interpositional spacer to prevent contact between the remaining distal ulna and the radius. The Darrach procedure is still recommended for cases of DRUJ arthritis with an unreconstructable TFC. Radioulnar fusion combined with proximal pseudarthrosis (Suave-Kapandji procedure) is another option for symptomatic arthritis.

3. Ulnocarpal abutment—***Ulnocarpal abutment*** is characterized by positive ulnar variance that leads to symptomatic overload of the ulnocarpal joint. Progressive degeneration of the TFC may result. ***This condition may develop after distal radius malunion.*** Treatment includes opening wedge (lengthening) radial osteotomy or shortening of the ulna (depending on the degree of malunion). Other treatment options are "wafer" resection of the distal pole of the ulna (open or arthroscopic) and Darrach excision.

4. Posttraumatic contracture of the DRUJ—Posttraumatic contracture leads to limited forearm rotation after DRUJ injury as a result of capsular fibrosis and contracture. More specifically, ***volar capsular contracture limits forearm supination, whereas dorsal contracture limits pronation***. Treatment includes partial or complete capsulectomy with preservation of the TFC.

5. ECU tendon dislocation—Tendon subluxation or dislocation can occur in association with injuries of the TFC. Alternatively, this condition may be confused with an isolated tear of the TFC because both conditions may cause painful clicking or snapping. Treatment of acute ECU dislocation is immobilization in pronation for 3 to 4 weeks. If this fails, tendon sheath reconstruction can be performed using a slip of the extensor retinaculum.

SUGGESTED READINGS

Classic Articles

Adams BA. Effects of radial deformity on distal radioulnar joint mechanics. *J Hand Surg.* 1993;18A:492–498.

Adams BD. Distal radioulnar joint instability. *Instr Course Lect.* 1998;47:209–213.

Agee JM. External fixation: technical advances based upon multiplanar ligamentotaxis, *Orthop Clin North Am.* 1993;24:265–274.

Alexander CE, Lichtman DM. Ulnar carpal instabilities. *Orthop Clin North Am.* 1984;15:307–320.

Altissimi M, Antenucci R, Fiacca C, et al. Long-term result of conservative treatment of fractures of the distal radius. *Clin Orthop.* 1986;206:202–210.

Axelrod TS, Paley D, Green J, et al. Limited open reduction of the lunate facet in comminuted intra-articular fractures of the distal radius. *J Hand Surg.* 1988;13A:372–377.

Barton JR. Views and treatment of an important injury to the wrist. *Med Examiner.* 1838;1:365.

Bartosh RA, Saldana MJ. Intra-articular fractures of the distal radius: a cadaveric study to determine if ligamentotaxis restores radiopalmar tilt. *J Hand Surg.* 1990;15A:18–21.

Beckenbaugh RD, Shives TC, Dobyns JH, et al. Kienböck's disease: the natural history of Kienböck's disease and consideration of lunate fractures. *Clin Orthop.* 1980;149:98–106.

Blatt G. Capsulodesis in reconstructive hand surgery: dorsal capsulodesis for the unstable scaphoid and volar capsulodesis following excision of the distal ulna. *Hand Clin.* 1987;3(1):81–102.

Bowers WH. Distal radioulnar joint arthroplasty: the hemiresection-interposition technique. *J Hand Surg.* 1985;10A:169–178.

Bruckner JD, Alexander AH, Lichtman DM. Acute dislocations of the distal radioulnar joint. *Instr Course Lect.* 1996;45:27–36.

Buterbaugh GA, Palmer AK. Fractures and dislocations of the distal radioulnar joint. *Hand Clin.* 1988;4(3):361–375.

Chen WS, Shih CH. Ulnar variance and Kienböck's disease: an investigation in Taiwan. *Clin Orthop.* 1990;255:124–127.

Colles A. On fractures of the carpal extremity. *Edinburgh Med Surg J.* 1814;10:182–186.

Cooney WP 3rd, Dobyns JH, Linscheid RL. Fractures of the scaphoid: a rational approach to management. *Clin Orthop Rel Res.* 1980;149:90–97.

Cooney WP, Berger RA. Treatment of complex fractures of the distal radius: combined use of internal and external fixation and arthroscopic reduction. *Hand Clin.* 1993;9:603–612.

Edwards HC. The mechanism and treatment of backfire fracture. *J Bone Joint Surg.* 1926;8:701–717.

Essex-Lopresti PA. Fractures of the radial head with distal radio-ulnar dislocation: report of two cases. *J Bone Joint Surg.* 1951;33B:244–247.

Fernandez DL. Correction of posttraumatic wrist deformity in adults by osteotomy, bone grafting and internal fixation. *J Bone Joint Surg.* 1982;64A:1164–1178.

Fernandez DL. Anterior bone grafting and conventional lag screw fixation to treat scaphoid nonunions. *J Hand Surg.* 1990;15A:140–147.

Frykman G. Fracture of the distal radius involving sequelae: shoulder-hand-finger syndrome, disturbance in the distal radio-ulnar joint and impairment of nerve function. *Acta Orthop Scand.* 1967;108:1–153.

Garcia-Elias M, Dobyns JH, Cooney WP, et al. Traumatic axial dislocations of the carpus. *J Hand Surg.* 1989;14A:446–457.

Gelberman, RH, Menon J. The vascularity of the scaphoid bone. *J Hand Surg.* 1980;5:508–513.

Gellman H, Caputo RJ, Carter V, et al. Comparison of short and long thumb spica casts for non-displaced fractures of the carpal scaphoid. *J Bone Joint Surg.* 1989;71A:354–357.

Green DP. The effect of avascular necrosis on Russe-bone grafting for scaphoid nonunion. *J Hand Surg.* 1985;10A:597–605.

Herbert TJ, Fischer WE. Management of the fractured scaphoid using a new bone screw. *J Bone Joint Surg.* 1984;66B:114–123.

Herzberg G, Comtet JJ, Linscheid RL, et al. perilunate dislocations and fracture dislocations: a multicenter study. *J Hand Surg.* 1993;18A:768–779.

Johnson RP. The acutely injured wrist and its residuals. *Clin Orthop.* 1980;149:33–44.

Jupiter JB. Fractures of the distal end of the radius. *J Bone Joint Surg.* 1991;73A:461–469.

Jupiter JB, Lipton H. The operative treatment of intraarticular fractures of the distal radius. *Clin Orthop.* 1993;292:48–61.

Jupiter JB, Fernandez DL, Toh CL, et al. The operative treatment of volar intra-articular fractures of the distal end of the radius. *J Bone Joint Surg.* 1996;78A:1817–1828.

Jupiter JB, Fernandez DL, Whipple TL, et al. Intra-articular fractures of the distal radius: contemporary perspectives. *Instr Course Lect.* 1998;47:191–202.

Kihara H, Palmer AK, Werner FW, et al. The effects of dorsally angulated distal radius fractures on distal radioulnar congruency and forearm rotation. *J Hand Surg.* 1996;21A:40–47.

Lichtman DM, Schneider JR, Swafford AR, et al. Ulnar midcarpal instability: clinical and laboratory analysis. *J Hand Surg.* 1981;6A:515–523.

Lichtman DM, Bruckner JD, Culp RW, et al. Palmar midcarpal instability: results of surgical reconstruction. *J Hand Surg.* 1993;18A:307–315.

Linscheid RL, Dobyns JH, Beabout JW, et al. Traumatic instability of the wrist: diagnosis, classification, and pathomechanics. *J Bone Joint Surg.* 1972;54A:1612–1632.

Mack GR, Bosse MJ, Gelberman RH. The natural history of scaphoid nonunion. *J Bone Joint Surg.* 1984;66A:504–509.

Mayfield JK, Johnson RP, Kilcoyne RK. Carpal dislocations: pathomechanics and progressive perilunar instability. *J Hand Surg.* 1980;5:226–241.

Melone CP Jr. Articular fractures of the distal radius. *Orthop Clin North Am.* 1984;15:217–236.

Melone CP Jr. Distal radius fractures: patterns of articular augmentation. *Orthop Clin North Am.* 1993;24:239–253.

Melone CP Jr, Nathan R. Traumatic disruptions of the triangular fibrocartilage complex, pathoanatomy. *Clin Orthop Rel Res.* 1992;275:65–73.

Mikic ZD. Galeazzi fracture-dislocations. *J Bone Joint Surg.* 1975;57A:1071–1080.

Palmer AK, Werner FW. The triangular fibrocartilage complex of the wrist: anatomy and function. *J Hand Surg.* 1981;6A:153–162.

Palmer AK, Werner FW. Biomechanics of the distal radioulnar joint. *Clin Orthop.* 1984;187:26–35.

Peltier LF. Eponymic fractures: Robert William Smith and Smith's fracture. *Surgery.* 1959;45:1035–1042.

Reagan DS, Linscheid RL, Dobyns JH. Lunotriquetral sprains. *J Hand Surg.* 1984;9A:502–514.

Ruby LK, Belsky MR. The natural history of scaphoid nonunion: a review of fifty-five cases. *J Bone Joint Surg.* 1985;67A:428–432.

Ruby LK. Carpal instability. *Instr Course Lect.* 1996;45:3–13.

Shaw JA. A biomechanical study comparison of scaphoid screws. *J Hand Surg.* 1987;12A:347–353.

Shaw JA, Bruno A, Paul EM. Ulnar styloid fixation in the treatment of posttraumatic instability of the radioulnar joint: a biomechanical study with clinical correlation. *J Hand Surg.* 1990;15A:712–720.

Smith D, Cooney WP 3rd, An K-N. The effects of simulated unstable scaphoid fracture on carpal motion, *J Hand Surg.* 1989;14A:283–290.

Strehle J, Gerber C. Distal radioulnar joint function after Galeazzi fracture-dislocations treated by open reduction and internal plate fixation. *Clin Orthop.* 1993;293:240–245.

Taleisnik J, Watson HK. Midcarpal instability caused by malunited fractures of the distal radius, *J Hand Surg.* 1984;9A:350–357.

Trousdale RT, Linscheid RL. Operative treatment of malunited fractures of the forearm. *J Bone Joint Surg.* 1995;77A:894–902.

Trumble TE, Bour CJ, Smith RJ, et al. Kinematics of the ulnar carpus related to the volar intercalated segment instability pattern, *J Hand Surg.* 1990;15A:384–392.

Viegas, SF, Bean JW, Schram RA. Transscaphoid fracture/dislocations treated with open reduction and Herbert screw internal fixation. *J Hand Surg.* 1987;12A(6):992–999.

Viegas SF, Patterson RM, Paterson PD, et al. Ulnar-sided perilunate instability: an anatomic and biomechanic study. *J Hand Surg.* 1990;15A:268–278.

Watson HK, Ballet FL. The SLAC wrist: scapholunate advanced collapse pattern of degenerative arthritis. *J Hand Surg.* 1984;9A:358–365.

Watson HK, Gabuzda GM. Matched distal ulna resection for posttraumatic disorders of the distal radioulnar joint. *J Hand Surg.* 1992;17A:724–730.

Watson HK, Hempton RF. Limited wrist arthrodesis. I. The triscaphoid joint. *J Hand Surg.* 1980;5:350–357.

Recent Articles

Anderson ML, Larson AN, Moran SL, et al. Clinical comparison of arthroscopic versus open repair of triangular fibrocartilage complex tears. *J Hand Surg Am.* 2008;33(5):675–682.

Buijze GA, Doornberg JN, Ham JS, et al. Surgical compared with conservative treatment for acute nondisplaced or minimally displaced scaphoid fractures: a systematic review and meta-analysis of randomized controlled trials. *J Bone Joint Surg Am.* 2010;92:1534–1544.

Chen NC, Jupiter JB. Management of distal radial fractures. *J Bone Joint Surg Am.* 2007;89:2051–2062.

Chung KC, Shauver MJ, Birkmeyer JD. Trends in the United States in the treatment of distal radius fractures in the elderly. *J Bone Joint Surg Am.* 2009;91:1868–1873.

Elhassan BT, Shin AY. Vascularized bone grafting for treatment of Kienbock's disease. *J Hand Surg Am.* 2009;34:146–154.

Gajendran VK, Peterson B, Slater RR Jr, et al. Long-term outcomes of dorsal intercarpal ligament capsa-lodesis for chronic scapholunate dissociation. *J Hand Surg.* 2007;32A:1323–1333.

Henry MH. Distal radius fractures: current concepts. *J Hand Surg.* 2008;33A:1215–1227.

McQueen MM, Gelbke MK, Wakefield A, et al. Percutaneous screw fixation versus conservative treatment for fractures of the waist of the scaphoid: a prospective randomised study. *J Bone Joint Surg Br.* 2008;90:66–71.

Orbay JL, Fernandez D. Volar fixed-angle plate fixation for unstable distal radius fractures in the elderly patient. *J Hand Surg.* 2004;29A:96–102.

Pollock PJ, Sieg RN, Baechler MF, et al. Radiographic evaluation of the modified Brunelli technique versus the Blatt capsulodesis for scapholunate dissociation in a cadaver model. *J Hand Surg Am.* 2010;35A:1589–1598

Pomerance J. Outcome after repair of the scapholunate interosseous ligament and dorsal capsulodesis for dynamic scapholunate instability due to trauma. *J Hand Surg.* 2006;31A:1380–1386.

Ram AN, Chung KC. Evidence-based management of acute nondisplaced scaphoid waist fractures. *J Hand Surg Am.* 2009;34:735–738.

Vinnars B, Pietrecanu M, Bodestedt A, et al. Nonoperative compared with operative treatment of acute scaphoid fractures. A randomized clinical trial. *J Bone Joint Surg Am.* 2008;90:1176–1185.

Waitayawinyu T, McCallister WV, Katolik LI, et al. Outcome after vascularized bone grafting of scaphoid nonunions with avascular necrosis. *J Hand Surg Am.* 2009;34:387–394.

Review Articles

Cooney WP, Dobyns JH, Linscheid RL. Arthroscopy of the wrist: anatomy and classification of carpal instability. *Arthroscopy.* 1990;6:133–140.

Fernandez DL. Fractures of the distal radius: operative treatment. *Instr Course Lect.* 1993;42:73–88.

Green DP. The effect of avascular necrosis on Russe Bone grafting for scaphoid nonunion. *J Hand Surg.* 1985;10A:597–605.

Peltier LF. Fractures of the distal end of the radius: a historical account. *Clin Orthop.* 1984;187:18–22.

Short WH. Wrist instability. *Instr Course Lect.* 1998;47:203–208.

Szabo RM. Extra-articular fractures of the distal radius. *Orthop Clin North Am.* 1993;24:230–232.

Wright TW, Dobyns JH, Linscheid RL, et al. Carpal instability nondissociative. *J Hand Surg.* 1994;19B:763–773.

Textbooks

Arnadio PC, Taleisnik J. Fractures of the carpal bones. In: Green DP, ed. *Operative Hand Surgery.* 3rd ed. New York, NY: Churchill Livingstone; 1993.

Berger RA. Anatomy and basic biomechanics of the wrist. In: *American Society for Surgery of the Hand: Hand Surgery Update.* Rosemont, IL: American Academy of Orthopedic Surgeons; 1996.

Bowers WH. The distal radioulnar joint. In: Green DP, ed. *Operative Hand Surgery*. 3rd ed. New York, NY: Churchill Livingstone; 1993.

Bruce JF. Hand. In: Miller MD, ed. *Review of Orthopaedics*. 2nd ed. Philadelphia, PA: WB Saunders; 1996.

Buterbaugh GA. Triangular fibrocartilage complex inquiry and ulnar wrist pain. In: *American Society for Surgery of the Hand: Hand Surgery Update*. Rosemont, IL: American Academy of Orthopaedic Surgeons; 1996.

Gellman H, ed. *Fractures of the Distal Radius*. Rosemont, IL: American Academy of Orthopaedic Surgeons; 1998.

Gileila LA. Imaging and evaluation. In: *American Society for Surgery of the Hand: Hand Surgery Update*. Rosemont, IL: American Academy of Orthopaedic Surgeons; 1996.

Green DP. Carpal dislocations and instabilities. In: Green DP, ed. *Operative Hand Surgery*. 3rd ed. New York, NY: Churchill Livingstone; 1993.

Havel DP. Volar plate fixation of distal radius fractures. In: Weiss AC, ed. *Atlas of the Hand Clinics*. Vol 2. Philadelphia, PA: WB Saunders; 1997.

Hendon JH, ed. *Scaphoid Fractures and Complications*. Rosemont, IL: American Academy of Orthopaedic Surgeons; 1994.

Jupiter JB. Scaphoid fractures. In: *American Society for Surgery of the Hand: Hand Surgery Update*. Rosemont, IL: American Academy of Orthopaedic Surgeons; 1996.

McMurtry RY, Jupiter JB. Fractures of the distal radius. In: Browner BD, Jupiter JB, Levine AM, et al, eds. *Skeletal Trauma: Fractures, Dislocations, Ligamentous Injuries*. Philadelphia, PA: WB Saunders; 1992.

Muller ME, Nazarian S, Koch P, eds. *Classification AO des Fractures: Les Os Longs*. Berlin: Springer-Verlag; 1987.

Palmer AK. Fractures of the distal radius. In: Green DP, ed. *Operative Hand Surgery*. 3rd ed. New York, NY: Churchill Livingstone; 1993.

Ruby L. Fractures and dislocations of the carpus. In: Browner BD, Jupiter JB, Levine AM, et al, eds. *Skeletal Trauma: Fractures, Dislocations, Ligamentous Injuries*. Philadelphia, PA: WB Saunders; 1992.

Saffer P. Current trends in treatment and classification of distal radius fractures. In: Saffer P, Cooney WP, eds. *Fractures of the Distal Radius*. London: Martin Dunitz; 1995.

Sanders WE. Distal radius fractures. In: *American Society for Surgery of the Hand: Hand Surgery Update*. Rosemont, IL: American Academy of Orthopaedic Surgeons; 1996.

Shuler TE. Trauma. In: Miller MD, ed. *Review of Orthopaedics*. 2nd ed. Philadelphia, PA: WB Saunders; 1996.

Trumble TE, Budoff JE, eds. *Hand Surgery Update IV*. Rosemont, IL: American Society for Surgery of the Hand; 2007.

Viegas SF. Carpal instability. In: *American Society for Surgery of the Hand: Hand Surgery Update*. Rosemont, IL: American Academy of Orthopaedic Surgeons; 1996.

Weiland AJ. Avascular necrosis of the carpus. In: *American Society for Surgery of the Hand: Hand Surgery Update*. Rosemont, IL: American Academy of Orthopaedic Surgeons; 1996.

Zabinski SJ, Weiland AJ. Fractures of the distal radius. In: Levine AM, ed. *Orthopedic Knowledge Update: Trauma*. Rosemont, IL: American Academy of Orthopaedic Surgeons; 1996.

CHAPTER 24

Injuries of the Hand

Thomas L. Mehlhoff, C. Craig Crouch, and James B. Bennett

I. Joint Injuries of the Hand
   A. Overview
      1. Anatomy (Figs. 24-1 through 24-4)—The small joints of the hand are hinged joints. The metacarpophalangeal (MCP) joints have a cam configuration, whereas the proximal interphalangeal (PIP) and distal interphalangeal (DIP) joints have a spherical shape. Stability depends on the articular contour, collateral ligaments, and volar plate. ***The volar plate has strong lateral attachments, but a weak distal attachment***.
      2. Small joint injuries—A partial or complete tear of the collateral ligaments, volar plate, or extensor tendon results in subluxation or dislocation of the finger joint. Intra-articular fractures, including avulsion fractures and fracture-dislocations, may be associated with these injuries.
      3. Evaluation—Swelling, tenderness, or ecchymosis of a finger should raise suspicion for a joint injury. Stress testing may reveal instability as a result of underlying fracture or ligamentous injury. Comparison stress testing to the noninjured opposite side is helpful in cases of ligamentous laxity. Limited motion of a joint may result from joint subluxation or a displaced articular fragment. Evaluation of these injuries requires excellent quality radiographs, including an anteroposterior (AP) X-ray view, a true lateral X-ray view centered on the injured articulation, and one or two oblique views. Tomograms may occasionally be necessary to obtain better visualization of a centrally depressed fracture.
      4. Treatment and outcome—Pain-free motion and joint stability are the treatment goals for these injuries. Treatment must correct subluxation and restore an acceptable joint surface. Studies suggest that ***pain and motion may improve for up to 1 year after injury to a small joint of the hand***.
   B. DIP Joint Injuries
      1. Mallet finger (Fig. 24-5)—A sudden forceful flexion to the DIP joint may rupture the extensor

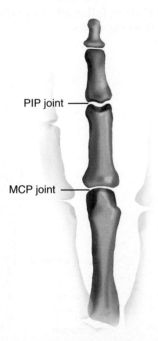

FIGURE 24-1 Metacarpophalangeal joints are unicondylar, and proximal interphalangeal joints are bicondylar, giving the PIP joints more stability.

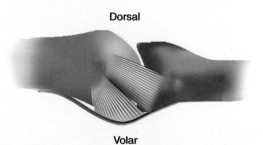

Dorsal

Volar

FIGURE 24-2 Collateral ligaments have a cordlike dorsal component and a fan-shaped volar component.

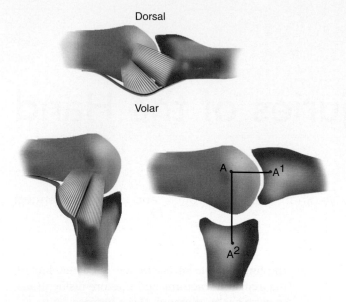

FIGURE 24-3 The shape of the metacarpal head is eccentric. This creates a cam effect that makes the collateral ligaments more taut in flexion than in extension (the distance from *A* to *A*1 is less than the distance from *A* to *A*2.

tendon from the distal phalanx, with or without a bone fragment. Large fracture fragments involving more than 30% of the articular surface are at risk for volar subluxation of the distal phalanx.
- Evaluation—Examination may reveal pain, swelling, and a dropped finger at the DIP

FIGURE 24-4 Structures about the MCP and interphalangeal joints.

joint. X-ray films demonstrate a flexed DIP joint and may demonstrate a fracture fragment still attached to the extensor tendon. Volar subluxation of the distal phalanx may accompany the fracture, particularly if the fragment is large.
- Classification of Mallet Finger
  - (a) Type I—It involves closed or blunt trauma with loss of tendon continuity, with or without a small chip fracture.
  - (b) Type II—It involves a laceration at or proximal to the DIP joint with loss of tendon continuity.
  - (c) Type III—It involves a deep abrasion with loss of skin, subcutaneous cover, and tendon substance.
  - (d) Type IV—It involves a physeal fracture in children, a hyperflexion injury with a fracture involving 20% to 50% of the articular surface, or a hyperextension injury with a fracture of the articular surface usually greater than 50% and with early or late volar subluxation of the distal phalanx.
- Treatment
  - (a) Closed treatment—Splinting or casting is indicated for mallet finger injuries with small fracture fragments that involve less than 30% of the articular surface or are displaced less than 2 mm. ***The mallet finger is treated in extension for 6 weeks full time***, followed by another 4 weeks at night (Fig. 24-6).

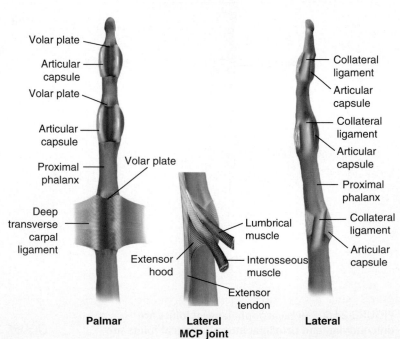

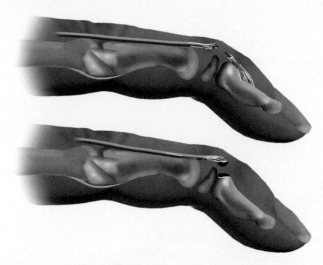

FIGURE 24-5   Mallet finger. Soft-tissue (terminal extensor tendon tear) mallet (*top*) and bony mallet (*bottom*).

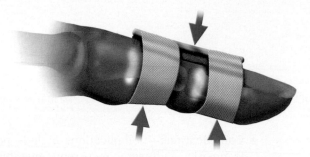

FIGURE 24-6   Extension splinting of the DIP joint for mallet injuries. The dorsal padded aluminum splint uses the three-point fixation principle (*arrows*).

(b) Surgery—***Mallet finger deformities require surgery when they are associated with fracture fragments greater***

than 30% of the joint surface, are displaced more than 2 mm, or are associated with volar subluxation of the distal phalanx. Volar subluxation of the DIP joint is the strongest indication for surgery. Open reduction with internal fixation (ORIF) of the fracture fragment is recommended to correct the volar subluxation of the DIP joint with a longitudinal K-wire in extension (Fig. 24-7); tendon repair is performed as needed. The use of a pullout button may lead to skin slough (beneath the button). Suture anchor fixation may be preferable.

• Complications—Complications include persistent mallet deformity, ***secondary swanneck deformity*** (Fig. 24-8), and traumatic arthritis of the DIP joint as a result of an incongruent joint or volar subluxation.

2. Dorsal dislocation of the DIP joint—A hyperextension force at the tip of the finger may disrupt the volar plate and the collateral ligaments, whereas the insertion of the profundus tendon remains intact. These injuries are frequently associated with a volar laceration (64% of cases), since the skin is firmly bound to the underlying bone.

• Evaluation

(a) Clinical examination—There is tenderness and deformity at the DIP joint. The patient is unable to flex or extend the joint.

(b) Radiographic evaluation—AP and true lateral X-ray studies should be taken before manipulation. Dislocations are usually dorsal and rarely lateral. Associated avulsion fractures should be identified.

FIGURE 24-7   **A.** X-ray film showing a mallet finger of bony origin. **B.** Postoperative film showing stabilization using a suture anchor and a Kirschner wire.

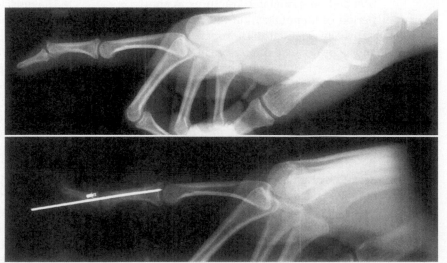

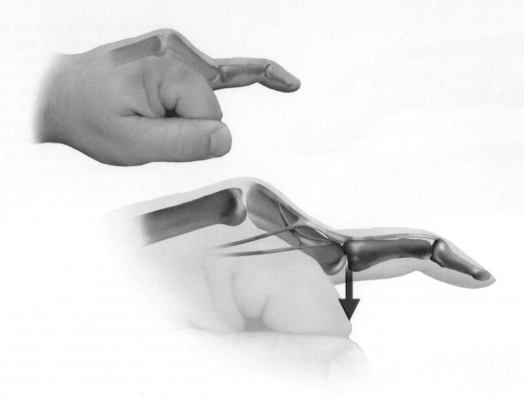

<u>FIGURE 24-8</u> Swan-neck deformity from dorsal subluxation of the lateral bands.

- Classification—Types include closed dislocation, open dislocation, and fracture-dislocation.
- Treatment
  - (a) Closed reduction—Gentle closed reduction is performed under metacarpal block anesthesia. The distal phalanx is extended and then reduced over the condyle. Stability after reduction should be assessed, although there is usually little tendency for redislocation. Postreduction X-ray studies should demonstrate a congruent reduction and no associated fractures. A short period of immobilization (10 to 14 days) is usually adequate. Thorough irrigation and debridement of any open laceration should be performed before reduction.
  - (b) Surgery—***Irreducible dislocations of the DIP joint may result from interposition of the volar plate, interposition of the profundus flexor tendon, or a displaced osteochondral fracture fragment***. In these cases, open reduction may be necessary to extract the interposed volar plate, sesamoid bone, or fracture fragment. ***Interposition of the profundus tendon should imply rupture of at least one collateral ligament***, and in this case, immobilization should be continued for 3 weeks.

- Complications—Complications include posttraumatic stiffness, recurrent instability, posttraumatic arthritis, and infection (septic arthritis and osteomyelitis).

C. PIP Joint Injuries
  1. Collateral ligament sprain of the PIP joint—An abduction or adduction force to the extended finger may result in tearing of the radial or ulnar collateral ligament at the PIP joint. ***The radial collateral ligament is injured more frequently than the ulnar collateral ligament***.
     - Diagnosis—Clinical examination demonstrates point tenderness over the specific site of injury. ***Ligament failure usually occurs at the proximal phalanx or less frequently, in the mid-portion of the ligament***. Stress testing should be performed with the joint in extension or 20° of flexion. Lack of a firm end point is diagnostic of a complete tear. Angulation greater than 20° on an AP stress X-ray film is also diagnostic of a complete tear. Small chip fractures may be noted at the origin of the collateral ligament. Digital block may facilitate examination.
     - Treatment
       - (a) Closed treatment—Partial tears and most complete tears can be treated with static splinting for 7 to 14 days, followed by

buddy-taping to the adjacent digit for 3 weeks. Active motion is encouraged from the outset. Residual joint discomfort and thickening of the collateral ligament as a result of underlying scar tissue formation are common, lasting for 3 to 6 months.

(b) Surgery—Indications for surgery include radiographic evidence of soft-tissue interposition, a displaced condylar fracture of the phalanx, or continued instability after 3 weeks of static splinting. Surgery for the radial collateral ligament to the index finger may be necessary to restore lateral key-pinch strength.

2. Volar plate injury of the PIP joint—Hyperextension injury to the PIP joint may cause the volar plate to tear from the middle phalanx, with or without a bone fragment.
   - Diagnosis
     (a) Clinical examination—There is fusiform swelling of the PIP joint, with point tenderness greatest over the volar plate.
     (b) Radiographic evaluation—Lateral X-ray films may show a small avulsion fracture fragment at the base of the middle phalanx, usually less than 10% of the joint surface. The PIP joint is usually reduced without subluxation.
   - Treatment—Closed management is indicated. Stable injuries are immobilized in a dorsal splint with 20° of flexion for 1 week, followed by an active range-of-motion program using buddy-taping.
   - Complications—Complications include posttraumatic flexion contracture, pain with limited range of motion, and *late swan-neck deformity*.

3. Dorsal dislocation of the PIP joint—One of the most frequently encountered articular injures of the hand is dorsal dislocation of the PIP joint. Hyperextension of the PIP joint forces the finger backward, resulting in dislocation of the middle phalanx dorsally relative to the proximal phalanx, *tearing the volar plate*.
   - Diagnosis
     (a) Examination—The finger usually has an obvious deformity as a result of the dislocation, unless it has already been reduced by a trainer or a bystander. Hyperextension stress testing determines residual instability. Collateral ligament stability may be satisfactory with a pure dorsal dislocation.
     (b) Radiographic evaluation—X-ray films demonstrate the dislocation of the PIP joint (Fig. 24-9). A small avulsion fracture from

the middle phalanx may be seen, identifying the distal location of the volar plate.
   - Treatment—Closed reduction is performed under a metacarpal block anesthesia with longitudinal traction. Most dorsal dislocations are easily reduced. *With stable reduction, range of motion may begin early with continuous buddy-taping for 3 to 6 weeks*. Less stable injuries may require an extension blocking splint to prevent the last 20° of extension for 3 weeks. If the volar fracture fragment contains more than 15% of the volar surface, operative intervention may be needed. Open dislocation should be thoroughly irrigated in the operating room, with extension of the skin lacerations if needed. *Rotational deformity of the finger may suggest entrapment of the middle phalanx condyle between the lateral band and the central slip*. This situation is often irreducible with closed traction and may require open reduction with repair of the extensor mechanism.
   - Complications—Complications include posttraumatic flexion contracture, pseudo-boutonnière deformity, and hyperextension instability.

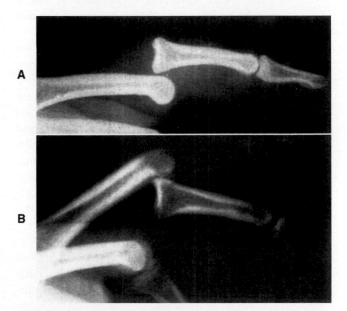

FIGURE 24-9 PIP joint dislocation. **A.** Dorsal dislocation (most common) can usually be treated by closed reduction and buddy-taping. Loss of reduction in extension may require extension block splinting. **B.** Volar dislocation (unusual) may require operative repair of the extensor tendon central slip. (Reprinted with permission from Green DP, Strickland JW. In: DeLee JC, Drez D Jr, eds. *Orthopaedic Sports Medicine: Principles and Practice.* Philadelphia, PA: WB Saunders; 1994.)

4. Volar dislocation of the PIP joint—The central slip insertion on the proximal phalanx is ruptured.
   • Diagnosis
     (a) Examination—Deformity and limited motion are usually obvious. If the joint has spontaneously reduced, lack of active extension of the middle phalanx against resistance should suggest rupture of the central slip. An irreducible dislocation can occur if the lateral bands or central slip becomes trapped under the head of the proximal phalanx.
     (b) Radiographic evaluation—X-ray films demonstrate volar dislocation of the PIP joint (see Fig. 24-9). A small avulsion fracture may be seen at the dorsum of the middle phalanx as a result of the ruptured central slip insertion.
   • Treatment—Closed reduction may be attempted with longitudinal traction and flexion of the MCP and PIP joints. The stability and strength of the central slip are tested after reduction. If the central slip is intact, a short period of immobilization can be followed by a carefully controlled range-of-motion program. *A disrupted central slip must be treated with static splinting in extension for 6 weeks or open operative repair of the disrupted central slip mechanism.*
   • Complications—Complications include extension contracture, PIP or DIP joint stiffness, and progressive boutonnière deformity. Failure to diagnosis the central slip rupture results in progressive volar subluxation of the lateral bands of the extensor mechanism and a resulting *boutonnière deformity* (Fig. 24-10). Global instability is another complication.
5. Fracture-dislocation of the PIP joint—Hyperextension, impaction, shear, and pilon fracture-dislocation may occur. These injuries are the most disabling PIP joint injuries.
   • Diagnosis
     (a) Examination—Swelling, pain, and limited motion, often without severe deformity, is seen. This injury is commonly mistaken as a sprain.
     (b) Radiographic evaluation—Radiographic evaluation is imperative. In a true lateral X-ray film centered on the injured joint, articular fracture fragments are seen; they range from a small fleck to up to 50% of the joint surface, with a variable degree of dorsal subluxation of the middle phalanx. A lateral view in flexion

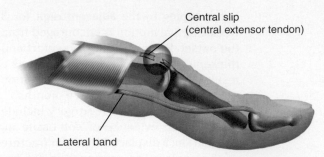

FIGURE 24-10 Central slip injuries, if left untreated, can result in volar displacement of the lateral bands and a *boutonnière deformity*. Volar dislocations of the PIP joint, although uncommon, can result in central slip injuries. Splinting the PIP joint (not the DIP joint) in extension and encouraging passive DIP flexion is the correct treatment for acute central slip injuries as long as the patient has active PIP joint extension to within 30° of full extension.

is helpful for assessing the relocation potential of the PIP joint in flexion.
   • Treatment—Effective treatment modalities may include dorsal extension block splinting, skeletal traction, ORIF, and volar plate arthroplasty.
     (a) Closed management—Stable PIP joints in flexion may be managed with dorsal extension block splinting. Full active flexion is allowed; progressively more extension is allowed over 4 weeks. Fracture fragments less than 30% of the articular surface are well suited to this approach.
     (b) Surgery
       • ORIF—Large fracture fragments involving 50% or more of the joint surface may be repaired with surgery, using a pullout wire, a Kirschner pin, or a compression screw. Pilon fractures with depressed joint surfaces may require elevation, bone grafting, and K-wire stabilization.
       • Volar plate arthroplasty—Comminuted fractures may require excision of the volar fragments and advancement of the volar plate to the middle phalanx to restore stability and resurface the damaged articular surface.
       • Skeletal traction—With highly comminuted fractures, there may be no option but continuous longitudinal distraction until the fracture has molded.
       • Complications—Complications include recurrent subluxation, limited joint motion (hinged motion on a subluxed PIP joint), and posttraumatic arthritis.
D. MCP Joint Injuries
   1. Thumb MCP ulnar collateral ligament injury—An injury to the ulnar collateral ligament of the

thumb is **also known as** gamekeeper's thumb or ski-pole thumb. **A competent ulnar collateral ligament of the MCP joint is critical for effective lateral key pinch.**

- Evaluation
    (a) Examination—Tenderness is noted over the ulnar aspect of the MCP joint. A palpable fullness may suggest **Stener's lesion** (interposition of the adductor pollicis aponeurosis between the torn end of the ulnar collateral ligament and the proximal phalanx). Stress testing of the ulnar collateral ligament with radial stress in some flexion should be compared with the opposite noninjured thumb. **Stress in some flexion tests the proper collateral ligament. Stress in extension tests the more volar accessory ligament. A poor endpoint in both flexion and extension confirms a complete tear of the ligament**, and an unstable joint. A digital block may be required before the examination.
    (b) Radiographic evaluation—Radiographs of the thumb should be taken before stress testing to look for associated fractures. Stress radiographs demonstrating more than 35° of opening should suggest complete tear of the ligament (Fig. 24-11).
- Treatment
    (a) Closed treatment—Partial tears of the ulnar collateral ligament that have good endpoints and do not open 35° with stress can be treated with cast immobilization or with a functional brace with the MCP joint held in slight flexion for 3 to 4 weeks.
    (b) Surgery—A complete tear of the ulnar collateral ligament associated with instability of the MCP joint (opening >35° with stress) or a displaced fracture fragment requires surgery to reattach the ulnar collateral ligament. In these cases, Stener's lesion is usually present and will not heal back to the proximal phalanx without surgery. Operative repair of the ligament can be performed with a suture anchor or a pullout button. Chronic injuries of the ulnar collateral ligament may require ligament reconstruction or advancement of the adductor pollicis to the proximal phalanx.
- Complications—Complications include residual instability with pain, decreased lateral key-pinch strength, volar subluxation of the MCP joint, and late arthritic changes.
2. Thumb MCP radial collateral ligament injury— Injury to the radial collateral ligament of the

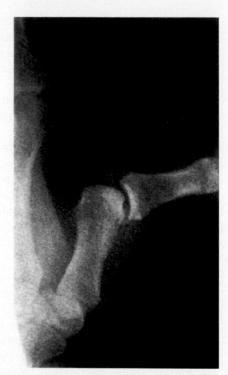

FIGURE 24-11   A thumb MCP ulnar collateral ligament stress test demonstrates significant radial deviation (and angulation) at the thumb MCP joint (as seen on this stress radiograph). (Reprinted with permission from O'Donoghue DH. *Treatment of Injuries to Athletes.* Philadelphia, PA: WB Saunders; 1986.)

MCP joint of the thumb is less common. However, the diagnosis is often missed, so treatment may be delayed.
- Evaluation
    (a) Examination—There is localized swelling and tenderness on the radial aspect of the thumb MCP joint. Stress testing elicits pain or demonstrates opening on the radial aspect of the joint. **Volar subluxation is commonly associated with radial collateral ligament injury of the thumb MCP joint.**
    (b) Radiographic evaluation—Two views of the thumb are needed to evaluate for an associated fracture. A small osteochondral fracture fragment from the metacarpal is frequently noted.
- Treatment
    (a) Cast—Almost all injuries of the radial collateral ligament can be treated conservatively with a cast or thumb spica splint for 4 to 6 weeks if diagnosed acutely. The cast must prevent volar subluxation of the MCP joint.
    (b) Surgery—If the MCP joint is unstable or has volar subluxation, surgery to repair

the radial collateral ligament may be required. ***The ligament is usually torn from the metacarpal head*** and requires repair with a suture anchor or a pullout button.

- Complications—Complications are the same as those listed for thumb MCP ulnar collateral ligament injury.

3. Finger MCP collateral ligament injury—Forced spreading into the web space may result in injury to the radial or ulnar collateral ligament of a finger MCP joint. The collateral ligament at the MCP joint usually fails at its attachment to the proximal phalanx and at times includes an avulsed bone fragment.

- Diagnosis
  - (a) Examination—Subtle swelling is noted in the web space between the two metacarpal heads. Local tenderness confirms the site of injury. Gentle stress testing to the MCP joint, in both extension and flexion, may reproduce pain or demonstrate instability.
  - (b) Radiographic evaluation—X-ray films may demonstrate a small avulsion fracture fragment from the metacarpal head.
- Treatment
  - (a) Closed treatment—The majority of collateral ligament injuries to the MCP joints of the fingers can be treated with conservative management. Buddy-taping of the fingers to protect the collateral ligament of the MCP joint is recommended, with intermittent use of a splint incorporating 50° or more of flexion for unstable injuries. Slow improvement in symptoms may be expected over 3 months.
  - (b) Surgery—Surgical treatment may be considered for an avulsion fracture fragment that involves 20% of the articular surface or is displaced more than 2 mm. ***Relative indications for surgical repair include injury to the radial collateral ligament of the index finger or the little finger.***
- Complications—Complications include instability, laxity, and weakness or pain. Chronic pain and secondary adhesions are more frequent sequelae than instability, and it is suggested that static splinting should not exceed 3 weeks. Extension contracture may also occur.

4. Dorsal dislocation of the MCP joint—MCP joint dislocations most often occur in a dorsal direction and most commonly involve the index finger, thumb, and little finger. Dorsal dislocation may be ***simple (reducible)*** or ***complex (irreducible).***

- Evaluation
  - (a) Simple dislocation—There is a notable deformity with marked MCP joint hyperextension. X-ray films demonstrate the proximal phalanx at 60° to 90° of hyperextension on the dorsum of the metacarpal head.
  - (b) Complex dislocation (Fig. 24-12)—Deformity is not as obvious, with the joint only slightly hyperextended. A common finding is a ***skin dimple*** (puckering) at the distal palmar crease. Radiographs demonstrate nearly parallel alignment of the proximal phalanx and the metacarpal. ***The presence of a sesamoid in a widened MCP joint indicates volar plate entrapment.***
- Treatment
  - (a) Simple dislocation—Gentle closed reduction should be performed by hyperextending the joint before pushing the proximal phalanx onto the metacarpal head. ***Straight longitudinal traction should be avoided because it may convert a simple to a complex dislocation.***
  - (b) Complex dislocation—A single attempt at closed reduction may be performed, but most complex dislocations require open reduction in the operating room. Open reduction can be achieved through either a dorsal or a volar approach and ***requires extraction of the interposed volar plate.*** The radial digital nerve may be tented over the index metacarpal head, or the ulnar digital nerve may be tented over the metacarpal head of the little finger, when performing the volar approach. The volar plate can be split longitudinally to assist reduction of the joint if needed. The dorsal approach eliminates the risk of damage to the digital nerves and allows treatment of any associated metacarpal head fracture. After reduction, the MCP joint is typically stable and allows early active range-of-motion exercises with buddy-taping.
  - (c) Complications—Complications can include digital nerve damage, stiffness, and arthritis (if associated with a metacarpal head fracture).

E. Carpometacarpal (CMC) Joint Injuries
  1. Dislocation (and fracture-dislocation) of the CMC joint—The CMC joints of the index, middle, and ring fingers are stable (fixed) joints that allow minimal gliding motion and are classified as *arthrodial diarthroses*. The CMC joint of the little finger is more mobile and is similar to the thumb

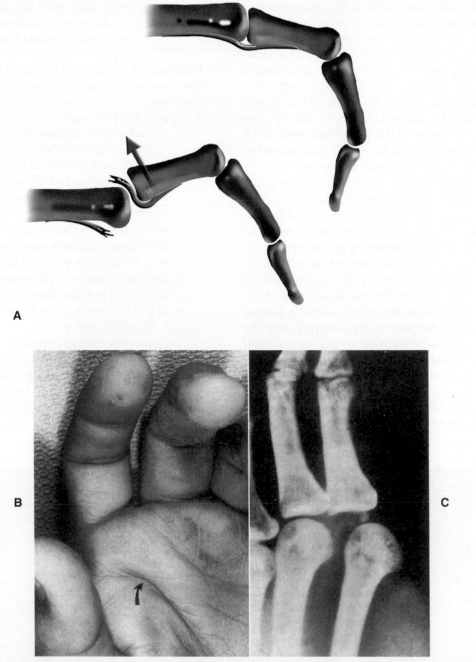

FIGURE 24-12 Complex dorsal dislocation of the MCP joint. **A.** Diagram demonstrating how the volar plate can become displaced dorsally, blocking reduction of the MCP joint dorsal dislocation. **B.** Clinical photograph demonstrating puckering (*arrow*) of the palmar skin. **C.** Radiograph showing entrapment of a sesamoid within the (widened) MCP joint. (**B** and **C** reprinted with permission from Green DP, Strickland JW. In: DeLee JC, Drez D Jr, eds. *Orthopaedic Sports Medicine: Principles and Practice*. Philadelphia, PA: WB Saunders; 1994.)

CMC joint. As a saddle joint, the CMC joint of the little finger allows motion not only in a gliding but also in rotation to allow its opposability to the thumb. The CMC joints are stabilized by very strong intermetacarpal and CMC ligaments that support the dorsal and volar aspects of the joint. Fracture-dislocation of the CMC joint occurs with severe force. Dislocation is generally in the dorsal direction (unless the dislocation results from a direct blow from the dorsal direction, causing a volar CMC dislocation). Volar dislocations are much rarer than dorsal dislocations but are relatively more common in the CMC joint of the little finger because of its increased mobility.

- Evaluation—Because of the overlap of the adjacent bone structures, X-ray interpretation of the CMC joint is often difficult, and various views are required for accurate interpretation. Radiographs demonstrate a subluxated or dislocated CMC joint (with or without a fracture fragment involving the CMC joint surface) (Fig. 24-13). Computed tomography (CT) may be indicated for more difficult diagnostic problems. *A 30° pronated view of the hand may be necessary for assessing the congruency of the joint surfaces*.
- Treatment—Closed reduction is easily obtained with longitudinal traction but cannot be maintained in a cast alone. *Percutaneous transarticular K-wire fixation, in addition to cast immobilization, is necessary.* Redislocation or incomplete reduction of the CMC joint often occurs in index- and little-finger CMC fracture-dislocations as a result of the pull of the *extensor carpi radialis longus tendon to the index metacarpal and the extensor carpi ulnaris to the metacarpal of the little finger*. Closed reduction and cast immobilization often result in recurrence of the CMC dislocation because of the instability and significant swelling that occur with these injuries.

- Complications—Complications include recurrent dislocation, pain, weakness, and arthritis. Posttraumatic arthritis of the CMC articulation can be effectively treated with arthrodesis.

II. Fractures of the Hand—Phalangeal and metacarpal fractures are common, comprising nearly 10% of all fractures.
  A. Phalangeal Fractures
    1. Classification—Extra-articular phalangeal fractures are described by location, including base, shaft, or neck for the middle and proximal phalanges, as well as tuft fracture for the distal phalanx. These injuries may be further described as displaced or nondisplaced, as open or closed, as associated with a rotational or angular deformity; they may have associated injuries to the skin, nerve, digital artery, or tendons.
    2. Deforming forces—The bony anatomy is an intercalated osseous chain. Fracture of a phalanx in this chain results in a predictable deformity.
      - Middle phalanx
        (a) *Fracture proximal to flexor digitorum superficialis (FDS) insertion causes the middle phalanx to angulate dorsally*.
        (b) *Fracture distal to the FDS insertion causes the middle phalanx to angulate volarly*.

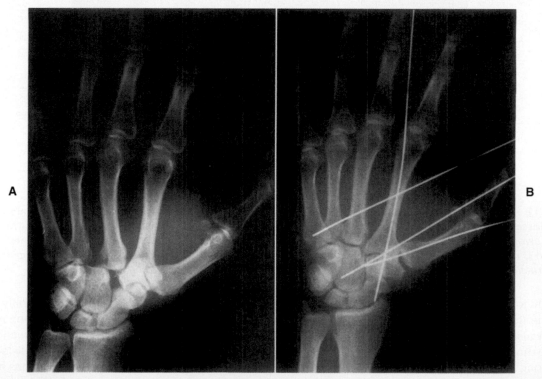

FIGURE 24-13 **A.** Injury film showing dislocation of the CMC joint of the index and long fingers. **B.** Postoperative film after reduction of the dislocations and stabilization with Kirschner wires.

- Proximal phalanx—***Interosseous attachments to the proximal phalanx flex the proximal fragment, whereas the central slip extends the distal portion, resulting in volar angulation at the fracture***.
3. Evaluation—Swelling, pain, limited motion, or deformity should suggest fracture and merit radiographic evaluation. Some 30% of phalangeal fractures may be open. Associated flexor tendon or digital nerve injuries should be identified. Nonunion and infection rates are higher with open fractures. A ***splay lateral X-ray study of the digits with various amounts of flexion is required to prevent overlap of the phalanges during radiographic examination.***
4. Treatment
   - General principles—Accurate fracture reduction is recommended, followed by remobilization of the injured finger as early as allowed by fracture stability. Uninvolved fingers should be mobilized early to prevent stiffness. ***The PIP joint is the most important joint for motion and function of the digit.***
   - Stable fractures—Stable phalangeal fractures with good radiographic alignment can be treated with buddy-tape, a splint, or a cast. X-ray studies should be repeated in 7 to 10 days.
   - Displaced fractures—Displaced fractures that can be reduced and converted to a stable position can be treated with closed management, including a cast or splint, followed by protected range-of-motion exercises. Percutaneous pinning may be necessary to prevent fracture displacement.
   - Unstable fractures—Fractures that cannot be reduced or have persistent instability despite attempted closed reduction require ORIF with skeletal fixation. Treatment options include K-wire fixation, intraosseous wiring, interfragmentary screws, and plate and screw fixation.
   - Segmental bone loss—Segmental bone loss is frequently associated with a severe soft-tissue injury. Primary treatment should include soft-tissue management with thorough irrigation and debridement, followed by open packing. These fractures are typically highly comminuted and may require external fixation to maintain length until definitive bony reconstruction can be performed with bone graft. Delayed flap coverage may be required as well.
5. Complications
   - Loss of motion—***Close adherence of the flexor and extensor tendons over the phalanges may lead to tendon adhesions to the bone***. Tenolysis may be required to improve motion after fracture healing. PIP flexion contracture is also common with phalangeal fractures. If not improved with therapy, joint release may be required.
   - Malunion—A closing wedge osteotomy of the phalanx may be needed to correct an angular deformity. Rotational deformity with overlap of the digits may require a transverse derotational osteotomy of the phalanx.
   - Infection
   - Nonunion
   - Symptomatic hardware—Exposed K-wires may be complicated by superficial pin-tract infection. ***Plate and screw fixation for a phalangeal fracture is often complicated by symptomatic hardware, requiring delayed removal after fracture healing, with tenolysis of the extensor mechanism***.

B. Metacarpal Fractures—Metacarpal fractures account for 36% of all fractures of the hand.
   1. Classification—Metacarpal fractures are described by location, including metacarpal head fractures, metacarpal neck fractures, metacarpal shaft fractures, and metacarpal base fractures. These fractures are typically further described as nondisplaced or displaced, as closed or open, or as associated with angulation, rotation, or a shortening deformity.
   2. Evaluation—X-ray studies define fracture alignment. The ***Brewerton X-ray view*** is particularly useful for evaluating metacarpal head fractures.
   3. Treatment
      - Metacarpal head fractures—Nondisplaced metacarpal head fractures can be treated with cast protection or buddy-taping. Displaced oblique fractures require ORIF with K-wires or small screws. Small osteochondral fractures may be excised. ***Avascular necrosis of the metacarpal head may occur after even a nondisplaced transverse fracture***.
      - Metacarpal neck fractures (Fig. 24-14)—Metacarpal neck fractures are also referred to as *boxer*, *fighter*, or *frustration fractures*. A direct blow on the metacarpal head of the little or ring finger may result in fracture with angulation at the metacarpal neck. ***If angulated less than 15°***, the fracture can be treated in an ulnar gutter splint for 2 weeks, followed by range-of-motion exercises. ***If angulated 15° to 40°***, the fracture should be reduced, followed by ulnar gutter splint treatment. ***If angulated more than 40° with unacceptable clinical deformity***, closed reduction

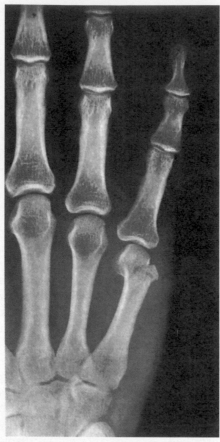

FIGURE 24-14 Boxer's fracture of the metacarpal neck of the little finger. (Reprinted with permission from Gartland JJ. *Fundamentals of Orthopaedics*. 4th ed. Philadelphia, PA: WB Saunders; 1987.)

and percutaneous pinning of the fracture is recommended. A total of 40° of dorsal angulation for a fracture of the metacarpal neck of the little finger can be accepted, with good resulting function, because of the compensatory motion at this metacarpal's CMC joint. *Residual angulation greater than 15° for metacarpal neck fractures of the index and long fingers is unacceptable because of the lack of compensatory CMC motion for these metacarpals.*

- Metacarpal shaft fractures—Transverse metacarpal shaft fractures are often caused by a direct blow, resulting in dorsal angulation. These fractures are often amenable to closed reduction, followed by cast treatment. *Spiral and long oblique fractures of the metacarpal shaft are inherently unstable with shortening and rotation. Rotational deformity manifests as overlap of the digits when making a fist* (Fig. 24-15). ORIF is recommended for metacarpal shaft fractures with *(a) malrotation, (b) dorsal angulation greater than 10° for the index and long finger metacarpals, (c) dorsal angulation greater than 20° for the ring and little finger metacarpals, and (d) any shortening greater than 3 mm.* Multiple displaced metacarpal shaft fractures are an indication for internal fixation as well. Treatment options

FIGURE 24-15 Assessment for rotational deformity of the fingers. **A.** Normally, the four flexed fingers converge at the scaphoid tubercle, and the nails are aligned. **B.** Rotational malalignment cannot be appreciated with the fingers extended. **C.** Same patient as in **(B)** with the fingers flexed. Note malrotation of the ring finger. (**B** and **C** reprinted with permission from Culver JE, Anderson TE. *Clin Sports Med.* 1992;11:101–128.)

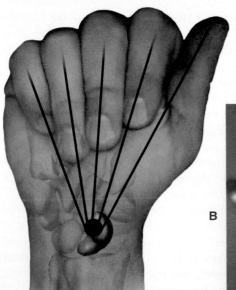

A

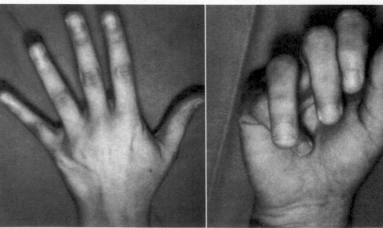

B

C

may include K-wires, interosseous wiring, interfragmentary screws, and screws and plates. ***Long oblique and spiral fractures are well suited to interfragmentary screw fixation. Short oblique and transverse fractures require a neutralization plate and screw fixation*** (Fig. 24-16). ***Open metacarpal fractures require treatment of the associated soft-tissue injuries and may require external fixation if highly comminuted or associated with segmental bone loss*** (Fig. 24-17).

- Metacarpal base fractures—Stable metacarpal base fractures can be treated with a cast alone. Displaced metacarpal base fractures require closed reduction and percutaneous pinning.

4. Complications
- Malunion—Dorsal angulation of a metacarpal shaft fracture may disturb the intrinsic or extrinsic tendon balance. Dorsal closing wedge osteotomy or volar opening wedge osteotomy may be necessary to correct this angular deformity. Derotational osteotomy through the base of the metacarpal corrects a rotational deformity. Other complications include nonunion, MCP joint contractures, intrinsic muscle contractures, and refracture.

C. Fractures at the Base of the Thumb Metacarpal—Fractures at the base of the thumb metacarpal can impair effective lateral key pinch and opposition of the thumb to the other digits.
1. Classification (Fig. 24-18)
   - Bennett's fracture—dislocation
   - Rolando's Y or T condylar fracture
   - Epibasal fracture
   - Comminuted fracture
2. Evaluation
   - Clinical examination—There is swelling and pain at the base of the thumb, often with bruising in the thenar region.
   - Radiographic evaluation—AP, lateral, and oblique views are obtained. Oblique views are necessary to assess for congruency of the CMC joint.
3. Treatment
   - Nondisplaced fractures—Nondisplaced well-aligned fractures can be treated with a cast for 4 weeks, followed by a removable splint.
   - Displaced fractures—Surgery is required for displaced fractures with an incongruent or a subluxed CMC joint. Only 1 to 3 mm of CMC joint incongruity can be accepted. A displaced Bennett's fracture-dislocation may be treated with longitudinal traction and percutaneous K-wire fixation if the volar ulnar fragment is small. A large bone

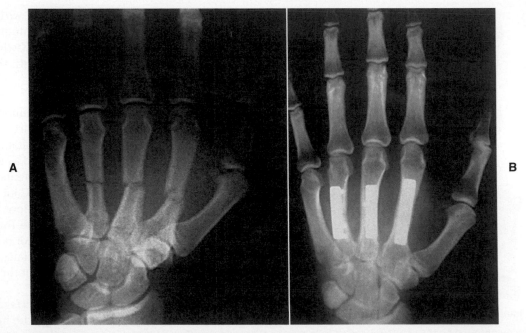

FIGURE 24-16   **A.** Injury film showing transverse/short oblique fractures of the index, long, and ring finger metacarpal shafts. **B.** Postoperative film after stabilization with plate and screw fixation. (Reprinted with permission from Jupiter J, Silver MA. In: Chapman M, ed. *Operative Orthopaedics*. Philadelphia, PA: J.B. Lippincott Company; 1988.)

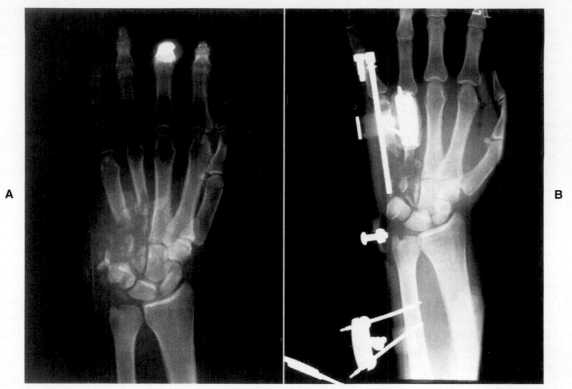

FIGURE 24-17 **A.** Injury film showing a comminuted fracture of the metacarpals of the ring and little fingers (also with involvement of the carpus) as the result of a handgun injury. **B.** Postoperative film showing stabilization with an external fixator.

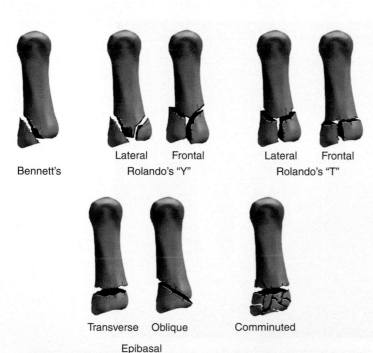

Bennett's   Lateral   Frontal   Lateral   Frontal
              Rolando's "Y"   Rolando's "T"

Transverse   Oblique   Comminuted
       Epibasal

FIGURE 24-18 Classification of fractures at the base of the thumb metacarpal.

fragment may require ORIF with K-wires or small lag screws. A comminuted fracture may require transarticular K-wires or external fixation to maintain length through indirect reduction.

4. Complications—Complications include malunion, nonunion, and posttraumatic arthritis. Accurate reduction of the articular surface minimizes posttraumatic arthritis. Up to 3 mm of incongruity may be accepted as long as a stable union of the fracture fragments is achieved without subluxation of the CMC joint.

D. Physeal Fractures in Children—More than 34% of hand fractures in children involve the epiphyseal growth plate. Common locations for such fractures are the base of the proximal phalanx, the base of the distal phalanx, and the base of the index, long, and ring finger metacarpals.

1. Classification—The *Salter-Harris* **classification** is used for physeal injuries of the hand.

   • Type I injuries are usually seen in early childhood and result from a shear injury. The prognosis is good.

- Type II injuries are usually seen after age 10, again as a result of a shear or angular force. The prognosis is also good.
- Type III injuries are also seen after age 10, although with intraarticular extension. This injury requires accurate reduction of the joint surface to avoid posttraumatic arthritis.
- Type IV injuries also have intraarticular extension but with associated metaphyseal displacement as well. Anatomic reduction of the fracture must be achieved. ***The prognosis is poor without anatomic alignment.***
- Type V injuries may occur at any age but are extremely rare in the hand. These fractures are thought to be the result of a severe axial load to the growth plate. ***The prognosis is poor and is not improved with surgery.***

2. Complications—Complications include malunion, traumatic arthritis, residual deformity, and growth plate arrest. Although growth disturbance may occur in a nondisplaced Salter-Harris Type II fracture, the worse prognosis is clearly found in Salter-Harris Types IV and V fractures.

III. Soft-Tissue Injuries of the Hand
  A. Flexor Tendon Injuries
    1. Anatomy—***Tendons are composed primarily of Type I collagen fibers.*** Most blood vessels to the flexor tendons are located in the epitenon, which is continuous with the endotenon surrounding individual bundles of collagen within the tendon. The FDS splits around the flexor digitorum profundus (FDP) to insert onto the middle phalanx. The FDP tendon inserts onto the distal phalanx. Excursion of the FDS tendon at the mid palm is 26 mm and over the proximal phalanx is 16 mm with composite flexion. FDP excursion is 23 mm at the mid-palm, 17 mm over the proximal phalanx, and 5 mm over the middle phalanx with composite flexion. In the distal palm and digits, the flexor tendons are enclosed within a synovial sheath. The ***visceral synovial layer*** covers the flexor tendons, and a ***parietal layer*** is continuous with the annular and cruciate pulleys. A fibroosseous tunnel extends from the MCP joint to the distal phalanx to ensure efficient digital flexion. The ***annular pulleys*** provide mechanical stability, and the cruciate pulleys permit flexibility at the joints (Fig. 24-19). ***It is imperative to preserve the A2 pulley over the proximal phalanx and the A4 pulley over the middle phalanx to prevent a bowstringing deformity*** (Fig. 24-20). The A1, A3,

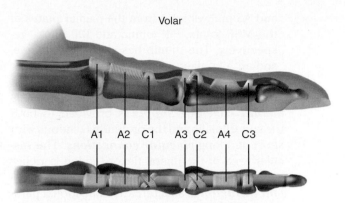

Volar

A1 A2 C1 A3 C2 A4 C3

FIGURE 24-19 Flexor tendon pulley system—there are five annular (A1, A2, A3, A4, A5) and three cruciate (C1, C2, C3) pulleys. Note that A2 and A4 are the most important pulleys to preserve. The odd-numbered annular pulleys overlie joints: A1 (first annular pulley) overlies the MCP joint, A3 (third annular pulley) overlies the PIP joint, A5 (fifth annular pulley) overlies the DIP joint (not shown). The even-numbered annular pulleys and the cruciate pulleys overlie the phalanges, A2 (second annular pulley) overlies the proximal phalanx, A4 (fourth annular pulley) overlies the middle phalanx, C1 (first cruciate pulley) is distal to A2 on the proximal phalanx, C2 and C3 (second and third cruciate pulleys) are proximal (C2) and distal (C3) to the A4 pulley on the middle phalanx.

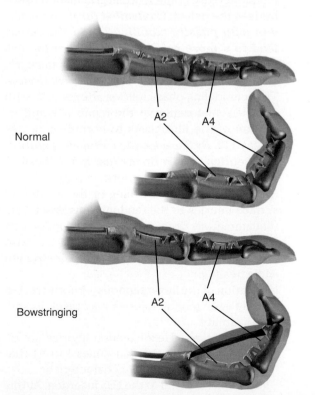

Normal

A2 A4

Bowstringing

A2 A4

FIGURE 24-20 Bowstringing of the flexor tendons may result from disruption of the A2 and A4 pulleys.

and A5 pulleys arise from the palmar plates of the MCP joints, PIP joints, and DIP joints, respectively. The thumb has an A1, an oblique, and an A2 pulley.

2. Nutrition—Tendon nutrition is via both a direct vascular supply and synovial diffusion. A **segmental vascular supply** is provided to both the superficialis and the profundus tendons with short and long **vincular connections**. The vascular area of the digital flexor tendon is richer on the dorsal aspect than the volar aspect. **Synovial diffusion** is an alternative nutritional pathway for flexor tendons and may function more rapidly and completely than vascular perfusion. Nutrients of the synovial fluid are pumped into the tendon by **imbibition** through conduits in the tendon surface, enhanced by tendon gliding.

3. Flexor tendon healing—Flexor tendons have both an intrinsic and an extrinsic ability to heal. The healing process involves an **inflammatory phase**, a **fibroblastic (or collagen-producing) phase**, and a **remodeling phase**. The inflammatory phase predominates during the first 3 to 5 days. During this phase, the strength of the repair is almost entirely that imparted by the suture itself. The fibroblastic, or collagen-producing, phase begins on day 5 and extends to day 21. During this phase, the strength of the repair increases rapidly while granulation tissue bridges the defect. **Controlled forces on a tendon with passive mobilization in this phase lead to a more rapid realignment of the collagen fibers with greater tensile strength, fewer adhesions, and improved excursion**. The remodeling phase follows after day 21, with complete maturation at the repair site and reversion of the fibroblasts to normal tenocytes by day 112. **By 8 weeks, the collagen is mature and realigned in a linear fashion**. Adhesions around the flexor tendon form in proportion to the extent of tissue crushing or the number of surface injuries to the tendon. Nonsteroidal antiinflammatory drugs (ibuprofen and indomethacin) decrease adhesion formation but also create a significant reduction in repair strength while healing.

4. Laceration of the flexor tendons—Poorly treated digital flexor tendon injuries may result in serious disability.
   • Classification—Flexor tendon injuries are divided into zones (Verdan Zones I to V) that have a specific anatomic characteristic.
      (a) Zone I is distal to the FDS insertion. At this level, only the profundus flexor tendon is contained within the fibroosseous tunnel.
      (b) Zone II is within the fibroosseous tunnel. Both the FDP and the FDS tendons are contained within one tight fibroosseous tunnel. **This area is the most difficult in which to obtain a good result; hence it was referred to as "no man's land" by Dr. Sterling Bunnell.**
      (c) Zone III is the palm. At this level, although both tendons may be injured, direct repair has a good prognosis because of the absence of fibroosseous pulleys.
      (d) Zone IV includes the carpal tunnel. Flexor tendon injuries are frequently protected by the carpal bones but are often complicated by injury to the median or ulnar nerve.
      (e) Zone V includes the wrist and forearm. Proximal to the carpal ligament, the flexor tendons are less constrained and are surrounded by loose areolar tissue, so repairs in this zone also have a more favorable prognosis. Associated injuries to major peripheral nerves and vessels are also common in this zone.
   • Examination—The resulting posture of the digits should be observed. The tenodesis effect of intact tendons can be demonstrated with wrist flexion and extension. Isolated testing of the FDS and FDP tendon with gentle blocking should be performed (Fig. 24-21). Pain on resisted motion may suggest partial laceration.
   • Treatment
      (a) Surgery—**Primary surgical repair is indicated for nearly all flexor tendon lacerations, even when in Zone II**.
   • Timing—Primary or delayed primary repair may be performed. Repair requires a tidy wound. Appropriate soft-tissue coverage should be available at the repair site. The repair is performed as soon after the injury as feasible, although it may be delayed as long as 2 or 3 weeks without compromising the ultimate result. Associated fractures are not a contraindication to flexor tendon repair. Tetanus prophylaxis must be considered for all penetrating injuries of the hand; see Chapter 1 for further details regarding tetanus prophylaxis.
   • Technique—Wound-extending incisions are necessary, since the tendon retracts from the injury site. The muscle pulls the proximal end, whereas extension of the digit pulls the distal end. Bruner zig-zag or midlateral incisions are used. Atraumatic technique during

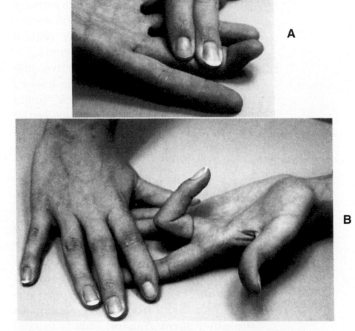

<u>FIGURE 24-21</u>   Testing finger flexors. **A.** The FDP can be tested by holding the PIP joint in extension and testing for DIP joint flexion. In this example, the FDP is intact. **B.** The FDS can be tested by holding the adjacent digits in extension and testing for PIP joint flexion of the affected digit. In this example, the FDS in intact. (Reprinted with permission from Rettig AC. *Clin Sports Med.* 1992;11:77–99.)

flexor tendon repair is imperative, since damage to the epitenon stimulates adhesions. The flexor tendon sheath is preserved, and it is imperative to maintain the A2 and A4 pulleys for composite flexion without a bowstringing deformity. Suture technique uses a 3–0 or 4–0 nonabsorbable synthetic suture as a core suture to prevent gapping during the early postoperative period. A circumferential suture is then added to the core suture to smooth the tendon surface. Sheath repair may also improve tendon gliding and the initial synovial tendon nutrition, although this remains controversial at this time.

- Repair by zone
  - (a) Zone I—The FDP tendon is advanced for direct repair. If less than 1.0 cm of tendon is still attached to the distal phalanx, the tendon is reinserted to the bone with a pullout button. The tendon should not be advanced more than1.0 cm.
  - (b) Zone II—Simultaneous repair of both the FDS and the FDP tendons is attempted

to retain independent finger motion and stronger flexor power. Repair of the superficialis prevents the occasional hyperextension deformity at the DIP joint and provides a smooth gliding bed for the FDP.

- (c) Zone III—Multiple flexor tendons may be injured and may be complicated by a vascular injury to the superficial palmar arch or an injury to the common palmar digital nerves. In selected cases with a heavily contaminated wound or a crush injury, repair of only the FDP tendon may be preferable to repair of both tendons.
- (d) Zone IV—Although uncommon, stab wounds to this zone may result in flexor tendon and median nerve injury. Surgical exploration may be necessary to diagnose partial laceration of the flexor tendons.
- (d) Zone V—Slash injuries to this level commonly involve multiple flexor tendons, as well as the median and ulnar nerves and the radial or ulnar arteries; an injury to this zone is also known as the spaghetti wrist.
- (e) Thumb—The thumb has only one extrinsic flexor tendon. Surgical repair is somewhat simpler, except for a Zone III repair, where the flexor pollicis longus (FPL) tendon is difficult to access because of the thenar musculature. This often requires a separate incision at the carpal tunnel to safely retrieve the retracted flexor tendon.
- Prognostic factors—A clean laceration has a better prognosis than a crush injury. Associated injuries such as fracture or skin loss worsen the prognosis. Zone II injuries carry the worst prognosis. Younger patients generally have a better prognosis than have older patients, although children present special management problems because of the small size of the injured structures and the patient's ability to cooperate.
- Flexor tendon rehabilitation protocol—Postoperative management includes a dorsal hood splint and controlled mobilization for 6 weeks. Complete immobilization may be appropriate for the young or uncooperative patient. The wrist is held in 35° of flexion and the MCP joint in 45° of flexion, with the interphalangeal joints extended. Controlled mobilization may limit the formation of restricting adhesions. Early mobilization programs include passive motion (***Duran's program***)

or a combined gentle passive/active tendon excursion with rubber bands *(Kleinert's program)*. This program is usually initiated 3 to 5 days after surgical repair. Active flexion and extension exercises may begin 4 to 6 weeks after repair. Isolated blocking exercises or electric stimulation of the flexors is delayed for 6 weeks. *For smaller children, rehabilitation of flexor tendon repairs should begin with cast immobilization for 4 weeks*.

- Results—In spite of ongoing improvement in flexor tendon repair, the restoration of normal function is difficult to achieve. Good results often follow surgical repair in Zones I, III, IV, and V. Functional results are much less certain in Zone II. Results are often reported in terms of *total active motion (TAM)*, which sums total active flexion for the MCP, PIP, and DIP joints minus the total extension deficit in degrees for these same three joints.

- Partial lacerations—Unrecognized partial lacerations may lead to mechanical triggering or rupture. *Tendon lacerations involving less than 25% of the cross-sectional area can be treated with resection of any oblique flap. Lacerations involving up to 50% of the cross-sectional area can be treated with a running suture around the periphery. Lacerations greater than 50% of the cross-sectional area should be repaired with a core suture and a running circumferential stitch*.

- Secondary repair—Delayed primary repair may no longer be possible later than 4 weeks after injury. Secondary repair may require flexor tendon grafting or staged tendon reconstruction with a Silastic Hunter rod, including possible pulley reconstruction. Patients with multiple surgical failures may be poor candidates for staged reconstruction and may require PIP joint arthrodesis or even amputation.

- Complications
  (a) Adhesions—Adhesion may limit active flexion despite normal passive range of motion. Tenolysis of the flexor tendons may improve active motion. *Tenolysis should rarely be performed before 3 months from the injury, and requires a motivated patient*. Local anesthesia is recommended when possible to evaluate gains in motion as the procedure progresses. If general anesthesia is used, an additional proximal incision may be required for traction/excursion check of the tendon. Immediate active range of motion should begin within 24 hours after tenolysis.

  (b) Tendon rupture—*Tendon rupture after primary repair should undergo immediate re-repair when identified*. The results may still approach those of a primary repair. Rupture of a flexor tendon during or after tenolysis surgery may require staged reconstruction with free grafts.

  (c) Quadriga effect—Decreased active motion in an uninjured digit may result when the digit has a common muscle origin to an adjacent injured digit, such as the FDP tendons to the fingers. Verdan explains this effect with the analogy of a Roman chariot in which the reins of all four horses are controlled in unison. The four FDP tendons have a common muscle belly, and therefore DIP flexion of any finger normally results in DIP flexion of the other three fingers. A *limitation of DIP flexion in any finger (such as from excessive shortening of the FDP tendon following repair of amputation) results in a limitation of DIP flexion in the other three fingers*. This is in contrast to the FDS, which maintains independent muscle function to each finger.

5. FDP rupture
  - Overview—Avulsions of the FDP occur most frequently in young adult men playing football and rugby. The ring finger is affected in most cases. The rupture occurs when the finger is forcefully extended during maximal contraction of the profundus muscle. The pathognomonic feature of this diagnosis is the *inability to actively flex the DIP joint of the injured finger*.

  - Classification—Avulsions of the FDP insertion have been classified by *Leddy and Packer*.
    (a) Type I—The FDP tendon retracts all the way into the *palm* and is held there by the lumbrical origin. Both vincula have ruptured, and therefore a substantial portion of the blood supply to the profundus tendon is lost.
    (b) Type II—The FDP tendon retracts to the level of the *PIP joint*, leaving the long vinculum to the FDP tendon intact, preserving more of the blood supply and retaining more of the length. Occasionally, a small bony flake can be seen at the level of the PIP joint on a lateral radiograph.
    (c) Type III—The FDP tendon ruptures with a large bone fragment, holding the FDP tendon out to length distal to the *A4 pulley*. The large fragment may be associated

with a comminuted intraarticular fracture of the DIP joint.

- Treatment—Surgical repair of the FDP tendon is recommended as soon as the diagnosis is made, preferably less than 2 weeks from injury.

    (a) Type I—Surgical repair should be undertaken within 7 to 10 days, advancing the FDP tendon to the distal phalanx with a pullout button. If treatment is delayed, the tendon becomes *contracted and necrotic as a result of loss of its nutritional supply, and it can no longer be advanced to the distal phalanx*.

    (b) Type II—Surgical repair of the FDP tendon to the distal phalanx is recommended. In contrast to Type I injuries, these injuries *can be reinserted at a later date, possibly 4 weeks or longer, because of the better blood supply* and preservation of length of the tendon.

    (c) Type III—*ORIF of the bone fragment is necessary to restore a congruent DIP joint and to reinsert the flexor tendon*. In rare instances, the profundus tendon may also be ruptured from the large bone fragment, and will need to be advanced as with a Type I or II injury (Fig. 24-22).

    (d) Neglected injury—Cases seen too late for reinsertion may best be left alone or may require excision of the retracted profundus tendon, with tenodesis or arthrodesis of the DIP joint if unstable.

- Complications—Misdiagnosis of this injury as a sprained or jammed finger delays treatment and substantially jeopardizes the result. Despite repair, flexor tendon adhesions may still limit composite flexion. A 10° to 15° loss of extension at the DIP joint is common after readvancement of the profundus tendon. Rehabilitation must be carefully supervised to avoid creating a PIP flexion contracture, especially after delayed advancement for a ruptured tendon.

B. Extensor Tendon Injuries

1. Anatomy (Fig. 24-23)—Extension of the fingers is a complex and more intricate motion than finger flexion, incorporating both (a) *extrinsic extensor tendons* and (b) *intrinsic muscles* of the hand. The extensor tendon is stabilized over the MCP joint by the *sagittal bands*, which insert on the proximal phalanx and volar plate of the MCP joint. The *extensor digitorum communis* tendon divides into three slips distal to the MCP joint, with the *central slip* extending onto the middle phalanx to actively extend the PIP joint. The two lateral slips diverge to meet the interossei and lumbrical bands and then form the *lateral bands* to *the terminal slip (terminal extensor tendon)*, which inserts on the distal phalanx for DIP joint extension. *Over the proximal phalanx, the common extensor tendon is particularly prone to adherence after fracture or laceration. The lateral bands are similarly vulnerable to adherence over the middle phalanx after fracture or laceration*. The interosseous muscles include *four dorsal interossei* that abduct the index, middle, and ring fingers, as well **as three volar interossei** that adduct the index, ring, and little finger. *All interossei pass volar to the axis of the MCP joint, providing effective MCP joint flexion and interphalangeal joint extension*. All interossei are innervated by the deep branch of the ulnar nerve. Retinacular ligaments also assist digital function. The *transverse retinacular ligament* proceeds from the flexor tendon sheath to the lateral edges of the conjoint

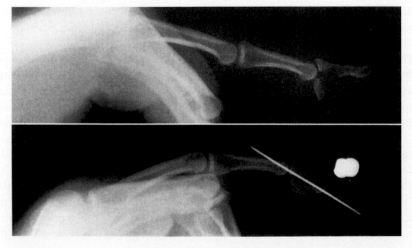

A

B

FIGURE 24-22 A. Injury film slowing an avulsion fracture (Leddy and Packer Type III injury) from an FDP avulsion. **B.** Postoperative film showing reduction and stabilization of the bony fragment with a Kirschner wire and a pullout wire.

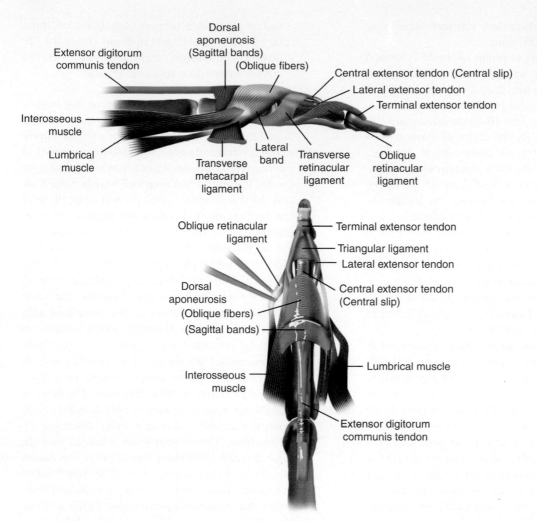

FIGURE 24-23 Extensor apparatus.

lateral band, serving to prevent excessive dorsal shift of the lateral bands. The ***oblique retinacular ligament*** runs from the volar crest of the proximal phalanx to the lateral terminal extensor tendon, linking the motion of the PIP and DIP joints. The ***triangular ligament*** holds the lateral bands over the middle phalanx, preventing excessive volar shift of the lateral bands. ***Grayson's ligament*** is volar to the neurovascular bundle, holding it in place and preventing bowstringing of the digital artery and nerve when the fingers flex, and ***Cleland's ligament*** is dorsal to the neurovascular bundle.

2. Extensor tendon lacerations—Management of lacerations to the extensor mechanism requires the same amount of skill and knowledge as flexor tendon injuries.
   - Classification—Extensor tendon lacerations have been classified according to injury Zones I to IX.
     (a) Zone I is the DIP joint.
     (b) Zone II is the middle phalanx.
     (c) Zone III is the PIP joint.
     (d) Zone IV is the proximal phalanx.
     (e) Zone V is the MCP joint.
     (f) Zone VI is the metacarpal.
     (g) Zone VII is the dorsal wrist retinaculum.
     (h) Zone VIII is the distal forearm.
     (i) Zone IX is the mid and proximal forearm.
   - Diagnosis and examination—Limited active extension after traumatic laceration should suggest partial or complete extensor tendon injury.
   - Treatment
     (a) Zone I—Laceration of the terminal slip at the DIP joint results in a mallet deformity. Although passive extension is present, active extension is lost. Hyperextension of the PIP joint may be observed as a result of unopposed central slip tension and PIP volar plate laxity. Open tendon lacerations should be repaired with undyed suture and with internal K-wire fixation of the DIP joint in extension, followed by a supplemental splint. Limited motion may begin at 6 weeks, although a

night splint should still be used for perhaps another 2 months. Deep abrasions with loss of skin, subcutaneous tissue, or tendon substance may require a tendon graft or arthrodesis of the DIP joint. (Closed tendon avulsion of the terminal slip is discussed in the next section.)

(b) Zone II—Injuries to the extensor mechanism over the middle phalanx usually result from laceration rather than avulsion. Partial laceration of the tendon is common because of the wide expanse and curved shape of the tendon over the middle phalanx. Partial lacerations (<50% of the tendon) can be treated with skin wound care, followed by gentle active motion in 7 to 10 days. Complete lacerations require suture repair and static splinting in full extension for 6 weeks, possibly with K-wire fixation of the DIP joint in extension.

(c) Zone III—Disruption of the central slip of the extensor tendon at the PIP joint results in volar migration of the lateral bands and a *boutonnière deformity* (see Fig. 24-10). Compensatory hyperextension may occur at the DIP joint. Open tendon lacerations should be repaired with suture, with internal fixation of the PIP joint with a K-wire in extension but not hyperextension, and with supplementary splinting for up to 6 weeks. The DIP joint is left free for flexion to maintain excursion of the lateral bands. After K-wire removal, continued splinting is advised, and range of motion begins. Techniques to augment the central slip repair with portions of the lateral band have been described. (Closed tendon avulsion of the central slip is discussed in the next section.)

(d) Zone IV—These extensor tendon lacerations are similar to those in Zone II in that they are usually partial lacerations as a result of the tendon width and underlying curvature of the osseous phalanx. Lacerations of an isolated lateral band can be repaired, followed by immediate protected motion. Complete lacerations require direct repair, with stabilization of the PIP joint in the extended position for 6 weeks, either with a static splint or with a K-wire. Dynamic traction may be used in some patients.

(e) Zone V—Lacerations over the MCP joint require open repair of the extensor mechanism and hood, followed by dynamic splinting. The sagittal bands must be repaired to the extensor tendon, or the tendon may sublux from the dorsum of the joint, and the finger will still exhibit loss of active extension. Injuries of the extensor mechanism at the **MCP joint may often be secondary to a human bite wound**. A high index of suspicion should be present when examining lacerations in this area. Human bite wounds are at high risk for wound infection, septic arthritis, and laceration of the extensor tendon. This wound must be irrigated and debrided, the extensor tendon repaired, and the patient given appropriate antibiotics. If heavily contaminated, the tendon laceration may have to be repaired secondarily 5 to 7 days later. Dynamic splinting is particularly effective in managing lacerations at the MCP joint level.

(f) Zone VI—Extensor tendon lacerations of the dorsal aspect of the hand have a better prognosis than finger lacerations. Tendons in Zone VI are located in the subcutaneous tissues without close relationship to the metacarpal bones, have a sufficient cross-sectional diameter to accept buried core-type sutures, and are effectively rehabilitated with dynamic splinting because of greater tendon excursion. Dynamic splinting may begin 3 to 5 days after repair.

(g) Zone VII—Injures to the extensor mechanism at the wrist level are associated with injuries to the extensor retinaculum. Limited excision of portions of the retinaculum may be needed to facilitate tendon exposure and prevent mechanical triggering or adhesions after repair. Preserving a portion of the retinaculum prevents bowstringing in the mobile wrist. Again, early dynamic splinting has demonstrated excellent results.

(h) Zone VIII—Repair of extensor tendon lacerations over the distal forearm may require approximation of the distal tendon to the proximal muscle belly. A fibrous tissue raphe in the muscle belly should be repaired with multiple sutures and without strangulation of the muscle. Postoperative management may require static immobilization of the wrist in 45° of extension for 4 to 5 weeks if a significant muscle belly repair has been required.

(i) Zone IX—Lacerations of the extensor tendon in the proximal forearm may be complicated by injury to the radial nerve. If the injury involves only the muscle belly, a careful repair of the muscle belly is performed; tendon weaving with the palmaris longus may be an effective technique for muscles with more than 50% of their substance lacerated. The radial nerve should be explored and repaired if injured. After surgery, the wrist is immobilized in 45° of extension, and the elbow is immobilized in 90° of flexion if the injured muscles originate above the lateral epicondyle. Immobilization is continued for 4 weeks, followed by protective range of motion for another 4 weeks.

3. Extensor tendon ruptures (closed injuries)
   - **Terminal slip rupture (mallet finger)** (see Fig. 24-5)—Closed injury or blunt trauma may avulse the extensor tendon from the distal phalanx, resulting in a mallet deformity. This injury may be referred to as a *mallet finger, baseball finger,* or *dropped finger*.
     (a) Evaluation—Extensor droop is noted at the DIP joint, although full passive extension is present. Hyperextension of the PIP joint may be observed, particularly in cases with PIP volar plate laxity. Microvascular anatomy of the distal digital extensor tendon reveals a deficient blood supply over the DIP joint, explaining vulnerability to rupture and poor results with open suture repair of the ruptured tendon or inappropriately applied splints.
     (b) Treatment—Closed tendon avulsion of the extensor tendon at the PIP joint is treated with **external splinting to maintain the DIP joint in the extended (not hyperextended) position for 8 weeks, followed by gradual splint removal over the next 4 weeks**. Excellent-to-good results are anticipated in 80% of cases when treatment is provided early. Fair or poor results follow delayed treatment or improper wearing of splints. Direct repair of tendon injuries without a bone fragment is not indicated. A buried transarticular K-wire may be used for 6 weeks in patients who cannot wear a splint, such as a dentist, surgeon, or professional athlete, although a splint may still need to be worn the majority of the time to protect the pin from breakage. Operative treatment for mallet fingers with fracture fragments involving

more than 30% of the joint surface is discussed earlier in this chapter under the section Joint Injuries of the Hand.
(c) Complications
   - Complications of splinting—Complications after splint treatment for a mallet finger may be as high as 40%, usually including transient skin problems such as dorsal maceration, skin irritation, or tape allergy. Other complications can include transverse nail grooves, pain while wearing the splint, or skin necrosis if the DIP joint is hyperextended. A residual extensor lag may result and may require longer full-time splinting.
   - Complications of surgery—*A greater than 50% complication rate has been noted in patients treated surgically for mallet finger*. Complications include permanent nail deformity, joint incongruities, infection, pin or pullout wire failure, posttraumatic arthritis, subluxation, and residual extensor lag. In one series, additional surgery was required in 7 out of 45 patients, including arthrodesis in 4 and amputation in 1.
   - Swan-neck deformity (see Fig. 24-8)—*A mallet finger deformity that coexists with PIP volar plate laxity allows the PIP joint to hyperextend, resulting in a swan-neck deformity*. Correcting the mallet finger deformity usually restores the correct balance to the central slip at the PIP joint and the terminal slip at the DIP joint. One technique for correcting this problem is a spiral oblique retinacular ligament reconstruction using the palmaris longus tendon. Alternatively, a Fowler extensor tendon central slip release may be considered to rebalance the extensor mechanism.
   - Neglected mallet deformity—Management of chronic mallet deformity seen late may include arthrodesis or secondary extensor tendon reconstruction. If a satisfactory joint is present without arthritis, *the extensor tendon can be advanced 2 to 3 mm, followed by stabilization of the DIP joint in the extended position with a K-wire for 6 weeks*. If significant degenerative arthritis is present, the only viable surgical option is arthrodesis.
- **Central slip rupture (boutonnière finger)** (see Fig. 24-10)

(a) Overview—Closed injury that ruptures the central slip at the PIP joint results in a boutonnière deformity as the lateral bands migrate in a volar direction. There is loss of extension of the PIP joint, with compensatory hyperextension at the DIP joint. An acute forceful flexion at the PIP joint may cause this injury. Volar dislocation of the PIP joint may also result in avulsion of the central slip.

(b) Evaluation—Initially, the PIP joint has swelling, with perhaps only a mild extensor lag. The boutonnière deformity may not be apparent until 10 to 21 days after injury. A 15° to 20° extensor loss at the PIP joint, or weak extension against resistance, should suggest rupture of the central slip.

(c) Treatment

- Closed acute injury—An acute central slip rupture that has not yet developed volar subluxation of the lateral bands can be treated with static splinting of the PIP joint in full extension for 6 weeks. Active and passive DIP joint flexion exercises are encouraged to centralize the lateral bands, prevent oblique retinacular ligament tightness, and advance the central slip. A variety of means are available to maintain extension of the PIP joint, including a static splint, a cast, or a transarticular Kirschner wire. If the central slip has been avulsed with a bone fragment over the PIP joint, open repair is indicated, with excision of the bone fragment or repair of the central slip to the middle phalanx; the PIP joint is transfixed with a K-wire for 2 to 6 weeks.

- Delayed treatment—Delayed treatment for an established boutonnière deformity begins with stretching and splinting. Any tendon procedure is best done after the joint has regained full passive extension. Stiffness that does not respond to splinting may require capsular contracture release, followed by repair or advancement of the central slip. Surgical treatment is considered only after failure of prolonged conservative treatment. Surgical options include central slip advancement to the middle phalanx (**Kilgore**), lateral band transfers (**Matev**), and extensor tenotomy over the middle phalanx (**Fowler**). Poor results are associated with a PIP contracture greater than 30° at the time of the

initial evaluation, failure to achieve full PIP extension before surgery, or a patient age greater than 45 years.

- *Traumatic Dislocation of the Extensor Tendon* (Rupture of the Sagittal Band)-*Rupture of the radial sagittal band at the MCP joint may result in subluxation or dislocation of the extensor tendon off the metacarpal head*. The long finger is most commonly involved.

  (a) Evaluation—The extensor tendon usually dislocates in an ulnar direction, associated with incomplete finger extension and ulnar deviation of the involved digit. With extension, the extensor tendon may realign once again over the dorsal metacarpal head, only to sublux again with attempted active flexion.

  (b) Treatment—*Acute tears are satisfactorily repaired by primary suture of the defect. If primary repair is not possible, then a distally based slip of the extensor tendon from the ulnar side may be passed to the radial collateral ligament to stabilize the extensor tendon*, as described by Carroll. Several case reports of successful closed treatment by cast immobilization with the MCP joint in extension for 4 weeks have been described. Conservative treatment is more likely to be successful with treatment instituted immediately after injury.

C. Nerve Injuries

1. Anatomy—Peripheral nerves are composed of motor, sensory, and sympathetic nerve fibers. Digital nerves contain primarily sensory and sympathetic fibers. Connective tissue supports the neural tissue. The *external epineurium* forms the outer covering of the peripheral nerve. The extension of this connective tissue into the nerve that separates the fascicular groups is called the *internal epineurium*. The *perineurium* is the connective tissue that wraps the fascicles, and the *endoneurium* is the fine connective tissue between nerve fibers. Segmental nutrient vessels supply longitudinally oriented nerves through the epineurium. An intrinsic longitudinal blood supply facilitates the safe elevation of a nerve from its tissue bed over a long distance.

2. Nerve regeneration—When the axon is severed, the distal nerve undergoes *Wallerian degeneration*. Schwann cells proliferate and phagocytize the axon and myelin debris in the distal nerve segment. This process clears the degraded myelin from the Schwann cell tube, providing a

favorable environment for regenerating axons. The cell body responds to injury by increasing in size, migrating the nucleus to the periphery of the cell, and producing materials required for neurotransmitter function and repair of the nerve. The production of growth-associated proteins is increased 100-fold. *Axonal sprouting* occurs at the site of injury up to 24 hours after laceration. Most sprouts are generated at the most distal intact *node of Ranvier.* Multiple collateral sprouts from each axon then advance distally as a regenerating unit, which then may enter separate and often unrelated Schwann cell tubes in the distal nerve stump. Once entered, the repair pathway follows the neural tube to the end organ. The growth cone at the tip of the regenerating axon samples the surrounding terrain and pulls the axon into its most suitable environment. The Schwann cell is critical to growth cone elongation. Several products contribute to growth cone elongation, including *laminin* in the Schwann cell membrane.

3. Classification—Several classification systems have been described. *Seddon's* classification includes neurapraxia, axonotmesis, and neurotmesis. *Sunderland's* classification includes first-, second-, third-, fourth-, and fifth-degree injury. *Mackinnon's* classification adds sixth-degree, or mixed, nerve injury.

   - *Neurapraxia,* or first-degree injury, represents a bruise or contusion to the nerve. The prognosis for recovery is excellent without surgery. *There is a local conduction block with no axonal disruption.* Treatment is observation, awaiting recovery over several days to 12 weeks.

   - *Axonotmesis* or second-degree injury—Axonal injury has occurred with Wallerian degeneration distally. However, the neural tube is still intact. Axonal sprouting occurs within the appropriate endoneural tube. Excellent recovery is anticipated without surgery; however, the rate of recovery is slower, perhaps 1 inch per month.

   - *Third-degree injury*—Axonal injury occurs, with varying degrees of scarring within the endoneurium. Recovery varies from complete recovery to no recovery depending on the degree of endoneurial scarring and mismatching of the regenerating sensory and motor fibers.

   - *Fourth-degree injury*—The nerve is physically intact, but scar tissue prevents any nerve regeneration across the area of injury. This represents a *neuroma-in-continuity.* No recovery can occur without excision of the scar tissue and nerve repair or nerve graft.

   - *Neurotmesis, or fifth-degree injury, represents complete transection of the nerve.* Direct nerve repair or nerve graft is necessary to obtain recovery. Without repair, there will be no functional recovery.

   - *Mixed Injury, or sixth-degree injury,* combines the various patterns of injury from fascicle to fascicle within a nerve and varies along the length of the nerve as well.

4. *Evaluation*—Preoperative evaluation after laceration is critical to planning surgery. Static or moving two-point discrimination demonstrates sensory deficits. The absence of sweating demonstrates the interruption of sympathetic nerve function. Digital nerve function should be tested, not at the tip of the finger but over the proximal third of the distal phalanx. Palmar cutaneous nerve branches of the median nerve can be tested near the thenar eminence. Dorsal cutaneous branches of the ulnar nerve should be tested over the dorsal ulnar surface of the hand. Radial nerve function should be tested over the dorsal first web space. Median nerve function can be tested over the pulp of the thumb and index finger. Ulnar nerve function can be tested over the pulp of the little finger.

5. Treatment

   - Nerve repair

     (a) Technique—Microsurgical technique with appropriate magnification, instrumentation, and suture material is required for successful nerve repair. The nerve repair must be tension free. If not, an interposition nerve graft or collagen conduit may need to be considered. *Primary repair of the nerve provides the best results.* The proximal and distal extent of the nerve should be mobilized, appropriate scar tissue is resected from the ends of the damaged nerve to visualize the fascicles, and the nerve is repaired without tension. *Extreme postural positioning of the extremity to facilitate end-to-end repair should be discouraged. Epineural repair is satisfactory for most mixed sensory nerves in the hand.* Group fascicular repair is not indicated for these sensory nerves, since increased surgical manipulation of fascicles may result in more scarring than epineural repair alone.

     (b) Timing—The majority of acute nerve injuries should be repaired primarily when a skilled surgeon and appropriate instrumentation are available and the patient is medically stable with an adequate nothing-by-mouth status. Delayed primary repair of the nerve is still possible after 3 or more weeks with mobilization of the nerve, but becomes progressively more difficult.

(c) Rehabilitation—After completion of the repair, the amount of movement allowed by the digit is noted (intraoperatively) and is incorporated into the postoperative plans for protected motion. Postoperative motor and sensory reeducation maximizes the potential surgical result.

- Nerve graft—When nerve repair without tension is not possible, a nerve graft should be considered. Potential donor sites for a nerve graft include the *sural nerve* for reconstructing a large peripheral nerve and the *medial antebrachial cutaneous nerve* for digital nerve defects. The clinical role of vascularized nerve grafts has not been established.

- *Neuroma-in-continuity*—Intraoperative evaluation of the neuroma-in-continuity is helpful with decision making. After neurolysis of the neuroma, a disposable nerve stimulator is used to identify motor function distal to the neuroma. *Working motor fibers are protected, and silent sensory fascicles can be resected and reconstructed with nerve graft if needed. If the sensory fascicles are intact and motor function is absent, tendon transfers may be more appropriate.*

- Closed nerve injuries—A patient with a closed injury to a nerve is treated with expectant observation for 3 months. If there is no evidence of clinical recovery, surgical exploration may be warranted, especially if localized to an area of nerve entrapment, which may benefit from early decompression of the nerve.

6. Results—The results of nerve repair and nerve grafting have improved since World War II. Although results can be variable, patients can expect sensory recovery of S3 or greater in 86% of cases with nerve repair and S3 sensory recovery in 80% of cases with nerve grafting (Hyatt's method of end result evaluation; S3 indicates return of superficial cutaneous pain and tactile sensibility [proprioception and sensation]). Furthermore, children have better neurologic recovery following nerve injuries than adults; *age is the best prognostic indicator of recovery*.

D. Vascular Injuries

1. Anatomy (Fig. 24-24)—The ulnar artery generally is more dominant than the radial artery and provides the primary arterial contribution to the *superficial palmar arch*. The radial artery passes deep in the snuffbox between the thumb and index metacarpals to form the deep palmar arch. Regarding the digital arteries, the ulnar digital artery is generally larger than the radial digital artery, except for the little finger.

2. Evaluation

- History—Presenting signs for ischemia may be pain, pallor, and absence of pulse. The patient may note a pulsatile mass at the previous

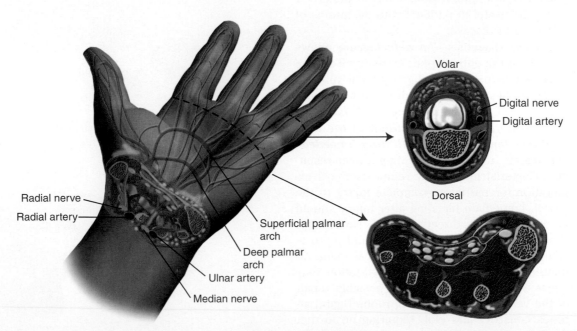

Volar

Digital nerve

Digital artery

Dorsal

Radial nerve

Radial artery

Superficial palmar arch

Deep palmar arch

Ulnar artery

Median nerve

FIGURE 24-24 Anatomy of the arteries and nerves of the hand. The digital nerves are the terminal branches of the median and ulnar nerves and are volar to the digital arteries in the fingers.

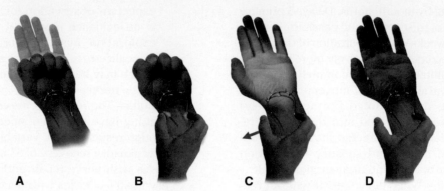

A   **B**   **C**   **D**

FIGURE 24-25   Allen's test. **A.** The patient is instructed to open and close the hand several times and squeeze tightly. **B.** The examiner occludes both the radial and ulnar arteries. **C.** The patient is instructed to open the hand, and one of the arteries is released. **D.** If the artery is competent, normal color will return to the hand. Both arteries should be selectively tested. If one artery allows quicker return of normal color, the patient may be classified as radial or ulnar dominant.

site of laceration or may experience cold intolerance, ulceration, or symptoms of Raynaud's disease. Exposure to vibratory tools and known collagen diseases should be sought.

- Physical examination—The limb should be observed for color, capillary refill, or possible splinter hemorrhages in the nailbed. The peripheral pulses are palpated, and **Allen's test** is performed for the radial and ulnar arteries at the wrist (Fig. 24-25), as well as for the digital vessels (Fig. 24-26). Areas of tenderness or any pulsatile mass are noted.

- Noninvasive diagnosis—A **Doppler scan** is performed to map out arterial topography and to record pulse volume. A cold stress test may be useful in patients with symptoms of Raynaud's disease.

- Invasive diagnosis—An **arteriogram** allows study of the entire upper extremity from the axillary artery to the digits. Digital subtraction studies provide good detail with a smaller amount of contrast. **Tolazoline (Priscoline) or urokinase can be instilled at the time of arteriogram for vasodilation if needed**.

3. Penetrating trauma—Penetrating trauma resulting in arterial injury may require surgical exploration for partial or complete injury to the vessel. Immediate bleeding after injury should be managed with direct pressure. No attempt should be made to probe the wound or to ligate a vessel in the emergency department. Attempted ligation with poor visualization may injure a nerve or compromise possible repair of the vessel in the operating room. Digital arteries constrict and clot, requiring no further treatment, except for associated injuries to the digital nerves or tendons.

4. False aneurysm—Partial injury of an arterial wall may lead to the formation of a false aneurysm. The false aneurysm may present as a pulsatile mass. An arteriovenous fistula may also result from partial injury to an artery. A false aneurysm should be resected, with or without arterial reconstruction, as dictated by the distal circulation.

5. Cannulation injury—Direct injury to the vessel wall during arterial cannulation may occur with needles, such as when drawing an arterial blood gas or placing a radial artery catheter. Distal ischemia of the hand may be a problem if the ulnar artery is hypoplastic or absent.

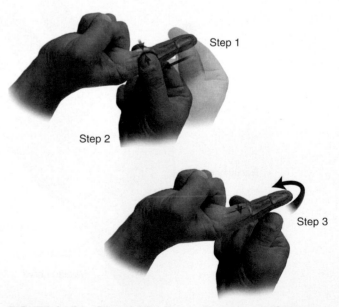

Step 1

Step 2

Step 3

FIGURE 24-26   Digital Allen's test. Note the similarity to Allen's test at the wrist (see Fig. 24-25).

Treatment may require vasodilators, stellate ganglion block, or surgery to repair the artery and thrombectomy with a Fogarty catheter.

6. Acute injection injury—Spasm and occlusion of a major vessel may occur with intraarterial injection. Pharmacologic management includes intraarterial urokinase at the time of arteriogram, systemic vasodilators, or stellate ganglion block. Persistent clots may require removal with a Fogarty catheter.

7. Ulnar artery thrombosis—Repetitive trauma in the hypothenar region of the palm may result in thrombosis of the ulnar artery. The thrombosis may present with a tender hypothenar mass, cold intolerance, and possible vascular insufficiency to the fingers. The ulnar artery demonstrates no flow with Allen's test. A Doppler study or an arteriogram confirms the diagnosis. Treatment options include sympathectomy, resection without reconstruction, and possible interposition vein graft for the ulnar artery.

8. Ring avulsion injuries—Urbaniak has classified ring avulsion injuries.
   - Class I—Circulation is adequate. Standard bone and soft-tissue treatment is sufficient.
   - Class II—Circulation is inadequate, but bones, tendons, and nerves are intact. Vessel repair will preserve viability. Revascularization is recommended for the arteries, with vein grafting if needed.
   - Class III—Complete degloving or a complete amputation injury occurs. *These injuries have the worst prognosis for replantation and are often best managed with surgical amputation of the digit.* If the amputation is distal to the superficialis insertion, vein and nerve grafts may be indicated for replantation. If the PIP joint is damaged or the proximal phalanx is fractured, amputation is recommended.

E. Replantation
1. Overview—Technical advances in microvascular surgery now make it possible to reattach parts of a digit at almost any level, provided that it has been sharply amputated.
   - Replantation—Replantation is the reattachment of a body part that has been totally severed from the body without any soft-tissue attachment.
   - Revascularization—Revascularization is the repair or reconstruction of blood vessels that have been damaged to restore circulation to a body part that has had an incomplete amputation.
   - Ischemia time—Replantation is usually not recommended if the **warm** ischemia time is greater than 6 hours for an amputation proximal to the carpus or greater than 12 hours for an amputated digit, whereas **cold** ischemia times for amputated parts can be extended to 10 to 12 hours for an amputation proximal to the carpus and 24 hours for a digit (because they have no muscle).

2. Indications—Factors that influence the decision to attempt replantation include the level of amputation; the type of injury (such as sharp, crush, avulsion, or the presence of a segmental injury); length of warm or cold ischemia time; the age, general health, and occupation of the patient; and the potential for rehabilitation. *Good indications for replantation include* (a) *the thumb at almost any level* (since a successful replantation is superior to any other method of reconstruction after amputation), (b) *individuals with multiple digit amputations* (in whom less severely damaged digits can often be replanted), (c) *metacarpal amputations through the palm* (since replantation will have a better outcome than that achieved with a prosthesis), (d) *almost any body part of a child*, and (e) *individual digit amputations distal to the superficialis insertion*. The patient must understand that the functional and cosmetic limitations of the amputated part will persist despite successful replantation of the digit.

3. Contraindications—Contraindications for replantation include severely crushed or mangled parts, amputations with a prolonged warm ischemia time, and amputations with multiple levels of injury. Furthermore, patients with serious arteriosclerotic disease or patients who are mentally unstable are not good candidates. *Replantation of individual finger amputations proximal to the FDS insertion in the adult, particularly for the index finger, do not improve hand function, and the patient may be better served with a ray resection*.

4. Emergency department—The amputated parts should not be placed directly on ice and should not be frozen. The digits should be placed in a sterile plastic specimen cup filled with physiologic lactated Ringer solution, and then the entire container placed on ice. The patient's medical condition is evaluated and stabilized in the emergency department. The amputated part is taken to the operating room for initial dissection and tagging of structures.

5. Surgical technique
   - Shortening of the bone—Bone shortening of 0.5 to 1.0 cm in the digit will enable primary repair of the arteries and veins. Fixation can be obtained with crossed K-wires, intraosseous wires, or plates.
   - Repair of the extensor tendons.
   - Repair of the flexor tendons—A Tajima or a modified Kessler technique is suggested.
   - Anastomosis of the digital arteries—At least one artery should be repaired for each digit. A vein graft may be required for a significant segmental defect.
   - Repair of the digital nerves.
   - Anastomosis of the veins—Two dorsal veins should be anastomosed in each digit.
   - Skin repair—Loose approximation of the wound is performed. Skin coverage may be achieved with split-thickness skin grafts or local rotation flaps if necessary.
6. Postoperative management—The extremity is elevated. The patient remains in bed in a quite, **warm room**; the patient should be **well hydrated** and should **not have any nicotine or caffeine products**. Anticoagulants such as aspirin, dipyridamole (Persantine), low–molecular-weight dextran, or heparin may be used. The replant is monitored. The first step if there is decreased skin temperature postoperatively is to loosen the bandage and inspect for any constriction. Venous congestion may require treatment with **medical leeches**. A failing replant requires careful evaluation. If not improved in 4 to 6 hours, a **return to the operating room may be required to evaluate and revise the anastomoses**. Technical problems may include a back wall suture, thrombosis, or poor proximal inflow resulting from spasm. Technical problems are most successfully managed within the first 48 hours after surgery. Revision of the anastomosis may often require vein grafting.
7. Results—An 85% viability rate can be expected with modern microsurgical technique. Sensation may not be normal, but protective sensation with two-point discrimination of 10 mm or less is seen in 50% of adults. Although cold intolerance symptoms are common, symptoms improve in 2 to 3 years. Range of motion is not normal, but patient acceptance of the digit after replantation is good. Best results are seen in replantations distal to the FDS insertion. Epiphyseal plates in children remain open and continue to grow.

F. Amputation—Amputation may be necessary when a digit is not salvageable. Patients with severely mutilated digits may be best served by early amputation, shortening the period of recovery, and earlier return to function.
   1. Principles—Amputation should strive to preserve functional length while maintaining function and cosmesis. Stabile and nontender soft-tissue coverage is necessary, with **sensibility (proprioception and sensation)**. Symptomatic neuromas must be avoided. Early mobilization of the proximal joints minimizes adjacent contractures. Physical therapy and a psychologist for selected patients may be necessary for early acceptance of the injury and return to independence.
   2. Level of amputation
      - Distal phalanx (fingertip amputations are discussed later)—If traumatic amputation occurs through the DIP joint, the bone may be shortened and contoured for primary closure. The digital nerves are resected away from the cutaneous scar to prevent neuroma. **The flexor tendon should not be sutured to the extensor tendon. A volar skin flap is preferable.**
      - Middle phalanx—The bone is shortened and contoured for primary closure. The superficialis insertion is preserved for active PIP flexion and strength.
      - Proximal phalanx—The bone is shortened and contoured for primary closure. The intrinsics control flexion of the MCP joint. Ray resection may be considered, especially for the index finger if the thumb readily transfers to the middle finger for function.
      - Ray resection—If the amputation includes the MCP joint, ray amputation may be indicated primarily. Ray amputation can also be performed later as an elective procedure if desired by the patient. The cosmetic result of a ray amputation is often less conspicuous than a short amputated digit, especially for the index finger.
   3. Thumb amputation
      - Overview—The opposable thumb provides 50% of hand function. Any shortening of the thumb results in greater impairment.
      - Treatment
        (a) Replantation—Replantation of an amputated thumb should be performed whenever possible, since alternative reconstruction is inferior in cosmesis and function. The viability for replantation of a sharply amputated thumb ranges from 75% to 90%, whereas the viability rate for replantation of an avulsion amputation falls to 40%. Aggressive debridement of injured tissue and the use of vein grafts have improved thumb replantation survival.

    (b) Amputation—Only patients with an amputation distal to the interphalangeal joint can demonstrate normal key-pinch activity. If replantation is not an option, the bone should not be shortened, and sensate stable coverage should be provided.

    (c) Pollicization—If the thumb metacarpal is traumatically absent, pollicization of the index finger to the thumb position provides an opposable digit.

    (d) Toe-to-thumb transfer—For amputation at the MCP joint, with an absent proximal phalanx, microsurgical transfer of a great toe or the second lesser toe to the thumb will provide an opposable structure for grasping.

IV. Fingertip and Nailbed Injuries—Fingertip and nailbed injuries are common hand injuries that may lead to significant disability. The goals of treatment are to maintain adequate sensibility without hypersensitivity and to recover a normal range of motion for the finger. The clinician should consider age, gender, occupation, and the involved digit when making treatment decisions.

  A. Fingertip Injuries

    1. Classification
- Simple laceration—The skin and dermis are affected.
- Tissue loss—There is loss of tissue with or without bone involvement.
  - (a) Transverse—The injury is straight across.
  - (b) Oblique dorsal—The tissue loss is primarily dorsal.
  - (c) Oblique palmar—The tissue loss is primarily palmar.

    2. Treatment
- Simple laceration—Treatment should include local wound cleansing with appropriate debridement, followed by direct closure. In adults, the clinician should normally use a 5–0 nonabsorbable suture to minimize scar formation. In children, an absorbable suture is appropriate.
- Tissue loss—It is always important to adequately clean and debride the wound.
  - (a) Open treatment—Open treatment is preferred in adults with a defect less than 1 cm^2 and in children with slightly larger defects. This technique allows direct epithelization, with resultant scar contracture that reduces the area and gives excellent results. The disadvantage of this technique is the length of time to complete healing.
  - (b) Direct closure—For direct closure to be successful, the wound must not have any tension on closure. If necessary, the bone is trimmed and shortened. The nail matrix should not extend past the bone or a hooked nail results. The main advantage of this technique is that it is a one-stage procedure.
  - (c) Skin grafting
    - Split-thickness skin graft—Split-thickness skin graft gives coverage over soft tissue and contracts to reduce wound size with healing. This graft is easy to obtain from the forearm or wrist, but may leave a scar at the donor site; it is not useful over exposed bone.
    - Full-thickness skin graft—Full-thickness skin graft is more durable than split-thickness skin graft but is more prone to failure. The donor site is usually better cosmetically. A full-thickness skin graft also cannot be used on exposed bone.
    - Composite graft—A composite graft is best reserved for use in children but still remains unpredictable and may delay more definite treatment. It provides excellent results if it works.
  - (d) Replantation—Replantation has the best outcome for amputations between the FDS insertion and the DIP joint. It has the potential for normal appearance and good sensibility but can result in cold intolerance, hypersensitivity, or a hypotrophic tip. Replantation is more expensive with a much longer recovery period.
  - (e) Local and regional flaps
    - V–Y advancement—The lateral (***Kutler***) and palmar (***Atasoy***) flaps are technically demanding but provide innervated coverage *for transverse and dorsal oblique skin and soft-tissue loss*. These flaps usually work for less than 1 cm of advancement. It is important not to devascularize the flap during dissection.
    - Volar advancement—The ***Moberg*** flap is used only for the thumb. It can be used to cover approximately a 1.5-cm deficit but may cause a flexion contracture. The biggest complication is necrosis of the tip of the flap if the vascularity is damaged.
    - Cross finger flap—This flap can cover *oblique palmar defects on the finger*, **especially the volar surface**, and

is very reliable. This flap may also be innervated. Its disadvantages are that it may cause stiffness and an unsightly donor site.
- Thenar flap—The thenar flap is especially useful in children and young adults but is less useful in older adults because of joint stiffness. The flap is limited in donor site availability.

B. Nailbed Injuries—The best results follow prompt treatment.
1. Classification
   - Subungual hematoma—After a crush injury, the patient complains of throbbing pain. Examination shows blood under the nail, with the nail intact.
   - Nailbed laceration—There is damage to the nailbed, but the matrix is still present.
   - Loss of the nail matrix.
2. Treatment
   - Subungual hematoma—The subungual hematoma exceeding 50% of the nailbed should be drained with a drill, cautery, or hot needle to relieve pressure. This should be followed by soaks, and then it is allowed to drain. Treatment should be performed using sterile technique because the injury could be associated with an exposed bone tuft fracture of the distal phalanx.
   - Nailbed lacerations—Nailbed lacerations include any laceration or a crushed nailbed. The nail should be removed and the nailbed repaired with a 6–0 plain absorbable suture. The nail can be reapplied as a protective cover.
   - Loss of the nail matrix—The wound associated with loss of the nail matrix should be irrigated, cleaned, and repaired if possible. It usually requires a nailbed graft from another finger or toe.
3. Complications—Complications include split nail, nonadherent nail, ingrown nail, osteomyelitis, ridging, and hypersensitivity.

V. Burns—Burns are the nonmechanical destruction of tissue, by heat, electricity, or chemicals.
A. Thermal burns—Thermal burns are most effectively treated by realizing the extent of destruction early and treating the wound appropriately.
1. Classification
   - First-degree burns—First-degree burns are superficial burns associated with erythema and often a few small blisters. These burns are quite painful.
   - Second-degree burns—Second-degree burns involve partial-thickness injury to the skin.

There is deep erythema and extensive blistering. These burns are painful and have a higher risk of infection.
   - Third-degree burns—With third-degree burns, there is loss of the complete thickness of skin. The skin is anesthetic, **and hence it is not painful**. It may appear to have a dirty cream to charred color.
2. Treatment
   - First-degree burns—First-degree burns should be treated with cool water, gentle cleaning, and localized treatment as for a sunburn.
   - Second-degree burns—Second-degree burn treatment includes an anti-infection agent such as 1% Silvadene cream. (The blisters should be allowed to rupture spontaneously.) The wound should be cleaned daily and covered with a protective dressing. Early range of motion, as well as splinting, is necessary to minimize contractures.
   - Third-degree burns—***Third-degree burns require debridement, escharectomy, and soft-tissue coverage***. The prognosis depends on the extent and depth of thermal injury. Occasionally, a split-thickness skin graft is required if no healing occurs over 2 weeks; this helps to prevent scar formation.
3. Complications
   - Early—Early complications include fluid loss and compartment syndrome.
   - Late—Contractures of the fingers, wrist, or elbow can result in the need for surgical release. Heterotrophic bone formation at the elbow is another late upper-extremity complication.

B. Electrical Burns—It is important to distinguish between the thermal component (heat) and the electrical injury caused by the passage of current. The extent of injury is determined by the amount of current, the type of current, the pathway, and the duration of exposure to the current.
1. Diagnosis—The severity of injury is always the greatest at the entrance and the exit wounds, which are usually "charred" with a zone of intact but necrotic tissue. It is usually difficult to assess the extension of tissue necrosis, since the ***current flows along the pathway of least resistance with nerve having the least resistance and bone having the most***.
2. Treatment—Initial treatment is debridement of obvious nonviable tissue, with fasciotomy and nerve decompressions as indicated. This should be followed by a "second-look" operation at 48 hours (for a second debridement). The clinician may see progressive necrosis, which requires

further debridement. When the patient's condition is stable, definitive treatment, including flaps or even amputation, may be required.

C. Chemical Burns—The severity of a chemical burn is determined by the concentration, duration of contact, amount, mechanism of action, and penetrability of the chemical. Tissue destruction continues until removal or neutralization of the material. Therefore, the first course of treatment of any chemical burn is water irrigation (i.e., running tap water). The recommendations for specific chemical burns are shown in Table 24-1.

VI. High-Pressure Injection Injuries—These commonly occur in young men in a new job and most commonly involve the nondominant hand.

A. Evaluation—The initial examination reveals an innocuous-looking entrance wound with the patient complaining of a variable amount of pain. Swelling is related to the site, amount, and time since the injection. There can be both physical distention and chemical irritation.

B. Prognosis

1. Material—The type of material injected is most commonly paint or grease. Paint causes necrosis and grease causes fibrosis. ***There is a 60% amputation rate with paint and a 25% amputation rate with grease***.

2. Pressure—The pressure involved with injections may range from 3,000 to 10,000 psi. ***If greater than 7,000 psi, there is a 100% amputation rate***.

3. Site involved—The digits have a poorer prognosis than the palm.

4. Amount—The amount injected bears a direct relationship to a worsening prognosis.

5. Time—The longer the time to treatment, the worse the prognosis.

C. Treatment

1. Emergency department

(a) Radiographic evaluation—X-ray studies can show the extent of soft-tissue involvement or proximal infiltration of the substance, especially if it has a metallic component.

(b) Antibiotics and tetanus prophylaxis

(c) Steroids

2. Operating room—These patients must go to the operating room for thorough debridement, copious irrigation, and nerve and forearm decompression if necessary.

3. Postoperative treatment—Postoperative treatment includes safe positioning in the intrinsic plus position to prevent or minimize contracture, sympathetic blocks for pain control and circulation, and a second-look procedure for further debridement. These cases commonly require multiple operative procedures.

VII. Infections of the Hand—Most hand infections are surgical rather than medical problems. Antibiotics are an adjunct to surgical management. For any infection, a history as to the underlying cause, as well as contributor factors such as diabetes, infection by the human immunodeficiency virus, gout, or systemic infections, is important. The clinician should be aware that the deep lymphatics drain to the palm, whereas the superficial lymphatics drain dorsally and palmarly. ***The epitrochlear nodes drain the ulnar side of the hand, and the axillary nodes drain the radial side of the hand***. All of these nodes should be checked.

A. Paronychia—Paronychia is a common infection of the periungual tissue. Paronychia is commonly associated with nail biting and manicuring. The most common organism is Staphylococcus aureus. (Anaerobes are also common.) If the diagnosis is made early, this infection may respond to appropriate antibiotics and soaks.

1. Diagnosis—Findings include pain, redness, and swelling about the nail.

2. Treatment—Drainage, either by incision or by nail elevation, is followed by soaks and antibiotics.

3. Complications—Complications include nail deformity and the possibility of osteomyelitis.

4. Other considerations—Individuals who are frequently in contact with the oral mucosa of others (dentists, anesthesiologists, wrestlers) are at increased risk of developing paronychia from the herpes simplex virus (herpetic whitlow). These patients have vesicles that contain clear fluid. The treatment of choice is acyclovir; there is no need to debride the vesicles. Individuals who engage in activities that involve prolonged immersion in water (such as dishwashers) are at increased risk of developing an infection from Candida organisms.

TABLE 24-1

Recommendations for Chemical Burns

Chemical	Treatment
Acid	Dilute topical sodium bicarbonate
Alkali	Dilute topical acetic acid
Phenol	Topical ethyl alcohol
Hydrofluoric acid	10% calcium gluconate by local injection

The treatment for such an infection is topical clotrimazole.

B. Felon—Felon is a deep infection in the pad of the finger and is usually associated with a history of a puncture wound or another open injury.
1. Diagnosis—There is intense, throbbing pain at the tip of the finger, with a swollen pad that is tight and tender on palpation.
2. Treatment—The treatment involves incision and drainage, making sure to open the septa that compartmentalize the infection. *The incision should be made midlateral to avoid the pad, unless the abscess is pointing superficially*. Once again, treatment after incision and drainage includes soaks and antibiotics.

C. Tendon Sheath Infections—Tendon sheath infections are usually the result of a penetrating wound, frequently an innocuous puncture.
1. Diagnosis—The patient has a painful and swollen finger with positive *Kanavel's sign*, which include symmetric swelling along the flexor tendon sheath, tenderness and erythema along the flexor tendon sheath, semi-flexed position of the finger, and *severe pain on passive extension of the finger*. This last sign is the most diagnostic of tendon sheath infections. This infection may also extend into the mid palmar space.
2. Treatment
   • Surgical drainage
      (a) Midlateral incision technique—The midlateral incision technique allows the scar to be off the palmar surface and still obtains full exposure. This incision can be left open and allowed either to heal or to be closed secondarily later.
      (b) Limited incision with catheter irrigation—With limited incision with catheter irrigation, the sheath is opened over the middle phalanx and then in the distal palm. A catheter is placed to irrigate the tendon sheath with 5 mL of saline every 2 hours for 48 hours.
   • Intravenous antibiotics—Intravenous antibiotics are administered pending culture and sensitivity tests.
   • Range of motion—Range of motion is started early.
   • Atypical infections—If the infection does not respond, an atypical infection, including mycobacterium, fungus, or anaerobes, should be considered.
   • Human bites—Infection from human bites usually has a rapid onset and should be treated aggressively.

D. Palmar Space Infections
1. Diagnosis—The mid palmar and thenar spaces can develop an abscess after penetrating trauma. The *mid palmar space* is the potential space between the flexor tendons and the metacarpals on the ulnar aspect of the hand. The *thenar space* is the potential space between the index finger and the thumb. The main symptoms are pain and swelling in these areas. Deep palmar space infections require incision and drainage.
2. Treatment—Incision and drainage are performed; care should be taken to avoid neurovascular structures in the palm. Antibiotics are administered intravenously.
3. Complications—The most common complication is incomplete drainage of the space without going deep into the area, such as for a buttonhole abscess, in which the presenting abscess is superficially drained, but the palmar space infection is not.

E. Septic Arthritis—Septic arthritis may occur secondary to penetrating trauma or bloodborne sepsis. The most notorious inoculation is the human bite, usually after a fist-to-mouth injury to an MCP joint.
1. Diagnosis—Signs and symptoms include erythema, tenderness in the joint, and pain with motion. X-ray studies may show bony changes.
2. Treatment—Treatment includes aspiration of the joint for diagnosis and culture, incision and drainage, and culture and sensitivity tests, followed by the intravenous administration of appropriate antibiotics (for 3 to 6 weeks).
3. Complications—Complications include joint destruction, stiffness, and osteomyelitis.

VIII. Reflex Sympathetic Dystrophy (Regional Pain Syndrome)
A. Overview—Reflex sympathetic dystrophy (RSD) is a catchall term that covers a wide spectrum of dystrophic responses to trauma. There is no physiologic basis for these dystrophies, but all appear to be a normal response of prolonged duration. The natural history is poorly understood but may result in permanent disability. The departure from the expected recovery for an injury or surgery with associated pain, stiffness, and anatomic dysfunction are early clinical hallmarks of RSD. Chronic regional pain syndrome (CRPS) Types I and II have been introduced to replace the term RSD. *CRPS Type I corresponds to the classic RSD without an identifiable nerve injury*. CRPS Type II occurs after an identifiable nerve injury. Either type may be sympathetically mediated or sympathetically independent.

B. Evaluation
   1. Classification
      - First stage—The first stage is the first 3 months and is sometimes referred to as the *acute stage*.
      - Second stage—The second stage is from 3 to 12 months, and is referred to as the *dystrophic stage*.
      - Third stage—The third stage is longer than 1 year and is called the *atrophic stage*.
   2. Examination—Although RSD has a variable presentation, there is always a history of trauma, although this may be very mild. Signs and symptoms include *pain out of proportion to what is expected, stiffness, delayed recovery, trophic skin changes, and autonomic dysfunction*.
   3. Diagnostic tests
      - Plain X-rays—Plain X-ray studies may be diagnostic in established RSD, showing juxta-articular osteopenia.
      - Bone scan—A three-phase bone scan is recommended, although the significance is still being debated (unknown prognostic significance).
      - Stellate ganglion blocks—Stellate ganglion blocks are an important diagnostic tool. Significant relief in the presence of a confirmed block is diagnostic for sympathetically mediated pain.
   4. Treatment
      - Early intervention—The key to treatment is early diagnosis. Some 80% of cases treated in the first 12 months show improvement, whereas only 50% of cases starting treatment in the second year show improvement.
      - Therapy—Therapy involves active and passive range of motion, below the threshold of pain, with splints and stimulation, as well as stress loading (Watson).
      - Medications—The clinician may administer amitriptyline, a corticosteroid, nifedipine, or phenytoin.
      - Stellate ganglion blocks—A series of stellate ganglion blocks can sometimes break the RSD cycle.
      - Sympathectomy—Sympathectomy is especially useful when a good, but temporary, response is noted after a stellate ganglion block.
      - Psychotherapy

IX. Late Effects of Traumatic Injuries
   A. Intrinsic-Plus Deformity (Fig. 24-27)—Intrinsic-plus deformity is caused by foreshortening of the intrinsic muscles. Treatment involves operative soft-tissue release.
   B. Intrinsic-Minus Deformity (see Chapter 22, Fig. 22-4)—Intrinsic-minus deformity is due to an injury to the ulnar nerve (with or without a median nerve injury) that causes a claw-hand deformity (hypertension of the MCP joint and flexion at the PIP joint). This results from loss of the intrinsic muscles that are normally responsible for flexion at the MCP joint and extension at the PIP joint and the unopposed action of the extrinsic muscles (FDS, FDP, and extensor digitorum communis). Treatment typically includes tendon transfers that re-route a functional tendon to correct the deformity.
   C. Extrinsic Tightness (Fig. 24-28)—The PIP joint can passively flex with the MCP joint held in extension but is unable to do so with the MCP joint held in flexion because the extensor digitorum communis is scarred to the bone or retinaculum

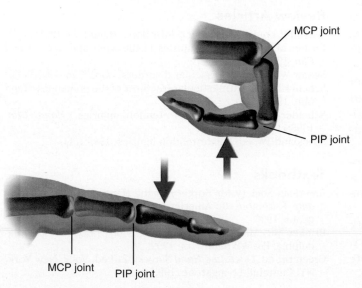

MCP joint

PIP joint

MCP joint   PIP joint

FIGURE 24-27 Test for intrinsic tightness. Note that the PIP joint cannot be flexed with the MCP joint held in extension when there is intrinsic muscle tightness.

FIGURE 24-28 Test for extrinsic tightness. Note that the PIP joint cannot be flexed with the MCP joint held in flexion when there is extrinsic muscle tightness.

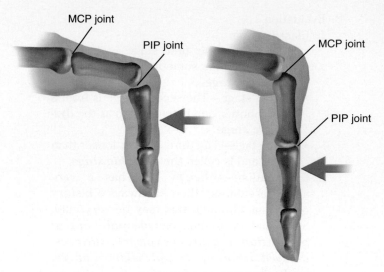

FIGURE 24-29 Lumbrical-plus deformity. With the MCP joint in extension and the PIP joint in flexion, active flexion of the MCP joint will cause paradoxical extension of the PIP joint.

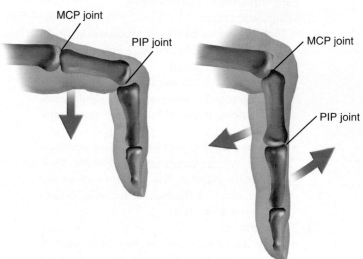

at the wrist or the dorsal metacarpal; this tendon lacks the necessary excursion to allow simultaneous flexion of both the MCP and the PIP joints.

D. Lumbrical-Plus Deformity (Fig. 24-29)—Lumbrical-plus deformity is caused by lumbrical tightness. It can occur as a late effect of an FDP laceration distal to the lumbrical origin. Physical examination reveals paradoxical extension of the PIP joint when he MCP joint is actively flexed (with the PIP joint beginning in the flexed position) (see Fig. 24-29). Treatment is operative soft-tissue release and repair.

E. Boutonnière Deformity (see Fig. 24-10)—Boutonnière deformity can occur as a late effect of a central slip injury. Treatment is discussed in the prior sections.

F. Swan-Neck Deformity (see Fig. 24-8)—Swan-neck deformity can occur as a late effect of a mallet injury, a volar plate injury of the PIP joint, or an FDS rupture. Treatment is discussed in the prior sections.

SUGGESTED READINGS

Review Articles

Jebson P, Louis D, eds. Hand Infections. *Hand Clin.* 1998;14(4).

Posner M, ed. Ligament injuries in the wrist and hand. *Hand Clin.* 1992;8(4).

Schaw Wilgis EF, ed. Vascular disorders. *Hand Clin.* 1993;9(1).

Schenck RR, ed. Intraarticular fractures of the phalanges. *Hand Clin.* 1994;10(2).

Scheider LH, ed. Extensor tendon injuries. *Hand Clin.* 1995;11(3).

Strickland JW, ed. Flexor tendon injuries. 1985;1(1).

Textbooks

American Society for Surgery of the Hand. *Hand Surgery Update.* Rosemont, IL: American Academy of Orthopaedic Surgeons; 1996.

Brinker MR, Miller MD. *Fundamentals of Orthopaedics.* Philadelphia, PA: WB Saunders; 1999.

Green DP, ed. *Operative Hand Surgery.* 3rd ed. Vol 2. New York, NY: Churchill Livingstone; 1993.

CHAPTER **25**

Spinal Cord and Related Injuries

Michael Fehlings, Marcus Timlin, and Nicolas Phan

I. Introduction—Few conditions are as devastating as spinal cord injury (SCI). Patients with SCI usually face several medical problems related to their initial immobilization, prolonged rehabilitation periods, significant readjustment in their lifestyle, and potential complications in the chronic stages of their disease. The earliest description of SCI as an entity was reported by the Egyptians in 1700 BC. Even at that time, patients were described with injuries so severe that they were considered to harbor an "ailment not to be treated." At the beginning of the century, the mortality of SCI was around 90%. At the end of World War I, special care of the urinary tract, respiratory system, and skin of patients with SCI led to a significant improvement of their survival. Despite this improved survival, patients were left with significant disabilities, and their recovery did not seem to benefit from any kind of therapy. Early studies on dogs by Allen showed that the spinal cord's secondary response to injury was responsible for a progression of the tissue damage created by the initial insult and that in certain cases, active early treatment such as decompression, could improve the neurological recovery. Goals of SCI treatment in recent decades have therefore been focused toward early aggressive treatment and prevention of secondary injury mechanisms.

II. Epidemiology—The incidence and prevalence of SCI in North America have been studied in detail over the past two decades (Table 25-1). The exact figures are difficult to determine because of inherent methodological limitations. For example, multiple admissions

of a single patient may overestimate the actual rate while misclassification of SCI when the patient presents with multiple injuries may underestimate it. The incidence of SCI, defined as the number of new cases in a given population in a discrete geographical region within a specific time frame is estimated to be around 40 per million per year. The prevalence of SCI, that is, the number of individuals with SCI within a specific population at a specific point in time, averages 70 per 100,000 or approximately 200,000 to 250,000 total patients in the United States.

As in most traumatic injuries, the incidence of SCI is significantly higher in males than in females (75% of cases occurring in males). The average age for both males and females at the time of injury is around 35 years old. Peak age of incidence is 20 to 24 for males compared with 25 to 29 for females. The incidence among males increases dramatically after age 15, declines after age 30, and increases again steadily in the later decades. The initial peak for

TABLE 25-1

Epidemiology of Spinal Cord Injury in North America

Parameter	Value
Incidence (cases/million/yr)	40
Prevalence (cases/100,000)	70
Male–female ratio	3:1

TABLE 25-2

Causes of Spinal Cord Injury in North America

Etiological Factor	Frequency (%)
Motor vehicle accidents	50
Falls	20
Violent assaults	15–20
Sports and recreational activities	10–20

females is approximately 5 years later than it is for males.

The causes of acute SCI are varied but have remained relatively consistent over the past two decades (Table 25-2). Motor-vehicle accidents are still the most frequent etiology of SCI, accounting for approximately 50% of all cases. Falls, either accidental or from suicide attempts, also account for a significant proportion of SCI cases at approximately 20%. Violent assaults in urban areas have increased dramatically over the past 15 years and are now estimated to be the etiological factors in 15% to 20% of SCI. The vast majority of penetrating injuries of the spinal cord involve firearms. Acute SCI occurs in the context of sports and recreational activities in approximately 10% to 20% of cases. *Diving injuries account for two-thirds of these injuries*. Because of widespread awareness campaigns and media coverage, sports-related SCI has been steadily decreasing since 1975.

In addition to the significant physical and psychological impact of SCI, the financial burden related to hospitalization, rehabilitation, and environment modification of victims is tremendous. The lifetime costs for SCI range from $600,000 to $1 million, depending on its cause. Based on the incidence of SCI, total direct costs for all causes of SCI in the United States are as high as $8 billion.

III. Anatomy of the Spinal Cord
  A. Meningeal Layers—The adult spinal cord lies in the vertebral canal and extends from the foramen magnum, where it is continuous with the medulla, to the first lumbar vertebra (Fig. 25-1). Three meningeal layers cover it. The *spinal dura*, the outermost layer, is a tubular continuation of the meningeal layer of the cranial dura. In contrast to its cranial counterpart, the spinal dura is separated from the inner periosteum of adjacent vertebrae by the *epidural space*. This space contains a variable amount of loose areolar tissue (epidural fat) and the internal vertebral venous plexus. The *pia mater* is adherent to the surface of the spinal cord and forms a triangular-shaped condensations on each side, at regular interval, which attach the

cord to the inner surface of the dural tube. These structures are called denticulate ligaments. The *arachnoid matter* is located between the dura and the pia mater, and extends to the proximal roots of spinal nerves. The space between the pia and arachnoid is termed *subarachnoid space*. It is in this space that the cerebrospinal fluid circulates. The spinal cord has two enlargements situated at the cervical and lumbar areas, which are associated with the spinal roots innervating the upper and lower limbs. The termination of the spinal cord has a conical shape and is termed *conus medullaris*. The conus is attached to a condensation of pia mater, the filum terminale. The filum extends caudally until it becomes invested by the end of the dural sac and forms the coccygeal ligament, which continues to the coccyx where it becomes continuous with the periosteum.

  B. Blood Supply—The arterial blood supply to the spinal cord consists of descending branches of the vertebral arteries and multiple radicular arteries derived from segmental blood vessels. *There are two posterior spinal arteries, each arising from its respective vertebral artery posteriorly*. They descend on the posterior surface of the spinal cord, just medial to the dorsal roots. They receive a variable amount of supply from the segmental posterior radicular arteries along the way down, forming two plexiform channels. Together, they supply the posterior third of the spinal cord. Paired anterior spinal arteries unite caudally just after they branch off their respective vertebral artery and descend as a single vessel that enters the anterior median fissure of the spinal cord. Branches from anterior radicular arteries anastomose with the anterior spinal arteries at different levels in order to form one continuous vessel, although it may become discontinuous or very small at certain levels. The anterior spinal artery supplies the anterior two thirds of the spinal cord. The radicular arteries arise from segmental vessels such as the ascending cervical, deep cervical, intercostal, lumbar and sacral arteries. Once it enters the intervertebral foramen, a radicular artery becomes an anterior radicular or posterior radicular artery or divides into both branches. Radicular arteries usually arise from the left side in the thoracic and lumbar region, while both sides supply the cervical cord equally. *The thoracic cord has the greatest distance between each of its supplying radicular arteries, rendering it more prone to ischemia in the event of an occlusion of one of these vessels*. The artery of Adamkiewicz is an anterior radicular artery found in the thoracolumbar area and is appreciably larger

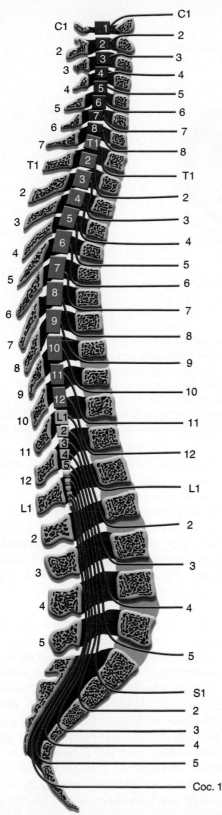

C1

2

3

4

5

6

7

T1

2

3

4

5

6

7

8

9

10

11

12

L1

2

3

4

5

S1

2

3

4

5

Coc. 1

<u>FIGURE 25-1</u> Human spinal cord in vertebral column seen in mid-sagittal section. Note the position of the spinal cord segments with reference to the bodies and spinous processes of the vertebrae. Locations of entrance and exit of spinal roots are indicated.

than all others. It usually arises between T8 and L2, mostly from the left.

C. Segmental Anatomy—An understanding of the segmental anatomy of the spinal cord is essential in order to interpret the different neurological syndromes that patients with SCI present with. A complete anatomical description is beyond the scope of this chapter, and only the relevant structures and pathways will be described. Figure 25-2 illustrates a transverse section of the spinal cord. The gray matter consists of a symmetrical butterfly-shaped structure in the middle of the cord. The dorsal horn is in the posterolateral position and contains mainly sensory neurons that receive afferents from sensory fibers whose cell bodies are located in the ipsilateral dorsal root ganglion. The anterior horn contains motoneurons that send axons to respective segmental skeletal muscle fibers and to intrafusal muscle fibers via the ventral root. In the thoracic cord, there is a lateral horn, which extends from C8 to L2. It consists of preganglionic sympathetic neurons. The sympathetic fibers from these cell bodies exit with the anterior root at the T1 to L2 levels and give white rami to sympathetic chain nuclei located on each side of the spine. There they synapse with postganglionic sympathetic neurons and the sympathetic fibers travel with blood vessels to the viscera and vascular beds they innervate.

1. Sensory pathways—Two main pathways carry sensation. The discriminative touch pathway carries sensations for two-point discrimination, proprioception, and vibration via large fibers in the dorsal root. Most of the fibers enter the cord and ***ascend immediately in the ipsilateral dorsal columns*** located in the posterior midline of the cord. They synapse with second-order neurons in the brainstem and then cross the midline, course cranially, and synapse in the contra-lateral thalamus. The third-order neurons in the thalamus send their projections to the somatosensory cortex. The pain and temperature pathway carries sensations of nociception, heat, cold and simple (primitive) touch via smaller fibers in the dorsal root. The fibers enter the cord and synapse with second-order neurons located in the dorsal horn. The axons of the second order neurons, after ascending or descending one or two segments, ***cross the midline within the spinal cord***. The crossing fibers form the anterior commissure, ventral to the central canal, and reach the spinothalamic tract located in the ventro-lateral aspect of the cord. They then ascend to synapse with third-order neurons in the contralateral thalamus.

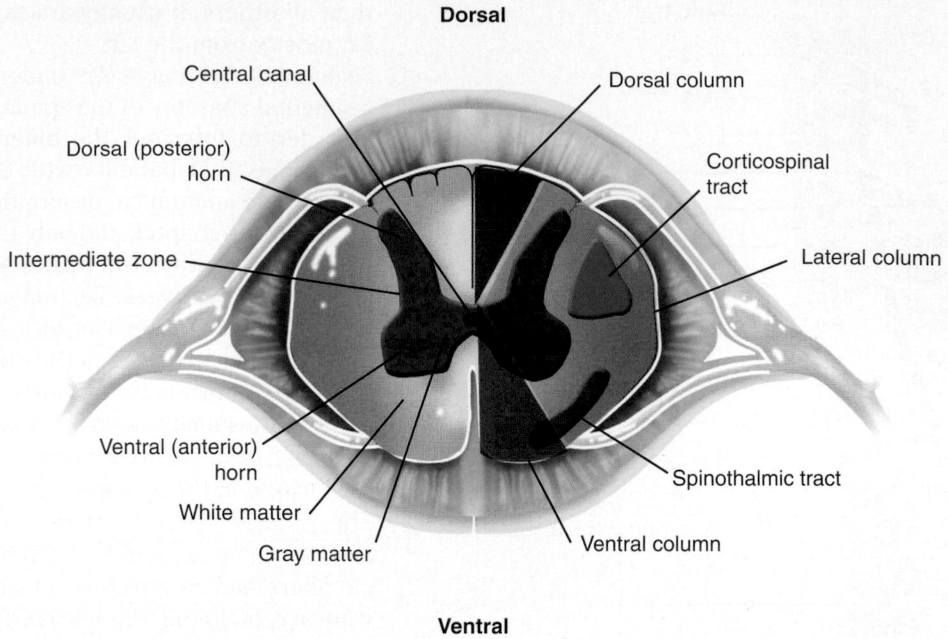

Dorsal

Central canal

Dorsal column

Dorsal (posterior) horn

Corticospinal tract

Intermediate zone

Lateral column

Ventral (anterior) horn

Spinothalmic tract

White matter

Gray matter

Ventral column

Ventral

FIGURE 25-2 Segmental anatomy of the spinal cord. The white matter is organized in three columns (dorsal, lateral and ventral) running in the log axis of the cord. The dorsal columns are involved in touch, proprioception and vibration sensation and the spinothalmic tracts, located ventrolaterally are involved in pain and temperature sensation. The corticospinal tracts, located laterally, carry the axons of upper motor neurons. The central gray matter is divided into the dorsal horn, comprising sensory cells, and the ventral horn, which contains motoneurons. The intermediate zone, between the dorsal and the ventral horns contains the preganglionic neurons of the sympathetic (thoracic cord) and sacral parasympathetic systems. The main components of the central gray matter and the surrounding white matter are illustrated.

The third-order neurons in the thalamus send their projections to the somatosensory cortex. Since the first pathway crosses the midline above the spinal cord and the second within the cord, dissociate sensory loss may occur in partial cord syndromes where only one side of the cord is affected (see later section).

2. Motor pathway—The motor pathway originates in the cerebral motor cortex, as well as from deeper extra pyramidal nuclei. The bulk of the fibers travel caudally in the internal capsule and enter the brainstem, where they form the corticospinal tracts located ventrally. In the medulla, the fibers form the pyramids, which are located ventrally. In the lower medulla, approximately 80% of the fibers cross the midline just before entering the spinal cord. The corticospinal tract in the spinal cord is located in the mid-lateral position and its fibers synapse with motoneurons of the ventral horn at appropriate levels.

3. Lamination of fibers—Fibers in the different tracts of the spinal cord are organized in a specific pattern. Figure 25-3 illustrates the location of the axons supplying the arms and legs in the dorsal columns and spinothalamic tracts. Although this lamination of fibers helps understanding the clinical presentation of certain incomplete syndromes in SCI, it is now

clear that such a somatotopic organization may not exist in the corticospinal tract (see later section).

4. Dermatomes and myotomes—Each segment of the spinal cord innervates a certain sensory area of the body called **dermatome** and specific groups of skeletal muscles called **myotome**. Figure 25-4 illustrates the major myotomes and all dermatomes of the human body.

IV. Classification of SCI—*Consensus in classification of SCI based on neurological examination is essential to determine prognosis as well as for follow-up examinations and longitudinal studies. The most recent classification, The International Standards for Neurological and Functional Classification of Spinal Cord Injury was developed in 1992 by the American Spinal Injury Association (ASIA) and the International Medical Society of Paraplegia (IMSOP). This system is now widely used internationally by all teams involved in the treatment of SCI (Table 25-3 and Fig. 25-4).*

A. ASIA/IMSOP Impairment Scale—The ASIA/IMSOP impairment scale shown in Table 25-3 consists of five grades of impairment. Grade A is defined as complete injury, while Grades B, C and D represent varying degrees of incomplete injuries, and

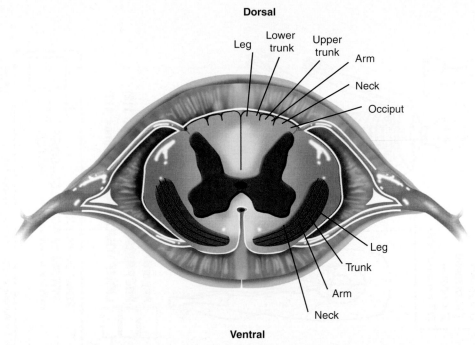

FIGURE 25-3 Segmental anatomy of the spinal cord illustrating the lamination of fibers in the main white matter tracts. The dorsal columns and the spinothalamic tracts are somatotopically organized.

Grade E denotes a normal neurological examination. ***Complete SCI is defined as an absence of motor and sensory function in the lowest sacral segments, S4 and S5***. As can be seen in Figure 25-4, this system requires the examination of 10 key muscle groups on the left and right as well as 28 dermatomes on the left and 28 on the right. The scoring system for the motor function uses the MRC scale from 0 to 5 (see Fig. 25-4), with a maximum possible score of 100. The sensory examination is based on a scale of 0 to 2 for pinprick with a maximum possible score of 112.

In order to determine if a lesion is complete, the sensory and motor functions of the lowest sacral segments S4 and S5 have to be tested. Sensory function is assessed at the perianal region and at the musculocutaneous junction while deep anal sensation and voluntary contraction of the external anal sphincter must be examined during digital rectal examination. Determination of the completeness of a lesion needs to be made early because the prognosis for recovery is much better in incomplete injuries.

The neurological level of a *SCI* is determined by both the sensory and the motor exam, on both sides of the body. ***The sensory and the motor levels are defined as the most caudal (lowest) segment with normal sensory or motor function, respectively***. The 1992 classification defined normal motor function as Grade 4

or 5. This statement led to some confusion in interpreting the neurological level in certain patients, especially those with incomplete injuries. A revision to the classification was thus made in 1996 where the motor level is defined as the lowest key muscle that has a *grade of at least 3*. Since the motor and sensory examination may differ on each side of the body, there may be up to four different levels identified. If dermatomes and myotomes remain partially innervated below an identified level, they are classified as a zone of partial preservation.

B. Spinal Shock—***Spinal shock is defined as the loss of somatic motor, sensory, and sympathetic autonomic function after SCI***. The loss of somatic motor function results in flaccid paralysis and areflexia. Sensory loss may be complete to all modalities. ***The loss of autonomic function, mainly sympathetic innervation, can manifest in hypotension, bradycardia as well as skin warmth and hyperemia***. The severity and duration of spinal shock varies, but it correlates with the severity of the SCI and the level of the injury. Thus, is it usually most severe in complete cervical and upper thoracic cord injuries, less severe in incomplete injuries, and minimal in lumbar injuries. ***In its most severe form, the loss of sympathetic tone (to the heart and vasculature) results in sustained hypotension and bradycardia which leads to neurogenic***

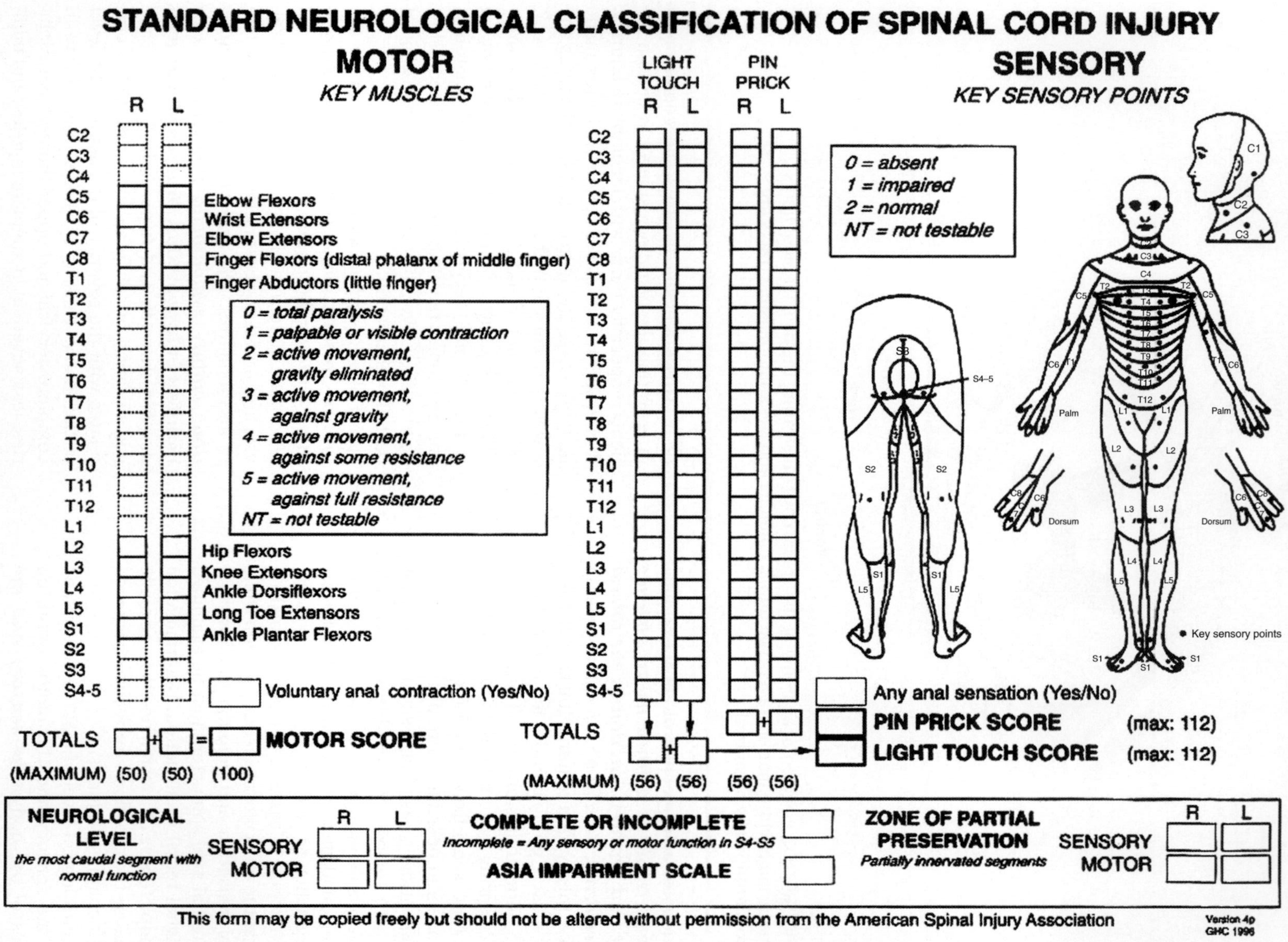

FIGURE 25-4 ASIA/IMSOP classification of SCI. The diagram illustrates the principal information about motor, sensory and sphincter function required for accurate classification and scoring of acute spinal cord injuries. The 10 key muscle groups to be tested are shown on the left along with the MRC grading system, and the 28 dermatomes to be tested on each side for the sensory examination are shown on the right. (Courtesy: American Spinal Injury Association, International Medical Society for Paraplegia: International standards for neurological and functional classification of SCI, revised 1996, Chicago, 1996, The Association and The Society.)

shock. The etiology of spinal shock is unknown, although suspected mechanisms include imbalances in transmembrane ionic concentrations and permeabilities secondary to local tissue trauma, such as an increase in extracellular potassium concentration resulting in inhibition of local neuronal excitability. ***The presence of spinal shock can cause a significant amount of confusion in the initial neurological assessment of the patient***. It is therefore recommended to assume that its effect on the somatic motor and sensory exam have resolved by 1 hour after the initial injury and that the autonomic and reflex dysfunctions may persists for days to weeks.

Acute SCI has been associated with pulmonary edema in a number of cases. Its mechanism is uncertain but it is suspected that massive sympathetic discharge at the time of injury results in a catecholamine surge. The rapid rise in catecholamines leads to acute left ventricular failure from a sudden increase in afterload as well as fluid shifts from the periphery to the pulmonary vasculature.

V. Incomplete Spinal Cord Syndromes—***When there is preservation of sensation or motor function in the lowest sacral segments S4 and S5, a SCI is said to be incomplete***. It therefore falls in the B, C, or D category of the ASIA/IMSOP classification. Patients with incomplete SCI often present with specific patterns of neurological deficits. ***The incomplete syndromes are generally classified according to the anatomic location of the injury in the transverse section of the spinal cord***. This classification is useful in understanding the pathophysiology and mechanisms involved in specific types of injury, which can help direct treatment in the early phase. Since the potential for neurological recovery differs for different syndromes, this classification also helps in the assessment of prognosis upon presentation.

A. Cervicomedullary Syndrome—This syndrome occurs in cervical spinal injury, where the high cervical cord and medulla are involved, although it can extend caudally as far as C4 and rostrally to the pons. It is caused either by direct injury to the cord or medulla or concomitant disruption of the vertebral arteries during cervical spine trauma. Other terms have been used for this presentation such as "bulbar-cervical dissociation." In its most severe form, this syndrome results in respiratory arrest, hypotension, tetraplegia and anesthesia, usually below C4. ***Without immediate first-aid treatment, death occurs shortly after the initial injury from cardiopulmonary arrest***. Improved on-site emergency airway management and cardiac resuscitation has led to an increase in

TABLE 25-3

Classification of SCI Based on the International Standards for Neurological and Functional Classification of SCI by the ASIA/IMSOP

ASIA/IMSOP Impairment Scale		
Grade A	Complete	No motor or sensory function is preserved in the sacral segments S4–S5.
Grade B	Incomplete	Sensory but not motor function is preserved below the neurological level and extends through the sacral segments S4–S5.
Grade C	Incomplete	Motor function is preserved below the neurological level, and the majority of key muscles below the neurological level have a muscle grade less than 3.
Grade D	Incomplete	Motor function is preserved below the neurological level, and the majority of key muscles below the neurological level have a muscle grade greater than or equal to 3.
Grade E	Normal	Motor and sensory function is normal.

patients presenting with this syndrome due to an increase in survivors. ***The mechanism of injury usually consists of traction on the high cervical cord and medulla caused by dislocation or anteroposterior compression from a displaced fracture or intervertebral disc rupture***. The vertebral artery enters the transverse foramen of C6, ascends vertically through each vertebral foramen, exits at C2, and courses over the lateral mass of C1. Entrapment at any point along its way may occur during cervical spine injury. It is particularly susceptible in cases of fracture-dislocation and acute torsion of the upper cervical spine. ***The clinical presentation of the cervicomedullary syndrome has two important characteristics***.

1. Dejerine pattern of anesthesia—Patients can present with the classic ***Dejerine pattern of anesthesia of the face*** (anesthesia of the outer periphery of the face with sparing of the middle portions including the nasal alae to the vermilion border of the lips). This peculiar presentation occurs because the sensory fibers of the face course downward in the spinal trigeminal tract after entering the brainstem and synapse with the spinal trigeminal nucleus as low as C4.

The fibers supplying the periphery of the face travel the furthest down while those supplying the center of the face synapse almost immediately after entering the brainstem, which explains why they are spared when the injury is at the level of the cervical cord. Anesthesia is present below the level of injury but there can be sparing of the collar area supplied by C2 to C4. This is thought to be due to the fact that the sensory fibers from these levels are carried via two different pathways; the classic lateral spinothalamic tract and the spinal trigeminal tract, which ascends caudally before crossing in the brainstem. The second tract may be spared from injury because of the difference in the level of crossing. A complete sensory exam, including the face, is thus essential in the assessment of all patients with cervical spinal injuries in order to recognize this pattern.

2. Cruciate paralysis of Bell—Cervicomedullary syndrome may also mimic central cord syndrome in producing more significant weakness in the arms than the legs. This form of weakness pattern is termed **cruciate paralysis of Bell**. The neuroanatomical explanation proposed to account for this syndrome was outlined in 1901 by Wallenberg. He suggested that the somatotopic organization of the corticospinal fibers in the pyramids resulted in different decussation locations for the leg fibers compared with the arm fibers. However, no neuroanatomic evidence has ever been presented to support this but the theory prevailed. It is now thought, based on several lines of evidence, that the reason why hand function is more affected is that the corticospinal tracts are more important for hand function. Detailed studies of the corticospinal tract organization confirm that a somatotopic organization is lacking. Marchi degeneration studies as well as modern neuroanatomic tracers have shown that the corticospinal fibers serving the upper and lower extremities are diffusely distributed within the pyramids and their decussation and within the corticospinal tract of the spinal cord. In his review of spinal cord syndromes, Schneider found that the pyramids are susceptible to compression by the odontoid process during fracture of the odontoid or atlantooccipital and atlantoaxial dislocations, or other lesions in the vicinity of this structure, such as tumors. Localized injury to the pyramids could explain the disproportionate hand weakness of cruciate paralysis of Bell. In a review of 14 patients with a clinical diagnosis of cruciate paralysis, Dickman and coworkers reported fractures of

the upper cervical spine (C1 to C3) in eight patients. In each of the eight patients with fractures, the C2 vertebra was involved. Of the seven patients who had MRI studies performed, three demonstrated contusions or edema localized to the anterior or anterolateral segments of the cervicomedullary junction and superior cervical cord; this supports the concept that the injury must be mild to moderate, damaging motor function (subserved by the corticospinal tracts in the pyramids) yet preserving life.

B. Central Cord Syndrome—This syndrome was also described initially by Schneider. It is **characterized by a disproportionately greater loss of motor power in the upper extremities than in the lower extremities**, bladder dysfunction usually in the form of urinary retention, and a varying degree of sensory loss below the lesion. Pathological reports of patients presenting with this condition who succumbed after the initial injury revealed that the spinal column and ligaments were intact and that the cord often had a central area of hemorrhage. Taylor has shown that it is possible to have compression of the spinal cord without damage to the vertebral column. He performed cervical myelography on cadavers with their necks in different positions and demonstrated that in the forced extension position, there were a series of indentations on the posterior surface of the spinal column at the level of the interlaminar spaces. These indentations appeared to be caused by inward bulging of the ligamentum flavum, resulting in a narrowing of the spinal canal by as much as 30%. The narrowing was even more marked when osteophytic protrusion in the posterior vertebral bodies were present. **It is thus believed that the major mechanism of injury involved in central cord syndrome consists of hyperextension of the cervical spine resulting in acute anteroposterior compression of the spinal cord**. In his analysis of spinal cord segments of patients with central cord syndrome, Holmes found a significant amount of edema in the tissue located at the level of the injury.

Schneider postulated that the syndrome is caused by hematomyelia and surrounding edema in the central cord and suggested that the discrepancies in arm and leg weakness is due to the lamination of fibers in the corticospinal tracts. He also postulated that the involvement of anterior horn cells in the cervical cord could account for the more pronounced weakness of the arms. As explained earlier, modern studies have failed to show a somatotopic organization of the corticospinal tracts in the spinal cord. An alternative explanation may be that the function of the corticospinal tract in the human is more important for hand and arm function than it is for lower extremity use. Several studies examined the effect of discrete lesioning of the corticospinal tracts. Most of them involved sectioning the medullary pyramids. The common results were surprising. There were relatively few motor deficits and the animals showed significant recovery with time. The most consistent and specific motor deficit was the production of substantial hand dysfunction, which was more prominent than arm and leg dysfunction. The motor recovery was similar to what is seen in humans with central cord syndrome (i.e., the recovery began in the proximal musculature and progressed to the distal musculature as the lower extremities usually recovered before the upper extremities). A recent radiological study investigated MRIs of patients diagnosed with acute central cord syndrome. None showed the MRI features characteristic of hemorrhage. Three post-mortem specimens were available for histological study, ranging from 3 days to 7 weeks after the injury. Again, there was no evidence of blood or blood products within the parenchyma of the spinal cord. The primary finding was diffuse disruption of axons, especially within the lateral columns of the cervical cord in the region occupied by the corticospinal tract. Moreover, 10 out of the 11 patients showed evidence of a prior underlying bone or disc abnormality leading to narrowing of the cervical spinal canal.

The syndrome of central cord syndrome is important to recognize because its prognosis is usually good compared with other syndromes. There have been some cases of rapid complete spontaneous recovery. *The recovery usually follows a specific pattern. Motor power returns in the lower extremities first, bladder function recovers next, and finally movement in the upper extremities returns. Hand and finger motion are the very last to return, and may not recover completely, while sensory recovery occurs in a non-specific pattern.* Because of the spontaneous recovery, treatment is usually conservative but cases have to be examined individually. If instability or persisting compression are present, early surgical management may be indicated in order to optimize recovery.

C. Anterior Cord Syndrome—This syndrome, also described initially by Schneider, *consists of paralysis and hypalgia below the level of the lesion with sparing of discriminative touch, proprioception and vibration sense.* The cases he described had either ruptured cervical discs, fracture dislocations, or both causing anterior compression of the spinal cord. Initial theories on the mechanism of tissue damage in these injuries suggested that they resulted from anterior spinal artery compression and insufficiency. However, the lack of pathological correlation made it less plausible. Kahn originally postulated a mechanism for chronic myelopathy from anterior cord compression secondary to calcified disc protrusion. He proposed that chronic traction on a cord fixed in place by the dentate ligaments was responsible for the clinical presentation of affected patients consisting in *hyperreflexia, spasticity, gait disturbance, weakness more severe in the lower extremities and subjective sensory disturbances.* He believed that the corticospinal tracts were more susceptible to this stress compared with the spinothalamic tracts because of their larger fibers. He also thought that the lateral fixation of the cord from the dentate ligaments caused a form of lateral sclerosis within its substance, thereby affecting the corticospinal tracts to a greater extent. Schneider applied this theory to the acute setting of anterior cord compression in order to explain the clinical findings. He also recommended that patients presenting with this syndrome be considered for early surgical management. The recovery from anterior cord syndrome varies considerably for both the sensory and motor functions.

D. Brown-Séquard Syndrome—The *syndrome of Brown-Séquard, or hemisection syndrome, is characterized by loss of one lateral half of the spinal cord functions.* In its pure form, there is *loss of the motor function, discriminative touch, proprioception and vibration senses ipsilaterally to the injury and loss of pain and temperature sensation on the opposite side.* Mechanisms of injury include hyperextension injuries, compression fractures, herniated discs, and penetrating injuries. It occurs more frequently in the cervical cord than the thoracic cord and conus medullaris. It is often seen in combination with other incomplete syndromes and may be apparent only days after the initial presentation of an incomplete injury. Although a significant number of patients presenting with the Brown-Séquard syndrome become ambulatory, prognosis for neurological recovery varies widely.

E. Conus Medullaris Syndrome—The conus medullaris comprises the tapering distal end of the spinal cord. The lower segments of the spinal cord are condensed in the region of the conus. Indeed, almost all of the lumbar segments are opposite to the vertebral body of T12 while most of the sacral segments are opposite the vertebral body of L1 (see Fig. 25-1). *The change in spinal anatomy, from the stiff thoracic spine to the more mobile lumbar spine, makes the thoracolumbar area prone to instability when submitted to severe stresses. Burst fractures and fracture-dislocations are common at the T11 to T12 and T12 to L1 area, which puts the conus medullaris at a greater risk of direct injury. The syndrome is characterized by a combination of lower motoneuron deficits causing flaccid paralysis of the lower extremities, and sphincter dysfunction. Sensory deficits are variable.* In the chronic phase, upper motor neuron findings may develop, such as spasticity, hyperreflexia and extensor plantar response. *The prognosis is usually not very good*; this may be related to the destruction of the lower motor neurons cell bodies located in the conus, which do not have the potential to regenerate.

F. Cauda Equina Syndrome—The spinal cord terminates at the L1 to L2 disc space. The cauda equina consists of the roots of the lumbar and sacral segments extending caudally below the termination of the cord. Injury below the L1 to L2 disc space will therefore affect the cauda equina. Like spinal cord injuries, cauda equina injuries can be classified as complete or incomplete according to the same criteria. Mechanisms of injuries include fracture-dislocation, burst fracture and acute disc herniation. *Acute central disc herniation causes damage to the more centrally placed sacral roots, often sparing the lumbar and the S1 roots.* The resulting clinical picture consists of perianal anesthesia, sphincter dysfunction, normal leg strength and the absence of radicular pain. The sacral roots are very susceptible to injury and tend not to recover after prolonged compression. *Urgent surgical decompression* is therefore mandated with this particular presentation. In general, however, cauda equina injuries usually have a better prognosis than spinal cord injuries because of the greater regenerative potential of lower motor neuron axons and their relative resilience to trauma and secondary injuries.

VI. Chronic Posttraumatic Syndromes—Patients who have suffered spinal cord injuries can also develop a number of important syndromes in the subacute and chronic stages (Table 25-4). A complete analysis of these syndromes is beyond the scope of this chapter and thus only brief descriptions will be

made. After an acute injury, the spinal cord undergoes changes in its epicenter. If the injury is severe, a central cavitation develops after hemorrhagic necrosis and ischemia of the cord.

A. Syringomyelia—*Syringomyelia refers to a cavitation in the spinal cord tending to extend in a longitudinal direction.* The syndrome of syringomyelia manifests itself in approximately 3% of SCIs. The time of onset varies from months to years (as long as 30 years), and usually presents with some type of deafferentation pain. This is followed by progressive loss of sensory and motor function, on top of the already existing deficit from the original injury. The deficits are somewhat similar to the central cord syndrome with the spinothalamic tracts affected to a greater degree than the dorsal columns. The motor deficit usually involves the lower motor neurons at the level of the injury or above. The exact mechanism by which the syrinx expands is not known. Abnormal transmission of intraspinal CSF pressures during periods of increased pressure such as during a Valsalva maneuver may cause the fluid cavity to expand. Obstruction of normal intraspinal CSF flow by arachnoiditis is also thought to play some role in the progression of a syrinx.

B. Microcystic Myelomalacia—Post-traumatic microcystic myelomalacia has a similar clinical presentation to post-traumatic syringomyelia. *The cord shows microcystic degeneration without a continuous cavity like in syringomyelia.* The first reports of "myelomalacic cores" at the level of injury expanding caudally and rostrally, were described at the beginning of the century in patients with gunshot wounds to the spine and experimental models of SCI. The cystic lesions can extend for several levels above and below the injury and their continuity can be interposed by segments of normal cord. Microcystic degeneration is sometimes difficult to distinguish from syringomyelia, even with MRI, and it too has been associated with arachnoiditis.

C. Arachnoiditis—Arachnoiditis can occur after any type of SCI, of any severity. It *consists of connective tissue adhesions between the spinal cord and its surrounding arachnoid*, often involving the dura. Neurological deterioration associated with arachnoiditis can be step wise or gradual. Tethering of the spinal cord, vascular congestion, ischemia due to fibrosis of arachnoid vessels, as well as obstruction of intraspinal CSF flow have been postulated to explain the mechanism by which arachnoiditis causes neurological deterioration.

D. Deafferentation Pain Syndromes—Deafferentation pain syndromes can affect as much as 25%

TABLE 25-4

Chronic Posttraumatic Syndromes after SCI

Syringomyelia
Microcystic myelomalacia
Arachnoiditis
Deafferentation pain

of SCIs patients in the chronic stage and are the result of abnormal nociceptive impulses generated at different levels such as injured nerve roots, spinal cord, and brain after injury.

VII. Sports-Related SCI—Sports-related SCI is an important group because of its predilection for specific activities and the significant role that prevention plays in reducing the number of such injuries. Sports considered to bear the highest risk include auto and motorcycle racing, diving, hand gliding, football and gymnastics. Other high-risk sports include horseback riding, ice hockey, mountain climbing, parachuting, ski jumping, snowmobile, trampoline and wrestling. The incidence of severe SCI associated with sports has declined dramatically over the past 20 years. In 1977, the National Collegiate Athletic Association (NCAA) provided funding to initiate a national survey of catastrophic football injuries. This was expanded in 1982 to include all sports for both men and women.

   A. Football-Related Injuries—Of the school sports, football is associated with the greatest number of catastrophic injuries. However, its incidence has been considerably reduced when compared with early 1970s data (cervical spine injuries 4.1 per 100,000, permanent quadriplegia 1.58 per 100,000). Evaluation of the data provided by surveys at that time led to the conclusion that one of the main contributing factors was the helmet redesign performed to provide better head protection. As a result of the improved helmet design, players started using the head as a major contact point for blocking and tackling, leading to an increase in cervical spinal cord injuries. This provided the primary incentive for the NCAA to ban the use of the head as an offensive weapon in football. The incidence of spine injuries and quadriplegia then decreased significantly and has remained relatively stable (1.3 per 100,000 and 0.4 per 100,000, respectively).

   B. Hockey-Related Injuries—In the mid-1970s, a significant increase in hockey-related spine injuries was observed and led to the formation of the Canadian Committee on the prevention of Spine and Head injuries Due to Hockey. The Committee found that there were virtually no reported cases of spinal injuries in hockey from 1948 to 1973 whereas it became the second most common cause of SCI in sports and recreational activities from 1977 to 1981. It was found that most cases resulted from a direct blow to the vertex of the head from being pushed or checked against uncushioned boards. Based on these findings, several modifications such as better enforcement of rules against boarding and crosschecking, rules against checking from behind, neck muscle conditioning programs, player education, and helmet redesign, led to an overall decrease of SCI in hockey by 50% since 1984.

   C. Pathophysiology—The pathophysiology of sports-related SCI appears to be similar regardless of the sport involved. The vast majority of cases involve the cervical spine and this is best illustrated by the fact that in football-related SCI, all documented cases have occurred in the cervical spine. Careful analysis of these injuries by Torg and coworkers clearly demonstrated that the ***most common mechanism of injury involves axial loading to the cervical spine***. Indeed, the normal lordosis of the cervical spine allows for absorption of the energy transmitted during axial loading as well as transmission and dissipation of this energy via the neck muscles. When the neck is slightly flexed, the cervical spine becomes straight and loses this ability to absorb and transmit mechanical energy efficiently, and the load is mainly transmitted to the bones, ligaments and intervertebral discs. If the tolerance of the bones, ligaments or discs is exceeded, they fail, resulting in various types of SCIs. The validity of this mechanism of injury has been emphasized by many authors and can be applied to almost any sports or recreational activities such as hockey and diving. Understanding the pathomechanics of cervical spine injury in these activities allows for better training, physical conditioning, and preventive measures that limit the occurrence of severe SCIs.

VIII. Early Treatment of Patient with SCI
   A. Acute Medical Interventions—Every patient with any type of SCI, with or without other associated trauma, has to be treated promptly by both the on-site primary care team and the medical team in the emergency room. The absolute primacy of the ABCs cannot be overemphasized. Adequate perfusion and oxygenation of injured tissue are essential for optimal recovery. Even brief periods of hypoperfusion can increase mortality and decrease the neurological recovery of patients with SCI. Stabilization of the spine during extrication, transportation, and transfer of any patient with a history of significant trauma is done with the assumption that the victim has a spinal column injury until proven otherwise. Complete immobilization of the entire spine from the beginning is essential to prevent further injury to an already damaged spinal column/cord. If endotracheal intubation is required, the cervical spine is maintained in position without extension by applying gentle in-line traction. These important

measures have contributed to a reduction in the ratio of quadriparesis to paraparesis in multiple trauma patients.

Restoration of any systemic hypotension to normotension is an emerging principle of first aid management in SCI based on the recognition that there is vascular compromise of the injured cord by local microcirculatory events including vasospasm and small vessel thrombosis. Initial resuscitation in hypotensive patients consists of volume replacement with a balanced electrolyte solution (e.g., Ringer's lactate) and blood replacement if persistent bleeding is suspected. Hypotension from spinal shock is much less common than hypovolemia, even in patients with SCI, and is considered only after adequate volume replacement has been achieved and potential sources of ongoing bleeding have been ruled out. Treatment of hypotension in this case involves the use of vasopressor agents, such as dopamine, dobutamine and noradrenaline. Early and aggressive medical management (volume resuscitation and blood pressure augmentation) of patients with acute spinal cord injuries has been shown to optimize the potential for neurological recovery after sustaining trauma.

B. Concept of Primary and Secondary Injury in Acute SCI (Table 25-5)—The spinal cord is damaged after SCI by a primary mechanical injury and by a secondary injury involving a series of molecular and cellular events which cause further tissue destruction.

1. Primary injury—The primary injury involves one or more of the following forces: compression, contusion, distraction, laceration, sheer, or missile injury. The primary injury then sets in motion a cascade of secondary injury as summarized in Table 25-5. Following an acute injury, the spinal cord undergoes a series of changes including hemorrhage, edema, axonal and neuronal necrosis, apoptosis (genetically programmed cell death), demyelination, and cavitation. By 24 to 48 hours after major trauma, the injury site is necrotic, especially the central zone previously occupied by hemorrhage. Following several days, the hemorrhagic zone shows cavitation and the adjacent areas demonstrate patchy necrosis. These cavitations are the result of coagulative necrosis.

2. Secondary injury—The secondary injury mechanisms include ischemia, intracellular calcium influx, free-radical-associated lipid peroxidation, and glutaminergic toxicity. In particular, studies of glutamate cytotoxicity

TABLE 25-5

Primary and Secondary Injury mechanisms of acute SCI

Primary Injury Mechanisms
Acute compression
Impact
Missile
Distraction
Sheer

Secondary Injury Mechanisms
Systemic events
Systemic hypotension
Neurogenic shock
Hypoxia
Hyperthermia
Vascular changes
Loss of autoregulation
Hemorrhage
Loss of microcirculation
Reduction in blood flow
Vasospasm
Thrombosis
Electrolyte changes
Increased intracellular calcium
Increased extracellular potassium
Increased sodium permeability
Biochemical changes
Neurotransmitter accumulation
Catecholamines (noradrenaline, dopamine)
Exitotoxic amino acids (glutamate)
Arachidonic acid release
Free-radical production
Eicosanoid production (prostaglandins)
Lipid peroxidation
Endogenous opioids
Cytokine excess
Edema
Loss of energy metabolism
Decreased ATP production
Apoptosis

in neuronal cultures, reports of hypoxic white matter injury and white matter compression injury, ultrastructural studies of calcium accumulation in axons after spinal cord trauma and confocal imaging studies provide strong support for the calcium hypothesis of neural injury. Apoptosis is a form of programmed cell death seen in a variety of circumstances such as immune cell selection and development. Apoptosis has very recently been observed after traumatic SCI in both animal models and human studies, suggesting that active cell death may mediate damage after CNS injury. This type of cell death has been observed in both neuronal and non-neuronal cells, such as oligodendrocytes which are responsible for myelinization of the CNS axons.

C. Pharmacological Therapies for Patients with Acute SCI—*Patients with SCI, even when complete, usually have some preservation of neural elements at the site of injury*. Recordings of somatosensory evoked potentials through the cord of patients with complete SCI have led to the hypothesis of a "discomplete" SCI syndrome where anatomical and functional elements are preserved. It is therefore conceivable that limiting secondary injury to nervous tissue after the initial insult can enhance neurological recovery after SCI. It has been shown that an increase in neural tissue survival of 10% to 20% may be sufficient to allow return of clinically significant neurologic function. The aim of pharmacological agents is thus to alter the response of nervous tissue to injury in order to improve its survival. Only a few agents have been subjected to clinical trials to date and only one has made it to routine clinical use.

1. National Acute Spinal Cord Injury Study I (NASCIS I)—The first National Acute Spinal Cord Injury Study (NASCIS I) was completed in 1984 and compared the effect of two different regimens (high-dose and low-dose) of methylprednisolone after SCI. There was no statistical difference in the neurological recovery between the two groups, but the study was criticized because (a) the dose of methylprednisolone was too low based on the 30 mg per kg dose-relationship already established and (b) the lack of a placebo arm.

2. NASCIS II—The NASCIS II was thus initiated, comparing methylprednisolone 30 mg per kg bolus followed by 5.4 mg/kg/hour for 23 hours, naloxone 5.4 mg per kg bolus followed by 4.0 mg/kg/hour for 23 hours, and placebo. The results were published in 1990. *It was found that patients treated with methylprednisolone within eight hours of injury showed evidence of statistically significant recovery of both sensory and motor function compared with naloxone and placebo, regardless if the injury was initially complete or incomplete.*

3. NASCIS III—The latest study, NASCIS III, which was published in 1997, compared two regimens of methylprednisolone, the standard 30 mg per kg bolus followed by 5.4 mg/kg/hour for 24 hours, and 30 mg per kg bolus followed by a 48-hour infusion of 5.4mg/kg/hour. A third arm was added with patients receiving a 30 mg per kg bolus of methylprednisolone followed by tirilazad mesylate bolus infusions of 2.5 mg per kg every 6 hours for 48 hours. For patients receiving the initial bolus within 3 hours of injury, there was no difference in neurological recovery between the three groups. *For patients who received the bolus between 3 and 8 hours after injury, the group receiving the 48 hours infusion of methylprednisolone had a statistically significant better neurological recovery than the 24-hour infusion group*. Patients receiving the tirilazad showed similar recovery to the 24-hour methylprednisolone infusion group. *This study thus stressed the importance of starting the initial bolus as soon as possible after the injury, and that for patients receiving the initial bolus between 3 and 8 hours of injury, an infusion of 48 hours of methylprednisolone should be administered*. The protocol is summarized in Table 25-6. Since the benefits in neurological recovery after methylprednisolone occur mostly below the level of injury, it is thought that it exerts its beneficial effect by limiting damage to the major long tracts of the spinal cord. The mechanism of action is likely related to suppression of lipid peroxidation and hydrolysis of neuronal and endothelial membranes by free radicals.

The NASCIS trials have received intense criticism over the last number of years. It should be noted that the guidelines committee of the American Association of Neurological Surgeons and Congress of Neurological Surgeons Joint Section on Disorders of the Spine and Peripheral Nerves on reviewing the evidence regarding the use MPSS in the treatment of acute SCI in adults concluded that the use of this medication could only be supported at the level of a treatment option (AANS/CNS, 2002). However, it is the authors' view that the intense criticism directed at the NASCIS II

TABLE 25-6

Methylprednisolone Therapy for Acute Spinal Cord Injury Based on Time of Presentation (NASCIS II and III Protocol)

Time of Presentation after Injury	Initial Bolus	Maintenance Infusion
<3 h after injury	30 mg/kg	5.4 mg/kg/h × 24 h
3–8 h after injury	30 mg/kg	5.4 mg/kg/h × 48 h

and III trials must be balanced by the current lack of alternative neuroprotective strategies for acute SCI. Moreover, the modest therapeutic benefit demonstrated by MPSS may potentially prove to impart a major benefit on cervical SCI patient's functional independence and quality of life.

D. Emerging Drugs for SCI—A number of promising pharmacological therapies are currently under investigation for neuroprotective abilities in animal models of SCI. These include the sodium channel blocker riluzole, the tetracycline derivative minocycline, the fusogen copolymer polyethylene glycol (PEG), and the tissue-protective hormone erythropoietin (EPO). Moreover, clinical trials investigating the putative neuroprotective and neuroregenerative properties ascribed to the Rho pathway antagonist, Cethrin® (Bio-Axone Therapeutic, Inc.), and implantation of activated autologous macrophages (ProCord®; Proneuron Biotechnologies) in patients with thoracic and cervical SCI are now underway. We anticipate that these studies will harken an era of renewed interest in translational clinical trials.

IX. Timing of Surgical Intervention after SCI—Despite the widespread use of surgery in patients with SCI in North America, the role of this intervention in improving neurological recovery remains controversial because of the lack of well-designed and executed randomized controlled trials. Early decompression and stabilization of spinal column fractures has several potential advantages: (a) allows early patient mobilization in order to prevent systemic complications of prolonged immobilization such as pulmonary infections, decubitus ulcers, thrombophlebitis, and pulmonary embolism; (b) improves neurological recovery after SCI, especially in patients with incomplete SCIs; (c) reduces hospital stay; and (d) improves rehabilitation.

Prompt stabilization of long bones and pelvic fractures in multiple trauma victims has been shown to significantly reduce patient morbidity and mortality. Recent studies comparing early versus delayed spinal surgery on patients with complete and incomplete SCI did not show any increase in medical complications in the early group. Some studies have shown a trend toward a decrease in systemic complications. There has also been a trend toward shorter hospital stay and earlier rehabilitation in patients treated with aggressive surgical therapy.

Although it seems intuitive that early decompression after SCI may improve neurological recovery, the question remains for the most part unanswered. Animal studies have shown that mechanical factors are important in the pathogenesis of SCI. MRI

investigation of SCI patients has demonstrated that the degree and extent of spinal cord compression is the most important predictor for neurological recovery. Guttman, using postural techniques and bedrest to achieve reduction and spontaneous fusion, first advocated conservative management of patients with SCI. At that time, it was believed that surgical intervention after SCI in the form of laminectomy led to a higher incidence of neurological complications. Spontaneous improvement in neurological status after conservative management has been observed in many studies. Most of the studies on nonoperative management are limited to non-controlled, retrospective analyses and thus provide limited evidence. Furthermore, laminectomy alone as a treatment for SCI often fails to decompress the spinal cord completely and can lead to spinal instability and subsequent neurological deterioration.

Modern medical intensive care management and surgical techniques in the treatment of SCI have evolved considerably over the years and have allowed earlier surgery to be performed with minimal hemodynamic and systemic complications. Although some studies have shown a trend toward better neurological recovery when surgery is performed early, there is no good statistical data supporting this approach. Most studies are indeed retrospective, case series with historical controls. Review of these studies reveals no clear consensus as to the appropriate timing of surgery after SCI, nor is there significant evidence that decompression affects neurological recovery after SCI. There is only one randomized prospective control trial reported to date regarding the timing of surgical decompression in SCI. This was a single center trial in which 62 patients were randomized to either early or late surgery. Early surgical treatment was defined as less than 72 hours after the initial trauma, with a mean time of decompression of 1.8 days. The late group was defined as surgical decompression later than 5 days after injury, and had a mean of 16.8 days. There was no difference in motor recovery at approximately 1-year follow up. Also, the investigators did not find any differences between the groups in the length of ICU stay or in-patient rehabilitation time. However, 20 of the 62 patients were lost to follow up.

Contemporary studies have shown that early surgery for SCI does not increase the systemic complication rate compared with delayed surgery. Based on this assumption, early decompression and stabilization may provide patients with SCI an optimal window for early mobilization and rehabilitation. The question regarding neurological recovery in early versus late surgical decompression in SCI thus far remains unanswered. This question is being addressed with the Surgical Treatment for Acute

Spinal Cord Injury Study (STASCIS) study, a multi-centre prospective randomized trial. Early data presented by the senior author at the Canadian Spine Society in 2008 suggests a benefit to early surgical decompression of the spinal cord. Neurological worsening associated with persistent spinal cord compression by disc and bone fragments is a widely accepted indication for early surgery.

X. Recovery after SCI

A. Somatic Motor Recovery—***Neurological improvement always occurs after SCI, even when it is complete***. In complete SCI, recovery occurs mainly at the zone of injury and continues for up to 2 years. It has been shown that when some strength is present in the spinal segment below the level of injury, recovery to Grade 4 or 5 occurs in 80% to 90% of patients. When no strength is present in that segment, only 25% to 35% show recovery to Grade 3 to 5. If the injury remains complete for longer than a week, there is usually no useful neurological recovery below the zone of partial preservation. In an extensive review of neurological recovery of complete cases, Hansebout found that approximately 1% of complete cases recover the ability to ambulate. Stover and coworkers found the best recovery in the B and C categories of incomplete injuries in which 30% to 50% of patients improved one grade. Presently, 50% to 60% of patients have incomplete injuries. Patients with incomplete cervical lesions usually recover sooner at the zone of injury as well as distal to the site. Over 80% of patients who have any voluntary movement in the lower extremities distal to the injury will recover useful motor function (ASIA class D or better).

B. Functional Status of Patients after SCI—***Paraplegia is defined as the neurological state when the most rostral muscle with no contraction is below the first dorsal interosseus (C8-T1) with no muscle contraction distally***.

   Quadriplegia is defined as the neurological state when the most rostral muscle with no contraction is the first dorsal interosseus (C8-T1) or higher.

   1. Paraplegia—Paraplegic patients are usually able to stand if sufficient strength is generated in the arms to bring them to an upright position with crutches. If quadriceps strength is less than Grade 3, orthoses for knee stabilization during standing are required. Gait is then assisted with crutches in a swinging motion. Gait assisted with crutches in paraplegic patients requires a significant amount of energy and is not practical. Most patients will prefer the wheelchair. If hip and knee strength is greater than Grade 3, patients are able to stand and only require foot orthoses to stabilize the foot and ankle. Crutches are usually required to assist gait and patients can walk only for a limited duration; a wheelchair is required for long distances.

   2. Quadriplegia—The exact level of function is critical in quadriplegic patients. Lesions above the C4 level often create respiratory impairment and if patients survive, they remain ventilator dependent. If diaphragm paralysis results from an upper motor neuron impairment, phrenic nerve stimulators may allow the patient to use their own diaphragm for ventilation. Patients can operate in wheelchairs onto which respiratory equipment is attached and they can perform desktop assisted tasks with the use of a mouth-stick. Ventilation is provided via a tracheotomy, allowing the patients to talk with exhalation.

   Table 25-7 illustrates muscle functions corresponding to functional levels below C4 in quadriplegic patients. At the *C5* level, the deltoid and elbow flexors allow shoulder and elbow flexion. An orthosis fixing the wrist allows grasp between the thumb and other fingers via a passive closing mechanism. ***Patients can then feed themselves independently***.

   The acquisition of *C6* musculature provides a major increment in the functional status of quadriplegic patients. Wrist extensors allow patients to ***propel themselves in a wheelchair, transfer from bed to chair manually, and live independently***. A wrist-hand orthosis can be used in order to improve wrist extension if the wrist extensors are weak. Another wrist orthosis linking the wrist to the metacarpophalangeal joints drives finger flexion when the wrist is extended, allowing active grasp between the thumb and fingers.

   C7 level function gives patients the use of their triceps. ***All patients with intact C7 functions should be able to transfer and live independently***. Wrist flexion and extension, as well as some finger extension are also preserved. Thumb and finger flexion is absent. The key muscles at the *C8* functional level are the thumb and finger flexors, and enable ***gross grasp and lateral pinching between the thumb and index finger***.

C. Autonomic Recovery after SCI

   1. Bladder and bowel function—***Because of the initial period of spinal shock, which can last between days to weeks, it is usually impossible to predict bladder and sexual function recovery after SCI***. After spinal shock subsides, reflex activity and spasticity may appear in the lower extremities, and

TABLE 25-7

Functional Levels of Quadriplegia

Functional Level	Key Muscles Innervated	Functional Capacity
C5	Deltoid Biceps	Shoulder and elbow flexion Arm lifting Feeding and grasping with orthoses
C6	Brachioradialis Extensor carpi radialis longus and brevis Pronator teres	Wrist extension Wheelchair propelling Transfers Grasping with orthoses Independent living possible
C7	Triceps Extensor digitorum communis Flexor carpi radialis	Full transfers Independent living
C8	Flexor digitorum profundus	Fine grasping
T1	Intrinsic hand muscles	Intrinsic hand muscle function

reflex bladder and bowel function may return. If reflex sacral activity returns after a complete injury, reflex bladder emptying will be retained in most patients. Triggering of reflex bladder emptying can be done by maneuvers such as suprapubic taping, stroking of the thighs, and Valsalva maneuver. An areflexic bladder can void by application of pressure on the bladder either externally or by Valsalva maneuver. Residual volumes can be high despite reflex bladder emptying and this can be facilitated by anticholinergic drugs that decrease smooth muscle spasm of the internal sphincter at the bladder neck, or antispasmodic drugs that decrease skeletal muscle tone in the external sphincter. External sphincter spasticity sometimes necessitates sphincterectomy to allow proper bladder emptying. Indwelling catheters are usually contraindicated because they lead to bladder constriction, which in turn leads to the formation of renal calculi and early renal failure. For the male, external condom catheter is the method of choice while in women, padding or diapering is recommended.

2. Sexual function—For a long time, patients who lost sexual function after SCI were thought to remain asexual for the rest of their life. Recent advances in the understanding of sexual neurological mechanisms and methods to enhance sexual activity have led to a significant improvement in sexual function, especially in men, after SCI. Erection in men is mainly mediated via the parasympathetic system located in segments S2 to S4. It is reflexogenic in nature, requiring an intact reflex arc, and can be induced by cutaneous or mucous membrane stimulation from areas below the level of the lesion. A complete erection is obtainable when the lesion is above T11. If the injury is below T11, only the corpora cavernosa will be involved, and not the corpus spongiosum. Psychogenic erection is thought to be mediated by a cortically activated sympathetic system located in segments T11 to L2 and can be induced by visual, auditory, olfactory or psychic stimuli. This type of erection is maintained with injuries below L2, but results only in swelling of the penis without rigidity thereby preventing coitus. When the lesion is between L2 and S2, mixed types of erections can be induced. The return of erection after SCI ranges between 54% and 95% after 2 years but its quality is usually not as good as in normal subjects. This is illustrated by a poorer successful coitus rate (5% to 75%). Patients with cervical and thoracic SCI tend to have a higher and quicker rate of recover than patients with lumbar injuries. Several methods can be utilized to enhance erection in patients with SCI such as vacuum devices, intracavernous or cutaneous injections of vasoactive drugs, penile prosthesis, and sacral anterior root stimulators.

3. Ejaculation—In men, ejaculation is mediated by the sympathetic, parasympathetic, and somatic pathways. A sympathetic center located in T11 to L2 is responsible for seminal emission from the vasa deferentia, seminal vesicles, and prostate, as well as closure of the bladder neck. The parasympathetic center located at S2 to S4 supplies the prostate and

helps in the formation of seminal fluid. The somatic center at S2 to S4 is responsible for the clonic contractions of the bulbospongiosus and ischiocavernosus muscles, leading to the projectile release of semen from the urethra. A lesion at this center prevents ejaculation proper, resulting only in dribbling. The frequency of ejaculation is usually higher in men with incomplete SCI compared with complete, lower motor neuron lesions compared with upper motor neuron, and lower lesions compared with higher ones. Methods used to enhance ejaculation or obtain semen for procreation include vibratory stimulation of the penis, electroejaculation from electric stimulation delivered from a probe, and surgical aspiration from the vas deferens.

SUGGESTED READINGS

Classic Articles

Agrawal SK, Fehlings MG. Mechanisms of secondary injury to spinal cord axons in vitro: role of Na+, Na(+)-K(+)-ATPase, the Na(+)-H+ exchanger, and the Na(+)-Ca2+ exchanger. *J Neurosci.* 1996;16:545–552.

Agrawal SK, Fehlings MG. The effect of the sodium channel blocker QX-314 on recovery after acute spinal cord injury. *J Neurotrauma.* 1997;14:81–88.

Agrawal SK, Fehlings MG. Role of NMDA and non-NMDA ionotropic glutamate receptors in traumatic spinal cord axonal injury. *J Neurosci.* 1997;17:1055–1063.

Agrawal SK, Theriault E, Fehlings MG. Role of group I metabotropic glutamate receptors in traumatic spinal cord white matter injury. *J Neurotrauma.* 1998;15:929–941.

Albin MS, Aronica MJ, Black WA, et al. Report, spinal cord injury task force, health advisory council, Dept. of Health, Commonwealth of Pennsylvania. *Penn Med.* 1978;81:29–54.

Allen AR. Surgery of experimental lesion of spinal cord equivalent to crush injury of fracture dislocation of spinal column: a preliminary report. *JAMA.* 1911;57:878–880.

Anthes DL, Theriault E, Tator CH, et al. Ultrastructural evidence for arteriolar vasospasm after spinal cord trauma. *Neurosurgery.* 1996;39:804–814.

Association ASI, Paraplegia IMSo. *International Standards for Neurological and Functional Classification of Spinal Cord Injury.* Chicago: ASIA/IMSOP; 1992.

Association ASI, Paraplegia IMSo. *International Standards for Neurological and Functional Classification of Spinal Cord Injury.* Chicago: ASIA/IMSOP; 1996.

Balentine JD, Spector M. Calcification of axons in experimental spinal cord trauma. *Ann Neurol.* 1977;2:520–523.

Barnard J, Woosley C. A study of localization in the corticospinal tracts of monkey and rat. *J Comp Neurol.* 1956;105:25–50.

Bell HS. Paralysis of both arms from injury of the upper portion of the pyramidal decussation: "cruciate paralysis." *J Neurosurg.* 1970;33:376–380.

Biering-Sorensen F, Sonksen J. Penile erection in men with spinal cord or cauda equina lesions. *Semin Neurol.* 1992;12:98–105.

Bohlman HH, Bahniuk E, Raskulinecz G, et al. Mechanical factors affecting recovery from incomplete cervical spinal cord injury: a preliminary report. *Johns Hopkins Med J.* 1979;145:115–125.

Bone LB, Johnson KD, Weigelt J, et al. Early versus delayed stabilization of femoral fractures. A prospective randomized study. *J Bone Joint Surg Am.* 1989;71:336–340.

Bracken MB, Collins WF, Freeman DF, et al. Efficacy of methylprednisolone in acute spinal cord injury. *JAMA.* 1984;251:45–52.

Bracken MB, Freeman DH, Hellenbrand K Jr, et al. Incidence of acute traumatic hospitalized spinal cord injury in the United States, 1970–1977. *Am J Epidemiol.* 1981;113:615–622.

Bracken MB, Holford TR. Effects of timing of methylprednisolone or naloxone administration on recovery of segmental and long-tract neurological function in NASCIS 2 [see comments]. *J Neurosurg.* 1993;79:500–507.

Bracken MB, Shepard MJ, Collins WF, et al. A randomized, controlled trial of methylprednisolone or naloxone in the treatment of acute spinal-cord injury. Results of the Second National Acute Spinal Cord Injury Study [see comments]. *N Engl J Med.* 1990;322:1405–1411.

Bracken MB, Shepard MJ, Holford TR, et al. Administration of methylprednisolone for 24 or 48 hours or tirilazad mesylate for 48 hours in the treatment of acute spinal cord injury. Results of the Third National Acute Spinal Cord Injury Randomized Controlled Trial. National Acute Spinal Cord Injury Study. *JAMA.* 1997;277:1597–1604.

Breasted JH. *The Edwin Smith Papyrus.* Vol 1. Chicago: University of Chicago Press; 1930.

Brisman R, Kovach RM, Johnson DO, et al. Pulmonary edema in acute transection of the cervical spinal cord. *Surg Gynecol Obstet.* 1974;139:363–366.

Brodkey JS, Miller CF, Harmody RM Jr, et al. The syndrome of acute central cervical spinal cord injury revisited. *Surg Neurol.* 1980;14:251–257.

Cantu RC. Head and spine injuries in the young athlete. In: Micheli LJ, ed. *Injuries in the Young Athlete.* Philadelphia, PA: WB Saunders; 1988:459–472.

Comarr A, Kaufman A. A survey of the neurological results in 858 spinal cord injury. A comparison of patients treated with and without laminectomy. *J Neurosurg.* 1956;13:95–106.

Coxe WS, Landau WM. Patterns of Marchi degeneration in the monkey pyramidal tract following small discrete cortical lesions. *Neurology.* 1970;20:89–100.

Crowe MJ, Bresnahan JC, Shuman SL, et al. Apoptosis and delayed degeneration after spinal cord injury in rats and monkeys [published erratum appears in *Nat Med.* 1997;3(2):240]. *Nat Med.* 1997;3:73–76.

DeVivo MJ. Causes and costs of spinal cord injury in the United States. *Spinal Cord.* 1997;35:809–813.

Dickman CA, Hadley MN, Pappas CT, et al. Cruciate paralysis: a clinical and radiographic analysis of injuries to the cervicomedullary junction. *J Neurosurg.* 1990;73:850–858.

Dimitrijevic MR. Residual motor functions in spinal cord injury. *Adv Neurol.* 1988;47:138–155.

Ditunno JF Jr, Stover SL, Freed M, et al. Motor recovery of the upper extremities in traumatic quadriplegia: a multicenter study. *Arch Phys Med Rehabil.* 1992;73:431–436.

DuBoulay GH. Pulsatile movements in the CSF pathways. *Brit J Radiol.* 1966;39:255.

Emery E, Aldana P, Bunge MB, et al. Apoptosis after traumatic human spinal cord injury. *J Neurosurg.* 1998;89:911–920.

Eyster EF, Watts C. An update of the National Head and Spinal Cord Injury Prevention Program of the American Association of Neurological Surgeons and the Congress of Neurological Surgeons. Think first. *Clin Neurosurg.* 1992;38:252–260.

Farmer JC, Vaccaro AR, Balderston RA, et al. The changing nature of admissions to a spinal cord injury center: violence on the rise. *J Spinal Disord.* 1998;11:400–403.

Fehlings MG, Tator CH. The relationships among the severity of spinal cord injury, residual neurological function, axon counts, and counts of retrogradely labeled neurons after experimental spinal cord injury. *Exp Neurol.* 1995;132:220–228.

Fine PR, Kuhlemeier KV, DeVivo MJ, et al. Spinal cord injury: an epidemiologic perspective. *Paraplegia.* 1979;17:237–250.

Folman Y, el Masri W. Spinal cord injury: prognostic indicators. *Injury.* 1989;20:92–93.

Frankel HL, Hancock DO, Hyslop G, et al. The value of postural reduction in the initial management of closed injuries of the spine with paraplegia and tetraplegia. I. *Paraplegia.* 1969;7:179–192.

Goris RJ, Gimbrere JS, van Niekerk JL, et al. Early osteosynthesis and prophylactic mechanical ventilation in the multitrauma patient. *J Trauma.* 1982;22:895–903.

Graham PM, Weingarden SI. Victims of gun shootings. A retrospective study of 36 spinal cord injured adolescents. *J Adolesc Health Care.* 1989;10:534–536.

Griffith ER, Tomko MA, Timms RJ, et al. Sexual function in spinal cord-injured patients: a review. *Arch Phys Med Rehabil.* 1973;54:539–543.

Gunby I. New focus on spinal cord injury. *JAMA.* 1981;245:1201–1206.

Hadley MN, Fitzpatrick BC, Sonntag VK, et al. Facet fracture-dislocation injuries of the cervical spine. *Neurosurgery.* 1992;30:661–666.

Hall ED, Braughler JM. Acute effects of intravenous glucocorticoid pretreatment on the in vitro peroxidation of cat spinal cord tissue. *Exp Neurol.* 1981;73:321–324.

Harvey C, Rothschild BB, Asmann AJ, et al. New estimates of traumatic SCI prevalence: a survey-based approach. *Paraplegia.* 1990;28:537–544.

Holmes G. Spinal injuries of warfare. *Brit Med J.* 1915;2:769–774.

Hussey RW, Stauffer ES. Spinal cord injury: requirements for ambulation. *Arch Phys Med Rehabil.* 1973;54:544–547.

Johnson KD, Cadambi A, Seibert GB, et al. Incidence of adult respiratory distress syndrome in patients with multiple musculoskeletal injuries: effect of early operative stabilization of fractures. *J Trauma.* 1985;25:375–384.

Kahn EA. The role of the dentate ligaments in spinal cord compression and the syndrome of lateral sclerosis. *J Neurosurg.* 1947;4:191–199.

Kalsbeek WD, McLaurin RL, Harris BS 3rd, et al. The National Head and Spinal Cord Injury Survey: major findings. *J Neurosurg.* 1980;(suppl.):S19–S31.

Koyanagi I, Tator CH, Lea PJ. Three-dimensional analysis of the vascular system in the rat spinal cord with scanning electron microscopy of vascular corrosion casts. Part 2: Acute spinal cord injury. *Neurosurgery.* 1993;33:285–291; discussion 292.

Kraus JF, Franti CE, Riggins RS, et al. Incidence of traumatic spinal cord lesions. *J Chronic Dis.* 1975;28:471–492.

Krengel WF 3rd, Anderson PA, Hanley MB, et al. Early stabilization and decompression for incomplete paraplegia due to a thoracic-level spinal cord injury. *Spine.* 1993;18:2080–2087.

Kurtzke JF. Epidemiology of spinal cord injury. *Exp Neurol.* 1975;48:163–236.

Lawrence DG, Kuypers HG. The functional organization of the motor system in the monkey. I. The effects of bilateral pyramidal lesions. *Brain.* 1968;91:1–14.

Lazorthes G, Géraud J, Espagno J, et al. Syndrome de Brown-Séquard et hernie discale cervicale. *Neurochirurgie.* 1961;7:228–231.

Levi L, Wolf A, Rigamonti D, et al. Anterior decompression in cervical spine trauma: does the timing of surgery affect the outcome? *Neurosurgery.* 1991;29:216–222.

Liu C, Chambers W. An experimental study of the corticospinal system in the monkey (*Macaca mulatta*). *J Comp Neurol.* 1964;123:257–284.

Liu XZ, Xu XM, Hu R, et al. Neuronal and glial apoptosis after traumatic spinal cord injury. *J Neurosci.* 1997;17:5395–5406.

Lou J, Lenke LG, Ludwig FJ, et al. Apoptosis as a mechanism of neuronal cell death following acute experimental spinal cord injury. *Spinal Cord.* 1998;36:683–690.

MacDonald RL, Findlay JM, Tator CH, et al. Microcystic spinal cord degeneration causing posttraumatic myelopathy. Report of two cases. *J Neurosurg.* 1988;68:466–471.

Maroon JC, Steele PB, Berlin R. Football head and neck injuries—an update. *Clin Neurosurg.* 1979;27:414–429.

McVeigh JF. Experimental cord crushes, with special reference to the mechanical factors involved and subsequent changes in the areas of the cord affected. *Arch Surg.* 1923;7:573.

Meguro K, Tator CH. Effect of multiple trauma on mortality and neurological recovery after spinal cord or cauda equina injury. *Neurol Med Chir (Tokyo).* 1988;28:34–41.

Pappas CT, Gibson AR, Sonntag VK, et al. Decussation of hind-limb and fore-limb fibers in the monkey corticospinal tract: relevance to cruciate paralysis. *J Neurosurg.* 1991;75:935–940.

Quencer RM, Bunge RP, Egnor M, et al. Acute traumatic central cord syndrome: MRI-pathological correlations. *Neuroradiology.* 1992;34:85–94.

Regan RF, Choi DW. Glutamate neurotoxicity in spinal cord cell culture. *Neuroscience.* 1991;43:585–591.

Rivlin AS, Tator CH. Effect of duration of acute spinal cord compression in a new acute cord injury model in the rat. *Surg Neurol.* 1978;10:38–43.

Scher AT. Vertex impact and cervical dislocation in rugby players. *S Afr Med J.* 1981;59:227–228.

Schneider RC. A syndrome in acute cervical injuries for which early operation is indicated. *J Neurosurg.* 1951;8:360–367.

Schneider RC. Concomitant craniocerebral and spinal trauma, with special reference to the cervicomedullary region. *Clin Neurosurg.* 1970;17:266–309.

Schneider RC. Traumatic spinal cord syndromes and their management. *Clin Neurosurg.* 1973;20:424–492.

Schneider RC, Cherry GL, Pantek H, et al. The syndrome of acute central cervical spinal cord injury. *J Neurosurg.* 1954;11:546–577.

Schneider RC, Thompson JM, Bebin J, et al. The syndrome of the acute central cervical spinal cord injury. *J Neurol Neurosurg Psychiatr.* 1958;21.

Schwartzman RJ. A behavioral analysis of complete unilateral section of the pyramidal tract at the medullary level in Macaca mulatta. *Ann Neurol.* 1978;4:234–44.

Sonksen J, Biering-Sorensen F. Fertility in men with spinal cord or cauda equina lesions. *Semin Neurol.* 1992;12:106–114.

Stys PK, Waxman SG, Ransom BR, et al. Ionic mechanisms of anoxic injury in mammalian CNS white matter: role of Na+ channels and Na(+)-Ca2+ exchanger. *J Neurosci.* 1992;12:430–439.

Tarlov IM, Klinger H. Spinal cord compression studies: II, time limits pre-recovery after acute compression in days. *Arch Neurol Psychiatry.* 1954;71:271–290.

Tator CH. Spine-spinal cord relationships in spinal cord trauma. *Clin Neurosurg.* 1983;30:479–494.

Tator CH, Carson JD, Edmonds VE. Spinal injuries in ice hockey. *Clin Sports Med.* 1998;17:183–194.

Tator CH, Duncan EG, Edmonds VE, et al. Comparison of surgical and conservative management in 208 patients with acute spinal cord injury. *Can J Neurol Sci.* 1987;14:60–69.

Tator CH, Edmonds VE. National survey of spinal injuries in hockey players. *Can Med Assoc J.* 1984;130:875–880.

Tator CH, Edmonds VE, New ML, et al. Diving: a frequent and potentially preventable cause of spinal cord injury. *Can Med Assoc J.* 1981;124:1323–1324.

Tator CH, Fehlings MG. Review of the secondary injury theory of acute spinal cord trauma with emphasis on vascular mechanisms [see comments]. *J Neurosurg.* 1991;75:15–26.

Tator CH, Rowed DW. Current concepts in the immediate management of acute spinal cord injuries. *Can Med Assoc J.* 1979;121:1453–1464.

Taylor AR. The mechanism of injury to the spinal cord in the neck without damage to the vertebral column. *J Bone Joint Surg.* 1951;33B:543–547.

Taylor AR, Blackwood W. Paraplegia in hyperextension cervical injuries with normal radiographic appearance. *J Bone Joint Surg.* 1948;30B:245–248.

Theodore J, Robin ED. Speculations on neurogenic pulmonary edema (NPE). *Am Rev Respir Dis.* 1976;113:405–411.

Torg JS. Epidemiology, pathomechanics, and prevention of football-induced cervical spinal cord trauma. *Exerc Sport Sci Rev.* 1992;20:321–338.

Torg JS, Pavlov H, Genuario SE, et al. Neurapraxia of the cervical spinal cord with transient quadriplegia. *J Bone Joint Surg Am.* 1986;68:1354–1370.

Torg JS, Vegso JJ, Sennett B, et al. The National Football Head and Neck Injury Registry. 14-year report on cervical quadriplegia, 1971 through 1984. *JAMA.* 1985;254:3439–3443.

Tower S. Pyramidal lesion in the monkey. *Brain.* 1940;63:36–90.

Tymianski M, Tator CH. Normal and abnormal calcium homeostasis in neurons: a basis for the pathophysiology of traumatic and ischemic central nervous system injury. *Neurosurgery.* 1996;38:1176–1195.

Vaccaro AR, Daugherty RJ, Sheehan TP, et al. Neurologic outcome of early versus late surgery for cervical spinal cord injury. *Spine.* 1997;22:2609–2613.

Vale FL, Burns J, Jackson AB, et al. Combined medical and surgical treatment after acute spinal cord injury: results of a prospective pilot study to assess the merits of aggressive medical resuscitation and blood pressure management. *J Neurosurg.* 1997;87:239–246.

Wallenberg A. Anatomischer Befund in einem als "acute bulbäraffection (embolie der Art. cerebellar. post. inf. sinistr?)" beschrieben Falle. *Arch Psych.* 1901;34:923–959.

Waxman SG, Ransom BR, Stys PK, et al. Non-synaptic mechanisms of Ca(2+)-mediated injury in CNS white matter. *Trends Neurosci.* 1991;14:461–468.

Wiberg J, Hauge HN. Neurological outcome after surgery for thoracic and lumbar spine injuries. *Acta Neurochir (Wien).* 1988;91:106–112.

Wilberger JE. Diagnosis and management of spinal cord trauma. *J Neurotrauma.* 1991;8(suppl. 1):S21–S28.

Wrathall JR, Choiniere D, Teng YD, et al. Dose-dependent reduction of tissue loss and functional impairment after spinal cord trauma with the AMPA/kainate antagonist NBQX. *J Neurosci.* 1994;14:6598–6607.

Yashimata Y, Takashi M, Matsuno Y, et al. Acute spinal cord injury: MRI correlated with myelopathy. *Br J Radiol.* 1991;64:201–209.

Yong C, Arnold PM, Zoubine MN, et al. Apoptosis in cellular compartments of rat spinal cord after severe contusion injury. *J Neurotrauma.* 1998;15:459–472.

Recent Articles

AANS/CNS. Pharmacological therapy after acute cervical spinal cord injury. *Neurosurgery.* 2002;50:S63–S72.

Baptiste MG, Fehlings MG. Pharmacological approaches to repair the injured spinal cord. *J Neurotrauma.* 2003;3; 318–324.

Fehlings MG. Editorial: recommendations regarding the use of methylprednisolone in acute spinal cord injury: making sense out of the controversy. *Spine.* 2001;26:S56–S57.

Review Articles

Fehlings M, Tator C. An evidence-based review of surgical decompression for acute SCI: rationale, indications, and timing based on experimental and clinical studies. *J Neurosurg Spine.* 1999.

Stover SL. Review of forty years of rehabilitation issues in spinal cord injury. *J Spinal Cord Med.* 1995;18:175–182.

Tator CH, Fehlings MG. Review of the secondary injury theory of acute spinal cord trauma with emphasis on vascular mechanisms. *J Neurosurg.* 1991;75:15–26.

Textbooks

Barnett HJM, Jousse AT. Postraumatic syringomyelia (cystic myelopathy). In: Vinken PJ, Bruyn GW, eds. *Handbook of Clinical Neurology.* Amsterdam, New York: North-Holland; 1976:113–157.

Braakman R, Penning L. Injuries of the cervical spine. In: Vinken PJ, Bruyn GW, eds. *Handbook of Clinical Neurology.* Amsterdam, New York: North-Holland; 1976:227–380.

Breasted JH. *The Edwin Smith Papyrus.* Vol 1. Chicago: University of Chicago Press; 1930.

Brown-Séquard CE. *Course of Lectures on the Physiology and Pathology of the Central Nervous System.* Philadelphia, PA: Collins; 1860.

Burstein AW, Otis JC, Torg JS, et al. Mechanisms and pathogenics of athletic injuries in the cervical spine. In: Torg JS, ed. *Athletic Injuries to the Head, Neck and Face.* Philadelphia, PA: Lea & Fibiger; 1982:119–149.

Cantu RC. Head and spine injuries in the young athlete. In: Micheli LJ, ed. *Injuries in the Young Athlete.* Philadelphia, PA: WB Saunders; 1988:459–472.

Carpenter MB. *Core Text of Neuroanatomy.* Baltimore, MD: Williams & Wilkins; 1991.

Collins JG. Types of injuries and imapirments due to injuries. Vital and Health Statistics. Vol 159: DHHS Publication (PHS) 87–1587.

Guttmann L. Initial treatment of traumatic paraplegia and tetraplegia. In: Harris P, ed. *Spinal Injury Symposium.* Edinburgh: Morrison & Gibb, Ltd., Royal College of Surgeons; 1963:80–92.

Guttmann L. *Spinal Cord Injuries. Comprehensive Management and Research.* Oxford, England: Blackwell; 1976.

Hansebout R. A comprehensive review of methods of improving cord recovery after spinal cord injury. In: Tator C, ed. *Early Management of Acute Spinal Cord Injury.* New York, NY: Raven Press; 1982:181–196.

Kiss ZHT, Tator CH. Neurogenic shock. In: Geller ER, ed. *Shock and Ressuscitation.* New York, NY: McGraw-Hill; 1993:421–440.

Kraus JF. Epidemiological aspects of acute spinal cord injury: A review of incidence, prevalence, causes and outcome. In: Becker DP, Povlishock JT, eds. *Central Nervous System Trauma Status Report, 1985: NINCDS.* 1985:313–322.

Narayan RK, Wilberger JE, Povlishock JT. *Neurotrauma.* New York, NY: McGraw Hill; 1996.

Thron A, Rossberg C, Mironov A. *Vascular Anatomy of the Spinal Cord: Neuroradiological Investigations and Clinical Symptoms.* New York, NY: Spinger-Verlag, Wien; 1988:114.

Woburn M. Factsheet No. 2: Spinal Cord Injury Statistical Information: National Spinal Cord Injury Association; 1992.

CHAPTER 26

General Principles of Vertebral Bony, Ligamentous, and Penetrating Injuries

Robert Greenleaf, Jory D. Richman and Daniel T. Altman

I. Cervical Spine
   A. Clinical Anatomy
      1. Occipitoatlantoaxial complex—The cervical spine consists of two atypical vertebrae, the **atlas (C1) and axis (C2)**, and five lower cervical vertebrae. The occipitoatlantoaxial complex functions as a unit, being composed of synovial joints surrounding the articulations and devoid of any intervertebral discs. The atlas consists of an anterior and posterior arch and two lateral masses. *The superior surfaces of the lateral masses articulate with the occipital condyles, allowing 25° of flexion and extension and 5° of lateral bending and rotation. The inferior aspect of the lateral masses of C1 articulates with the superior facets of C2, allowing rotation.* Approximately 50% of the rotatory movement of the entire cervical spine occurs at the atlantoaxial articulation. In the upper cervical spine, flexion is limited by bony anatomy, and extension is limited by the tectorial membrane. Rotation and lateral bending are restricted by the contralateral alar ligament. The axis, or second cervical vertebrae, consists of a vertebral body, an odontoid process (dens), pedicles, laminae, and a spinous process. The synchondrosis between the dens and the body of the axis generally closes by age 6 years, but may persist into adulthood as a thin sclerotic line that may resemble a nondisplaced fracture.
      2. Odontoid process—The odontoid process (dens) with its attached ligamentous structures is the major stabilizer of the atlantoaxial articulation. The atlantoaxial joint depends on a complex of ligaments for stability (Fig. 26-1). The dens is held against the anterior arch of the atlas by the strong **transverse ligament**, which inserts on the lateral masses of C1. The **alar ligaments** originate from the occipital condyles, attach to the tip of the dens, and limit excessive lateral flexion and rotation. The **apical ligament** originates at the ventral surface of the foramen magnum and inserts on the tip of the odontoid. It is only a minor stabilizer of the craniocervical junction. The odontoid may fracture alone or occasionally in combination with ligamentous disruption. Isolated rupture of the transverse ligament, although common in patients with rheumatoid arthritis, is relatively uncommon, secondary to trauma. *At the C1–C2 level the space available for the spinal cord is greater than at any other level of the cervical spine. Steel's rule of thirds states that the area inside the atlas is equally occupied in thirds by the dens, spinal cord, and space. The space is primarily occupied by cerebrospinal fluid. This accounts for the low incidence of spinal cord injuries associated with C1 and C2 fractures.* Complete spinal cord injuries at this level are rarely survivable events.
      3. Anatomy of the subaxial cervical spine—The subaxial cervical vertebrae (C3 to C7) are relatively uniform in their morphologic characteristics. The vertebral body is connected posteriorly to the neural arch by the **pedicles**. The pedicles connect the vertebral body to the lateral masses. Within the lateral masses are **superior and inferior facets**, which form diarthrodial joints. The facet joints are oriented 45° in the sagittal plane and neutrally in the coronal plane. The superior articular facet (of the lower vertebrae) is anterior and inferior to the inferior

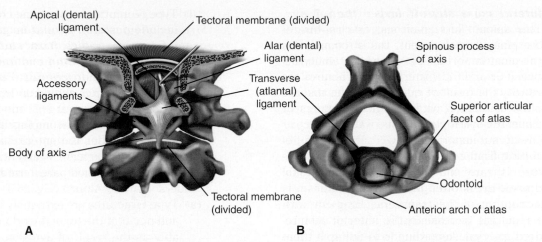

FIGURE 26-1 Atlantoaxial joint and cranium (the occipitoatlantoaxial complex). **A.** Posterior coronal view. Note the alar, transverse, and apical ligaments. **B.** Superior view of the atlantoaxial articulation.

articular facet of the vertebra above. The **uncinate processes** are small, bony ridges that project from the posterolateral aspect of the superior end plate of the vertebral body. They articulate with indentations on the inferior surface of the adjacent vertebral body, which form the **uncovertebral joints of Luschka**. The **transverse foramina** from C2 to C7 are surrounded by the pedicles, transverse processes, and facets. Spinous processes from C2 to C6 are usually bifid. The C7 spinous process is usually nonbifid and the most easily palpable. The vertebral arteries originate from the first branch of the subclavian arteries and usually enter the spine at the foramen transversarium of C6. The artery passes through the foramen of C1 and then turns sharply medially and superiorly into the foramen magnum. Although rare, fractures of the transverse process or fracture-dislocations of the cervical spine may cause injury to the vertebral artery.

4. Stability of the subaxial cervical spine—The lower cervical spine has little intrinsic bony stability. Spinal ligaments include the anterior and posterior longitudinal ligaments, the ligamentum flavum, and the supraspinous, interspinous, and intertransverse ligaments. The **anterior longitudinal ligament** covers the anterior surface of the vertebral body and resists extension moments to the vertebral column. The **posterior longitudinal ligament** is narrower than the anterior longitudinal ligament and is continuous with the tectoral membrane. It covers the posterior surface of the vertebral body and resists hyperflexion moments. The interspinous and supraspinous ligaments insert on the spinous processes and limit flexion. The

intervertebral discs between the bodies of the vertebrae consist of a central nucleus pulposus and a strong outer annulus fibrosis, which also provides stability and limits motion at each level of the subaxial cervical spine.

B. Injuries of the Cervical Spine
1. Injuries involving the occiput, atlas, and axis
   • Atlanto-occipital dislocation—Atlanto-occipital dislocation usually results from a high-energy injury in a patient with concomitant head trauma; the injury is often fatal. These rare injuries are often associated with significant delays in diagnosis.
   • Occipital condyle fractures—Anderson and Montesano classified occipital condyle fractures seen on CT based on mechanism of injury.
   (a) Type I injuries are impaction fractures of the condyle secondary to an axial load.
   (b) Type II injuries are basilar skull fractures associated with fractures of the condyle.
   (c) Type III injuries are avulsion fractures of the alar ligaments. This type of injury represents a more unstable injury with a higher association with atlanto-occipital dissociation.
   • Atlas (C1) fractures—Atlas (C1) fractures are generally felt to be secondary to an axial load. Fracture of the C1 ring can involve the anterior arch, the posterior arch, the lateral masses, or most commonly the anterior and posterior arches **(Jefferson's fracture). Fractures of the atlas are usually not associated with neurologic symptoms and most are stable. Injuries are considered radiographically unstable if the open-mouth AP radiograph reveals a combined**

lateral mass step-off larger than 7 mm. This amount of step-off suggests rupture of the transverse ligament, the strongest and the most important ligament for stability between C1 and C2. Posterior arch fractures are usually the result of extension forces and are often associated with odontoid fractures or traumatic spondylolisthesis of C2.

- C1–C2 subluxation—C1–C2 subluxation resulting from acute transverse ligament rupture is rare and as with atlanto-occipital dislocation is often fatal. The mechanism is disruption of the transverse ligament with a resultant increase in the anterior atlanto-dens interval. According to Fielding, if there is less than 3 mm of anterior displacement the transverse ligament is intact; if there is 3 to 5 mm of anterior displacement the transverse ligament is ruptured; and if there is more than 5 mm of anterior displacement the transverse and alar ligaments are likely ruptured. Further, if the ADI is greater than 7 mm, there is probable rupture of the tectorial membrane.
- Atlantoaxial rotatory subluxation—Atlantoaxial rotatory subluxation is often difficult to diagnose, which may cause a delay in treatment. In adults, the injury is usually related to motor-vehicle trauma and may be associated with fracture of the lateral mass as a result of flexion and rotation. In children, the injuries are usually self-limited and are the result of a viral illness. Fielding divides rotatory subluxation into four types (Fig. 26-2).
  - (a) Type I injuries are the most common. Radiographic findings reveal fixed rotational deformities without anterior displacement or disruption of the transverse ligament.
  - (b) Type II injuries demonstrate transverse ligament insufficiency with 3 to 5 mm of anterior displacement of the atlas.
  - (c) Type III injuries have more than 5 mm of anterior displacement of the atlas. The transverse ligament is typically ruptured.
  - (d) Type IV injuries are the least common and include posterior displacement of the atlas and associated rotatory subluxation.
- Odontoid fractures—Odontoid fractures may occur when flexion forces cause anterior displacement or when extension forces cause posterior displacement of the odontoid. These motions result in impingement of the dens against either the anterior arch of the atlas or the transverse ligament. The classification system most often used is that by Anderson and D'Alonzo (Fig. 26-3).
  - (a) Type I fractures are extremely uncommon and occur at the tip of the odontoid, probably as the result of avulsion of the alar ligaments. Type I fractures may be associated with craniocervical dislocation and must be ruled out radiographically and clinically.
  - (b) Type II fractures are the most common and occur at the junction of the base of the odontoid and the body of C2. The fracture does not extend into the C1–C2 articulation. Type II fractures have a high rate of nonunion and pseudoarthrosis because the blood supply to the cephalad fragment is disrupted.
  - (c) Type III fractures occur within the cancellous bone of the body of the axis.
- Traumatic spondylolisthesis of the axis—Traumatic spondylolisthesis of the axis (hangman's fracture) is usually a combined hyperextension and axial loading injury, causing fracture of the C2 pars interarticularis. As with other fractures of the upper cervical spine, traumatic spondylolisthesis of the axis tends to decompress the neural canal, and thus neurologic involvement is uncommon. The most widely used classification is by Levine and Edwards and is based on a lateral cervical spine radiograph (Fig. 26-4).
  - (a) Type I fractures are usually secondary to hyperextension and axial loading with less than 3 mm of displacement of C2 on C3.

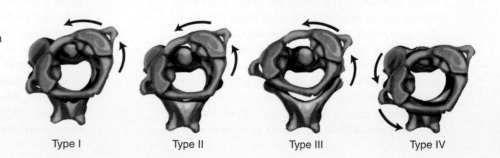

FIGURE 26-2 Four types of atlantoaxial rotatory subluxation according to Fielding.

Type I   Type II   Type III   Type IV

Type I   Type II   Type III

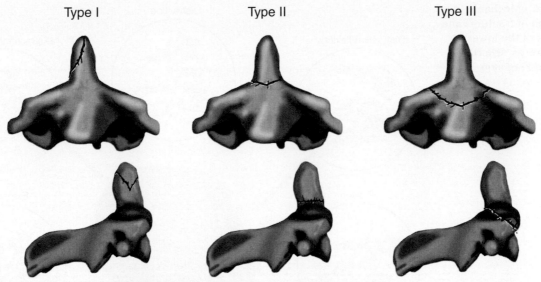

FIGURE 26-3   Anderson and D'Alonzo classification of odontoid fractures.

Type I   Type II   Type IIa   Type III

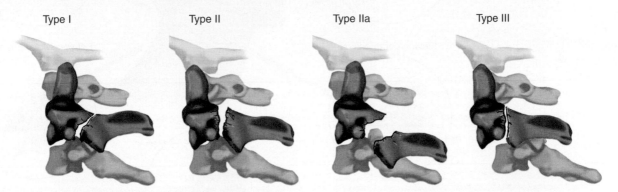

FIGURE 26-4   Classification of traumatic spondylolisthesis of the axis as described by Levine and Edwards.

(b)   Type II injuries also result from hyperextension and axial loading but have significant angulation, translation, or both. Type IIa fractures are the result of a flexion force and have minimal translation but severe angulation.

(c)   Type III fracture-dislocations are secondary to a flexion force and result in severe angulation and displacement as well as concomitant unilateral or bilateral facet dislocations at C2–C3. Type III injuries are the pattern most commonly associated with neurologic deficits.

(d)   Stability—Type I fractures are stable, whereas Types II, IIa, and III are unstable disruptions of the C2–C3 motion segment.

2.   Injuries involving the lower cervical spine— The lateral cervical spine radiograph is important to evaluate for gross bony or ligamentous injury by ensuring continuity of the longitudinal "lines" (Fig. 26-5). A comprehensive classification system of closed fractures and dislocations of the lower cervical spine based

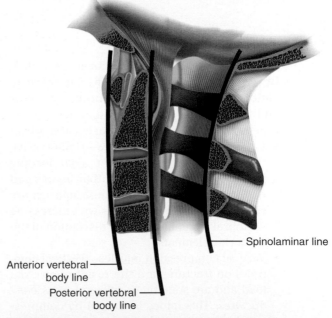

Spinolaminar line

Anterior vertebral
body line

Posterior vertebral
body line

FIGURE 26-5   Radiographic lines seen on the lateral cervical spine film to evaluate for bony or ligamentous injury. The facets appear as stacked blocks or parallelograms.

FIGURE 26-6 Mechanistic classification of fractures and dislocations of the lower cervical spine as described by Allen and Ferguson.

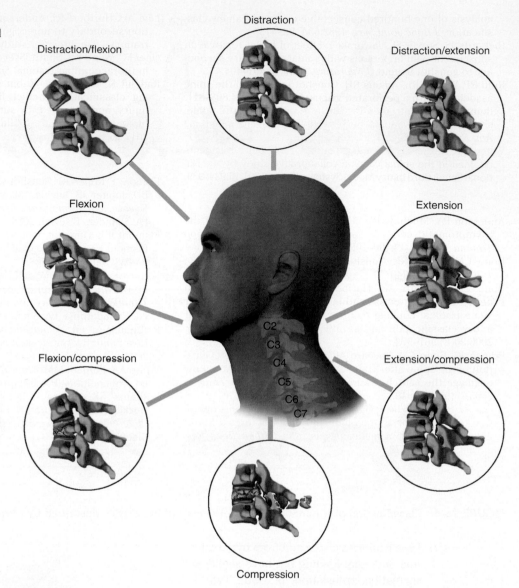

Distraction/flexion

Distraction

Distraction/extension

Flexion

Extension

Flexion/compression

Extension/compression

C2
C3
C4
C5
C6
C7

Compression

on mechanism of injury has been described by Allen and Ferguson (Fig. 26-6). This classification describes both the major injury vector and the position of the head and neck at the time of injury. There are six basic categories.

- Compressive flexion injuries—Compressive flexion injuries result from axial loading forces such as diving and football injures and motor-vehicle accidents. These injuries are subclassified into five stages with increasing vertebral comminution and disruption of the posterior elements.

- Vertical compression injuries—Vertical compression fractures are the result of an axial load and are sometimes referred to as *burst fractures*. This injury is caused by compression to the vertebral body with the posterior ligaments remaining intact.

- Distractive flexion injuries—Distractive flexion injuries usually result in posterior ligamentous disruption without fracture. These injuries occur most often from motor-vehicle accidents or falls and produce distractive or tensile forces on the posterior ligamentous structures.

  (a) Stage I injuries are simple flexion sprains.

  (b) Stage II injuries usually occur with rotation and result in unilateral facet dislocation and approximately 25% translation of the vertebral body.

  (c) Stage III injuries produce a bilateral facet dislocation and have approximately 50% translation. Prior to reduction in the obtunded or anesthetized patient, an MRI is often necessary to evaluate for concomitant disc herniation.

(d) Stage IV injuries demonstrate 100% vertebral body translation.

- Compressive extension injuries—Compressive extension injuries result from a frontal force to the head or face and are frequently associated with maxillofacial trauma. These injuries have been subdivided into five stages based on the degree of disruption of the posterior elements and vertebral body translation.

- Distractive extension injuries—Distractive extension injuries are less common than compressive extension injuries. The mechanism of injury causes a failure of the anterior longitudinal ligament or a transverse fracture of the vertebral body. These injuries may be difficult to diagnose because they primarily involve soft tissue and may spontaneously reduce when the head is in a neutral position. Distractive extension injuries are frequently associated with *central cord syndrome* in the elderly patient with preexisting spondylolysis and central canal stenosis.

- Lateral flexion injuries—Lateral flexion injuries are the least common injuries and are caused by asymmetric compression of the vertebral body. There may be an associated fracture of the neural arch.

II. Thoracolumbar Spine
  A. Clinical Anatomy
    1. Thoracic spine—The thoracic spine consists of 12 vertebrae. The facet joints are oriented 60° in the sagittal plane and 20° posterior in the coronal plane.
    2. Lumbar spine—The lumbar spine consists of five vertebrae (Fig. 26-7). The facet joints are oriented 90° in the sagittal plane and 45° anterior in the coronal plane.
    3. Superior articular facet—In both thoracic and lumbar spines, the superior articular facet (from the lower vertebrae) of the facet joint is anterior and lateral to the inferior articular facet of the vertebra above.
    4. Supporting ligaments of the thoracic and lumbar spines (Fig. 26-8).
      - Entire length of the spine
        (a) Anterior longitudinal ligament
        (b) Posterior longitudinal ligament
        (c) Supraspinous ligament
      - Each level of the spine
        (a) Ligamentum flavum
        (b) Interspinous ligament
  B. Injuries of the Thoracolumbar Spine
    1. Classification—Several classifications exist for thoracolumbar injuries; they are based on fracture morphology, fracture mechanism, or both factors. With improved imaging techniques, classification schemes have been further defined to address the issue of spine stability. White and Panjabi have defined *spinal instability* clinically as the loss of the ability of the spine to maintain structure under physiologic conditions. In Holdsworth's initial two-column model of the spine, the integrity of the posterior ligamentous complex determined the stability of the spine. *Denis further classified the spine into a three-column model* with the use of computed tomography (Fig. 26-9). The *anterior column* includes the anterior longitudinal ligament and the anterior half of the vertebral body and disc. The *middle column* consists of the posterior longitudinal ligament and the

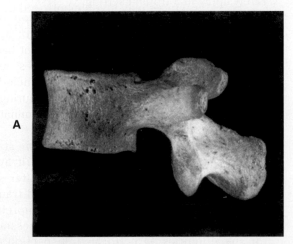

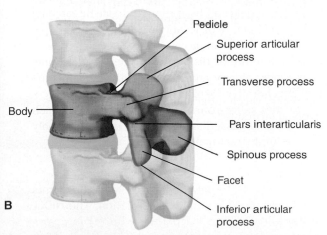

Pediole

Superior articular process

Transverse process

Body

Pars interarticularis

Spinous process

Facet

Inferior articular process

A

B

FIGURE 26-7 Lateral view of a lumbar vertebra **(A)** and a schematic drawing **(B)** demonstrating the superior and inferior articular processes (and facets). (**A,** reprinted with permission from Weissman BNW, Sledge CB. *Orthopedic Radiology.* Philadelphia, PA: WB Saunders; 1986.)

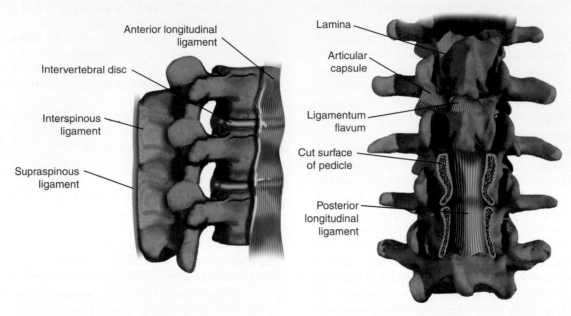

FIGURE 26-8   Supporting ligaments of the spine.

posterior half of the vertebral body and disc. The ***posterior column*** includes the bony neural arch (pedicles, lamina, facets, and spinous process) and the associated ligamentous structures, including the facet capsules, ligamentum flavum, and spinous ligaments.

2. Mechanism of injury—The thoracolumbar junction is the most frequently affected area for vertebral fractures because it is the transitional zone between the rigid thoracic spine and the more flexible lumbar spine. In addition, axial forces are concentrated at the thoracolumbar junction, since the sagittal alignment of the spine is neutral between thoracic kyphosis and lumbar lordosis. The most common mechanisms associated with thoracolumbar injuries are axial compression, flexion, shear, and flexion-distraction. Denis developed a classification system that categorizes

major spinal injuries into four different groups: compression fractures, burst fractures, flexion-distraction injuries, and fracture-dislocations. Gertzbein has introduced a comprehensive classification with three broad mechanistic patterns: compression, distraction, and multidirectional with translation. Each of these is further divided by fracture pattern (Fig. 26-10).

• Compression fractures—Compression fractures by definition involve the anterior column and typically result from a flexion force to the spine. If compression of the vertebral body exceeds 50%, the posterior ligamentous structures may be disrupted. Denis classified compression fractures into four types. Fractures may involve both end plates (Type A), the superior end plate (Type B), the inferior end plate (Type C), or central

FIGURE 26-9   Denis three-column model of the thoracolumbar spine with involved structures.

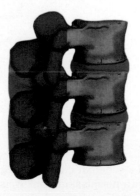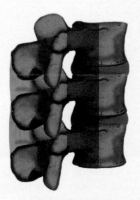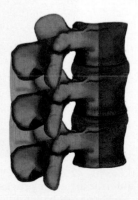

Posterior column   Middle column   Anterior column

FIGURE 26-10 Gertzbein classification of thoracolumbar fractures. Type A involves compression of the vertebral body. Type B involves distraction with anterior and posterior element injury. Type C involves anterior and posterior element injury with translation and rotation. (From Gertzbein SD. *Fractures of the Thoracic and Lumbar Spine.* Baltimore, MD: Williams & Wilkins; 1992, with permission.)

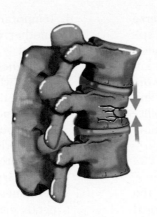 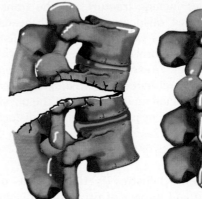 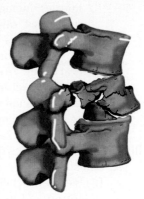

Type A   **Type B**   **Type C**

failure of the body with both end plates intact Type D). Type B injuries are the most common. Compression fractures are common in the elderly population, especially in osteoporotic postmenopausal women. Short tau inversion recovery (STIR)-weight MRI is the best method to evaluate for an acute compression fracture. The presence of an intravertebral vacuum cleft on plain radiographs and a high T2 signal on MRI suggest nonunion of the vertebral fracture with osteonecrosis.

- Burst fractures—Burst fractures cause disruption of the anterior and middle columns and most frequently occur at the thoracolumbar junction. They are caused primarily by an *axial loading mechanism.* Approximately 50% of patients with burst fractures have neurologic deficits. Attempts have been made to classify these fractures into stable and unstable based on the integrity of the posterior ligamentous structures.

- Flexion-distraction injuries—Flexion distraction injuries are caused by a flexion force that results in distractive failure of all three vertebral columns and may occur through bone, soft tissues, or both structures. These injuries are sometimes referred to as *seat belt injuries or chance fractures* and have classically occurred in passengers restrained by a lap belt without a shoulder harness. The "seat belt" sign, an abdominal ecchymosis caused by the lap belt, may be present and should raise suspicion for an underlying abdominal injury. Injuries with primarily ligamentous involvement may create chronic instability, whereas flexion-distraction injuries with predominantly bony involvement have an excellent capacity for healing.

- Translational injuries (fracture-dislocation)— Translational injuries are highly unstable,

involve all three columns, and often cause neurologic deficit. These injuries may result from combined compression, tension, rotation, or shear forces (Fig. 26-11). Often, the injury presents as a fracture-dislocation of the spine, and less commonly, a pure dislocation (ligamentous injury without fracture) may occur. Radiographic signs of translational

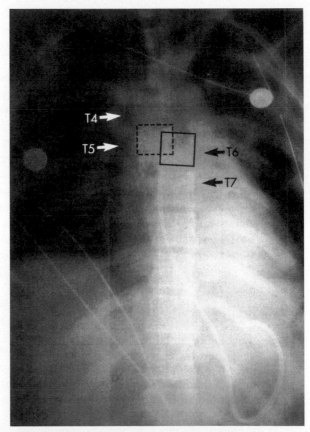

FIGURE 26-11 Anteroposterior radiograph demonstrating an unstable translational injury at T5–T6 as a result of a motor-vehicle accident.

injuries include fractures of the transverse processes, dislocation of the rib heads, spinous process widening, and subtle listhesis of the vertebral bodies, especially with lateral offset. ***These complex injuries have the highest incidence of neurologic deficit*** and the physician must be alert to the possibility of a reduced or partially reduced dislocation.

III. Penetrating Injuries of the Spine
  A. Ballistics
    1. Overview—Ballistics is the science of the motion and impact of projectiles discharged from firearms. ***The damage created by a projectile depends on mass, velocity, and bullet composition and design***. The amount of tissue damage caused by a bullet depends on its kinetic energy (KE), which is defined by the formula $KE = \frac{1}{2} MV^2$, where M is mass and V is velocity. Low velocity generally refers to a firearm that can project a bullet at 1,000 ft per second or slower. High-velocity bullets travel at velocities in excess of 2,000 ft per second. There has been a gradual blurring of the distinction between civilian and military firearms, and an increasing percentage of civilian firearm injuries are caused by high-velocity weapons. Most handgun injuries, however, should be considered low-velocity ballistic trauma.
    2. Wounding capacity—***The composition and design of a bullet affect its wounding capacity***. Military ammunition, under international law, must be fully jacketed with a hard metal such as copper to prevent expansion and unnecessary deformation of the projectile. Jacketed bullets are designed for maximal penetration and minimal deformation. Civilian weapons and many of those used by law enforcement officials are not under the same constraints. Nonjacketed, hollow-tipped, or soft-nosed bullets deform significantly on impact, imparting more tissue damage than comparable jacketed bullets of similar mass and velocity.
    3. Secondary missiles—A bullet striking the body creates ***secondary missiles*** such as bone fragments or articles of clothing, which may also impart significant tissue damage. Shattered bone fragments can cause more damage to neural elements in the spinal canal than the actual bullet because their course is erratic and unpredictable. Bullets fired at high velocity have a tendency to yaw or tumble, which also increases the probability of fragmentation on impact.

    4. Temporary and permanent cavitation—Another critical element of wound ballistics concerns the mechanism of ***temporary and permanent cavitation***. Temporary cavitation occurs when a high-velocity projectile accelerates the tissues forward and sideways, causing an expanding cavity that enlarges on passage of the bullet. The cavity formed is at subatmospheric pressure, which sucks air and material into the entrance and exit wounds. The temporary cavity rapidly collapses to form the permanent cavity, which is the tissue permanently macerated or crushed by the projectile. Temporary cavitation explains why nerves and blood vessels at a distance from the immediate bullet path can incur significant damage. Temporary cavitation is more dramatic in high-velocity injuries, whereas lower velocity injuries involve more of a crushing mechanism.
    5. Shotgun injuries—Shotgun injuries differ from gunshot wounds in that the mass of the projectile is far greater, releasing much more kinetic energy when fired at close range. In addition to the pellets, shotgun charges contain wadding, which often becomes embedded in the wound, complicating wound management. This wadding material, consisting of paper or plastic particles, must be thoroughly debrided to prevent secondary infection and wound necrosis.
  B. Epidemiology—Approximately 14% of spinal cord injuries are caused by penetrating trauma, although this figure is higher in many urban trauma centers. Gunshot wounds are now the second leading cause of spinal cord injuries after motor-vehicle accidents. In a recent study, male victims outnumbered female victims by nearly 10 to 1. Unfortunately, most victims of penetrating spinal cord trauma are young, with a peak incidence in the third decade of life. ***More than half of spinal cord injuries caused by penetrating trauma are complete injuries***.
  C. Patient Evaluation—A patient with a suspected gunshot wound to the spine should be evaluated according to standard trauma protocols. Spinal immobilization is essential until clinical and radiographic assessment is made of the vertebral column.
    1. History—The history should determine, if possible, the type of weapon that caused the injury. The conscious and alert patient should be questioned for the presence of paresthesias or numbness. A complaint of transient paralysis after the injury is highly significant.
    2. Physical examination—The physical examination should begin with inspection of the entrance and exit wounds. The presence of a

large wound should alert the physician to the probability of significant wound cavitation. A detailed neurologic examination is performed to assess motor function, reflexes, and sensation. ***Any deficits must be documented and reassessed at frequent intervals*** for possible worsening or progression to a more cephalad level. A rectal examination with assessment of the bulbocavernosus reflex should be performed to determine whether spinal shock is present. Priapism is a poor prognostic sign for neurologic recovery when it is present.

3. Radiographs—AP and lateral radiographs of the vertebral column are obtained to assess the degree of missile and bone fragmentation. Significant bullet fragmentation indicates a large permanent cavity. A CT scan is recommended for assessing the extent of spinal canal encroachment by bone or bullet fragments of the three spinal columns. Other imaging studies such as barium swallows, arteriography, and intravenous pyelography may be necessary to assess the integrity of adjacent visceral or vascular structures.

D. Treatment of Gunshot Wounds to the Spine

1. Wound management—Penetrating wounds to the chest, thorax, and abdomen require immediate surgical exploration if there is evidence of vascular, tracheal, esophageal, or visceral injury. Large or contaminated wounds to the torso, especially shotgun injuries, may require surgical debridement. Empiric antibiotic treatment is begun with a first or second-generation cephalosporin for 48 to 72 hours for uncontaminated wounds without hollow viscus perforation. Grossly contaminated wounds, especially if the bullet may have traversed the colon, should be treated aggressively with 1 to 2 weeks of parenteral antibiotics with broad-spectrum coverage for intestinal organisms.

2. Assessment of spinal stability—Civilian gunshot wounds to the spine rarely cause spinal column instability. For cervical spine injuries, immobilization with an orthosis is recommended if the anterior spinal column or posterior facets are injured. Halo-vest immobilization may be required for both-column injuries. For thoracolumbar spinal injuries, the anterior, middle, and posterior columns as described by Denis are evaluated with CT imaging. A rigid orthosis is recommended for injuries that destabilize two or more columns. An additional potentially destabilizing injury involves a transverse path injuring the pedicles or facets. However, instability is unlikely when at least one pedicle and one facet remain intact. Surgery is rarely necessary for restoring spinal stability. Spinal arthrodesis may be indicated for two or three-column injuries when bullet removal is being contemplated for other reasons.

3. Treatment of bullets in the spinal canal and disc space

- Bullet removal—A multicenter review of 90 patients with retained bullets in the spinal canal revealed that ***bullet removal had a positive effect on neurologic outcome for gunshot wounds between T12 and L4***. For lesions between T1 and T11, there was no significant difference in outcomes for patients with either complete or incomplete injuries whether or not the bullet was removed. Similarly, in the cervical spine, bullet removal does not appear to affect the ultimate neurological outcome. Removal of bullets in the cervical spinal canal may be indicated to improve neurologic function of the exiting nerve root, similar to removing bone or disc fragments in patients with cervical spinal cord injury from other causes.

- Timing of surgery—The timing of surgery for spinal cord or cauda equina injury remains controversial. Emergent surgery is indicated only for the rare cases with neurologic deterioration in the presence of cord compression from an enlarging hematoma or retained fragments of bone, disc, or foreign bodies. For patients whose results of neurologic examination are stable, bullet removal, if indicated, should be performed after a delay of several days or longer. This delay allows for more complete trauma resuscitation and evaluation and also simplifies the repair of dural lacerations. ***In the absence of a deteriorating neurologic picture, there is no indication for emergent surgery to remove retained bullet fragments.***

- Lead poisoning—Retained bullets or fragments in an intervertebral disc may be observed. Lead poisoning has been reported from retained bullets in a disc or synovial joint. For that reason, baseline serum lead levels should be obtained. If serum lead levels rise or if clinical signs of plumbism develop, bullet removal should be performed. If the disc is compromised, consideration should be given to concomitant arthrodesis. ***Bullet removal and spinal fusion are also indicated if the patient develops symptomatic mechanical back pain refractory to conservative measures.***

E. Complications of Gunshot Wounds to the Spine

1. Cerebrospinal fluid-cutaneous fistulas—A cerebrospinal fluid-cutaneous fistula complicates approximately 6% of spinal gunshot wounds if laminectomy, debridement, and bullet removal are performed. Fistulas are quite rare in the absence of surgical intervention. If a surgical debridement or bullet removal is performed, a watertight repair of the dura is important to avoid development of this complication. Consideration should also be given to the use of a fibrin glue or a lumbar subarachnoid drain to supplement dural repair.

2. Infection—Spinal infections, including osteomyelitis, discitis, and meningitis, have all been reported after gunshot wounds to the spine that are complicated by perforation of the pharynx, esophagus, or colon. ***Bullets that traverse the colon are particularly likely to cause spinal infections and should be considered highly contaminated.*** Aggressive management of the visceral injury is required and may include diversionary drainage. Broad-spectrum parenteral antibiotic coverage for 1 to 2 weeks is recommended. Surgical treatment of spinal infections is indicated for progressive neurologic deficit or increasing deformity. ***Bullets should be removed if an infection develops, since eradication of an established infection is difficult in the presence of a retained foreign body.*** Discitis or osteomyelitis should be treated with at least 6 weeks or parenteral antibiotics after sensitivities have been obtained.

3. Chronic pain—Dysesthetic chronic pain is particularly common in patients who have sustained spinal cord injury secondary to penetrating trauma. Removal of the bullet and decompressive procedures has not been shown to have a positive benefit. Medical management remains the mainstay of treatment. The use of implantable morphine pumps or dorsal root entry zone procedures may be of some benefit if medical management fails. A permanent implantable spinal cord stimulator may also be considered. If pain or neurologic deficit progresses to a more cephalad level, a MRI or myelography should be performed to evaluate for the presence of a posttraumatic syrinx. The presence of a chronic infection must also be excluded.

F. Stab Wounds of the Spine—Stab wounds or impalement injuries causing spinal cord injuries are relatively uncommon. The most common incomplete spinal cord injury seen with stab wounds is ***Brown-Séquard syndrome***, which has a greater chance for neurologic recovery than is seen in other incomplete spinal cord injuries. Radiographs must be obtained to exclude the presence of any retained foreign bodies. ***Strong consideration should be given to the removal of foreign bodies from stab wounds, since the incidence of wound contamination is higher than for gunshot wounds.*** Patients with spinal impalement injuries should undergo surgical debridement if the wound is large. Wound infections and cerebrospinal fluid-cutaneous fistulas are more common with stab wounds than gunshot wounds and should be managed aggressively with surgical debridement and prolonged parenteral antibiotics.

SUGGESTED READINGS

Classic Articles

Allen BL Jr, Ferguson RL, Lehmann TR, et al. A mechanistic classification of closed, indirect fractures and dislocations of the lower cervical spine. *Spine*. 1982;7:1–27.

Anderson LD, D'Alonzo RT. Fractures of the odontoid process of the axis. *J Bone Joint Surg*. 1974;56A:1663–1674.

Anderson PA, Henley MB, Rivara FP, et al. Flexion distraction and chance injuries to the thoracolumbar spine. *J Orthop Trauma*. 1991;5:153–160.

Anderson PA, Rivara FP, Maier RV, et al. The epidemiology of seatbelt-associated injuries. *J Trauma*. 1991;31:60–67.

Benzel EC, Hadden TA, Coleman JOE. Civilian gunshot wounds to the spinal cord and cauda equine. *Neurosurgery*. 1987;20:281–285.

Cammisa FP, Eismont FJ, Green BA. Dural laceration occurring with burst fractures and associated laminar fractures. *J Bone Joint Surg*. 1989;71A:1044–1052.

Denis F. The three-column spine and its significance in the classification of acute thoracolumbar spine injuries. *Spine*. 1983;8:817–831.

Ferguson RL, Allen BL Jr. Mechanistic classification of thoracolumbar spine fractures. *Clin Orthop*. 1984;189:77–88.

Fielding JW, Hawkins RJ. Atlanto-axial rotatory fixation: fixed rotatory subluxation of the atlanto-axial joint. *J Bone Joint Surg*. 1977;59A:37–44.

Fredrickson BE, Edwards WT, Rauschning W, et al. Vertebral burst fractures: an experimental morphologic, and radiographic analysis. *Spine*. 1992;17:1012–1021.

Fredrickson BE, Mann KA, Yuan HA, et al. Reduction of the intracanal fragment in experimental burst fractures. *Spine*. 1988;13:267–271.

Gertzbein SD, Court-Brown CM. Flexion distraction injuries of the lumbar spine: mvechanisms of injury and classification. *Clin Orthop*. 1988;227:52–60.

Holdsworth FW. Fractures, dislocations and fracture-dislocations of the spine. *J Bone Joint Surg*. 1963;45B:6–20.

Holdsworth FW. Fractures, dislocations and fracture-dislocations of the spine. *J Bone Joint Surg*. 1970;52A:1534–1551.

Keenen TL, Antony J, Benson DR. Non-contiguous spinal fractures. *J Trauma*. 1990;30:489–491.

Levine AM, Edwards CC. The management of traumatic spondylolisthesis of the axis. *J Bone Joint Surg*. 1985;67A:217–226.

Levine AM, McAfee PC, Anderson PA. Evaluation and emergent treatment of patients with thoracolumbar trauma. *Instr Course Lect*. 1995;44:33–45.

McAfee PC, Yuan HA, Fredrickson BE, et al. Value of the computed tomography in thoracolumbar burst fractures: an analysis of one hundred consecutive cases and a new classification. *J Bone Joint Surg.* 1982;65A:461–473.

Richards JS, Stover SL, Jaworski T. Effect of bullet removal on subsequent pain in persons with spinal cord injury secondary to gunshot wound. *J Neurosurg.* 1990;73:401–404.

Roffi RP, Waters RL, Adkins RH. Gunshot wounds to the spine associated with a perforated viscus. *Spine.* 1989;14:808–811.

Velhamos G, Demetriades D. Gunshot wounds of the spine: should retained bullets be removed to prevent infection? *Ann R Coll Surg Engl.* 1994;76:85–87.

Waters RL, Adkins RH. The effects of removal of bullet fragments retained in the spinal canal: a collaborative study by the National Spinal Cord Injury Model Systems. *Spine.* 1991;16:934–939.

Recent Articles

Anderson PA, Muchow RD, Munoz A, et al. Clearance of the asymptomatic cervical spine: A meta-analysis. *J Orthop Trauma.* 2010;24(2):100–106.

Bono CM, Heary RF. Gunshot wounds to the spine. *Spine J.* 2004;4(2):230–240.

Bono CM, Vaccaro AR, Hurlbert RJ, et al. Validating and newly proposed classification system for thoracolumbar spine trauma: Looking to the future of the thoracolumbar injury classification and severity score. *J Orthop Trauma.* 2006;20(8):567–572.

France JC, Bono CM, Vaccaro AR. Initial radiographic evaluation of the spine after trauma: when, what, where, and how to image the acutely traumatized spine. *J Orthop Trauma.* 2005;19(9):640–649.

Gnanenthiran SR, Adie S, Harris IA. Nonperative versus operative treatment for thoracolumbar burst fractures without neurologic deficit: a meta-analysis. *Clin Orthop Relat Res.* 2012;470(2):567–577.

Levi AD, Hurlbert RJ, Anderson P, et al. Neurologic deterioration secondary to unrecognized spinal instability following trauma—a mulitcenter study. *Spine.* 2006;31(4):451–458.

Öner FC, Wood KB, Smith JS, et al. Therapeutic decision making in thoracolumbar trauma. *Spine.* 2010;35(21S):S235–S244.

Radcliff K, Kepler CK, Rubin TA, et al. Does the load sharing classification predict ligamentous injury, neurologic injury, and the need for surgery in patients with thoracolumbar burst fractures? Clinical articles. *J Neurosurg Spine.* 2012;16(6):534–538.

Textbooks

Eismont F, Roper JG. Gunshot wounds of the spine. In: Browner BD, Jupiter JB, Levine AM, et al, eds. *Skeletal Trauma: Basic Science, Management, and Reconstruction.* 4th ed. Philadelphia, PA: Saunders Elsevier; 2008.

Eismont FJ. Gunshot wounds of die spine. In: Levine AM, Eismont FJ, Garfin SR, et al, eds. *Spine Trauma.* Philadelphia, PA: WB Saunders; 1988.

Kwon BK, AndersonPA. Injuries of the lower cervical spine. In: Browner BD, Jupiter JB, Levine AM, et al, eds. *Skeletal Trauma: Basic Science, Management, and Reconstruction.* 4th ed. Philadelphia, PA: Saunders Elsevier; 2008.

Reitman CA, ed. *Management of Thoracolumbar Fractures.* Rosemont, IL: American Academy of Orthopaedic Surgeons; 2004.

White AA, Panjabi MM. *Clinical Biomechanics of the Spine.* 2nd ed. Philadelphia, PA: JB Lippincott; 1990.

Williams SK. Thoracic and lumbar spinal injuries. In: Herkowitz HN, Garfin SR, Eismont FJ, et al, eds. *Rothman-Simeone the Spine.* 6th ed. Philadelphia, PA: Saunders Elsevier; 2011.

CHAPTER 27

Cervical Spine Trauma

Jens R. Chapman and Sohail K. Mirza

I. Overview
   A. Anatomy—For functional and anatomic reasons, the cervical spine can be divided into anatomic regions: the upper cervical spine (UCS) and the lower cervical spine (LCS).
      1. Upper cervical spine—The UCS (Fig. 27-1) extends from the skull base to the lower endplate of C2. It includes the occipital condyles and the bony aperture surrounding the foramen magnum, the C1 segment (atlas) and the C2 segment (axis). Conceptually, the C1 segment functions as a "washer" between the skull base and the C2 segment. The axis consists of the odontoid with its tip resting between the lateral masses of the atlas and its narrow waste. The superior articular processes of the atlas are convex and rest below the concave inferior facets of the atlas. They are connected through a bone bridge (pars interarticularis) on either side to the inferior articular processes. With its unique anatomic configuration, the UCS allows for extensive motion between its contributing segments and provides minimal intrinsic stability between the skull base and the LCS. Anatomic alignment of the bony segments of the UCS is maintained by several important ligamentous structures (Table 27-1; see Fig. 26-1). Occipito-cervical stability is provided by a few key ligaments, which are listed in Table 27-1 and are depicted in their functional arrangement in Figure 26-1. These ligaments allow for approximately half of the C-spine motion in rotation and flexion/extension while protecting the spinal cord and vertebral arteries. It is important to remember that these ligaments together form the functional unit of the UCS, with any bony or ligament injury to this area representing a more serious injury.
      2. Lower cervical spine—The LCS begins with the caudal half of the C2 vertebral body and ends with the T1 segment. Similar to the upper C-spine, the lower C-spine requires functional integrity of its soft-tissue components (Table 27-2)

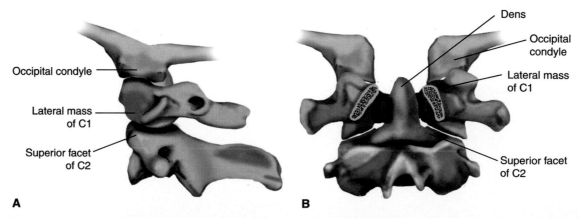

FIGURE 27-1 Osseous anatomy of the upper cervical spine. Note the functional unit that is formed by the occipital condyles and C2; C1 serves as an "intercalary washer." The bony elements offer no inherent stability toward one another. **A.** Important articulations as seen on a lateral projection plane. **B.** Posterior to anterior cutaway view with the posterior elements of C1 and C2 removed through the pedicles.

TABLE 27-1

Ligaments of the Upper Cervical Spine

Name of Ligament	Location	Function	Structural Contribution
Tectorial membrane	Clivus to posterior vertebral body of C2 (rostral continuation of ligamnetum flavum into skull base)	Resists traction and flexion	Key ligament
Alar ligament	(paired) Lateral aspect of odontoid tip to the medial aspect of the occipital condyle	Cranio-cervical rotation and lateral tilt	If bilateral injury, it is very concerning; isolated unilateral injury may not cause major instability
Transverse atlantal ligament (TAL); also known as Transverse ligament	Medial aspects of C1 lateral masses (left to right)	Locates the odontoid tip between C1 lateral masses while allowing its rotation	Key ligament
Anterior cranio-cervical membranes (deep and superficial)	Anterior skull base to anterior longitudinal ligament (ALL)	Prevents hyperextension	Key structure
Posterior occipito-cervical membrane & atlanto-axial membranes	Connects opisthion (posterior foramen magnum) to laminae of C1 and C2 (rostral continuation of ligamentum flavum)	Resists flexion	Accessory function
Apical ligament	Basion (anterior rim of the foramen magnum) to the tip of odontoid	Resists axial distraction	Residual ligament
Cruciate ligament	Attenuation to TAL and tectorial membrane (composite of TAL and Tectorial membrane fibers)	Multidirectional	Accessory function to TAL and tectorial ligament
Articular capsules (occipito-cervical and atlanto-axial—paired)	Joint capsules	Multidirectional	Accessory function

to maintain a balanced alignment and to protect neurological elements. A healthy C-spine has a lordotic alignment of approximately 20° between the inferior vertebral body of C2 and the inferior C7 vertebral body. This assures balanced distribution of loads between vertebral bodies and lateral masses (tripod concept). The uncovertebral processes are unique to the cervical spine. They arise out of the lateral margins of the superior aspects of the vertebral bodies and secure the spinal column against excessive lateral tilt. Well-functioning extensor muscles are necessary to provide active neck control and maintain balance. All together, the anatomic arrangements of the LCS allow for considerable motion while maintaining usually **_less than 11° flexion/extension_** and **_less than 3.5-mm translational motion_** between each adjacent segment.

B. Incidence and Injury Mechanism—The neck and its surrounding soft-tissue structures are more prone to injury than the lower thoracolumbar spine due its exposed location, permissiveness to an extensive range of motion, relatively small size, and proportionally frail ligamentous restraint structures. The relatively large mass of the head tethered to the rostral cervical spinal column exposes the cervical spine to injury due to indirect mechanisms. Important determinants of the type and magnitude of injury sustained are the position of the head at the time of impact and the direction and magnitude of the kinetic energy acting on the C-spine. A large number of variables contribute to the severity of the injury, including the age of the patient, bone mineral health, pre-existent ligamentous laxity, spinal ankylosis, and spinal canal size. In general, flexion and bursting type injuries affect the LCS most commonly in a younger more active age

TABLE 27-2

Important Soft-Tissue Structures of the Lower Cervical Spine

Name of Structure	Location	Function	Importance
Anterior longitudinal ligament (ALL)	Coats anterior vertebral bodies	Limits hyperextension	High
Longus colli muscles (paired)	Antero-lateral vertebral bodies	Flexion, lateral tilt, rotation	Intermediate, little structural limitations
Intervertebral discs	Connect vertebral bodies	Intervertebral cushion, alignment and centering structure	Key
Disco-vertebral ligaments	Connects lateral margin of the annulus fibrosus to the super-olateral margins of vertebral bodies. They are thicker in anterior and posterior regions.	Locks intervertebral disc to vertebral bodies, resists extension/flexion and lateral tilt depending upon location	Key
Posterior longitudinal ligament (PLL)	Coats posterior vertebral bodies within the spinal canal	Limits flexion	Low
Facet capsules	Connects posterior facets	Limits flexion	Moderate
Interspinous and supraspinous ligaments	Connects posterior interspinous processes	Limits flexion	High
Exensor muscles (several layers)	Skull base to various posterior and posterolateral bony elements of the LCS	Neck extension/rotation/tilt. Actively resists hyperflexion and rotation	High (active only—no passive component)
Nuchal ligament	Superficial thickening of the posterior extensor muscle fascia	Prevents hyperflexion	Low

group due to deceleration trauma, while elderly patients are more commonly affected by hyperextension injuries commonly sustained from ground level falls. Direct trauma to the cervical spine usually results from penetrating injuries, especially in North American urban regions. The spectrum of C-spine injuries ranges from mild soft-tissue sprains to life-threatening high-grade fracture dislocations. Some 2% to 5% of patients with blunt trauma can be expected to have sustained a fracture or dislocation of the cervical spine. Increasingly elderly and frail patients with concomitant degenerative C-spine disorders and multiple co-morbidities suffer from serious C-spine injuries, which can be easily missed and for which there commonly are no simple treatment options.

II. Evaluation
   A. Overview—Systematic clinical evaluation forms the basis of C-spine injury evaluation. The NEXT criteria identify that a patient who (a) *is cognitively unimpaired*, (b) has *not sustained a high kinetic injury mechanism* (i.e., motorized vehicle crash >35 mph, fall >4 ft, presence of acute cranio-cervical fractures, long-bone or pelvic fracture), (3) has a *nonfocal neurologic examination and nonpainful full neck range of motion does not require radiographic assessment*. Although these criteria have been shown to be highly predictive of absence of neck trauma, they rarely apply in a trauma setting.

   The basic principle in the evaluation of a trauma patient is to assume the presence of an unstable spinal injury and then to rule it out based on clinical evaluation and imaging studies. As in all trauma patients, spine precautions, including C-spine immobilization, are maintained during resuscitation and evaluation until a determination of spine stability has been made.
   B. Clinical Evaluation—Clinical evaluation starts with the history of injury mechanism (if available) and review of basic vital signs. After successful resuscitation using the advanced trauma life support ABC principles, a more comprehensive patient evaluation, including assessment for spinal injuries, is performed. Inspection and palpation of a traumatized patient's spine are performed from occiput to sacrum using a log-roll maneuver. Any manipulation of the neck is

avoided outside life-saving efforts. Particular attention is directed to areas of bruising, focal tenderness, or interspinous gaps along the posterior midline. In conscious and cooperative patients, a formal examination includes assessment of the Glasgow Coma Scale (see Table 1-1), cranial nerve function, and evaluation of extremity motor, sensory, and reflex function. Testing of these functions is performed according to the guidelines of the American Spinal Injury Association (ASIA) (see Fig. 25-4). In unconscious sedated patients, segmental motor and sensory testing should be attempted, but is commonly limited. Withdrawal responses and the presence of deep tendon reflexes and long tract signs are important components in the evaluation. Assessment for priapism in males, detailed rectal examination, and assessment of the bulbocavernosis reflex should be performed in patients with suspected spinal cord injury and in unconscious patients.

C. Radiographic Evaluation (Fig. 27-2 and Table 27-3)

1. Plain radiographs—Radiographic evaluation of the cervical spine is suggested in patients with neck pain after a significant injury mechanism,

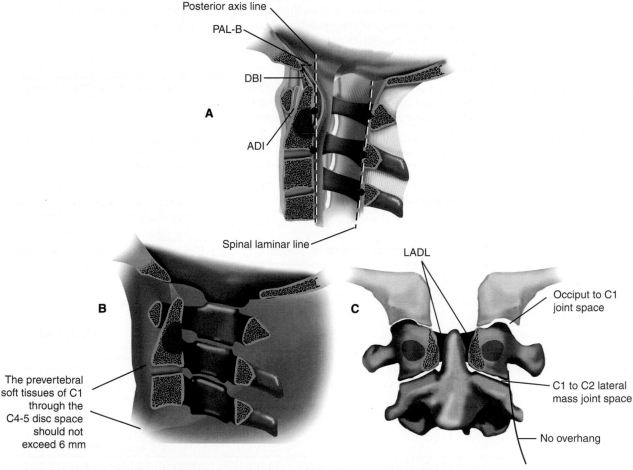

FIGURE 27-2 Accurate interpretation of the landmarks of the upper cervical spine is important for injury assessment in this region. **A.** On the lateral radiographic image the most posterior cortical margin of the bony spinal canal of C1, C2, and C3 should form a line **(spinal laminar line)** of which no point deviates more than 1 mm. The anterior cortex of the odontoid should lie in close proximity (and parallel) to the posterior cortex of the anterior arch of C1; this distance of atlas to dens is referred to as the *ADI* and should measure less than 3 mm in a normal adult and less than 5 mm in a normal child. The ADI is maintained primarily by the transverse atlantal ligament. Two important reference lines for the physiologic craniocervical articulation are the dens-basion interval (*DBI*), which should be less than 12 mm, and the distance of the basion to the posterior axis line (*PAL-B*), which should not exceed 12 mm, with the basion not protruding posteriorly beyond 4 mm. **B.** The prevertebral soft tissues of C1 through the C4 to C5 disc space should not exceed 6 mm of thickness (as seen on the lateral radiograph) in normal individuals. Artifacts may be caused by endotracheal or esophageal tubes and crying. **C.** On an open-mouth odontoid or coronal CT reformatted view the C1 lateral masses should not overhang C2. In addition, the occiput to C1 and the C1 to C2 joint spaces should be nearly uniformly equidistant (occiput to C1 joint space, 1 to 2 mm; C1 to C2 lateral mass joint space, 2 to 3 mm). The odontoid should be centered symmetrically between the C1 lateral masses. (The lateral atlas-dens interval [*LADI*] should not vary by more than 2 mm.)

TABLE 27-3

Radiographic Reference Lines for the Upper and Lower Cervical Spine

Reference Line	Location	Meaning
Upper cervical spine		
Harris lines	Measure from the clivus to the tip of the dens and from the clivus to a line running superiorly along a line along the posterior aspect of the dens (should be less than 12 mm for both)	Potential for cranio-cervical dissociation
Wackenheim's line	A line drawn along the posterior aspect of the clivus and assessed with respect to the tip of the dens. The line should lie essentially at the tip of the dens	Aids in assessing for cranio-cervical dissociation
Power's ratio	This is a ratio of the distance from the basion to the anterior aspect of the posterior ring of C1 compared to the distance from the anterior aspect of the ring of C1 to the opisthion (abnormal at values greater than 1)	Aids in assessing for cranio-cervical dissociation
Atlanto-Dens interval (ADI)	The gap between the posterior aspect of the C1 ring and the anterior aspect of the dens (should be <3 mm in adults and <4 mm in children)	Assessment for C1–C2 instability
Prevertebral soft-tissue swelling	Above C4 < 5 mm (variable due to screaming, age, intubation, infection)	Potential for hemorrhage (indirect injury sign)
Spinal laminar line (SLL)	Connects the anterior cortical margins of the laminae of each level.	There should be < 4 mm translation of each segment of this line. Presence of larger translation could indicate instability
Rule of Spence	On open mouth odontoid view or coronal CT reformat, the overhang of the sum of C1 lateral masses over the C2 lateral masses should be less than 7 mm	If greater than 7 mm, this is highly suggestive of a transverse alar ligament (TAL) disruption.
Lower cervical spine		
Prevertebral soft-tissue swelling	Above C4 < 5 mm (variable due to screaming, age, intubation, infection)	Potential for hemorrhage (indirect injury sign)
Anterior vertebral body line (AVBL)	Smooth continuous lordotic arch immediately anterior to the vertebral bodies	Assessment for step off between segments, reminds of prevertebral swelling
Posterior vertebral body line (PVBL)	Continuous lordotic line posterior to the vertebral bodies	Should be parallel to AVBL, runs along the posterior vertebral bodies and should be of smooth contour
Spinal laminar line (SLL)	Connects the anterior cortical margins of the laminae of each level.	There should be <4 mm translation of each segment of this line. Presence of larger translation could indicate instability
Interspinous process spacing (ISPS)	Absence of focal "gapping" between spinous processes. There are no specific degrees or distances described	Focal gapping at a single level could represent an interspinous ligament tear
Intervertebral distance (IVD)	Distance between vertebral bodies (anterior vs. posterior and from one to other)	Excessive gapping of one disc space compared to others could indicate a distractive injury. Focal kyphosis of one disc in contrast to others may indicate more advanced disc degeneration or segmental instability

Reference Line	Location	Meaning
Intervertebral angulation (IVA)	In general, adjacent vertebral endplates of the LCS should be parallel.	Focal angulation > 11° kyphosis is of concern regarding excessive instability or potential injury
Facet joint apposition	Each lateral mass should be in close and parallel alignment to the next higher and lower segment	Gapping or excessive unroofing of facet joints can represent instability due to injury
Torg/Pavlov ratio	Shortest AP distance of spinal canal (posterior vertebral body to anterior laminar cortex) expressed as ratio over shortest AP distance of the vertebral body in millimeters	Screening line, which can indicate spinal stenosis

in the presence of facial fractures, polytrauma, neurologic deficits, or symptoms, and in patients with altered mental status and a history of possible significant trauma. *The plain lateral C-spine radiograph remains the most important imaging test for identifying fractures and dislocations of the neck and ideally visualizes the skull base to the C7–Tl motion segment.* Due to common limitations of visualizing the cervico-thoracic junction, swimmer's views or shoulder pull-down views are necessary to assess the cervicothoracic junction on a lateral radiograph. Open-mouth odontoid views are used to assess the odontoid and the Cl lateral masses. An anteroposterior (AP) C-spine radiograph usually allows for assessment of the C3 segment to the UCS. Trauma oblique radiographs can be helpful in visualizing the neuroforamina and the facet joints of the LCS.

Due to their time- and resource-intensive nature, such plain radiographs have increasingly been replaced by helical CT-scan with coronal and sagittal reformatted views with comprehensive visualization of the entire C-spine from the skull base to the upper thoracic spine.

Among many subtle findings, a normal lateral cervical spine radiograph is expected to demonstrate maintenance of physiologic lordosis, absence of vertebral subluxation or kyphosis, symmetrically maintained disc heights, congruous, overlapping facet joints without subluxation, and a narrow prevertebral soft-tissue shadow. Although plain cervical radiographs are still used today, they are rapidly being surpassed by helical CT scans with reformats as a faster and more sensitive modality.

2. Lateral flexion-extension radiographs—Lateral flexion-extension radiographs remain a controversial but efficient way for assessing cervical spine stability. In awake, fully cooperative patients who are neurologically intact and

have normal plain radiographs, X-ray studies taken with maximum pain-free neck extension and flexion may provide helpful early determination of spinal stability. In patients who do not meet these prerequisites and have continued neck pain, delayed reevaluation with a second clinical and radiographic examination using flexion and extension radiographs on a delayed nonacute basis is mandated.

3. Computed tomography (CT)—*Noncontrast CTs of the neck have largely surpassed plain radiographs as the imaging modality of choice in assessing and diagnosing cervical spine injuries.* Helical CT scans with sagittal and coronal reformats can be rapidly obtained and are more sensitive than plain radiography. *Noncontrast head CT scans have become the common initial screening study for patients presenting with cognitive impairment.* Adding a cervical spine screening from the skull base to T4 is time- and cost-effective. It is also considered more sensitive and cost-effective than plain radiography, however, at higher radiation exposure. In an obtunded patient, a CT scan without any abnormality can also be used to clear the cervical spine without the addition of controlled flexion-extension radiographs or the addition of MRI.

4. Magnetic resonance imaging (MRI)—MRI is recommended for patients with spinal cord injury, especially in the presence of progressive or unexplained neurologic deficits or discrepant skeletal and neurologic injury. Controversy persists as to the timing of an MR scan relative to reduction attempts in a displaced spinal column injury. It is widely accepted to proceed with a closed reduction of a dislocated spinal column using sequential cranial traction in an awake patient before performing MRI; this approach is intended to minimize the duration of ongoing spinal cord compression and optimize chances for cord regeneration. If readily available, an

MRI scan can be considered in neurologically intact patients or in the presence of an unknown neurological status before reduction to rule out the presence of a large disc herniation, which may cause postreduction spinal cord compression. MRI can also detect posterior interspinous ligament and facet capsule injury, especially within the first 72 hours, and can allow differentiation of full-thickness tears and sprain. The additional cost and imaging time poses a limitation to this modality on a routine screening basis. MRI scans in the pediatric population are limited by lack of compliance issues. Usually monitored sedation or preferably general endotracheal intubation are required for a quality study. This should be duly considered prior to ordering a MRI in these patients. MRI may not be useful in the morbidly obese patient (who cannot fit into the MRI gantry), patients with significant fixed deformities due to inflammatory spinal conditions, and patients with pacemakers or implantable stimulators.

5. Bone scans—Bone scans are rarely used in the assessment of acute cervical spine trauma. They have a limited role in the evaluation of occult spine fractures, especially in skeletally immature patients. Typically, this modality is not useful until at least 48 hours after injury; further enhancement with single photon emission CT (SPECT) may be necessary to increase image resolution of the small bony structures of the cervical spine. With the advent of current technology and imaging resolution with CT and MRI imaging, bone scans are essentially obsolete in traumatic conditions.

6. Other tests—Noninvasive vascular tests can be of value in the assessment of vertebral artery injuries. CT angiography (CT-A) is recommended with fractures into the transverse foramina or in patients with significant post-traumatic malalignment or displacement as in the case of facet dislocation. CT angiography has largely displaced invasive arteriography as a screening tool. Transcranial Doppler tests and MR angiography are usually secondary-tier tests for patients with unclear CT-A or in the presence of unexplained mental status changes. Although the sensitivity of these tests is high, the specificity remains well below that of arteriography. Routine use of noninvasive vascular tests and treatment of suspected vertebral artery injuries remain in a state of evolution.

III. Injury Classifications—Injury classifications of the spine attempt to predict spinal stability by describing neurologic injury, bony injury, and disruption of disco-ligamentous structures. There are descriptive systems, which identify the injured anatomic components of the injured segment. Finally, there are systems that ascribe an injury mechanism to the imaging tests. Spinal cord injury classifications are described in Chapter 25. In the upper C-spine, there are level-specific well-established classifications. Unfortunately, there is no such consensus for the lower C-spine. Many variations of descriptive anatomic and mechanistic models continue to persist, thus impeding, among other things, study, and testing.

A. UCS Injuries
1. Occipital condyle fractures (Fig. 27-3)
The major classification scheme used to differentiate occipital condyle fractures is that of Anderson and Montesano described in 1988.
• Type 1—Impaction mechanism: comminution of the occipital condyle with an

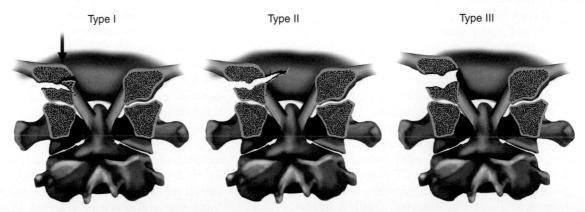

Type I   Type II   Type III

FIGURE 27-3 Occipital condyle fractures. The alar ligaments provide important structural support for the craniocervical junction. Type I injuries are relatively stable and demonstrate comminution of the occipital condyle. Type II injuries are basilar skull fractures extending into the occipital condyle; they are relatively stable. Type III injuries are potentially unstable avulsion injuries of the alar ligament with the tip of the occipital condyle.

impaction mechanism; these fractures are stable and are managed conservatively.

- Type II—Shear mechanism: basilar skull fracture with occipital condyle involvement; these fractures are stable and are usually managed in accordance with the basilar skull fracture.
- Type III—Distraction: avulsion of the alar ligament with the tip of the occipital condyle; these fractures may be unstable and an associated craniocervical dissocation (CCD) or atlantooccipital dissociation (AOD) must be ruled out.

2. AODs or CCDs (Fig. 27-4)

These injuries are always generally considered unstable. There are two main classifications used. The first is that described by Traynelis in 1986 and is descriptive of the position of the skull with respect to the C1 articulation.

- Type I—Anterior displacement of the occiput on the cervical spine (11%)
- Type II—Vertical displacement of the occiput on the cervical spine (3%)
- Type III—Posterior displacement of the occiput on the cervical spine (2%)
- Type IV—Oblique displacement of the occiput on the cervical spine (84%)

A more recent classification is the Harborview classification, which provides stratification based on the severity of ligament injury irrespective of location of the occiput with respect to the adjoining C1 articulations.

- Type I—Incomplete ligament injuries, such as unilateral alar ligament tears. There is sufficient biomechanical stability retained that these can be treated conservatively.
- Type II—Complete CCDs with initial lateral radiographs showing borderline screening measurement values. These injuries, however, feature a complete disruption of key ligaments of the craniocervical junction and are innately unstable. A spontaneous partial reduction of the cranium to its cervical location through some remaining residual ligamentous attachments may provide false reassurance to a reviewer.
- Type IIIa—Complete disruption of craniocervical ligaments with obvious major displacement on plain radiographs with survival of at least 24 hours.
- Type IIIb—Criteria as in IIIa with death from AOD in the first 24 hours following injury.

3. C1 ring fractures—Levine and Edwards (1991) used descriptive anatomic terms to differentiate between fracture subtypes.

- Posterior arch fracture—***stable***.
- Transverse process fracture—***stable***.
- Simple lateral mass fracture—A simple fracture is generally stable; however, a unilateral sagittal split fracture may progressively subluxate, leading to a "cock-robin type deformity."
- Anterior arch fracture—A segmental anterior arch fracture is ***unstable***.
- Comminuted lateral mass fracture—***Usually unstable***.
- Three- or four-part burst fracture (Jefferson fracture)—A three- or four-part burst fracture

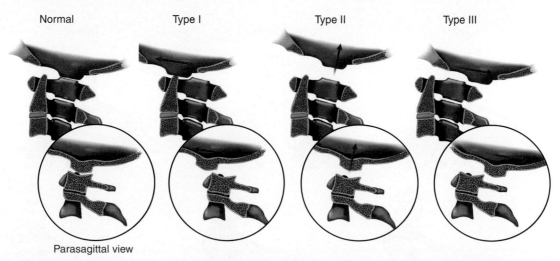

Normal   Type I   Type II   Type III

Parasagittal view

FIGURE 27-4 Classification of occipitocervical dissociation (*AOD*) according to Traynelis (the bottom row is a parasagittal representation). A Type I injury has anterior displacement of the occiput on the cervical spine. A Type II injury has vertical displacement, and a Type III injury has posterior displacement of the occiput on the cervical spine. Type IV injuries are the most common and display displacement in an oblique plane (not shown). Occult ligamentous damage has to be cautiously evaluated.

is unstable when the TAL is disrupted. ***This is typically the case if the lateral masses overhang those of C2 by a total of 7 mm or more on an open mouth odontoid view***. This well-known finding was originally described by Spence in 1970; although helpful, it was refuted by Dickman et al. in 1996, who showed that many injuries previously thought to be stable really are unstable.

4. Atlantoaxial instability—***Atlas-dens interval (ADI) in adults should be less than 3 mm***; 3 to 7 mm has the potential for a transverse ligament tear, and ***more than 7 mm is a complete tear***. ADI in children should be less than 3 to 5 mm; 5 to 10 mm is a transverse ligament tear; and with 10 to 12 mm, all ligaments have failed.
   • Transverse ligament injury
     (a) Type I—A Type I transverse ligament injury is a midsubstance or purely ligamentous tear. It usually requires surgical management with C1–C2 fusion.
     (b) Type II—A Type II injury is a bony avulsion. Nonoperative treatment is possible.
   • Atlantoaxial dissociation—Atlantoaxial dissociation represents a variant of AOD and is ***highly unstable.*** Usually, the dissociation occurs in a vertical direction and is accompanied by disruption of the alar ligaments.
   • Rotatory translation
     (a) Type A—ADI less than 3 mm and the TAL is intact
     (b) Type B—ADI 3–5 mm with the TAL insufficient
     (c) Type C—ADI greater than 5 mm with failure of the alar ligaments
     (d) Type D—Complete posterior displacement of the atlas

5. ***Fractures of the odontoid*** (Fig. 27-5)—Classification schemes for fractures of the odontoid are generally based on the level of the fracture as described by Anderson and D'Alonzo in 1974.
   • Type I—A Type I fracture occurs at the tip of the odontoid. It is an uncommon injury. ***Stability is questionable***. The clinician should rule out AOD. The differential diagnosis includes os odontoideum.
   • Type II—A Type II fracture occurs at the waist of the odontoid. It is the most common type and is easily missed. This fracture is ***usually unstable***. Clinically relevant variables include fracture pattern, displacement, distraction, angulation, and the age of the patient. There is an increased risk of nonunion with this fracture pattern.
   • Type III—A Type III fracture occurs through the cancellous body of the axis. This fracture can be ***relatively stable***.

6. C2 ring fractures (Hangman's fractures)—C2 ring fractures involve traumatic spondylolisthesis of the axis (Fig. 27-6). The classification scheme used was originally described by Effendi in 1981 and further modified by Levine and Edwards in 1985.
   • Type I—Type I fractures have less than 3 mm of displacement; there is no angulation. These fractures are ***relatively stable***.

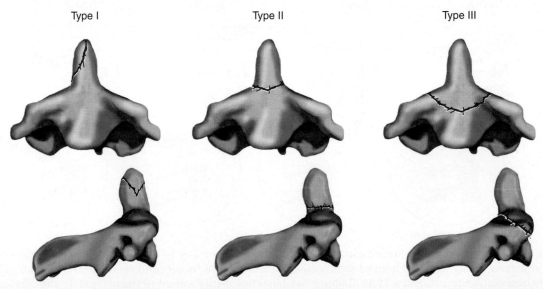

Type I   Type II   Type III

FIGURE 27-5 Classification of odontoid fractures (Anderson and D'Alonzo). *Type I,* avulsion of the tip (unstable); *Type II,* waist-line fracture (unstable); *Type III,* fracture through the vertebral body (conditionally stable).

Type I   Type II   Type IIa   Type III

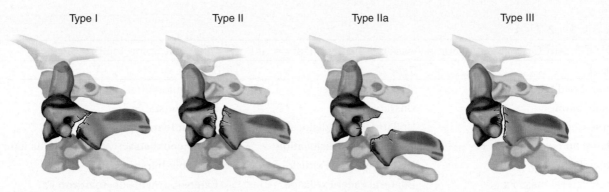

FIGURE 27-6   Levine classification of traumatic spondylolisthesis of the axis (see text for details).

- Type II—Type II fractures have more than 3 mm of displacement and angulation. They are ***potentially unstable***.
- Type IIa—Type IIa fractures are a variant of C2–C3 flexion-distraction injuries and have significant angulation. These fractures are ***unstable***.
- Type III—Type III fractures are facet fracture-dislocations. They are **highly unstable**.

B. LCS Injuries—As stated earlier, there is no universally accepted LCS injury classification system. Each system has inherent limitations and drawbacks. Familiarity with at least one descriptive anatomic system, one mechanistic model, and basic cervical spine stability concepts is suggested (Fig. 27-7).

1. Stability of the lower C-Spine—Lower C-spine stability is defined as the "ability of the spine to bear loads under physiologic conditions." A useful checklist for clinical instability of the lower C-spine as described by White and Panjabi in 1990 remains well accepted and includes the following factors:

- Anterior elements destroyed or unable to function (2 points)
- Posterior element destroyed or unable to function (2 points)
- Sagittal displacement radiographically of more than 3.5 mm (2 points)
- Sagittal angulation of more than 11° (2 points)
- Positive Stretch Test (2 points)
- Spinal cord damage (2 points)
- Nerve root damage (1 point)
- Abnormal disc space narrowing (1 point)
- Dangerous load anticipated (1 point)

   A cumulative point value of 5 or more suggests clinical instability of the cervical spine.

2. Descriptive anatomic (Table 27-4)
3. Mechanistic model—There are six basic injury types; stages have increasing instability. These were described by Allen and Ferguson in 1982.

- Distractive flexion (stages I to IV)—Ventral compression and dorsal disruption
- Vertical compression (stages I to III)—Axial load

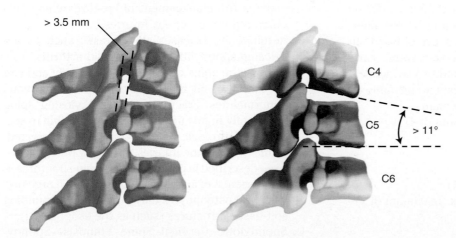

> 3.5 mm

C4

C5   > 11°

C6

FIGURE 27-7   Translational displacement greater than 3.5 mm or angulation greater than 11° on a flexion-extension lateral radiographs is associated with cervical spine instability.

TABLE 27-4

AO/ASIF and Orthopedic Trauma Association Classification of Lower Cervical Spine Injuries

Type A	Type B	Type C
"**A**xial" Load	"**B**ending" Injuries	"**C**ircumferential" injuries
Usually stable	Unstable	Highly unstable
Simple Compression Fx	Unilateral facet dislocation	Flexion teardrop
Isolated Spinous Process Fx	Bilateral facet dislocation	Displaced distractive ligamentous injury
Lamina Fx	Unilateral facet Fx/disloc	Unstable burst fracture
Simple lateral mass Fx	Bilateral Facet Fx/disloc	Extension/Avulsion Teardrop Fx
Extension/Avulsion Teardrop Fx		Unstable Extension Fx/Disloc

Note: Multiple subtypes of the basic three injury types exist and are listed in an alphanumeric system. These are not presented here for clarity sake and are unlikely to be the subject of test material.

- Compressive flexion (stages I to V)—Progressively worsening vertebral body comminution
- Compressive extension (stages I to V)—Posterior compression and ventral distraction
- Distractive extension (stages I and II)—Posterior compression and global distraction
- Lateral flexion (stages I and II)—Lateral compression

4. Cervical Spine Injury Severity Score—The Cervical Spine Injury Severity Score was described by Moore, Anderson, and coworkers in 2006; it uses a measuring scale for the two lateral columns and the anterior and posterior column to assess the amount of displacement of a fracture or distraction through the disc space or joints. This displacement is measured in millimeters for each column with a minimum of 0 mm and a maximum of 5 mm. The four columns are then added together giving a total possible score of 0–20 mm. A total score of greater than 7 is cause for concern regarding the possibility of an unstable injury.

5. Subaxial Cervical Spine Injury Classification System (SLIC)—The SLIC was published in 2007 by Vaccaro and consists of the sum of three different elements of the injury. A score of less than 4 merits consideration for conservative care, a score equal to 4 could go either way, while a score of greater than 4 suggests an unstable injury meriting surgical management.
   - Injury morphology (maximum of 4)
      (a) Compression (1)
      (b) Burst (2)
      (c) Distraction (3)
      (d) Translation/rotation (4)
   - Disco-ligamentous complex (maximum of 2)
      (a) Intact (0)
      (b) Indeterminate (1)
      (c) Disrupted (2)

- Neurological status (maximum of 4)
   (a) Intact (0)
   (b) Nerve root deficit (1)
   (c) Complete spinal cord injury (2)
   (d) Incomplete spinal cord injury (3)
   (e) Add on: persistent compression or stenosis with spinal cord injury (1)

   At this point of time, for practical purposes, it appears most advisable to be knowledgeable about the basic components of the AO/OTA system since it uses terms commonly used and provides relatively straightforward grouping of injuries into reproducible categories. However, scientifically validated severity scales, such as the SLIC score, will likely become increasingly prevalent in the near future due to their more systematic approach and comprehensive nature.

IV. Associated Injuries
   A. Penetrating Trauma—For penetrating trauma, the primary concern of the initial treating physicians is the management of life-threatening vascular and upper-airway injuries.
   B. Autoimmune Diseases—In diseases such as ankylosing spondylitis or rheumatoid arthritis, fractures of the spine can occur more readily and can be missed easily due to disease-specific osseous abnormalities. Fractures in an ankylosing spine are usually highly unstable and susceptible to secondary neurologic deterioration if left untreated. Primary traumatic injuries to the esophagus have been described in patients with C-spine fractures in the presence of ankylosing spondylitis. (Large prevertebral osteophytes may injure the surrounding soft-tissue structures [such as the esophagus]).
   C. Spondylotic Cervical Spine Stenosis—Spondylotic cervical spinal stenosis is associated with

an increased likelihood of spinal cord injury. "Spear-tackler's spine" identifies a clinical and radiographic condition consisting of loss of cervical lordosis and profound foraminal stenosis with propensity toward nerve root impaction in athletes who use the head for physical impact. Athletes with signs of a "spear-tackler's spine" or symptomatic cervical spondylotic myelopathy should abstain from athletic activities that place the head or neck at increased injury risk because of an increased risk of neurologic injury.

D. Vertebral Artery Injuries—Vertebral artery injuries have an estimated incidence of 5% to 30% in C-spine trauma. Presenting symptoms range from mental status changes to symptoms of severe stroke. Work-up and monitoring consist of CT angiography and if a vertebral artery injury is detected, then serial trans-cranial Doppler should be performed to assess for emboli. Treatment is based on the individual patient presentation and may consist of observation, aspirin administration, formal anticoagulation, or angiographic embolization.

V. Treatment and Treatment Rationale
A. Rogers' Rule—The tenets of care for spinal injuries follow Rogers' rules: reduction of deformity, decompression of impinged neural tissues, and prevention of further injury by immobilization of the injured segment.
B. Nonoperative Treatment
1. Overview—Most bony injuries to the cervical spine can be expected to heal with appropriate immobilization. External devices such as braces or a halo-vest assembly offer varying degrees of spinal column immobilization.
2. Unstable bony injuries—Nonoperative management of truly unstable bony injuries is not supported by clinical studies or basic science and is therefore not recommended. Thus, surgical fusion with bone graft and instrumentation is usually recommended for such injuries.
3. Unstable injuries of the ligaments and discs—In contrast to the appendicular skeleton, unstable injuries to the ligaments and discs of the cervical spine heal poorly with nonsurgical management, even with prolonged external immobilization. Surgical repair of disrupted ligaments of the spine is not supported by clinical studies or basic science and is therefore not recommended. Thus, surgical fusion with bone graft and instrumentation is commonly recommended for such injuries.
4. Soft neck collars—Soft neck collars offer no structural support or immobilization of the

cervical spine and are mainly intended for brief periods of symptomatic treatment for neck muscle soreness.
5. Rigid neck collars—Rigid neck collars reduce cervical spine motion in a limited fashion and are therefore indicated for minor fractures or injuries only; they can also be used as an adjunct to operative stabilization.
6. Cervicothoracic braces—Cervicothoracic braces, such as sternal–occiput–mandibular immobilization (SOMI) and Minerva devices, are the most effective external noninvasive devices in limiting cervical spine flexion and extension. Their efficacy relies on a close fit of the brace to the mandible and occiput as well as a snug fit of the vest to the torso. These braces can be considered as definitive treatment for patients with injuries such as minimally displaced atlas fractures, nondisplaced Type III odontoid fractures, and stable-appearing burst or facet fractures. Compliance with brace wear and a body habitus suitable for brace wear are further prerequisites for this treatment.
7. Skeletal traction—In patients with a spinal canal compromised by dislocation or retropulsed vertebral body fragments, indirect reduction by means of appropriately applied skeletal traction is highly successful and the most effective early intervention strategy at the disposal of the treating surgeon. Early closed reduction of fracture-dislocations or burst fractures of the C-spine for patients with acute spinal cord injury can lead to dramatic neurologic improvement. Therefore, patients with manifest spinal cord injury preferably are considered for early reduction using an established traction protocol. Contraindications to traction are certain skull fractures, distractive neck injuries, and ankylosing spinal disorders (traction may lead to secondary neurologic deterioration). A delay in fracture reduction may be associated with increased cord swelling, ischemia, and a widened zone of secondary cord injury. In patients with facet dislocations, case reports of neurologic deterioration after closed reduction, presumably resulting from dislodgment of a disc fragment into the spinal canal, have led to suggestions to perform an MRI scan before reduction efforts. The incidence of a herniated nucleus pulposus has been reported to be 13% in bilateral facet dislocations compared with 23% in unilateral facet dislocations. Hence, prereduction MR scans are recommended for unconscious patients and in cases of planned open reduction

under general anesthesia. In neurologically intact and conscious patients with facet dislocation, an MR scan can be considered before reduction if this study will not delay realignment efforts. There is, however, ongoing controversy surrounding prereduction MRIs due to inherent delays in getting these studies and necessary further manipulation during the additional patient transfers in the presence of a compromised spinal cord.

8. Halo ring—A halo ring relies on skull fixation using at least four pins tightened to 6 to 8 in/lb in adults and six to eight pins tightened to 2 to 6 in/lb, depending on size and age factors, for children. Correct halo pin placement is important. The anterior pins should be placed approximately one fingerbreadth above the lateral third of the eyebrows. (The patient's eyes should be closed during pin insertion.) The anterior pins should be located lateral to the supraorbital nerve and frontal sinus and anterior to the temporal fossa. The posterior pins are ideally placed diametrically opposed to the anterior pins (posterior to the ear lobe and superior to the mastoid process). *The biomechanical stability of a halo ring vest assembly is most significantly influenced by secure vest fit about the torso.* Halo vest assemblies limit rotation of the spine more effectively than cervical braces.

- Indications—A halo orthosis can be reasonably considered in most patients with stable occipitocervical injuries, unstable atlas fractures, hangman's fractures of the axis, Types II and III odontoid fractures, neurologically intact burst fractures, and some unilateral, anatomically reduced facet fractures. Nondisplaced cervical spine fractures in patients with ankylosing spondylitis require at least a halo vest assembly, if not treated with operative stabilization.

- Results of treatment—Loss of reduction has been reported in patients in whom the fracture reduction was achieved with a halo ring held in distraction to the vest. "Snaking" and other alignment changes have been reported at a frequency of 20% to 77% of patients treated with a halo vest.

- Contraindications—The application of cranial tong traction or a halo ring in patients with skull fractures can be dangerous and should usually be avoided. In general, the application of cervical traction is also contraindicated in patients with distractive or hyperextension injuries to the C-spine.

9. *Methylprednisolone*—The use of methylprednisolone given in high intravenous doses has been reported to improve neurologic outcomes in patients with spinal cord injury if given within 8 hours of injury according to the NASCIS trials. Current dose recommendations are as follows: *bolus, 30 mg/kg over 1 hour; followed by infusion at the rate of 5.4 mg/kg per hour for 23 hours if administered less than 3 hours from the time of the injury or for 48 hours if the bolus was administered 3 to 8 hours from the time of the injury.* Currently, the medical literature does not support the use of steroids if given more than 8 hours after injury; it also does not support their use for peripheral nerve injuries. An increased incidence of gastrointestinal bleeding and sepsis has also been reported as a side effect of high dose steroid treatments. In the recent years, the use of steroids for spinal cord injury have increasingly been called into question and are increasingly falling out of favor due to lack of a clear clinical benefit to patients. **At this time, the use of steroids is labeled as a "treatment option" based on a large-scale review of the scientific literature.**

10. Other treatments—Other pharmacologic agents such as naloxone, lazaroids (tirilizad), and gangliosides (GM-I) are investigational and are not the standard of care. Similarly, cooling of the spinal cord and anticoagulant treatment are not part of recommended care for spinal cord injuries. However, relatively straightforward trauma resuscitation measures are recommended for patients with spinal cord injury, such as maintaining normotension while avoiding secondary hypotension, maintaining a normal hematocrit and providing adequate oxygenation.

C. Operative Treatment

1. Indications—In general, surgical care is recommended for patients with neurologic injury, discoligamentous disruption (dislocations), highly comminuted burst fractures, displaced Type II odontoid fractures, and multisegmental spine fractures or multiple trauma in which stabilization of one or more spinal fractures can expedite mobilization and care of the patient. Usually surgical stabilization is also recommended for patients with concurrent neck deformities and ankylosing spine conditions due to the inadequacy of external bracing.

2. Anesthesia—General endotracheal anesthesia in a patient with an unstable cervical spine is preferably performed while avoiding neck manipulation. Manual inline traction has been recommended to minimize manipulation. However,

awake nasal intubation and fiberoptic intubation (while maintaining external neck immobilization) offer a chance at airway access with the least risk of inadvertent neck manipulation. However, this technique may not always be applicable. Monitoring spinal cord function with clinical checks or electrophysiologic monitoring is helpful to identify possible emerging neurologic deterioration.

3. Timing of surgery—The timing of surgery for cervical spine fractures remains controversial. Currently there is no consensus as to the definition of "early" surgery. Previously held beliefs that early surgical intervention for cervical spine trauma is potentially dangerous because of an increased risk of neurologic deterioration have largely been refuted. However, there is no consensus as to the benefits gained from early surgical intervention either with respect to neurological function. There is substantial evidence, however, that early fixation allows for early mobilization and decreased complications such as pulmonary complications and decubitus ulcers.

4. Emergent surgery—Emergent surgical intervention in the C-spine is usually indicated for patients with a cord compression due to a herniated nucleus pulposus or bone fragments, an expanding epidural mass (such as an epidural hematoma), an unreducible fracture-dislocation with spinal cord compression, and in the presence of cord swelling with a progressive neurodeficit (controversial).

5. Surgical approach—Surgical treatment options in C-spine trauma consist of an anterior, posterior, or combined anterior–posterior approaches. With present day techniques, most operatively treated C-spine injuries no longer require combined approaches, but are sufficiently treated with anterior or posterior approaches alone.

6. Bone graft—As in any arthrodesis, C-spine fusions generally require bone graft. This can be obtained from local, autologous, or allograft sources and can be of morsellized or structural nature as needed. For trauma, the use of xenografts or prosthetic devices is not considered standard of care.

7. Anterior approach—Anterior cord decompression via discectomy or corpectomy achieves a more complete and neurologically relevant decompression compared with posterior techniques for most conditions. This approach is relatively atraumatic and can be accomplished without manipulating the patient. However, it is more limited in its biomechanical fixation strength especially in the presence of osteopenia and unsuitable for highly unstable patients or patients with ankylosing spinal disorders as a stand-alone approach for fixation.

8. Posterior approach—The posterior approach offers the advantage of a more extensile exposure with access to the occiput and thoracic spine as needed. ***Posterior instrumentation systems usually offer more rigid stabilization than anterior instrumentation***.

9. Cervical laminectomy—Cervical laminectomy may be indicated for patients with depressed laminar fractures and foraminal obstruction from facet fractures. A cervical laminectomy, however, destabilizes the spine and does not lead to a meaningful anterior spinal cord decompression. It is therefore not recommended as a stand-alone procedure for patients with C-spine trauma, and therefore is usually combined with multisegmental posterior fixation and fusion.

10. Spinal instrumentation—The goal of spinal instrumentation is to maintain fracture reduction and column alignment while providing a stable environment for timely bony union. In surgically treated C-spine trauma, supplemental instrumentation is commonly used to achieve a predictable fusion result.

VI. Anatomic and Biomechanical Considerations and Operative Techniques
   A. Anterior Cervical Surgery
      1. Anterior exposure—Standard anterior exposure techniques usually allow for access from the base of C2 to the T1 vertebra.
         • Smith-Robinson approach—The concept that a left-sided Smith-Robinson approach can reduce the risk of a recurrent laryngeal nerve palsy because of the more predictable anatomic course of the nerve has remained debated, but is increasingly called in doubt. ***The recurrent laryngeal nerve is a branch of the vagus nerve.***
         • Landmarks—Along with radiographic confirmation, the carotid tubercle, which is located at the C6 segment, provides a useful bony landmark for level determination. The cricoid cartilage ring usually is anterior to the C6 segment as well. The thoracic duct enters the neck on the left side of the esophagus and runs posterior to the carotid sheath. The vertebral artery is located in the foramina transversaria from the C2 to C6 segments and is covered anteriorly by the longus colli muscle. The vagal nerve lays anterolateral to the longus colli muscle.
      2. Tricortical iliac crest autograft—Anterior fusions are most commonly accomplished with structural tricortical iliac crest autograft. Fusion

rates well above 90% have been reported with this technique. Segmental fibula allografts have been increasingly used as an alternative to iliac crest autograft in an effort to minimize donor site morbidity, but have slightly lower union rates as compared with autograft. Increasingly, structural cages made of a variety of biomaterials filled with bone graft material of allograft are being used to avoid the morbidity and time required for bone graft harvesting.

3. Anterior fusions performed for traumatic indications—In this setting, rigid supplemental fixation with a plate–screw construct has become a recommended treatment component in addition to an arthrodesis to (a) maximize chances for fusion, (b) maintain restored physiologic alignment, and (c) protect decompressed neural alignment. As previously stated, an anterior procedure offers a less traumatic chance to provide effective neural decompression and fixation with the patient in a supine position. There remain relatively few indications for combined anterior and posterior surgery. For instance, a patient with a locked facet dislocation and concurrent large disc herniation can pose a treatment challenge due to the risk of postreduction cord impingement. In this situation, an anterior discectomy with placement of an intervertebral bone graft is followed by open posterior reduction and instrumented fusion. Of course, an alternative to this treatment sequence would consist of an anterior discectomy with attempts at subsequent open reduction, followed by anterior fusion and stabilization with a locking plate.

4. Anterior implant biomechanics—Anterior instrumentation systems are typically less stiff than posterior instrumentation except in extension loading. This may be the reason for the slightly higher nonunion rates in cervical spine trauma, where the anterior approach is generally preferred (better patient recovery). Anterior approaches are also limited in terms of multilevel fixation and occipito-cervical as well as cervico-thoracic instrumentation options.

5. Anterior plate fixation—Currently, anterior plates are of a low-profile design and are usually made of titanium to minimize esophageal impingement. Screws featuring a locking mechanism allow for a unicortical screw design and minimize the risk of screw back-out or toggle loosening. The surface of the screw–plate construct should be devoid of any sharp edges or protuberances to facilitate unencumbered esophageal motility. There are few (if any) advantages for "dynamic" or compressible" anterior plates in the trauma setting due to instability concerns. Although these implants can be placed anywhere from the C2 to the T1 vertebral bodies, multilevel anterior fusion with these devices remains controversial and more prone to complications. Fortunately, the majority of LCS injuries requiring surgical stabilization do not require fusion beyond one or two motion segments. Translational plates are rarely indicated in the setting of trauma.

6. Anterior compression screw fixation—Anterior compression screw fixation has been described specifically for Type II odontoid fractures. This technique may be contemplated if nonoperative treatment with a halo vest seems unlikely to succeed and if a fusion of the C1–C2 segment is undesirable. Single screw fixation seems to afford sufficient fracture fixation compared with the more traditional two-screw construct. Anterior screw fixation is not recommended in patients with os odontoideum or delayed or established nonunions of odontoid fractures. There is also strong concern that in a debilitated elderly population, anterior screw fixation may have an increased complication rate due to dysphagia and there may be significant swallowing difficulties leading to aspiration. Because of these issues, many support posterior instrumentation so as to avoid any proximal anterior dissection.

7. Anterior C1–C2 fusion—Anterior C1–C2 fusion can be accomplished through the facet joints and stabilized with interfragmentary compression screws or an anterior plate placed through a transoral approach. While this procedure is a technical possibility, it is rarely used due to increased risk of dysphagia from retraction of the superior laryngeal plexus and retraction of the upper esophagus.

8. Anterior decompression of C1 or C2—Anterior decompression of C1 or C2 structures is very rarely indicated in the treatment of acute neck fractures in the absence of comorbid conditions. It may be considered for symptomatic malunions or nonunions of odontoid fractures.

B. Posterior Cervical Surgery
1. Posterior cervical fusion—Posterior cervical fusion for trauma is typically accomplished with autologous cancellous bone graft, allograft, and/or bone substitute extenders placed into the desired facet joints and along the laminae (if present). For trauma indications, supplemental, posterior instrumentation is recommended to promote a successful union with restored anatomic alignment.

2. Interspinous wire fixation—Interspinous wire fixation of the cervical spine, as popularized by

Rogers, can be an efficient technique for achieving posterior reduction and fusion over one or two motion segments in cases of facet dislocations. In trauma, interspinous wire fixation may be considered in patients with unstable facet injuries. Limitations of this simple and inexpensive instrumentation option are patients with laminar or spinous process fractures, laminectomies, multilevel fusion needs, severe osteoporosis, and rotationally unstable injuries. With the advent of today's modern instrumentation, there is rarely an indication for the use of interspinous wiring alone given the higher rate of nonunion and failure.

3. Posterior cervical segmental fixation—Posterior cervical screw and rod or plate fixation has become the preferred form of posterior fixation due to fixation strength and ability to provide stability in transition zones (occipito-cervical and cervico-thoracic regions) even in the presence of impaired posterior segments or across multiple levels. Screw purchase is obtained in a unicortical or bicortical fashion within the lateral masses of C3 to C6 using specific trajectories, such as those described by Roy Camille, Magerl, and others. Key structures to avoid include the spinal cord medially, the vertebral artery anteriorly, and the nerve roots laterally and inferiorly. At C2 and C7, and in the upper thoracic spine, the lateral masses are either absent or unsuitably small. In these vertebral segments, screws can be placed within the vertebral pedicle aiming toward or into the vertebral body as per the specific bony anatomy of these levels. Compared with interspinous wire fixation, segmental posterior cervical instrumentation offers increased rotational stiffness, and much improved fixation stiffness in all dimensions in cases of multilevel fixation. These instrumentation techniques require intricate knowledge of the spinal anatomy and therefore are preferably preformed by trained spine surgeons.

4. Posterior atlantoaxial fusion—*In cases of traumatic instability of the C1–C2 complex resulting from fracture or dislocation, a posterior atlantoaxial fusion with instrumentation is indicated*. A variety of techniques have been described.

   • Gallie and Brooks wiring techniques—The C1–C2 fusion techniques using wire or cable constructs basically employs either a Gallie or a Brooks technique, with many variations of each having been described. The Gallie technique consists of a sublaminar C1 wire loop secured to the C2 spinous process. This construct achieves only limited biomechanical rigidity. Fusion is accomplished with an autologous clothespin-shaped corticocancellous bone graft. The Brooks technique offers increased biomechanical stiffness, especially in flexion and translation, as compared to the Gallie technique. However, it requires one or two sublaminar wire passages on either side of the posterior arches of C1 and C2. Usually an oval corticocancellous bone graft is secured to either side of the spinous processes to allow for fusion.

   • Transarticular screws—A more stable form of C1–C2 stabilization can be achieved with transarticular screws placed bilaterally from posterior through the inferior articular process of C2 into the lateral mass of C1. If executed correctly, this technique offers satisfactory stabilization even in patients with deficient laminae at C1 and C2. Posterior fusion can be performed via a technique similar to the Gallie or Brooks technique or by means of a facet arthrodesis if the C1–C2 laminae are deficient or fractured. Improper drilling or screw passage may cause vertebral artery injury. Minimizing this risk requires preoperative evaluation of a fine-cut CT scan to look for an abnormally medialized vertebral foramen and placement of the screws by an experienced surgeon using an adequate C-arm technique. Approximately 15% of patients will have vertebral artery anatomy not conducive to safe placement of these screws.

   • Harms technique—Though initially described by Goelle, this technique is commonly referred to as the Harms technique. This technique consists of placement of C1 lateral mass screws linked via a rod to C2 pedicle screws. This technique is biomechanically equivalent to transarticular screws but allows for more versatility in patients with vertebral artery anatomy not conducive to transarticular screws. This technique can be used with deficient or traumatized lamina. Again, careful preoperative planning is indicated with careful evaluation of axial and sagittal CT scans.

5. Occipitocervical fusion—In exceptional circumstances, occipitocervical fusion may have to be considered if adequate C1–C2 stabilization cannot be achieved. Occipitocervical fusion is also the treatment of choice for any displaced occipitocervical dissociation. Surgical options consist of structural corticocancellous bone graft with stabilization using occipitocervical

plating or wire fixation with a halo. New constructs allow for the use of locking plates secured to the occiput and linked via a rod to top-loading, poly-axial screws in the UCS.

6. Sublaminar hooks and clamps—Sublaminar hooks and clamp constructs are generally contraindicated in the subaxial cervical spine because they can encroach on the spinal cord. In light of the high success rates with standard wire constructs or transarticular screws and in the absence of biomechanical advantages, posterior cervical clamps and compression claws are unnecessary.

VII. Complications of Cervical Spine Injuries
A. Missed C-Spine Injuries—Before CT, more than 33% of C-spine injures were missed on completion of the initial workup. In the C-spine, the main areas of concern for missed injuries are the transition zones (occipitocervical and cervicothoracic spine) and occult ligamentous injuries. Missed C-spine injuries may result from a variety of factors, including most commonly, failure to order a study, failure to visualize or recognize an injury, and less commonly, failure of the patient to report an injury. Neurologic deterioration after a missed C-spine injury occurs in about 30% of patients. A variety of patient conditions such as a short neck with a stout body habitus, radiographic osteopenia, skeletal immaturity, preexisting skeletal deformity or advanced degenerative changes, and an altered or diminished mental state can make the diagnosis of a C-spine injury very difficult.

1. Odontoid fractures—In the upper C-spine, odontoid fractures can be easily missed. An odontoid fracture may not be visible on an axial plane CT scan since the fracture is in the same plane as the study. Displaced Type II odontoid fractures that are left untreated are not expected to heal. The presence of osteophytes or an ostepenic skeleton can make a correct diagnosis challenging. A CT with reformatted sagittal and coronal views usually allows for reliable diagnosis.

2. Atlantooccipital injuries—Atlantooccipital injures are rare injuries and are missed 60% to 75% of the time. Spontaneous partial reduction and suboptimal radiographic visualization of the occiptocervical junction are potential causes. Severe neurologic deterioration has been reported in patients with missed atlantooccipital injures. Historically these patients did not survive, however, with increasing awareness of this injury many patients are now surviving. Careful scrutiny is necessary to accurately make the diagnosis

and treat these patients appropriately in an expeditious fashion.

3. Cervicothoracic injuries—Injuries in this transition zone have been missed or underestimated in severity in 50% to 70% of patients as a result of difficulties in visualizing the area with conventional radiographs. CT with reformatted views is helpful in visualizing this area.

4. Occult ligament injuries—Despite the advent of MRI, ligamentous injuries of the cervical spine continue to pose a diagnostic and treatment challenge. Upright lateral radiographs, lateral dynamic motion studies, and MRI may help in assessing the integrity of the cervical spine ligaments. In general, if a helical CT scan with axial, coronal, and sagittal reformats does not show any abnormalities, the cervical spine can be cleared. The difficulty with this algorithm is in patients with degenerative changes, and in these cases, MRI is helpful and indicated.

5. Presence of ankylosing conditions—The presence of ankylosing spondylitis or other ankylosing conditions make the spine, especially the neck, more prone to fractures. 90% of these injuries will be extension-type injuries with anterior widening or disruption, most commonly in the C5/6 or C6/7 region. Frequently, fracture lines follow unusual patterns and can be easily missed because of radiographic distortion caused by the underlying disease process. Most fractures in ankylosing spondylitis are inherently unstable. *If missed, a 75% incidence of secondary neurologic deterioration has been described*.

B. Neurologic Deterioration
1. Injury severity—A number of factors determine the occurrence of spinal cord injury in cervical spine trauma. The magnitude and direction of injury force are obvious contributing factors. Similarly, the duration of neural element compression may have some effect on the severity of neurologic deficit and recovery potential. Small spinal canal dimensions relative to the cord size have a high prognostic correlation with the occurrence of spinal cord injury. Further pathomechanisms include cord ischemia and cord swelling. *The severity of neurologic injury is related to the presence and magnitude of abnormal cord signal on early postinjury MRI*.

2. Mental status changes—Vertebral artery injuries may cause ongoing cranial infarction by embolization or can be associated with stroke or even death in the case of vertebral artery

flow obstruction in patients with an incomplete Circle of Willis.

C. Musculoskeletal Function—Neck sprains such as whiplash-type injuries are commonly associated with temporarily decreased motion and pain. The expected course of neck sprains in the absence of more serious structural trauma is benign. Persistent neck pain should prompt clinical and, if indicated, radiographic reevaluation such as flexion-extension radiographs or MRI. Patients who have sustained fractures or dislocations of the neck are overwhelmingly most affected by the neurologic injury and the extent of neurologic recovery. To date, there is no established correlation between injury severity, type of treatment, and the presence of neck pain in these patients.

VIII. Complications of the Treatment of Cervical Spine Injuries

A. Early Perioperative Neurologic Deterioration—This is a feared but fortunately rare complication. Regularly documented postoperative neurologic status checks are important for early recognition of neurologic deterioration. In the case of unexpected neurologic status deterioration, expedient further workup with neuroimaging such as plain CT or MRI with contrast is recommended. In the early postoperative phase (up to 2 to 3 weeks after surgery), a variety of possible causes should be considered. Causes of early postoperative neurologic deterioration include malreduction of the neural canal or foramina, hardware interference, loss of reduction, graft displacement, epidural hematoma, cord swelling, cord ischemia, and epidural infection. Cord ischemia can have lasting adverse effects on neurologic function and is commonly poorly understood.

B. Late Posttreatment Neurologic Deterioration—The onset of late neurologic deterioration begins on completion of injury healing, and should be investigated with neuroimaging studies. Causes of late neurologic deterioration include adjacent level stenosis, nonunion or malunion of the fracture (or fusion) with loss of alignment, syrinx, perineural cysts, loss of alignment, and osteomyelitis or discitis.

C. Halo Treatment—The most common complications of halo treatment are loss of reduction, pin tract loosening in 36%, pin tract infection in 20%, and loss of reduction in 15%. Despite the relatively common incidence of complications, halo vest assemblies maintain a key role in the nonoperative management of many cervical spine injuries in North America. Generally, the more common complications such as pin tract loosening or infection can easily be handled. With respect to loss of reduction, it is important to develop an understanding of which injury patterns can appropriately be managed with a halo and which ones will develop loss of reduction and are therefore better handled surgically from the start.

1. Loss of cervical spine alignment—Specific treatment recommendations for this scenario cannot be given here. The basic treatment concept of nonoperative care of the particular patient should be reevaluated; readjustment of the halo assembly can be considered. Alternatively, a return to closed reduction with recumbent traction care or surgical stabilization may be considered.

2. Pin tract infections—Pin tract infections are frequently associated with pin loosening. Prevention by insisting on antiseptic placement technique at correct skeletal locations and avoiding bunching of the skin are prerequisites. Correct daily pin care and patient education are very important. In the case of infection or loosening, local wound care, antibiotic treatment, and pin retightening should be considered. ***Pin retightening can usually be undertaken once (to 8 in/lb) if resistance is met within the first two turns. Recurrent loosening is preferably treated by pin removal and reinsertion at another safe site***.

3. Injury of the supraorbital nerve—The supraorbital nerve is the structure most commonly injured by improperly placed anterior halo pins. Anterior halo pins should be placed anterior to the temporalis fossa and temporalis muscle and lateral to the frontal sinus and the supraorbital nerve. The supratrochlear nerve is medial to the supraorbital nerve just above the eyebrow.

D. Anterior Cervical Surgery—Complications of anterior cervical spine surgery are mainly related to surgical exposure, patient comorbidity, and graft healing.

1. Anterior neck exposures—complications of anterior surgical neck exposures include hoarseness (recurrent laryngeal nerve palsy), dysphagia (esophageal laceration, excessive retraction, denervation), sympathetic plexus injury (Horner's syndrome), vascular injures (carotid arteries, vertebral arteries, jugular veins), and restrictive airway problems. All of these complications together are reported in less than 5% of patients.

- Injury of the recurrent laryngeal nerve—*Injury of the recurrent laryngeal nerve is the most common neurological complication after anterior cervical spine surgery*. The most common cause is a traction-induced neuropraxic injury. If hoarseness persists beyond 6 weeks after surgery, laryngoscopy is indicated. Surgical exploration is usually delayed for more than 6 months after surgery.
- Retropharyngeal hematoma—Retropharyngeal hematoma formation can occur in the early postoperative phase. Presenting clinical symptoms can range from swallowing difficulty to difficulty in breathing.

2. Anterior neck fusion—Complications of anterior neck fusion include graft migration, graft subsidence, hardware breakage, hardware pullout, nonunion, and malunion. In general, these complications occur in less than 5% of patients. Increasing complications rates may be expected in anterior treatment series with multilevel corpectomies without posterior fusion, in the presence of poor bone structure, or in patients with impaired bone healing.

E. Posterior Cervical Surgery—Complications of posterior cervical instrumentation are infrequent, with a 0.6% incidence of iatrogenic root injury and a 2.4% incidence of delayed union or nonunion associated with instrumentation failure. There is a trend toward higher surgical exposure-related musculoskeletal pain and decreased neurologic recovery in patients undergoing posterior cervical surgery as compared with anterior cervical surgery. Nonunions and iatrogenic vertebral artery injuries have been reported occasionally.

IX. Nonunion
A. Atlas—Nonunions of the atlas are uncommon and thus are infrequently a cause for concern. Splaying of the C1 lateral masses a total of 7 mm or more beyond the C2 lateral masses is usually associated with a transverse ligament injury and unacceptable atlantoaxial instability. Unilateral C1 lateral mass sagittal splits may also progress to a nonunion with settling of the occiput onto C2 causing C2 radicular symptoms and a cock-robin type deformity.
B. Odontoid—*Type II odontoid fractures are at an increased risk of nonunion with displacement of more than 5 mm*. Nonoperative treatment of these fractures usually requires closed reduction with a halo vest for at least 3 months. Nonunion

rates of 50% have been reported. Primary atlantoaxial (C1–C2) fusions have the lowest nonunion rates for Type II odontoid fractures. Mixed results have been reported with anterior internal fixation of odontoid fractures using compression screws. Increased nonunion rates of Type II odontoid fractures have been associated with poor technique, osteoporosis, elderly patients, segmental comminution, and reverse obliquity of the fracture line. A nonunion of an odontoid fracture usually requires an atlantoaxial fusion with instrumentation and autologus corticocancellous bone graft. An occipitocervical fusion can usually be avoided but remains an option.
C. Ring Fractures of the Axis—Nonunions of the axis (Hangman's fracture) are uncommon if the injury is identified and properly immobilized.
D. Lower C-Spine—Nonunions of lower C-spine fractures are relatively uncommon with nonoperative treatment.

X. Malunions and Deformities
A. Atlas—Intra-articular fracture extension can be associated with pain and loss of range of motion.
B. Odontoid—Regardless of treatment type, atlantoaxial rotational motion rarely returns to normal, even in the event of anatomic fracture union. Atlantoaxial rotation commonly remains diminished by at least 30% because of scarring and heterotopic bone formation within the atlantoaxial articulations.
C. Ring fractures of the Axis—Malunions without ligamentous instability after treatment of displaced hangman's fractures are usually well tolerated.
D. Lower C-Spine—*The most common type of posttraumatic malunion of the lower C-spine is cervical kyphosis*. Causes for kyphosis include compression fractures or burst injuries, and interspinous ligament failure. Unrecognized injury to the interspinous and supraspinous ligaments may result in interspinous widening, vertebral translation, and pain. The assessment of instability includes clinical evaluation, dynamic motion studies, and neural imaging. Instability parameters (see earlier section on lower C-spine stability) can be used as an aid in the decision-making process. If instability or unacceptable malalignment is identified, the suggested treatment usually consists of fusion and an attempt at deformity correction with posterior, anterior, or combined surgical techniques depending on the severity of displacement and the timing of presentation.

XI. Special Circumstances
A. Ankylosing Spondylitis and Diffuse Idiopathic Hyperostosis—Fractures in patients with ankylosing conditions occur more readily, are more

easily missed, and are inherently unstable. Given the patient population with this condition, these fractures are more prone to develop secondary complications, including spinal cord compromise. These patients will develop epidural hematomas in about 20% of cases and therefore an MRI is often indicated, particularly in the case of progressive neurological deterioration. Early surgical stabilization, usually involving posterior fusion and instrumentation with multilevel fixation, is the preferred treatment option, provided that the patient's medical status permits surgical intervention.

B. Spinal Cord Injuries without Radiographic Abnormalities (SCIWORA)—SCIWORA have been identified in patients with hypermobile spine segments (e.g., pediatric patients). This injury entity has become increasingly rare in light of MRI scans. The assessment of patients with unexplained neurologic deficit focuses on ruling out an occult fracture or ligamentous injury. If none are found, conservative care with immobilization lasting weeks to months is preferred.

SUGGESTED READINGS

Classic Articles

Anderson PA, Montesano PX. Morphology and treatment of occipital condyle fractures. *Spine.* 1988;13(7):731–736.

Anderson LD, D'Alonzo RT. Fractures of the odontoid process of the axis. *J Bone Joint Surg Am.* 1974;56(8):1663–1674.

Allen BL Jr, Ferguson RL, Lehmann TR, et al. A mechanistic classification of closed, indirect fractures and dislocations of the lower cervical spine. *Spine.* 1982;7(1):1–27.

Bracken MB, Shepard MJ, Halford TR, et al. Administration of methylprednisolone for 24 to 48 hours or urilized mesylate for 48 hours in the treatment of acute spinal cord injury: results of the Third national Acute Spinal Cord Injury Randomized Controlled Trial. *JAMA.* 1997;277:1597–1604.

Clark CR, White AA 3rd. Fractures of the dens: a multicenter study. *J Bone Joint Surg.* 1985;67A:1340–1348.

Effendi B, Roy D, Cornish B, et al. Fractures of the ring of the axis. A classification based on the analysis of 131 cases. *J Bone Joint Surg Br.* 1981;63-B(3):319–327.

Felding JW, Hawkins RJ. Atlanto-axial rotatory fixation (fixed rotary subluxation of the atlanto-axial joint). *J Bone Joint Surge.* 1977;59A:37–44.

Garfin SR, Botte MJ, Byrne TP, et al. Application and maintenance of the halo skeletal fixator. *Spinal Dis.* 1987;2:1–8.

Garfin SR, Botte MJ, Waters RL, et al. Complications in the use of the halo fixation device. *J Bone Joint Surg.* 1986;86A:320–325.

Graham B, Van Peteghem PK. Fractures of the spine in ankylosing spondylitis: diagnosis, treatment and complications. *Spine.* 1989;14:803–807.

Grant G, Mirza SK, Chapman JR, et al. Risk of early reduction in cervical spine subluxation injuries. *J Neurosurg.* 1999;90:1–18.

Grob D, Crisco JJ III, Panjabi MM, et al. Biomechanical evaluation of four different posterior atlantoaxial fixation techniques. *Spine.* 1992;17:480–490.

Harris JH Jr, Carson GC, Wanger LK, et al. Radiologic diagnosis of traumatic occipitovertebral dissociation: 2. Comparison of three methods of detecting occipitovertebral relationships on lateral radiographs of supine subjects. *AJR Am J Roentgenol.* 1994;162:887–892.

Herkowits HN, Rothman R. Subacute instability of the cervical spine. *Spine.* 1984;9:348–357.

Hunter T, Dubo H. Spinal fractures complicating ankylosing spondylitis. *Am Intern Med.* 1978;88:546–549.

Johnson RM, Harr DL, Simmons EF, et al. Cervical orthoses: a study comparing their effectiveness in restricting cervical motion in normal subjects. *J Bone Joint Surge.* 1977;59A:332–340.

Johnson RM, Own JR, Hart DL. Cervical orthoses: a guide to their selection and use. *Clin Orthop.* 1981154:34–45.

Levine AM, Edwards CC. Fractures of the atlas. *J Bone Joint Surg.* 1991;73A:680–691.

Levine AM, Edwards CC. The management of traumatic spondylolisthesis of the axis. *J Bone Joint Surg Am.* 1985;67(2):217–226.

Lieberman IH, Webb JK. Cervical spine injuries in the elderly. *J Bone Joint Surge.* 1994;76B:877–881.

Torg JS, Sennett B. Spear tackler's spine: an entity precluding participation in tackle football and collision activities that expose the cervical spine to axial energy inputs. *AM J Sports Med.* 1993;21:640–649.

Webb JK, Broughton RB, McSweeney T, et al. Hidden flexion injuries of the cervical spine. *J Bone Joint Surge.* 1976;58B:322–327.

White AA III, Johnson RM, Panjabi MM, et al. Biomechanical analysis of clinical stability of the cervical spine. *Clin Orthop.* 1975;109:85–96.

Recent Articles

Bransford RJ, Stevens DW, Uyeji S, et al. Halo vest treatment of cervical spine injuries: a success and survivorship analysis. *Spine.* 2009;34(15):1561–1566.

Harms J, Melcher RP. Posterior C1–C2 fusion with polyaxial screw and rod fixation. *Spine.* 2001;26(22):2467–2471.

Harris TJ, Blackmore CC, Mirza SK, et al. Clearing the cervical spine in obtunded patients. *J Spine.* 2008;33(14):1547–1553.

Johnson MG, Fisher CG, Boyd M, et al. The radiographic failure of single segment anterior cervical plate fixation in traumatic cervical flexion distraction injuries. *Spine.* 2004;29(24):2815–2820.

Mirza SK, Krengel WF 3rd, Chapman JR, et al. Urgent surgical stabilization of spinal fractures in polytrauma patients. *Clin Orthop.* 1999;359:104–114.

Moore TA, Vaccaro AR, Anderson PA. Classification of lower cervical spine injuries. *Spine.* 2006;31(suppl. 11):S37–S43.

Vaccaro AR, Hulbert RJ, Patel AA, et al. The subaxial cervical spine injury classification system: a novel approach to recognize the importance of morphology, neurology, and integrity of the disco-ligamentous complex. *Spine.* 2007;32(21):2365–2374.

Review Articles

Bohlman HH. Acute fractures and dislocations of the cervical spine: an analysis of three hundred hospitalized patients and a review of the literature. *J Bone Joint Surge.* 1979;61A:1119–1142.

Bono CM, Vaccaro AR, Fehlings M, et al. Measurement techniques for upper cervical spine injuries: consensus statement of the Spine Trauma Study Group. *Spine.* 2007;32(5):593–600.

Bono CM, Vaccaro AR, Fehlings M, et al. Measurement techniques for lower cervical spine injuries: consensus statement of the Spine Trauma Study Group. *Spine.* 2006;31(5):603–609.

Kwon BK, Vaccaro AR, Grauer JN, et al. Subaxial cervical spine trauma. *J Am Acad Orthop Surg.* 2006;14(2):78–89.

CHAPTER 28

Thoracolumbar Spine Fractures and Dislocations

C. Chambliss Harrod, Michael Banffy, and Mitchel B. Harris

I. Overview
   A. Anatomy—The kyphosis of the thoracic spine is produced and maintained by the wedge shape of the vertebral bodies (taller posteriorly than anteriorly). Normal kyphosis of the thoracic spine ranges from 20° to 50°. In contrast, the lordosis of the lumbar spine ranges from 40° to 70° (average 50°) and is principally created by the intervertebral disc configuration, taller anteriorly than posteriorly. Unique to the thoracic spine is its anatomic continuity with the rib cage and sternum; providing significant added stiffness and thus spinal cord protection. This stiffness contrasts with the mobile lumbar spine, and thus produces a transition zone at the thoracolumbar junction (T10–L2). This zone is marked with the loss of ribs, and a transition from a small thoracic spinal canal diameter to a larger lumbar canal diameter. Concurrently, the facet joint orientation transitions from coronal (thoracic) to sagittal (lumbar). This portion of the spine is distinctly "straight" from T10–T11 through L1 to L2.

   Of all fractures, 6% involve the spine and 90% involve the thoracic and lumbar regions. Most occur in the T10-L2 transitional area with 40% of these having a spinal cord injury. In the presence of high-energy mechanisms, there is a 6:1 ratio of complete/incomplete neurologic injuries.

   The spinal cord generally terminates around the L1 to L2 interspace; thus in addition to it being the structural transition area, the thoracolumbar spine is also a neurological transition area. Injuries at the conus medullaris and the cauda equina often have a more favorable prognosis than the more rostral spinal cord areas due to the presence of spinal nerves in addition to the terminal spinal cord. Spinal nerves are generally more resilient with improved capacity for recovery compared to the spinal cord. Due to this highly variable mix of spinal cord and spinal nerves, minimal correlation has been demonstrated between the degree of neurologic injury and the degree of canal compromise.

   B. Epidemiology—Most common site of vertebral fractures (T10–L2—50% all spinal fractures).
      1. Age—bimodal—most common <30 years old and geriatric
      2. *Motor vehicle accidents* (young) and falls (elderly)
      3. *Gunshot wounds* are increasing in frequency (Fig. 28-1)
      4. Gender—Males > Females
      5. Noncontiguous injuries—5-15%
      6. Other injuries—pulmonary injuries (20%), peritoneal and retroperitoneal bleeding (10%—liver/spleen)

   C. Mechanisms
      1. Axial compression—Axial loading produces compressive loading to the vertebral bodies. With sufficient loads, failure occurs initially at the end plates (end-plate impaction fractures—perhaps due to the intervertebral disc driven through the end plates). The common vertebral body *compression fractures* (wedge fractures—Figs. 28-2 and 28-3) occur anteriorly with relative sparing of the middle and posterior body portions. A transition to *burst fractures* (Figs. 28-3 and 28-4) occurs with further axial and, subsequent, flexion loading. A *pincer fracture* (Fig. 28-5) is a unique vertebral body fracture characterized by the same axial loading mechanism; however, *disc implosion through the vertebral body creates a coronal splint with separate anterior and posterior fragments.* The disc below and above the involved vertebrae is in contact. This combined disc and vertebral body injury creates poorer healing.
      2. Flexion—Tensile forces are created posteriorly while compressive forces act at the vertebral

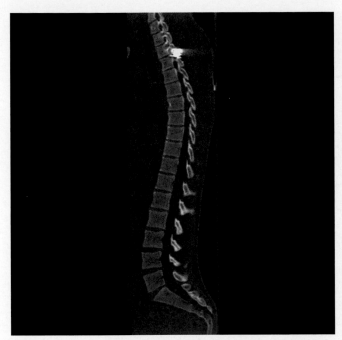

FIGURE 28-1 Sagittal computed tomography (CT) image demonstrating a missile (GSW) lodged in the right T3–T4 spinal canal. The patient had a Brown Sequard syndrome and the foreign body was removed via laminectomy.

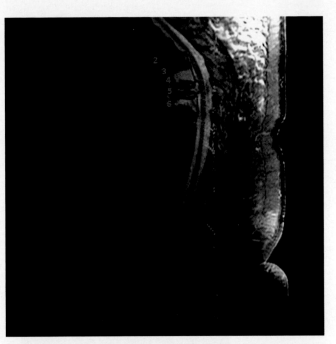

FIGURE 28-3 Midsagittal Short Tau Inverted Recovery (STIR)-weighted magnetic resonance image demonstrating multiple acute and chronic ***osteoporotic compression and burst fractures*** in a caucasian obese 70-year-old female on steroids for chronic lung disease. A chronic T3 burst, acute T4 compression (mild), acute T5 burst, and acute T6 compression fracture are noted with edema (increased signal intensity) denoting acute fractures.

body. When there is a loss of greater than 50% of the vertebral body height, the posterior ligamentous integrity needs to be carefully evaluated. With an intact posterior osteoligamentous complex, this injury pattern is deemed mechanically "stable." Failure to diagnose and treat posterior ligamentous injuries can result in

instability with angular deformity and potential neurologic injury. MRI is the study of choice to directly assess the integrity of these structures (T2 and STIR images).

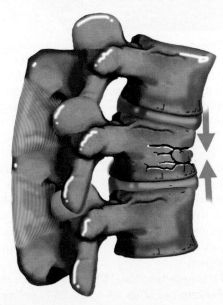

FIGURE 28-2 Vertebral compression fracture.

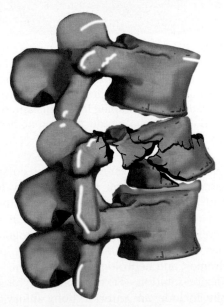

FIGURE 28-4 Vertebral burst fracture.

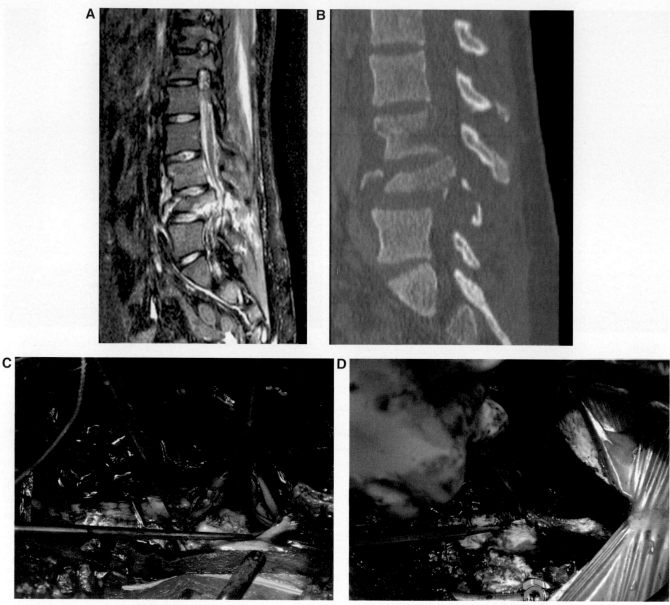

FIGURE 28-5 *Burst Fracture* with incomplete traumatic cauda equina syndrome, ventral and dorsal traumatic durotomies treated with posterior open reduction, decompression, and fusion with durotomy repair. MRI **(A)** and CT **(B)** demonstrate a *burst fracture with pincer morphology* with retropulsion, severe canal and cauda compromise, ligamentous injury, and lamina fracture. Operative photos demonstrate intradural fragments **(C, D)**, which after dural repair were reduced via tamping fragments anteriorly away from the neural elements. Post-reduction CT is seen in Figure 28-12B with adequate reduction and no need for anterior decompression with strut grafting.

3. Lateral compression—Lateral compression forces create lateral vertebral body fractures with or without contralateral or posterior ligamentous disruption. These are best seen on anteroposterior (AP) X-rays. Unrecognized injuries can lead to subacute deformity, pain syndromes, and neurologic deterioration.

4. Flexion-rotation—Flexion-rotation forces usually include an anterior bony injury with an increased probability of posterior ligamentous

and facet capsule failure. The resultant anterior and posterior column involvement typically makes these unstable injuries. Pure dislocation at the thoracolumbar level is uncommon due to facet orientation; when it does occur, it is usually associated with a significant spinal cord injury.

5. Flexion-distraction (FDI)—Also known as *"Chance Fractures"* (Figs. 28-6 and 28-7) or "seat belt injuries" are classically seen in patients wearing

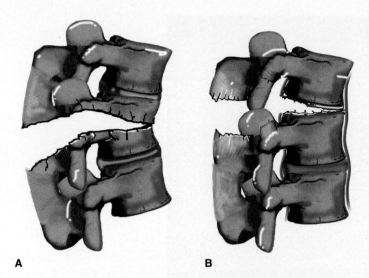

FIGURE 28-6 Flexion-distraction (Chance) injuries.
A. One-level injury with the injury through bone.
B. One-level injury with the injury through soft tissues.

only a lap belt during a motor vehicle collision. The generally accepted mechanism involves a flexion injury with the axis of rotation anterior to the spinal column creating posterior to anterior tensile (distractive) forces across the entire spinal segment with resultant posterior ligamentous or posterior bony avulsion injuries. Forces then continue anteriorly to create either injury to the disc, vertebral body, or both. Vertebral body injury usually exits into the adjacent disc spaces across the end plate ("osseoligamentous" chance fracture) or exits the anterior cortex of the body, creating a pure "bony" chance fracture. Isolated bony chance fractures, most common at L1 to L3, generally heal with proper immobilization while osseoligamentous injuries, most common at the thoracolumbar junction, heal significantly poorer. In addition, secondary axial loading thought to be related to deceleration forces with instantaneous displacement of the axis of rotation can produce vertebral body fractures on a continuum from compression to burst fractures as noted by Court Brown and Gertzbein who devised a flexion-distraction classification based on anterior or posterior fracture involving disk and soft tissue elements and/or bony elements.

6. Extension—Rare shearing injuries ("lumbarjack" injuries): extension and distraction (ED) have opposite injury patterns and mechanisms compared to flexion injuries. Anterior tensile failure with posterior compressive forces leads to posterior element fractures including laminae, facets, and/or spinous processes (Fig. 28-8). Retrolisthesis of cephalad on caudad vertebral body and anterior disc injury (due to tension) can lead to angular deformities. One must be

aware of these injury patterns and associated fractures in patients with stiff spines such as those with Diffuse Idiopathic Skeletal Hyperostosis (DISH) or Ankylosing Spondylitis (AS).

II. Evaluation
A. Associated Injuries—50% of patients with thoracolumbar fractures have non-spinal injuries. Forty-five percentage of flexion-distraction injuries have intraabdominal injuries (i.e., splenic or liver lacerations). Noncontiguous injuries occur 20% of the time. Head injuries and extremity injuries are also common in falls from a height.
B. Overview—The primary trauma survey should be conducted with the "ABCs" (airway, breathing, circulation) and Advanced Trauma Life Support (ATLS) with identification of life-threatening injuries, oxygen, and hypotension management. Cervical collar placement and full spine immobilization precedes the secondary survey.
1. History—Mechanism with likelihood of associated injuries may be determined. Witnesses are helpful as are full details of motor vehicle accidents (speed, location of impact, restraint use). Evaluation of neurologic symptoms may provide insight into spinal cord or neural element pathology.
2. Physical examination—"Log rolling" with full spine visualization and palpation for tenderness, spinal process step-offs or soft tissue defects, and crepitus. Concomitant rectal examination should be performed with notice of tone, perianal sensation, evaluation of anal wink and bulbocavernosus reflex. Fifty percentage of spinal injuries are missed on initial evaluation. Serial neurologic exams include motor and sensory testing, and reflex examination. Careful

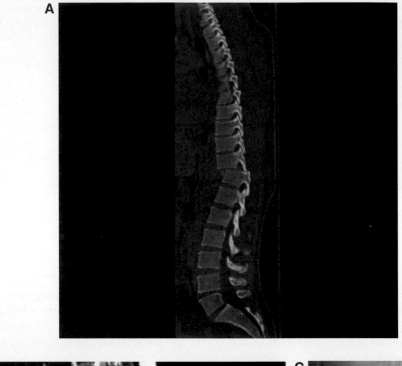

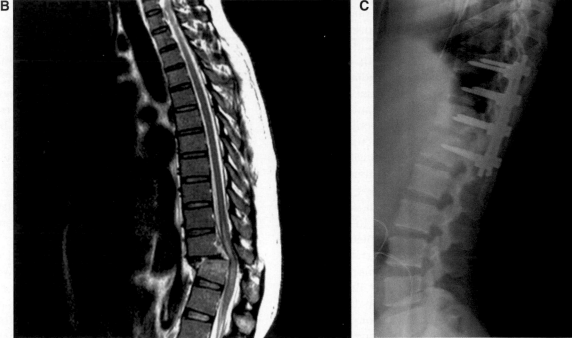

FIGURE 28-7   Parasagittal CT **(A)** image demonstrates a ***flexion-distraction injury*** with superior facet fracture with dislocation. Midsagittal MRI **(B)** demonstrates severe spinal cord compression with edema. This patient had a T9 ASIA B injury (see Table 25-3) with only sacral sparing. Treatment was via posterior open reduction with compression instrumentation **(C)** with iliac crest autograft.

evaluation of the trauma patient in shock is necessary to determine the etiology including consideration of spinal shock as causative. Abdominal tenderness and ecchymosis should raise suspicion for a "seatbelt" injury.

C. Clinical Evaluation and Steroid Use
   1. Spinal shock and complete versus incomplete injury—***Spinal shock*** is a physiologic spinal cord dysfunction occurring below the level of anatomic cord injury with

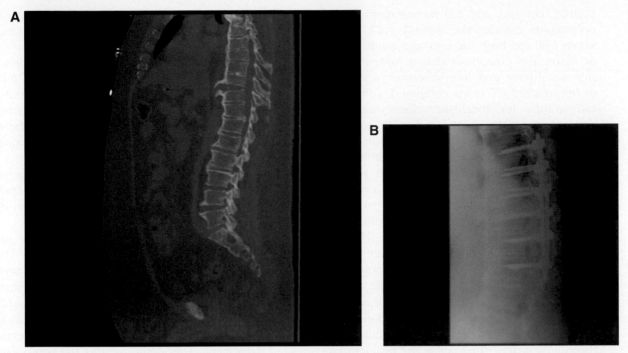

FIGURE 28-8   Midsagittal CT **(A)** and postoperative lateral radiograph **(B)** demonstrate an unstable T9–T10 *extension-distraction fracture* in a patient with Diffuse Idiopathic Skeletal Hyperostosis (DISH). MRI did not show epidural hematoma. Positioning on a Wilson frame on a Jackson table facilitated reduction in flexion followed by posterior compression instrumentation.

flaccid paralysis, areflexia, and absent sensory modalities resolving in 99% of cases by 48 hours. Re-examination with return of the bulbocavernosus reflex hails the end of spinal shock. Total absence of motor (Frankel system grades 0 to 5) and sensory function below the anatomic injury level denotes *complete neurologic injury* whereas *incomplete* injuries maintain residual cord or root function below the injury level. The American Spinal Injury Association (ASIA) has devised the standards for describing spinal cord injuries based on motor and sensory levels in addition to the presence or absence of sacral sparing.

2. Incomplete spinal cord injury patterns *(see Chapter 25)*

D. Steroids—(see Chapter 25)

E. Imaging—After clinical evaluation, multiple modalities can be utilized to effectively visualize thoracolumbar fractures. One must remember to image the entire spinal column once spinal fractures are found in order to avoid missing noncontiguous fractures (typically CT).

1. Radiographs—AP and lateral views combined with swimmer's views that are occasionally necessary to visualize the cervicothoracic junction tend to define vertebral anatomy. The lateral view allows vertebral, facet, spinous process, and intervertebral foramina alignment and assessment. Loss of vertebral body height (>50%) and cortical margins also denote compressive spinal injury patterns. Particular care should be noted to the posterior vertebral line or angle as this can differentiate burst (from compression) fractures with spinal canal compromise. AP views may demonstrate lateral compression fractures, spinous process and pedicular alignment or widening allowing diagnosis of posterior element injury and secondary evaluation of spinal *posterior ligamentous complex (PLC)* instability (>30° kyphosis). Lateral radiographs also allow Cobb measurements of sagittal kyphotic deformities, translation anteriorly or posteriorly (>2.5 mm). Close attention to the endplates on the AP view will also identify subtle injuries missed on lateral views. Plain films are becoming increasingly less popular due to low sensitivities and the utility of screening CT scans for chest, abdomen, and pelvis. However, stable fractures treated nonoperatively should have standing lateral radiographs in an orthosis to ensure a good baseline radiograph as well as no collapse or kyphosis once mobilized.

2. Computed tomography (CT)—CT allows ideal characterization of bony fracture patterns with

sagittal, coronal, and 3-D reconstructions. In polytrauma evaluations, screening CT scans serve well for both visceral and bony injury as Inaba and coworkers demonstrated superior sensitivity and interobserver variability of reformatted CT scans compared with plain radiographs for localizing, classifying, and delineating the thoracolumbar spinal injuries (25% injuries are missed on radiograph alone with gross underestimation of burst spinal canal compromise). Abdominal CT is recommended when a FDI is suspected to evaluate for intraabdominal injury.

3. Magnetic resonance imaging (MRI)—MRI is the modality of choice for visualization of disc herniation, epidural hematoma, ligament injury and SCI. Injury to ligamentous and neurologic structures can be characterized and classified regarding presence of disruption, edema, hematoma, traumatic disc herniation, and presence of cysts or syrinx. Discontinuity of the "black stripe" (classically the ligamentum flavum) with focal stripe of T2 fluid extending superficially indicates instability with tension band disruption. Spinal cord edema or hemorrhage can easily be seen on T2 or T1 weighted images. Use of MRI is controversial in GSW patients.

F. Spinal Stability
1. Injury classifications generally relate to the concept of spinal stability. White and Panjabi define clinical instability as "loss of the ability of the spine under physiologic loads to maintain relationships between vertebrae in such a way that there is neither damage nor subsequent irritation to the spinal cord or nerve roots and no development of incapacitating deformity or pain".

2. Holdsworth predominately identified the posterior ligamentous complex as the key structure(s) to thoracolumbar spinal stability. He classified fracture-dislocations and shear injuries as unstable, whereas all other fracture patterns were deemed stable. The two-column theory arose from belief that the vertebral body and disc were more important as a weightbearing column with a tension band column posteriorly (facet capsules and interspinous ligaments).

3. James et al. confirmed biomechanically the importance of the posterior (instead of middle) column in 1994 emphasizing nonoperative treatment in neurologically intact individuals without posterior column involvement. In vitro studies demonstrated that in addition to posterior ligamentous complex (PLC) disruption, a rotational torque or sectioning of the posterior aspect of the anterior column (posterior annulus) was needed to produce instability.

4. Denis proposed a three-column theory identifying a middle column injury to deem an injury unstable and needing operative intervention. The middle column is an osseoligamentous segment including the posterior half of the vertebral body, nucleus pulposus, annulus, and posterior longitudinal ligament (PLL).

5. Denis classified thoracolumbar spine fractures into four categories: (a) compression fractures, (b) burst fractures, (c) flexion-distraction injuries, and (d) fracture-dislocations.

6. Mechanical instability is defined as the presence of injuries to two or more of the three columns, which allows abnormal motion across the injured spinal segment. However, burst fractures involving the anterior and middle column can have an intact PLC, maintaining sufficient ligamentous integrity to allow nonoperative treatment. This demonstrates the weakness of the three-column approach.

7. Others such as Panjabi and White maintain a vague yet pragmatic method defining clinical stability present when under normal physiologic loading the spinal column can maintain its normal pattern without displacement creating any additional neurologic deficit, incapacitating pain or deformity.

III. Injury Classifications
A. Holdsworth Classification—This early classification system conceptualizes the spine as composed of two columns (anterior/posterior). Holdsworth believed that the PLC ultimately determined stability at each segment. All posterior column injuries were hence unstable.

B. Denis Classification—The three-column classification scheme involves structures of the ***anterior*** (ALL, anterior ½ body/disk/annulus), ***middle*** (posterior ½ body/disk/annulus, PLL), and ***posterior*** (all posterior bony and ligamentous structures including pedicles/laminae/facets/spinous process/ ligamentum flavum/spinous ligaments) columns. Injuries were described as minor (15% to 20% of fractures involving the spinous and transverse processes, pars interarticularis, and facet articulations) and major (compression fractures, burst fractures, flexion-distraction injuries and fracture-dislocations). Definitions of stability and instability are described above. Middle column injury essentially defined stability. Criticism has evolved due to lack of insight in determining stable/unstable injuries especially in light of modern biomechanical studies questioning middle column importance, advances in imaging modalities, and inability to direct fracture management.

C. McAfee Classification—McAfee's classification (wedge-compression, stable and unstable burst, Chance, flexion-distraction, and translational) arose in response to criticisms of Denis' classification by utilizing CT to describe the mode of failure of the middle column, and the classification emphasizes various injuries as stable/unstable with emphasis on the importance of the PLC. The "stable burst fracture" was coined by McAfee and involves the anterior and middle columns with compression fractures but an intact PLC whereas unstable burst fractures involve disruption of the PLC. Chance fractures consist of a horizontal vertebral avulsion injury with the axis of rotation anterior to the ALL. The other two modes include flexion-distraction and translational injuries.

D. AO/ASIF and OTA Classification (Magerl and coworkers)—The AO/ASIF classification is based on the three primary forces applied to the spine. Type A injuries are those caused by compressive loads, Type B injuries are distractive injuries, and Type C injuries are rotational and multidirectional. Each fracture type is divided into three subtypes depending on the severity of load applied and structure(s) compromised (bone vs. soft tissue). The classification provides rationale for determining treatment and prognosis but is limited due to its complex scheme yielding low interobserver reliability.

E. McCormack "Load Sharing"—Assesses vertebral body comminution, fragment displacement, and kyphosis to predict which injuries can be treated with nonoperative management, short-segment transpedicular constructs, or additional anterior column support. Total points greater than 6 require additional anterior column support. Biomechanical and clinical reports have validated its use.

F. Thoracolumbar Injury Classification and Severity Score (TLICS)—TLICS was developed by Vaccaro and coworkers as a practical comprehensive system to aid in decision making regarding operative versus nonoperative care in unstable injury patterns. TLICS is based on three injury characteristics: (1) injury morphology on radiographic appearance, (2) integrity of the posterior ligamentous complex, and (3) neurologic status of the patient. Each characteristic is assigned points and if the sum totals less than 3, nonoperative treatment is recommended. If the sum is greater than 5, surgical intervention is recommended. If the score is 4, injuries might be handled operatively or nonoperatively. In addition, TLICS guides the surgical approach to injuries as seen in Table 28-1. General principles include (a) anterior procedure for incomplete neurologic injuries in which neural elements are compressed from anterior spinal elements, (b) posterior procedure for PLC disruption, and (c) combined approaches for combined incomplete neurologic injury and PLC disruption.

1. Injury morphology—Fracture patterns are similar to the AO classification and described as compression, translation/rotation, and distraction.

TABLE 28-1

The Thoracolumbar Injury Classification and Severity Score (TLICS)

Parameter	Points
Morphology	
Compression	1
Burst	2
Translational/ rotational	3
Distraction	4
Neurologic status	
Intact	0
Nerve root injury	2
Spinal cord/conus medullaris injury	
Complete	2
Incomplete	3
Cauda equina	3
Posterior ligamentous complex	
Intact	0
Indeterminate	2
Disrupted	3
Treatment Recommendations	
Total Score	*Treatment*
≤3	Nonoperative
4	Indeterminate (nonoperative vs. operative)
≥5	Operative

From Vaccaro AR, Lehman RA Jr, Hurlbert RJ, et al. A new classification of thoracolumbar injuries: the importance of injury morphology, the integrity of the posterior ligamentous complex, and neurologic status. *Spine*. 2005;30:2325–2333, with permission.

- Compression (1 point, 2 points for burst)—Compression fractures include axial, flexion, and lateral compression or burst fractures secondary to vertebral body failure under axial loading.
- Rotation/translation (3 points)—These fracture patterns include translation/rotation compression or burst fractures, and unilateral or bilateral facet dislocations with or without compression or burst characteristics. These patterns generally occur under torsional and shearing forces.
- Distraction injuries (4 points)—Distraction injuries are subdivided into flexion or extension injuries with or without compression or burst components. Distraction injuries generally leave one part of the spinal column separated by a space between another area of the spinal column.
  2. Integrity of the posterior ligamentous complex—The PLC or "posterior tension band" protects the spine from flexion, rotation/translational, and distraction forces and heals poorly generally necessitating surgical treatment. Plain radiographs, CT, and MRI imaging are useful in determining whether the PLC is intact (0 points), suspected/indeterminate (2 points), or disrupted (3 points).
  3. Neurologic status—Neurologic injury denotes severe spinal injury and neurologic status in increasing severity can be classified as intact (0 points), nerve root or complete (ASIA A) cord injuries (2 points), or incomplete (ASIA B, C, and D) cord or cauda equina injuries (3 points).

IV. Nonoperative Management
  A. Overview—TL fracture management goals are to restore spinal stability, correct coronal or sagittal deformities, optimize neurologic recovery, decrease pain, and allow early rehabilitation.
  B. Indications for Nonoperative Treatment—In general, fractures without neurologic compression or instability. Also, neurologically and ligamentously intact burst fractures, and some bony FDI (bony Chance) fractures.
  C. Contraindications for Nonoperative Treatment—Ligamentous FDI, fracture-dislocations, fractures with neurologic deficits. Note most AS or DISH patients with subtle appearing extension distraction (most often) fractures can actually have significant three-column injuries requiring stabilization. Late neurologic decline after hospitalization is not uncommon as epidural hematoma in addition to instability can cause neurologic injury.

D. General Guidelines
  1. Typically orthoses are worn for 12 weeks.
  2. Nonoperative cases must still be followed for progressive deformity, nonunion, late neurologic compression, and chronic pain, which may necessitate late surgical management.
  3. Standing lateral radiographs are recommended after orthosis fitting to diagnose physiologic instability which would indicate a fracture requiring surgical stabilization.
  4. Orthoses—Plaster casts or jackets have been replaced.
  5. Jewett (Hyperextension appliances)—resist flexion but are less effective in resisting rotation or lateral bending.
  6. Thoracolumbosacral orthosis (TLSO)—"Clamshell" orthosis.
     - Prefabricated or custom fit—TLSO reduces motion in multiple planes.
     - Limited to T6 and below.
  7. Leg extensions—Addition of leg extensions is indicated when L5-S1 immobilization is required.
  8. Cervicothoracic orthoses (CTO)—TLSO with a CTO extension is indicated in fractures above T5.

V. Spinal Decompression—Decision Making, Timing, Techniques
  A. General Surgical Treatment Pearls
    1. Goals—Spinal stability, deformity correction, neurologic decompression, early rehabilitation, minimization of medical complications (pneumonia, deep vein thrombosis, decubitus ulcers).
    2. Indications—Patients with unstable fractures with progressive kyphosis or translation, incomplete neurologic deficits with persistent cord compression or PLC disruption benefit from surgical management.
    3. Early surgical management—Early surgical management (<72 hours) has been shown to minimize ventilator and ICU days and maximize respiratory function.
    4. Obese patients (unable to tolerate bracing) and polytrauma patients often benefit from surgical treatment to allow early mobilization and rehabilitation.
    5. Ligamentotaxis—distraction instrumentation can aid in canal clearance in patients with greater than two-third canal compromise with an intact posterior annulus attached to bony fractures. Postoperative CT scans and postop neurologic assessments can aid in determining the need for additional anterior decompression.

B. Decision Making—Surgical intervention depends on the mechanical stability/alignment of the fracture, the neurologic status, and general medical condition. General surgical principles of thoracolumbar fracture management tend to maximize function, shorten hospital stay, improve nursing care, and prevent deformity, instability, and pain. Specific surgical goals focus on reconstructing spinal alignment and stabilization of unstable fractures in addition to decompressing neural structures in the setting of neurological deficits. TLICS has been useful at not only classifying and guiding operative versus nonoperative management but also suggesting the surgical approach required.

1. Operative Versus nonoperative treatment
   • TLICS less than 4—nonoperative treatment indicated (exceptions: AS, DISH, neurologic deficit)
   • TLICS equal to 4—nonoperative versus operative treatment based on surgeon experience
   • TLICS greater than 4—operative treatment indicated

2. Anterior Versus Posterior Surgical Approach
   • Posterior approach
     (a) Fracture reduction, malalignment realignment, decompression of epidural hematoma, and biomechanically superior (increased axial, rotational, and pull-out strength) transpedicular instrumentation are the major benefits of the posterior approach.
     (b) Disruption of PLC—requires restoration of the tension band is best done posteriorly (see Figs. 28-7C and 28-8B).
     (c) FDI, Facet dislocations, translational injuries.
     (d) Nerve root injuries are associated with lamina fractures in burst injuries in addition to traumatic dural tear and require posterior decompression. (Figs. 28-5 C & D, 28-9).
     (e) Kyphotic deformities—best treated with a posterior approach within 3 to 5 days of injury (prior to fracture consolidation) with compression instrumentation (distraction instrumentation increases the rate of nonunion).
     (f) Osteoporotic patients—longer constructs with cement augmentation or transpedicular bone grafting can decrease construct failures.
     (g) Complete SCI—best managed via posterior only approach to minimize future deformity, achieve solid fusion, and allow early rehabilitation.

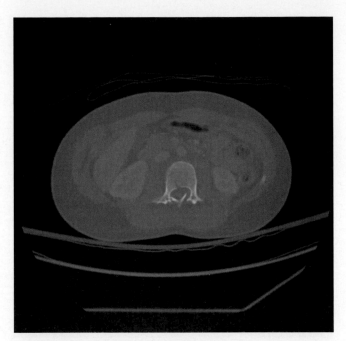

FIGURE 28-9 Axial CT image demonstrates a lamina fracture associated with burst fractures. This patient did have an entrapped root with lacerated dura, which was repaired via open posterior approach.

   • Anterior approach (Fig. 28-10)
     (a) Most other patients with neurologic compression require anterior decompression.
     (b) Anterior-only decompression and reconstruction can be performed in nonosteoporotic burst fractures with neurologic compromise whose posterior ligaments remain intact (TLICS 4 or 5).
     (c) Patients with severe deformity or loss of anterior column support require anterior interbody strut grafting or cage placement.
     (d) Subacute fractures (>5 to 7 days) often require anterior treatment as reduction and ligamentotaxis is often not possible at this point.
   • Posterolateral approach
     (a) Recently, transpedicular, costotransversectomy, and the lateral extracavitary approach has allowed simultaneous superior posterior reduction, instrumentation with anterior decompression and reconstruction via an all posterior approach.

C. Timing of Surgery—Urgent decompression is indicated in injuries with progressive neurologic deficits and mechanically unstable fracture patterns with cord compression.

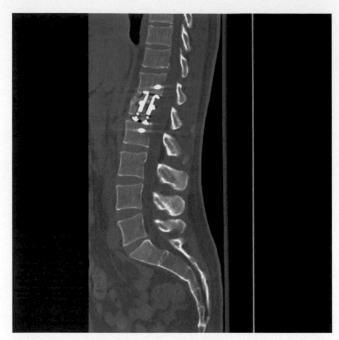

FIGURE 28-10 Postoperative CT midsagittal image following anterior L1 corpectomy with expandable interbody cage placement with anterior bicortical screw-rod instrumentation for a burst fracture with neurologic deficit but without PLC disruption.

1. Animal studies demonstrate recovery of electrophysiologic function if spinal cord decompression occurs within 1 to 3 hours suggesting a possible critical window of opportunity though not corroborated in human studies.
2. Gaebler and coworkers found in one retrospective study greater return of neurologic function when treated surgically less than 8 hours from injury.
3. McLain and Benson found that urgent (<24 hours) spinal stabilization is safe and appropriate in polytrauma patients (ISS > 26 in their study) when there is progressive neurologic deficit, thoracoabdominal trauma, or fracture instability. They reported no venous thromboses, pulmonary emboli, neurologic injuries, decubiti, deep wound infections, or episodes of sepsis in patients undergoing urgent or early (24 to 72 hours) treatment. Chipman and coworkers found similar decreased complications and shorter hospitalizations when treated within 72 hours.
4. Bohlman and coworkers found that late (average 4.5 years from injury) anterior decompression in patients with chronic pain and evidence of spinal cord and cauda equina compression can still have substantial pain relief and neurologic improvement (>1 Frankel grade).

D. Techniques—Indirect, anterior, posterolateral, combined
1. Indirect reduction (Fig. 28-11)—Indirect reduction utilizes a posterior approach through ligamentotaxis via application of distractive forces via segmental instrumentation. Laminectomy alone has been shown to be ineffective in alleviating anterior compression unless an isolated laminar fracture exists with neurologic deficit from a suspected fracture. Indirect reduction requires an intact annulus and maintains that infringing fracture fragments can be reduced to near pre-injury state if done within 2 days with removal of fragments from the spinal canal. If performed late (>10 to 14 days), minimal reduction occurs. Gertzbein and coworkers showed that posterior distraction can provide effective canal clearance when carried out in the first 4 days with initial canal compromise of between 34% and 66%. The extent of canal clearance was notably less in patients with initial compromise less than 33% or greater than 67% and in patients whose operation was done after 4 days from injury.
2. Anterior (see Fig. 28-10)—Anterior approach is the most direct and consistently successful approach for decompression. Corpectomy with direct removal of offending bone/soft tissue fragments is usually performed. The key benefit is minimal neural tissue manipulation with excellent load sharing reconstructive options. Approaches are usually right sided for injuries above T6 due to the location of the heart and great vessels, and are left sided for thoracoabdominal approaches (vena cava, liver). Anterolateral approaches via transthoracic (T4–T9), thoracoabdominal (T10-L1), or retroperitoneal (T12-L5) usually involve resection of the rib at the level or one to two levels above the injured vertebral body for visualization. After resection of the rib, the parietal pleura is incised over the vertebral body with radiographic confirmation of level. Segmental vessels are ligated as needed with subperiosteal exposure of the vertebral body. Diskectomies above and below are performed with subsequent pedicle removal and nerve root identification. The root can be traced to the thecal sac. Removal of the vertebral body occurs with rongeours, curettes, and burs down to the PLL and to the medial border of the contralateral pedicle, which completes the anterior decompression. A portion of the anterior wall is left to protect against graft displacement. Reconstruction can then be undertaken.

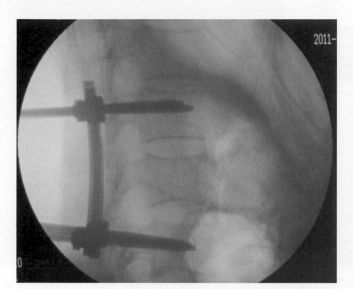

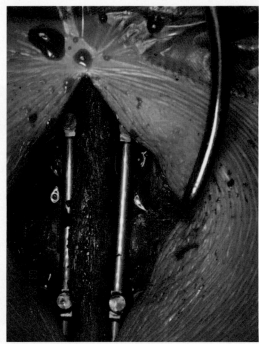

FIGURE 28-11   Burst fracture without neurologic deficit but 35° of kyphosis preoperatively is treated with posterior open reduction with instrumentation with *distraction ligamentotaxis* without fusion.

3. Posterolateral (Fig. 28-12)—Decompression can be undertaken with segmental posterior instrumentation without need for a subsequent anterior procedure. Preoperative axial CT images allow localization of the side and degree of canal compromise. Direct posterior approaches have a high incidence of iatrogenic neurologic injury due to inability to decompress ventral dura without manipulation of the spinal cord. After midline or paramedian skin incision, instrumentation typically extends 2 to 3 levels above and below the injured level; distractive reductive forces can then be applied to assist with reduction. Transpedicular decompression after hemilaminectomy and facetectomy at the injured level is then undertaken after pedicle boundaries are identified. While protecting the nerve root with a Penfield instrument, superior and lateral then inferior and medial cortices are removed via burring then rongeuring with curetting to access the posterolateral vertebral body. Fragments can then be excised or anteriorly translated into the vertebral bodies. Costotransversectomy or lateral extracavitary approaches can be utilized with more lateral exposure to allow more room for anterior decompression and reconstruction though pleural violation is more common. The major drawback is difficulty assessing intraoperative canal decompression. Ultrasound can identify the canal and neural elements from the posterior viewpoint. Postoperative CT scan with/without myelography (or MRI as hardware artifact has decreased with higher resolution scans) remains the procedure of choice for assessing adequacy of decompression, and the potential need for subsequent anterior corpectomy. With the posterolateral approach, reconstruction with placement of an expandable cage is often utilized when the anterior column is significantly destabilized.

4. Combined—Combined anterior and posterior approaches are useful in the treatment of displaced fracture-dislocations with incomplete injury as initial reduction is accomplished posteriorly with subsequent anterior decompression and fusion. Combined procedures are useful when initial posterior realignment and stabilization fails to provide adequate decompression or when open spinal fractures, ankylosing spondylitis or diffuse idiopathic skeletal hyperostosis are present.

VI. Spinal Reconstruction and Instrumentation
   A. Anterior Surgery and Instrumentation
      1. Indications—Indications for anterior surgery include unstable fractures with significant compromise (>50%) of the anterior column

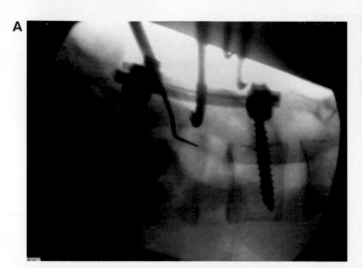

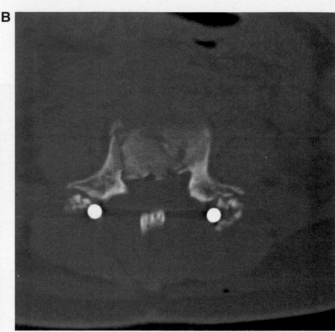

FIGURE 28-12 Direct posterior reduction is demonstrated intraoperatively with fluoroscopy **(A)** and on postoperative CT imaging **(B)** from the patient in Figure 28-5.

support, spinal cord compression via fracture fragments or discs, unstable burst fractures with neurologic injury, and to preserve motion segments.

- Advantages—Safest and most effective method to address cord compression. Anterior surgery allows for optimal biomechanical reconstruction (approximately 80% of axial load is transmitted through the vertebral body). Direct access for cage or interbody device placement allows for improved sizing and fit with lower rates of displacement and subsequent injury/deformity.
- Reconstructive devices—Reconstruction of the anterior column usually combines allograft or autograft with metallic or polyetheretherketone (PEEK) interbody or vertebral body spacers. Structural allografts include tricortical iliac crest, and femoral or humeral shaft. In general, autograft provides higher fusion rates but allograft gives initial increased structural stability without associated harvest site morbidity. Additional internal fixation with plates and screws or dual rods decreases rates of nonunion, resultant deformity and graft dislodgement rates. Current implants are now low profile and rates of great vessel injury are declining.

B. Posterior Surgery and Instrumentation
  1. Indications—Posterior surgery allows spinal realignment and indirect reduction via ligamentotaxis. Long segment constructs typically provide the best fixation. McCormack and coworkers identified the best candidates for short segment pedicle screw constructs (one level above and below injury) to include flexion-distraction or lower lumbar burst fractures with less than 2 mm of fracture fragment displacement, less than 10° of kyphosis, and less than 30% body comminution.
     - Advantages—Significant reduction forces can be applied via posterior instrumentation. Pedicle screw systems facilitate improved realignment relative to earlier hook-rod or sublaminar wiring techniques.
     - Disadvantages—Multiple motion segments must be fused to ensure stable constructs with pedicle screws. Short segment fixation has been associated with increased construct failures in osteoporotic patients as well as those with significant anterior comminution or kyphotic deformities.

C. Minimally Invasive Techniques
  1. General
     - No prospective evidence demonstrates benefit over open approaches.
     - Concept is decreased tissue disruption, less blood loss, shorter hospitalizations, which will lead to improved long-term outcomes.
     - Steep learning curves are expected.

- Relative contraindications—significant canal compromise with incomplete neurologic injuries.
2. Endoscopically-assisted thoracoscopic corpectomy
3. Lateral access approaches—Lateral access approaches (Far-lateral transthoracic or retroperitoneal approaches) via mini-open expandable or tubular retractors (Fig. 28-13).
4. Cement augmentation (Figs. 28-13 and 28-14)
   - Concept—Cement infiltration into fractured vertebral bodies for restoration of anterior support with improved weight-bearing capacity of the anterior column used with or without supplemental fixation.
   - Concern—Cement extravasation through posterior vertebral wall defects can cause iatrogenic neurologic injury as well as respiratory embolization with hypotension and hemodynamic compromise.
   - Vertebroplasty—transpedicular insertion of cement.
   - Balloon-assisted kyphoplasty—vertebral height and angulation are attempted to be

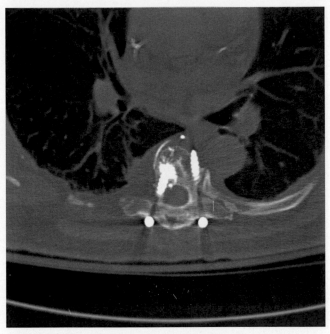

FIGURE 28-14 *Pedicle screw augmentation with cement.* Note the left pedicle screw lateral breach brushing the descending thoracic aorta.

restored with balloon reduction then cement infiltration.

VII. Complications
   A. Medical
      1. GI related—Ileus, gastroesophageal reflux disease, constipation.
      2. Thromboembolic disease—Deep vein thrombosis and pulmonary embolism (up to 2% symptomatic in SCI patients).
         - Consider mechanical compression devices, TED stockings, chemical anticoagulation or vena cava filter placement in SCI patients.
      3. Prolonged hospitalization, pneumonia, decubitus ulcers, malnutrition.
   B. Surgical
      1. Iatrogenic neurologic injury—1% with posterior operations.
      2. Hardware malposition (Fig. 28-15)—visceral, vascular, neural, and dural injuries.
      3. Infection—10%.
      4. Cerebrospinal fluid leaks—primary watertight repair is best although subarachnoid lumbar drain placement with bedrest for 5 days typically allows resolution.
      5. Pseudarthrosis—Pseudarthrosis with construct pullout or failure (see Fig. 28-15), recurrent deformity, unrelenting pain. Revision surgery is often required.

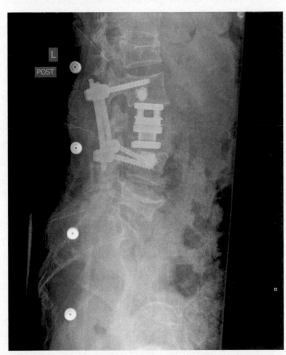

FIGURE 28-13 A 65-year-old woman with severe rheumatoid arthritis on steroids with multiple chronic osteoporotic compression fractures sustained a L3 burst fracture with ligamentous disruption and was treated with an anterior *minimally invasive direct lateral retroperitoneal approach* with L3 corpectomy, expandable cage placement, L2 and L4 vertebroplasty (with cement) to augment endplate strength, and anterior and posterior fusion with percutaneous posterior fixation.

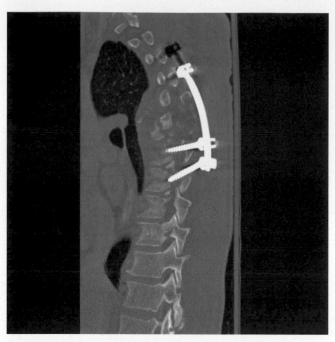

FIGURE 28-15 *Construct failure* with caudal T8 pedicle screw pullout. The laterally placed right T7-8 screws were inadequate to stabilize the T5 and T6 burst fractures in this neurologically intact patient with a ligamentous injury. Revision posterior fixation with extension in addition to anterior column strut grafting was subsequently performed.

 6. Anterior approach related complications—pneumothorax, poor respiratory function, intercostal neuralgia.

VIII. Treatment of Specific Thoracolumbar Injuries
 A. Outcomes
  1. Classic measures—Fusion rate, sagittal alignment, return to work
  2. Patient-centered outcomes
   • General health—SF-36, SF-12: allow a utility score/cost effectiveness analysis.
   • Disease-specific—Oswestry-Disability Index (ODI)—allows identification of lumbar function and disability.
 B. Compression Fractures—A compression fracture is a failure of the anterior column with an intact middle column. Mechanism is axial loading with or without flexion and lateral bending moments. PLC integrity determines treatment but is usually intact. Compression fractures with greater than 50% anterior column height loss or kyphosis greater than 30° have a higher likelihood of an associated PLC injury (strain, attenuation or true disruption). General treatment principles using the following criteria have been recommended.

1. Nonoperative treatment—Nonoperative treatment is recommended for less than 50% height loss and less than 30° of kyphosis. Treatment with orthotics typically includes thoracolumbosacral orthosis (TLSO) or Jewett type hyperextension orthosis. Cervical extension to the brace should be added if cephalad to T7. Activity can be as tolerated while wearing the brace and treatment generally takes 3 months. Brace weaning and PT then proceeds. Interval AP and lateral radiographs taken at approximately 12 weeks determines motion segment stability and the presence of a kyphotic deformity. If early follow up films shows increasing angular deformity or the patient experiences unrelenting pain, increased consideration for surgery should be given.

2. Operative treatment—Operative treatment is usually not indicated in compression fractures without PLC injury unless significant anterior column deficiency or incomplete neurologic injury exists in which case anterior decompression and reconstruction is the procedure of choice. Compression fractures with PLC injury are treated primarily with posterior segmental instrumentation with a combination of pedicle screws and rods. Constructs typically span 2 or 3 levels above and below the injured motion segment as short segment constructs typically have increased rates of loss of fixation and postoperative deformity. After internal fixation, the use of a hyperextension orthosis or body cast for 3 months is optional but should be considered particularly in the setting of compromised bone quality.

3. High versus low energy compression fractures—Differentiation between low energy osteoporotic fractures (elderly) and high energy fractures is important as low energy fractures rarely require operative intervention due to an intact PLC.

4. Contiguous compression fractures—Contiguous compression fractures "act differently" than singular fractures. Total percentage loss of anterior column height should be measured as deformity across contiguous levels can dictate operative intervention of injuries that would be amenable to bracing if occurring in isolation.

C. Burst Fractures—The integrity of the PLC and neurologic status are the driving factors for treatment of thoracolumbar burst fractures. In neurologically intact patients, treatment is near identical to compression fracture management regardless of the presence of retropulsed fragments. With less than 20° of kyphotic deformity, less than 50% anterior vertebral body height loss, no facet subluxation or posterior interspinous widening and intact neurologic exam, brace treatment with full contact orthosis for 12 weeks including early ambulation is reasonable. Bedrest for initial pain relief may be necessary preceding ambulation and bracing.

1. Neurologic status—***Neurologically intact individuals with burst fractures with an intact PLC can be treated nonoperatively. Neurologic injury remains the key factor guiding management of thoracolumbar burst fractures***. Neurologic deficits may manifest as subtle bowel or bladder changes and dysfunction instead of gross sensorimotor deficits. Loss of anal sphincter function, perirectal or perineal sensation or residual urine volume (<50 mL is normal) may be the only noted signs of a subtle neurologic (conus) injury. Incomplete neurologic injuries in the presence of imaging documentation of spinal cord compression provide significant impetus for surgical decompression. Anterior decompression and reconstruction with instrumentation is usually sufficient without evidence of injury to the PLC. Patients with significant PLC disruption should be decompressed and stabilized anteriorly with a strong consideration for additional posterior stabilization. Anterior decompression, reconstruction and stabilization can successfully address this global instability pattern while simultaneously restoring sagittal alignment as shown by Sasso and McGuire. Late anterior decompression (up to 4.5 years after injury) of incomplete injuries in patients in whom acute decompression of the spinal cord or cauda equina was not performed has been shown (by Bohlman and coworkers) to improve neurological function (>50%) and relieve chronic pain (>90%).

2. Posterior ligamentous complex—The PLC is the second key determinant in thoracolumbar burst fracture management. Complete injury to the PLC in neurologically intact individuals is a relative surgical indication. Neurologically intact individuals with less than 50% loss of height are generally treated via posterior reconstruction effecting a reliable return to premorbid sagittal contour. Neurologically intact individuals with significant anterior injury (>50% height loss) can be treated via anterior reconstruction or combined anterior and posterior reconstruction (typically short segment posterior construct) with more severe PLC injuries.

3. Treatment—As described and outlined above with either nonoperative bracing (or casting for noncompliant patients) versus operative intervention with variable approaches. Studies by Cantor and coworkers and Reid and coworkers (prospective) evaluated thoracolumbar burst fractures treated with TLSO bracing and noted no significant change in sagittal alignment at an average of 19 months followup in 18 and 21 patients, respectively. Progression of kyphosis was noted to range between 1° and 4.6° with loss of vertebral height at 6%. Pain was noted to be minimal and the vast majority of patients returned to pre-morbid activities. Nicholl, McAfee, Mumford, and Weinstein, demonstrated that residual sagittal deformity and canal compromise do not correlate with functional outcomes, pain scores, and ability to work. In cadaveric studies, Oda and Panjabi found that near anatomic reduction typically can be accomplished with a combination of distraction (5 mm) and lordosis/extension (6°) applied through posterior pedicle screw-rod constructs. Controversy still persists with regard to optimal management of burst fractures regarding decompression of neurologically complete injuries.

D. Flexion-distraction injuries—These injuries are better known as "seat belt injuries" and typically involve one or two levels. As the mechanism implies, these injuries involve posterior column disruption with some intact anterior elements acting as a hinge or fulcrum with the axis of rotation generally anterior to the spine. However, secondary axial loading often occurs with deceleration and the axis of rotation can exist within the vertebral body. Flexion-distraction injuries can occur through bone only, soft tissue only, or multilevel injuries through a combination of bony and ligamentous/disk elements. ***Management typically is nonoperative for pure bony injuries (as excellent healing typically occurs) and operative for ligamentous or combined injury due to slow and unpredictable healing rates. Stabilization is typically performed via posterior instrumented*** *techniques involving the level above and below the injury.*

1. Nonoperative treatment—Nonoperative treatment of bony flexion-distraction injuries consists of initial bedrest followed by mobilization in a TLSO molded in hyperextension. In the initial postop period, it is important to remember the association of seat-belt injuries with retroperitoneal visceral injuries; therefore, serial abdominal examinations with possible general surgical consultation should be standard. The abdominal injury often dictates the period required before braced ambulation is initiated. After the acute phase has passed, standard nonoperative follow up is initiated with serial standing AP and lateral radiographs. After 3 months, the injury should be re-evaluated with standing AP and lateral films as well as flexion and extension views. If the segment does not heal, the fracture should be surgically stabilized with a short segment posterior compression construct as noted above.

2. Operative treatment—Treatment of flexion-distraction injuries concentrates on identifying compromised column(s) and neutralizing the injury forces. *Short segment (usually one level above and below) posterior stabilization usually suffices with compressive constructs to address injury mechanism.* Evaluation of the middle column and epidural space is important as an associated herniated disk or burst fracture may exacerbate cord or cauda compression with further retropulsion. In the setting of a burst fracture, a *neutralization construct* is more appropriate to realign but not compress the middle column. In the setting of a herniated disk, a hemilaminectomy and a decompression prior to reduction and posterior instrumentation is recommended. Anterior surgery is rarely required to manage injuries seen with this mechanism.

E. Fracture-dislocations—By definition, these are severe injuries with three column involvement and an associated high incidence of neurologic deficits. Nearly all patients are managed operatively. Due to the combined instability, posterior segmental reduction and stabilization will be necessary whereas additional anterior intervention may be indicated depending on the particular injury pattern. Incomplete neurologic injuries in association with fracture-dislocation may benefit from urgent surgery to realign, decompress and stabilize the spine. Safe monitoring while the patient is positioned is possible with awake intubation and prone positioning with close monitoring of the neurologic status prior to anesthesia. Identification of shear injuries is a necessity as management does not involve distraction.

SUGGESTED READINGS

Classic Articles

Albert TJ, Levine MJ, An HS, et al. Concomitant noncontiguous thoracolumbar and sacral fractures. *Spine (Phila Pa 1976)*. 1993;18:1285–1291.

American Spinal Injury Association/International Medical Society of Paraplegia: International standards for neurological and functional classification of spinal cord injury patients. Chicago, ASIA; 2000.

Bohlman HH, Kirkpatrick JS, Delamater RB, et al. Anterior decompression for late pain and paralysis after fractures of the thoracolumbar spine. *Clin Orthop Relat Res.* 1994;300:24–29.

Bracken MB, Shepard MJ, Collins WF, et al. A randomized controlled trial of methylprednisolone or naloxone in the treatment of acute spinal cord injury: results of the Second National Acute Spinal Cord Injury Study. *N Engl J Med.* 1990;322:1405–1411.

Bracken MB, Shepard MJ, Holford TR, et al. Administration of methylprednisolone for 24 or 48 hours or tirilazad mesylate for 48 hours in the treatment of acute spinal cord injury. results of the third national acute spinal cord injury randomized controlled trial. national acute spinal cord injury study. *JAMA.* 1997;277:1597–1604.

Bradford DS, Akbarnia BA, Winter RD, et al. Surgical stabilization of fractures and fracture-dislocations of the thoracic spine. *Spine.* 1977;2:185–196.

Bradford DS, McBride GG. Surgical management of thoracolumbar spine fractures with incomplete neurologic deficits. *Clin Orthop.* 1987;218:201–216.

Cammisa FP Jr, Eismont FJ, Green BA. Dural laceration occurring with burst fractures and associated laminar fractures. *J Bone Joint Surg Am.* 1989;71:1044–1052.

Cantor JB, Lebwohl NH, Garvey T, et al. Nonoperative management of stable thoracolumbar burst fractures with early ambulation and bracing, *Spine.* 1993;18:971–996.

Chance GQ. A note on flexion injuries of the spine. *Br J Radiol.* 1948;21:452–453.

Delamarter RB, Sherman JE, Carr JB. Cauda equine syndrome: neurologic recovery following immediate, early or late decompression. *Spine.* 1991;16:1022–1029.

Denis F. The three column spine and its significance in the classification of acute thoracolumbar spinal injuries. *Spine.* 1983;8:817–831.

Dommisse GF. The blood supply of the spinal cord: a critical vascular zone in spinal surgery. *J Bone Joint Surg.* 1974;56B: 225–235.

Edwards CC, Levine AM. Early rod-sleeve stabilization of the injured thoracic and lumbar spine. *Orthop Clin North Am.* 1986;17:121–145.

Eismont FJ, Green BA, Berkowitz BM, et al. The role of intraoperative ultrasonography in the treatment of thoracic and lumbar spine fractures. *Spine.* 1984;9:782–787.

Ferguson RL, Allen BL. A mechanistic classification of thoracolumbar spine factures. *Clin Orthop.* 1984;189:77–88.

Fidler M. Remodeling of the spinal canal after burst fractures. *J Bone Joint Surg.* 1988;59A:143–149.

Fredrickson BE, Edwards WT, Rauschning W, et al. Vertebral burst fractures: an experimental, morphologic, and radiographic study. *Spine.* 1992;17:1012–1021.

Garfin SR, Mowery CS, Guerra J Jr, et al. Confirmation of the posterolateral technique to decompress and fuse the thoracolumbar spine burst fractures. *Spine.* 1985;10:218–223.

Gertzbein SD, Crowe PJ, Schwartz M, et al. Canal clearance in burst fractures using the AO internal fixator. *Spine.* 1992;17:558–560.

Gertzbein SD. Scoliosis research society: multicenter spine fracture study. *Spine.* 1992;17(5):528–540.

Harris MB. The role of anterior stabilization with instrumentation in the treatment of thoracolumbar burst fractures. *Orthopedics.* 1992;15(3):357–367.

Holdsworth F. Fractures, dislocations, and fracture-dislocations of the spine. *J Bone Joint Surg.* 1970;52A:1534–1551.

James KS, Wenger K, Schlegel ID, et al. Biomechanical evaluation of the stability of thoracolumbar burst fractures. *Orthopedics.* 1992;15(3):357–367.

Kaneda K, Abumi K, Fujiya M. Burst fractures with neurological deficits of the thoracolumbar spine: results of anterior decompression and stabilization with anterior instrumentation. *Spine.* 1984;9:788–795.

Kostuik J. Anterior Fixation for burst fractures of the thoracic and lumbar spine with or without neurological involvement. *Spine.* 1988;13(3):286–293.

Magerl F, Aebi M, Gertzbein SD, et al. A comprehensive classification of thoracic and lumbar injuries. *Eur Spine J.* 1994;3:184–201.

McAfee PC, Bohlman HH, Yuan HA. Anterior decompression of traumatic thoracolumbar fractures with incomplete neurological deficit using a retroperitoneal approach. *J Bone Joint Surg.* 1985;67A:89–104.

McAfee PC, Yuan HA, Lasda N. The unstable burst fracture. *Spine.* 1982;7(4):365–373.

McCormack T, Karaikovic E, Gaines R. The load sharing classification of spine fractures. *Spine.* 1994;19:1741–1744.

McLain RF, Benson DR. Urgent surgical stabilization of spinal fractures in polytrauma patients. *Spine.* 1999;24(16):1646–1654.

McLain RF, Sparling E, Benson DR. Early failure of short segment pedicle instrumentation for thoracolumbar fractures: a preliminary report. *J Bone Joint Surg.* 1993;75A:162–167.

Osebold WR, Weinstein SL, Sprague BL. Thoracolumbar spine fractures: results of treatments. *Spine.* 1981;6(1):13–34.

Pope MH, Panjabi M. Biomechanical definition of spinal stability. *Spine.* 1985;10:255–256.

Weinstein JN, Collalto P, Lehmann TR. Thoracolumbar "burst" fractures treated conservatively: a long-term follow-up. *Spine (Phila Pa 1976).* 1988;13:33–38.

Wenger DR, Carolloa JJ. The mechanics of thoracolumbar fractures stabilized by segmental fixation. *Clinc Orthap.* 289.

Recent Articles

Acosta FL Jr, Aryan HE, Taylor WR, et al. Kyphoplasty-augmented short-segment pedicle screw fixation of traumatic lumbar burst fractures: initial clinical experience and literature review. *Neurosurg Focus.* 2005;18:e9.

Afzal S, Akbar S, Dhar SA. Short segment pedicle screw instrumentation and augmentation vertebroplasty in lumbar burst fractures: an experience. *Eur Spine J.* 2008;17:336–341.

Baptiste DC, Fehlings MG. Pharmacological approaches to repair the injured spinal cord. *J Neurotrauma.* 2006;23:318–334.

Bellabarba C, Fisher C, Chapman JR, et al. Does early fracture fixation of thoracolumbar spine fractures decrease morbidity or mortality? *Spine (Phila Pa 1976).* 2010;35:S138–S145.

Chapman JR, Agel J, Jurkovich GJ, et al. Thoracolumbar flexion-distraction injuries: associated morbidity and neurological outcomes. *Spine (Phila Pa 1976).* 2008;33:648–657.

Chipman JG, Deuser WE, Beilman GJ. Early surgery for thoracolumbar spine injuries decreases complications. *J Trauma.* 2004;56:52–57.

Eck JC, Nachtigall D, Humphreys SC, et al. Questionnaire survey of spine surgeons on the use of methylprednisolone for acute spinal cord injury. *Spine (Phila Pa 1976).* 2006;31:E250–E253.

Gaebler C, Maier R, Kutscha-Lissberg F, et al. Results of spinal cord decompression and thoracolumbar pedicle stabilisation in relation to the time of operation. *Spinal Cord.* 1999;37:33–39

Gnanenthiran SR, Adie S, Harris IA. Nonoperative versus operative treatment for thoracolumbar burst fractures without neurologic deficit: a meta-analysis. *Clin Orthop Relat Res.* 2012;470:567–577.

Harrop JS, Vaccaro AR, Hurlbert RJ, et al. Intrarater and interrater reliability and validity in the assessment of the mechanism of injury and integrity of the posterior ligamentous complex: a novel injury severity scoring system for thoracolumbar injuries. Invited submission from the joint section meeting on disorders of the spine and peripheral nerves, March 2005. *J Neurosurg Spine.* 2006;4:118–122.

Khoo LT, Beisse R, Potulski M. Thoracoscopic-assisted treatment of thoracic and lumbar fractures: a series of 371 consecutive cases. *Neurosurgery.* 2002;51:S104–S117.

Korovessis P, Hadjipavlou A, Repantis T. Minimal invasive short posterior instrumentation plus balloon kyphoplasty with calcium phosphate for burst and severe compression lumbar fractures. *Spine (Phila Pa 1976).* 2008;33:658–667.

Lee JY, Vaccaro AR, Schweitzer KM Jr, et al. Assessment of injury to the thoracolumbar posterior ligamentous complex in the setting of normal-appearing plain radiography. *Spine J.* 2007;7:422–427.

Marco RA, Kushwaha VP. Thoracolumbar burst fractures treated with posterior decompression and pedicle screw instrumentation supplemented with balloon-assisted vertebroplasty and calcium phosphate reconstruction. *J Bone Joint Surg Am.* 2009;91:20–28.

Radcliff K, Su B, Kepler C, et al. Correlation of posterior ligamentous complex injury and neurological injury to loss of vertebral body height, kyphosis, and canal compromise. *Spine (Phila Pa 1976).* 2011.

Sasso RC, Renkens K, Hanson D, et al. Unstable thoracolumbar burst fractures: anterior-only versus short-segment posterior fixation. *J Spinal Disord Tech.* 2006;19(4):242–248.

Shen WJ, Liu TJ, Shen YS. Nonoperative treatment versus posterior fixation for thoracolumbar junction burst fractures without neurologic deficit. *Spine (Phila Pa 1976).* 2001;26:1038–1045.

Siebenga J, Leferink VJ, Segers MJ, et al. Treatment of traumatic thoracolumbar spine fractures: A multicenter prospective randomized study of operative versus nonsurgical treatment. *Spine (Phila Pa 1976).* 2006;31:2881–2890.

Vaccaro AR, Baron EM, Sanfilippo J, et al. Reliability of a novel classification system for thoracolumbar injuries: The thoracolumbar injury severity score. *Spine (Phila Pa 1976).* 2006;31:S62,9.

Vaccaro AR, Lehman RA Jr, Hurlbert RJ, et al. A new classification of thoracolumbar injuries: the importance of injury morphology, the integrity of the posterior ligamentous complex, and neurologic status. *Spine.* 2005;30(20):2325–2333.

Vaccaro AR, Lehman RA Jr, Hurlbert RJ, et al. A new classification of thoracolumbar injuries: the importance of injury morphology, the integrity of the posterior ligamentous complex, and neurologic status. *Spine (Phila Pa 1976).* 2005;30:2325–2333.

Vaccaro AR, Zeiller SC, Hulbert RJ, et al. The thoracolumbar injury severity score: a proposed treatment algorithm. *J Spinal Disord Tech.* 2005;18:209–215.

Wood K, Buttermann G, Mehbod A, et al. Operative compared with nonoperative treatment of a thoracolumbar burst fracture without neurological deficit. A prospective, randomized study. *J Bone Joint Surg Am.* 2003;85-A:773–781.

Wood KB, Bohn D, Mehbod A. Anterior versus posterior treatment of stable thoracolumbar burst fractures without neurologic deficit: a prospective, randomized study. *J Spinal Disord Tech.* 2005;18 Suppl:S15–S23.

Reviews

Anderson PA. Nonsurgical treatment of patients with thoracolumbar fractures. *Instr Course Lect.* 1995;45:57–65.

Bohlman HH. Treatment of fractures and dislocations of the thoracic and lumbar spine. *J Bone Joint Surg.* 1985;67A:165–169.

Gertzbein SD, Court-Brown CM. Rationale for the management of flexion-distraction injuries of the thoracolumbar spine based on a new classification. *J Spinal Disord.* 1989;2(3):176–183.

Hurlbert RJ. The role of steroids in acute spinal cord injury: an evidence-based analysis. *Spine.* 2001;26(24 Suppl):S39–S46.

Inaba K, Munera F, McKenney M, et al. Visceral torso computed tomography for clearance of the thoracolumbar spine in trauma: a review of the literature. *J Trauma.* 2006;60(4):915–920.

Jacobs RR, Asher MA, Snider RK. Thoracolumbar spinal injuries: a comparative study of recumbent and operative treatment in 100 patients. *Spine.* 1980;5:463–477.

Levine AM, McAfee PC, Anderon PA. Evaluation and emergent treatment of patients with thoracolumbar trauma. *Instr Course Lect.* 1995;44:33–46.

McAfee PC, Levine AM, Anderson PA. Surgical management of thoracolumbar fractures. *Inst Course Lect.* 1995;44:47–55.

White AA. Spinal stability: evaluation and treatment. *Inst Course Lect.* 1981;30:457–483.

Willen J, Anderson J, Toomoka K, et al. The natural history of burst fractures at the thoracolumbar junction. *J Spinal Disord.* 1990;3(1):39–46.

Wood EG 3rd, Hanley EN Jr. Thoracolumbar fractures: an overview with emphasis on the burst fracture. *Orthopedics.* 1992;15(3):329–337.

Textbooks

Dick W. *Internal Fixation of Thoracic and Lumbar Spine Fractures.* Berne, Switzerland, Hans Huber, 1989.

Eismont FJ, Garfin SR, Abitbol JJ. Thoracic and upper lumbar spine injuries. In: Browner BD, Jupiter JB, Levine AM, et al, eds. *Skeletal Truama: Fractures, Dislocations, Ligamentous Injuries.* Vol 1. Philadephia, PA: WB Saunders; 1992.

Fredrickson B, Yuan H. Nonoperative treatment of the spine: external immobilization. In: Browner BD, Jupiter JB, Levine AM, et al, eds. *Skeletal Truama: Fractures, Dislocations, Ligamentous Injuries.* Vol 1. Philadephia, PA: WB Saunders; 1992.

Haher TR, Felmly WT, O'Brien M. Thoracic and lumbar fractures: Diagnosis and treatment. In: Bridwell KH, DeWald RL, eds. *The Textbook of Spinal Surgery.* 2nd ed. Vol 2. New York, NY: Lippincott-Raven; 1997.

Levine AM, Eismont FJ, Garfin SG, et al, eds. *Spine Trauma.* Philadelphia, PA: WB Saunders; 1998.

Kostuick JP, Huler RF, Esses SI, et al. Thoracolumbar spine fractures. In: Frymoyer JW, ed. *The Adult Spine: Principles and Practice.* Vol 2. New York, NY: Raven Press Ltd.

Stauffer ES, ed. *Thoracolumbar Spine Fractures Without Neurologic Deficits.* Rosemont, IL 1993. Thoracolumbar spine injuries. In: Errico TJ, Bauer RD, Waugh T, eds. *Spinal Trauma.* Philadelphia, PA: JB Lippincott; 1991.

White AA, Panjabi MM. *Clinical Biomechanics of the Spine.* 2nd ed. Philadelphia, PA: JB Lippincott; 1990.

SECTION III

Pediatric Trauma

CHAPTER 29

General Principles of Pediatric Trauma

William D. Murrell, Michael W. Wolfe, Fredric H. Warren, and Howard R. Epps

I. Child with Multiple Injuries
  A. Incidence of Injuries
    1. Trauma—Trauma is the most common cause of death in children and adolescents in the United States and costs over $1 billion annually. Traumatic injuries account for 20,000 deaths, 600,000 hospital admissions, and 16 million visits to the emergency room. Mechanisms of injury include child abuse, falls, and motor-vehicle accidents (either in them or hit by them). Head injury is the most common reason for death from trauma in children; the ratio of boys to girls is 2:1. Death occurs most often from blunt trauma. Alcohol plays an increasingly important role in the injury of adolescents.
    2. Fractures—Fractures are common in children with multiple injuries. About 9% of fractures in such children are open.
    3. Child abuse—The annual incidence of child abuse in the United States is 15 to 42 cases per 1,000 children; the incidence is increasing (or cases are being better recognized). More than 2 million children each year are victims of physical abuse or neglect, and over 150,000 suffer serious injury or impairment (Neglect is more common than physical abuse.) Children of all socioeconomic backgrounds suffer physical abuse or neglect; however, the incidence does appear to be related to family income. (Children in homes with a family income of less than $15,000 per year are 25 times more likely to suffer abuse compared with children in homes with a family income greater than $30,000 per year.)
       Children with the highest risk for abuse include first-born children, unplanned children, premature children, and stepchildren. Children with an increased risk for abuse include children in a single-parent home, children of parents who abuse drugs, children of parents who were abused, children of unemployed parents, and children of families of lower economic status.

Approximately one-third of abused children are eventually seen by an orthopaedic surgeon. A clear and thorough history and physical examination should be performed. Knowledge of a child's social environment, age, injury pattern, and stated mechanism of injury are all important factors in the evaluation.

Knowledge of injury patterns suggestive of nonaccidental trauma in children is essential. Child abuse must be suspected in all cases of multiple injuries in children younger than 2 years if there is no obvious witnessed explanation for the trauma. *Skeletal injuries that have a high specificity for child abuse include posterior rib fractures, sternal fractures, spinous process avulsion fractures, and scapular fractures. Skeletal injuries that have a moderate specificity for child abuse include multiple fractures, fractures in various stages of healing, vertebral compression fractures, and epiphyseal separations.* Long-bone fractures are commonly seen in cases of child abuse, but have a low specificity. Some authors have suggested that the most common fracture seen in child abuse is a single transverse fracture of the femur or humerus. (Other authors disagree.)

The differential diagnosis in cases of suspected child abuse includes true accidental injury, osteogenesis imperfecta, and metabolic bone disease.

A skeletal survey is a useful initial imaging modality and may be repeated 2 to 3 weeks after the child's initial presentation. Nuclear medicine bone scanning may be helpful when the skeletal survey is negative.

The most important aspect of management is the establishment of the diagnosis of child abuse. (The history of injury must be clearly detailed, documented, and understood.) An instrument for detection of nonaccidental trauma called the screening index for physical child abuse (SCIPA) has been validated; it can assist with diagnosis. By law, all suspected cases of child abuse must be reported to Child Protective Services.

B. Initial Resuscitation—Resuscitation can be cost effective and adequately provided at a general level I trauma center. The ABCs of trauma are the same as those for an adult.

1. Cervical spine—The cervical spine must be stabilized. Special transport spine boards are recommended for children younger than 6 years. *Other ("distracting") injuries such as long-bone fractures, abdominal injuries, and crush injuries can mask cervical spine injuries*.

2. Intravenous access—In the child, intravenous access may be difficult; intraosseous fluid infusion can be considered.

3. Blood pressure—A child's blood pressure must be maintained at an adequate level because *death is more common in children than in adults if hypovolemic shock is not quickly reversed*. (Injuries are usually internal.) Attention to volume administration in a child with a severe head injury is paramount unless hypotension is present from obvious internal or external blood loss. Adolescent girls with traumatic shock have significantly decreased risk of death as compared to boys.

4. Aggressive fluid replacement—Aggressive fluid replacement may lead to internal fluid shifts and thus decrease blood oxygenation levels secondary to interstitial pulmonary edema.

C. Evaluation and Assessment—After initial resuscitation and stabilization, a thorough check for other injuries is initiated.

1. Injury Severity Score (ISS)—The ISS is a valid, reproducible method for pediatric multitrauma. It classifies injuries as moderate, severe, serious, critical, and fatal for each of the five major body systems. Each level of severity is given a numerical code (1 to 5). Systems include general, head and neck, chest, abdomen, and extremities. The ISS is the sum of the squares of the three most injured body systems. The range of severity is from 0 to 75. The New Injury Severity Score (NISS) has been shown to be a better predictor of outcome in severely injured patients.

2. Glasgow Coma Scale (GCS)—Head injury is rated using the GCS. For further details, see Chapter 1.

3. Abdominal examination

4. Extremity examination—Every joint is palpated, and range of motion is assessed. A neurovascular examination is performed.

5. Open fractures
   - Assessment—The nature and extent of the open wound is assessed without probing. The patient should not be subjected to multiple examinations. The injury is then provisionally stabilized. Neurovascular status is checked after stabilization.
   - Treatment—If there is profuse bleeding, a compression dressing or a tourniquet should be applied. Tetanus prophylaxis and an initial dose of broad-spectrum intravenous antibiotics should be given to prevent early wound sepsis. After appropriate radiographic studies and other lifesaving measures have been performed, the patient should be quickly taken to the operating room for a formal irrigation and debridement and skeletal stabilization.

6. Imaging studies
   - Plain radiographs—In the trauma cervical spine series (lateral from C1 to the top of T1, anteroposterior [AP], open-mouth odontoid views), the clinician should watch for pseudosubluxation of C2 on C3 or of C3 on C4, which are normal variants. An AP chest, AP pelvis, and appropriate extremity films should also be obtained.
   - Computed tomography (CT)—CT of the head is performed without contrast if warranted.
   - Retrograde urethrography—Retrograde urethrography is performed if there is urethral obstruction. Urethral injury is common with pelvic fractures.
   - Magnetic resonance imaging (MRI)—If spinal cord injury is suspected, MRI can be valuable, especially in children who have signs and symptoms of compromise without radiographic abnormality.
   - Ultrasonography—Ultrasonography is a fast and accurate way of detecting hemoperitoneum. In some centers, it has replaced laparoscopy and diagnostic peritoneal lavage, but accuracy depends on user experience.

D. Nonorthopaedic Conditions
1. Head injury
   - Recovery—*Head injury is the leading cause of morbidity and mortality in pediatric trauma patients. Recovery from significant head injury, however, is substantially*

better in children than in adults. Even in children with severe head injuries, full functional recovery is likely. Poor oxygenation on arrival to the emergency department and a low GCS at 72 hours after head injury have been correlated with a poorer functional result and a greater neurologic deficit. Failure to treat orthopaedic injuries in a child with a head injury is inappropriate. It must be assumed that a full functional recovery will occur, and optimal orthopaedic care should be provided when the child is able to undergo surgery.

- Complications—Abundant callus forms in fractures of patients with head injuries. Other complications after head injury include spasticity, contractures, and the formation of heterotopic ossification.

2. Thoracic injuries—Thoracic trauma has a mortality rate of 25% in children less than 5 years of age. When there is concomitant head trauma, children with chest trauma have significantly higher morbidity and mortality. Rib fractures are less frequent due to their intrinsic flexibility, and chest contusions can occur without external evidence of trauma.

3. Injuries to abdominal viscera—Injuries to both solid and hollow abdominal viscera are often associated with multiple skeletal injuries. Liver and spleen injuries together comprise 75% of abdominal injuries in children. Multiple pelvic fractures correlate strongly (80%) with abdominal or genitourinary injury. Abdominal trauma should not delay fracture care if the child's medical condition is stable.

4. Fat embolism syndrome—Fat embolism syndrome is unusual in children, but it presents the same as it does in adults. Radiographic changes of pulmonary infiltrates that appear within several hours of a long-bone fracture, axillary petechiae, and hypoxemia should indicate the diagnosis, even in a child.

5. Nutritional requirements—Nutritional requirements can be determined based on the patient's weight and age. The daily nitrogen requirement in the acute phase of injury for a child is approximately 250 mg/kg.

E. Orthopaedic Management—Orthopaedic injuries are rarely life threatening in children, and skeletal stabilization is initially accomplished with a splint.

1. Closed fractures—Early skeletal stabilization can decrease the risk of acute respiratory distress syndrome in children with multiple injuries. Specific guidelines for operative fixation (e.g., intramedullary fixation, compression plate fixation, and external fixation) are beyond the scope of this chapter.

Skeletal injury should be stabilized to facilitate mobilization and management of the patient.

2. Open fractures
   - Classification (Table 29-1)
   - Treatment
   (a) Stages
      - Emergency treatment—Emergency treatment includes tetanus prophylaxis, appropriate antibiotics, a compression dressing to stop bleeding, and application of a splint.
      - Initial treatment in the operating room (OR)—Initial OR treatment includes adequate debridement of devitalized tissue and pulsatile lavage with saline solution with or without antibiotics. The wound is left open if markedly contaminated or if a large soft-tissue defect exists; if a more viable soft-tissue envelope is present, primary closure may be performed after adequate débridement.
      - Definitive treatment—Wound cultures are obtained at the second debridement. Local soft tissue is used to cover a neurovascular bundle, tendons, and exposed cortical bone. Wound debridement is repeated at 48- to 72-hour intervals until the wound can be closed or covered with

TABLE 29-1

Classification of Open Fractures

Type	Description
I	Open fracture with a wound <1 cm long and clean (usually inside out)
II	Open fracture with a laceration ≥1 cm long without extensive soft-tissue damage, flaps, or avulsions
III	Massive soft-tissue damage, compromised vascularity, severe wound contamination, and marked fracture instability
IIIA	Adequate soft-tissue coverage despite extensive soft-tissue laceration or flaps: high-energy trauma irrespective of the size of the wound (e.g., gunshot wound)
IIIB	Extensive soft-tissue injury or loss with periosteal stripping and bone exposure (usually associated with massive contamination) (e.g., farm injury)
IIIC	Open fracture associated with a vascular injury requiring repair

From Beaty J, Kasser J, eds. *Rockwood and Wilkins' Fractures in Children*. 6th ed. Philadelphia, PA: Lippincott Williams & Wilkins; 2006, with permission.

either a split-thickness skin graft or a local of free flap.

(b) Antibiotic treatment (Table 29-2)

(c) General principles of management—General principles of open fracture management include early skeletal stabilization allowing access to wounds for debridement, allowing weightbearing when appropriate, and allowing range of motion of the surrounding joints. Splints and casts can be used for most Type I and stable Type II open fractures with minimal soft-tissue damage. External fixation is usually the treatment of choice for Type II and III open fractures in children (allows easy access to the wound for debridement, allows flap reconstruction, and preserves the length of the injured limb while allowing mobilization and weightbearing). Open reduction with internal fixation is usually reserved for open intra-articular fractures. Hybrid external fixation may be used for fractures that involve the diaphysis and metaphysis.

(d) Bone loss—Bone loss can be managed by immediate or delayed bone grafting.

(e) Free flaps—*Free flaps are more problematic in children than in adults.*

II. Fractures in Children—Attempting to globally define the incidence of pediatric fractures is difficult because of many cultural, climatic, and age differences.

A. Incidence of Pediatric Fractures (Table 29-3)

B. Age Group—There is a linear increase in the annual incidence of fractures with age. The annual incidence of pediatric fractures peaks at age 12, with a decline until age 16.

C. Child Abuse—There is a high incidence of pediatric fractures resulting from nonaccidental trauma (such as battered child syndrome).

TABLE 29-2

Guidelines for Antibiotic Treatment of Open Fractures by Type in Children

Type	Description
I	First-generation cephalosporin for 48–72 h
II	Combination of a first-generation cephalosporin and an aminoglycoside for 72 h
III	Combination of a first-generation cephalosporin and an aminoglycoside for 72 h; for farm injuries (Type IIIB) add penicillin

From Beaty J, Kasser J, eds. *Rockwood and Wilkins' Fractures in Children.* 6th ed. Philadelphia, PA: Lippincott Williams & Wilkins; 2006, with permission.

TABLE 29-3

Incidence of Pediatric Fractures

Type	Percentage
Children sustaining at least one fracture up to 16 yr of age	
Boys	42
Girls	27
Children sustaining a fracture in 1 yr	1.6–2.1
Children who are hospitalized because of a fracture	
During the entire childhood (up to 16 yr of age)	6.8
Each year	0.43
Children with injuries (all types) who have fractures	17.8

From Beaty J, Kasser J, eds. *Rockwood and Wilkins' Fractures in Children.* 6th ed. Philadelphia, PA: Lippincott Williams & Wilkins; 2006, with permission.

Nonaccidental trauma is the leading cause of fractures in the first year of life. This high incidence extends to age 3.

D. Gender—More boys than girls sustain fractures. The ratio of boys to girls in all groups is 2.7:1. The incidence of fractures in girls peaks before adolescence and then decreases. The incidence of fractures from pedestrian versus motor-vehicle accident peaks in both boys and girls from 5 to 8 years of age. Again, the incidence of these injuries is higher in boys.

E. Side of the Body—Left-sided fractures are more common by a ratio of 1.3:1.

F. Frequency by Season—Fractures are more common during the summer. The most consistent climatic factor is the number of hours of sunshine.

G. Long-Term Trends
1. Increase in the number of cases of minor trauma (seen by physicians)—The increase in the number of cases of minor trauma can be attributed to the introduction of subsidized medical care. Expense is no longer a factor; parents are more inclined to seek medical attention for less serious problems.
2. Increase in child abuse—One study showed that the number of fractures from abuse increased almost 150 times from 1984 to 1989. This increase may be attributed to a combination of improved recognition, better social resources, and an increase in the number of cases of child abuse.

H. Specific Fractures
1. Supracondylar humerus fractures—Supracondylar humerus fractures are most common in the first decade of life, and their incidence peaks at age 7.
2. Femoral fractures—Femoral fractures are most common up to age 3 years.
3. Physeal fractures—Physeal fractures are most common just before skeletal maturity. The percentage of fractures that involve the physis is 21.7%.
4. ***Long-bone fractures*** (Table 29-4)
5. ***Specific fractures by anatomic site*** (Table 29-5)
6. Open fractures—The percentage of fractures in children that are open fractures is 2.9%.
7. Multiple fractures—The percentage of children with fractures that have multiple fractures is 3.6%.
I. Common Environments of Childhood Fractures—The percentage of fractures that occur at home is 37%, that occur during sports is 18% to 20%, and that occur during school is 5% to 10%. The number of fractures that occur in motor-vehicle accidents is very low.

III. General Fracture Management
A. Anatomic Features
1. Bone—Pediatric bone is more porous, is less dense (because of less mineralization), and has more vascular channels as compared with adult bone.
2. Periosteum—A child's periosteum is thicker and stronger than an adult's. In the metaphyseal–epiphyseal region, the physis is stabilized by the firm attachment of the periosteum.
3. Other differences—The physis (growth plate) and the secondary ossification center (epiphysis) are the other differences from adult bone.
B. Biomechanical Features
1. Bone—The modulus of elasticity of immature bone is lower than that of adult bone. There is greater plasticity of immature bone. Less energy is required to break immature bone. The bones of children can fail in tension or compression. Greenstick or incomplete fractures occur only in immature skeletons; other patterns of fractures include longitudinal, bowing, torus (compression), and stress. ***Comminuted fracture patterns are less commonly seen because pediatric bone breaks with far less energy applied***.
2. Epiphysis and physis—Epiphyseal fractures are rare in younger age groups, but as ossification occurs, epiphyseal fractures become more common. Intra-articular fractures, joint dislocations, and ligamentous disruptions are less common in children. The bone usually fails before the soft tissues. Fractures that involve physeal separations or the metaphyseal region are common because these areas are relatively weaker than the surrounding ligaments.
C. Physiologic Features
1. Healing—Children heal more rapidly than adults because of increased blood flow and increased cellular activity. Some fractures can be allowed to heal in an overlapped position because of the great remodeling potential found in children.
2. Periosteum—The periosteum has osteogenic activity that leads to rapid healing. An intact periosteal tube can regenerate lost bone. Periosteal damage or loss can lead to significant delays in fracture healing in children.
3. Healing rates and times—Younger children heal faster than adolescents and adults. The healing rate is related to the area of bone injured.

TABLE 29-4

Relative Frequency of Fractures of the Long Bones

Long Bone	Percentage
Radius	45.1
Humerus	18.4
Tibia	15.1
Clavicle	13.8
Femur	7.6

From Beaty J, Kasser J, eds. *Rockwood and Wilkins' Fractures in Children*. 6th ed. Philadelphia, PA: Lippincott Williams & Wilkins; 2006, with permission.

TABLE 29-5

Relative Frequency of Specific Fractures by Anatomic Site

Anatomic Site	Percentage
Distal radius (including physis)	23.3
Hand	20.1
Elbow	12.0
Radial Shaft	6.4
Tibial Shaft	6.2
Other	32.0

From Beaty J, Kasser J, eds. *Rockwood and Wilkins' Fractures in Children*. 6th ed. Philadelphia, PA: Lippincott Williams & Wilkins; 2006, with permission.

Physeal injuries heal faster than metaphyseal injuries, which heal faster than diaphyseal injuries. Nonunion in children is rare.

4. Remodeling—Perfect alignment is not necessary for good results in extraarticular fractures because of remodeling capabilities. Remodeling potential depends on growth remaining (more time for remodeling) and the location of the fracture. *The capacity to remodel is as follows: periphyseal better than metaphyseal better than diaphyseal.* Deformity is more acceptable in the plane of motion of the adjacent joint. Remodeling potential is greatest in areas at the end of the bones that contribute the most to longitudinal growth. Significant remodeling may be expected to occur in the proximal humerus (80% of longitudinal growth), distal femur (70% of longitudinal growth), distal radius (75% of longitudinal growth), and fractures of the elbow (which display less remodeling, so alignment must be kept within a narrower threshold). In general, children younger than 10 years of age have a far greater potential for remodeling than children 10 years or older have. In many anatomic sites, completely displaced and severely angulated fractures in young children can heal without a functional deficit. However, accepting fracture displacement in the young child must be tempered by parental concern regarding cosmetic deformity.

IV. Physeal Injury
   A. Physeal Anatomy
      1. Growth—The physis contains cells responsible for the growth of long-bone and is located at the end of all long bones. These cells are oriented perpendicular to the long axis. Longitudinal growth is the primary function of the physis and occurs through the process of *enchondral bone formation.* The periphery of the physis also produces latitudinal growth.
      2. Relationship to the capsule—*The physis and metaphysis of the proximal femur, proximal humerus, radial neck, and distal fibula are within their respective joint capsules. In all other locations, the physis and metaphysis are extracapsular.*
      3. Ultrastructure—There are *three distinct zones of the physis* (Fig. 29-1).
         • First zone—The first zone has abundant cartilage matrix and is relatively strong. It consists of the germinal or growth cells and is known as the *reserve zone.*
         • Second zone—The second zone is the *proliferative zone* and is where longitudinal growth occurs by the stacking of chondrocytes on one another.
         • Third zone—In the third zone *(hypertrophic zone),* chondrocytes hypertrophy as they begin the transformation from cartilage to bone matrix. (They have a decreased ability to resist shear forces). The hypertrophic zone may be divided into the zones of maturation, degeneration, and provisional calcification. The hypertrophic zone is strengthened by the mineralization process (zone of provisional calcification) but is still weaker than the first two zones. *Physeal fractures tend to occur in the third zone.*
   B. Statistics—The peak age of physeal injury is 11 to 12 years. Boys injure their physes twice as often as girls do. Only about 20% of all children's fractures involve the physis.
   C. Physeal Fractures
      1. Classification—The Salter-Harris classification is used (Fig. 29-2).
      2. Treatment considerations
         • Assessment—The fracture type must be properly identified. The fracture patterns that usually require operative intervention (i.e., Tillaux fracture, triplane fracture) must also be identified.
         • Technique—*Repeated reduction attempts may increase the incidence of growth plate disturbance. Internal fixation should not cross the physis whenever possible. The placement of compression screws across epiphyseal fragments, parallel to the physis, is an effective means of restoring stable articular congruity. When implants must cross the physis, the clinician should use the smallest pin feasible.*
   D. Physeal Arrest (Fig. 29-3)—Trauma is the most common cause of physeal arrest. Arrest occurs when a bridge of bone ("bony bar") forms between the metaphysis and the epiphysis. The magnitude of the resultant deformity is determined by the remaining growth of the child as well as the location of the bar.
      1. Types
         • Partial arrest—Three different patterns of partial physeal arrest may occur. Partial physeal arrest is most commonly recognized on plain radiographs 3 to 6 months after physeal injury. It may appear as a blurring and narrowing of the physis or as an area of reactive bone condensation.

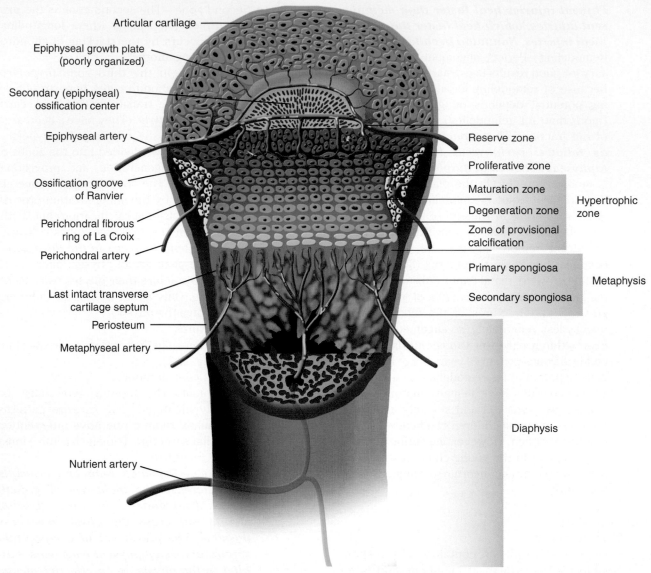

Articular cartilage

Epiphyseal growth plate (poorly organized)

Secondary (epiphyseal) ossification center

Epiphyseal artery

Ossification groove of Ranvier

Perichondral fibrous ring of La Croix

Perichondral artery

Last intact transverse cartilage septum

Periosteum

Metaphyseal artery

Nutrient artery

Reserve zone

Proliferative zone

Maturation zone

Degeneration zone

Hypertrophic zone

Zone of provisional calcification

Primary spongiosa

Secondary spongiosa

Metaphysis

Diaphysis

FIGURE 29-1 Structure and blood supply of a typical growth plate. (Redrawn from The CIBA Collection of Medical Illustrations, Vol 8, part 1, 1987. Illustrated by Frank H. Netter, with permission.)

(a) Peripheral bars—Peripheral bars produce an angular deformity; this is the most common pattern.

(b) Central bars—Central bars result in tenting of the physis and epiphysis and lead to articular surface distortion.

(c) Linear bars—Combined arrests (linear bars) are often the result of a Salter-Harris Type IV injury that has healed in a displaced position. Combined arrests lead to articular incongruity and angular deformity.

• Complete arrest—Complete arrest is usually seen after a crush-type injury to the growth plate (Salter-Harris Type V injury).

2. Common areas for growth arrest—The most common areas for growth arrest are the distal femur, distal tibia, proximal tibia, and distal radius.

3. Diagnosis—MRI and CT imaging are useful for diagnosing a physeal arrest.

4. Treatment

• Conversion of partial arrest into complete arrest—Partial physeal arrest can be converted into a complete arrest to prevent further angulation, but limb length discrepancy results if much skeletal growth remains.

• Contralateral limb epiphysiodesis—Contralateral limb epiphysiodesis is performed to prevent possible limb length discrepancy

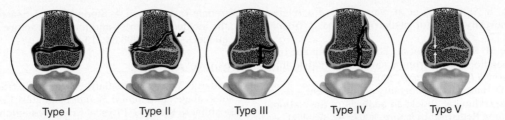

Type I   Type II   Type III   Type IV   Type V

FIGURE 29-2 Salter-Harris classification of physeal fractures. *Type I*, Transverse fracture through the physis. *Type II*, Fracture through the physis with a metaphyseal (Thurston-Holland) fragment (*arrow*). *Type III*, Fracture through the physis and into the epiphysis (intra-articular). *Type IV,* Fracture through the epiphysis, physis, and metaphysis. *Type V*, Crush injury of the physis. (Redrawn from Salter RB, Harris WR. *J Bone Joint Surg.* 1963;45A:587–622. From Tachdjian MO. *Pediatric Orthopedics.* 2nd ed. Vol 4. Philadelphia, PA: WB Saunders; 1990, with permission.)

or eliminate the need for lengthening of the shortened (arrested) limb.

- Bar resection—If more than 2 years of growth remains and less than 30% to 50% of the physis is damaged, bar resection can be considered.
- Surgical approaches
  (a) Peripheral bars—The overlying periosteum is directly approached and excised, and abnormal bone is removed until normal physeal cartilage is uncovered. Interpositional material such as fat or Cranioplast may be used to prevent recurrence. Corrective osteotomies should be performed to correct angular deformities that exceed 15° to 20°.

  (b) Central bars—The surgeon approaches through a metaphyseal window while preserving the periphery of the physis to maintain longitudinal growth.
- Results of treatment—Unfortunately, injured physeal plates tend to close prematurely, before the normal contralateral side, despite the successful restoration of growth. Bar recurrence and incomplete resection have been shown to be factors contributing to poor results.

SUGGESTED READINGS

Classic Articles

Beekman F, Sullivan J. Some observations on fractures of long bones in children. *Am J Surg.* 1941;51:722–741.

Bisgard J, Martenson L. Fractures in children. *Surg Gynecol Obstet.* 1937;65:464–474.

Compere E. Growth arrest in long bones as result of fractures that include the epiphysis. *JAMA.* 1935;105:2140–2146.

Curry J, Butler G. The mechanical properties of bone tissue in children. *J Bone Joint Surg.* 1975;57A:810–814.

Gustilo R, Anderson J. Prevention of infection in the treatment of 1,025 open fractures of long bones: retrospective and prospective analyses. *J Bone Joint Surg.* 1976;58A:453–458.

Hynes D, O'Brien T. Growth disturbance lines after injury of the distal tibial physis: their significance in prognosis. *J Bone Joint Surg.* 1988;70B:231–233.

Landin L. Fracture patterns in children. *Acta Orthop Scand.* 1983;54(suppl. 202):1–109.

Langenskiold A. Surgical treatment of partial closure of the growth plate. *J Pediatr Orthop.* 1981;1:3–11.

Lichtenburg R. A study of 2,532 fractures in children. *Am J Surg.* 1954;87:330–338.

Salter R, Harris W. Injuries involving the epiphyseal plate. *J Bone Joint Surg.* 1963;45A:587–622.

Recent Articles

Chang D, Knight V, Ziegfeld S, et al. The multi-institutional validation of the new screening index for physical child abuse. *J Pediatr Surg.* 2005;40:114–119.

Cross MB, Osbahr DC, Gardner MJ, et al. An analysis of the musculoskeletal trauma section of the Orthopaedic In-Training Examination (OITE). *J Bone Joint Surg Am* 2011;93:e49.

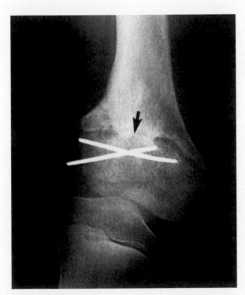

FIGURE 29-3 Physeal bar (*arrow*). (Courtesy Gary T. Brock MD. Fondren Orthopedic Group LLP, Texas Orthopedic Hospital, Houston. From Brinker MR, Miller MD. *Fundamentals of Orthopaedics.* Philadelphia, PA: WB Saunders; 1990, with permission.)

Cuff S, DiRusso, S, Sullivan T, et al. Validation of a relative head injury severity scale for pediatric trauma. *J Trauma.* 2007;63:172–177.

Galano G, Vitale M, Kessler M, et al. The most frequent traumatic orthopaedic injuries from a national pediatric inpatient population. *J Pediatr Orthop.* 2005;25:39–44.

Haider A, Efron D, Haut E, et al. Mortality in adolescent girls vs. boys following traumatic shock: an analysis of the National Pediatric Trauma Registry. *Arch Surg.* 2007;142:875–880.

Hasler C, Foster B. Secondary tethers after physeal bar resection: a common source of failure? *Clin Orthop Relat Res.* 2002;405:242–249.

Hennrikus W, Shaw B, Gerardi J. Injuries when children reportedly fall from a bed or couch, *Clin Orthop Relat Res.* 2003;407:148–151.

Lackey WB, Jeray KJ, Tanner S. Analysis of the musculoskeletal trauma section of the Orthopaedic In-Training Examination (OITE). *J Orthop Trauma* 2011;25:238–42.

Mendelson S, Dominick T, Tyler-Kabara E, et al. Early versus late femoral fracture stabilization in the multiply injured pediatric patient. *J Pediatr Orthop.* 2001;21:594–599.

Peterson D, Schinco M, Kerwin A, et al. Evaluation of initial base deficit as a prognosticator of outcome in the pediatric trauma population. *Am Surg.* 2004;70:326–328.

Sullivan T, Haider A, DiRusso S, et al. Prediction of mortality in pediatric trauma patients: new injury severity score outperforms injury severity score in the severely injured. *J Trauma.* 2003;55:1083–1087.

Thompson E, Perkowski P, Villarreal D, et al. Morbidity and Mortality of children following motor vehicle crashes. *Arch Surg.* 2003;138:142–145.

Wareham K, Johansen A, Stone M, et al. Seasonal variation in the incidence of wrist and forearm fractures, and its consequences. *Injury.* 2003;34:219–222.

Review Articles

Gladden P, Wilson C. Pediatric orthopedic trauma: principles of management. *Semin Pediatr Surg.* 2004;13:119–125.

Khoshhal K, Kiefer G. Physeal bridge resection. *J Am Acad Orthop Surg.* 2005;13:47–58.

Kocher M, Kasser J. Orthopaedic aspects of child abuse. *J Am Acad Orthop Surg.* 2000;8:10–20.

Legano L, McHugh M, Palusci VJ. Child abuse and neglect. *Curr Probl Pediatr Adolesc Health Care.* 2009;39(2):31.e1–26.

Stewart D Jr, Kay R, Skaggs D. Open fractures in children. Principles of evaluation and management. *J Bone Joint Surg.* 2005;87:2784–2798.

Textbooks

Abel M, ed. *Orthopaedic Knowledge Update: Pediatrics 3.* Rosemont, IL: American Academy of Orthopaedic Surgeons; 2006.

Beaty J, Kasser J, eds. *Rockwood and Wilkins' Fractures in Children.* 7th ed. Philadelphia, PA: Lippincott Williams & Wilkins; 2010.

Green N, Swiontkowski M, eds. *Skeletal Trauma in Children.* 3rd ed. Philadelphia, PA: Saunders; 2003.

Herring J, ed. *Tachdjian's Pediatric Orthopaedics.* 4th ed. Philadelphia, PA: Saunders Elsevier; 2008.

Morrissy R, Weinstein S, eds. *Lovell and Winter's Pediatric Orthopaedics.* Philadelphia, PA: Lippincott Williams & Wilkins; 2006.

CHAPTER 30

Pediatric Lower Extremity Injuries

Howard R. Epps

I. Introduction—Pediatric lower-extremity injuries occur much less frequently than upper extremity injuries. Long-bone fractures occur after high-energy trauma such as motor-vehicle accidents and sports injuries or after simple falls in younger children. Unfortunately, child abuse may be the etiology, particularly in younger children. The clinician must always consider this possibility. Sequelae of fractures, such as growth arrest, leg length discrepancy, malunion, neurovascular injury, and compartment syndrome, can profoundly affect the child's function. Attention to detail when managing lower-extremity injuries can lessen the frequency of these undesirable outcomes.

Because lower-extremity fractures can result from high-energy trauma, the patient must have a systematic evaluation. The primary survey is performed to exclude life-threatening injuries and is followed by the secondary survey. Management of specific musculoskeletal injuries depends largely on the age of the patient and the associated injuries.

Open fractures are irrigated and meticulously debrided in the operating room before skeletal stabilization. Prophylactic antibiotics are administered in weight-appropriate doses. Tetanus prophylaxis should be given if necessary. Depending on the mechanical stability and extent of soft-tissue damage, some fractures can be managed in a cast that is windowed for wound care. External fixation, internal fixation, or traction is used for more extensive injuries. As with adult patients, surgical (skeletal) stabilization is generally preferred in cases of pediatric multiple trauma and in cases of head injury.

II. Fractures of the Hip
   A. Overview—Hip fractures, defined as injuries to the portion of the femur proximal to the lesser trochanter, are rare. Such fractures represent less than 1% of all pediatric fractures. Approximately 85% of pediatric hip fractures result from high-energy trauma. The remaining 15% consist of pathologic fractures, usually through tumors. The capital femoral epiphysis appears between 4 and 6 months of age, and the physis fuses between 14 and 16 years of age. ***The proximal femur contributes 13% of the length of the leg, or 3 to 4 mm per year. The blood supply is tenuous and therefore susceptible to injury***.
   B. Evaluation—The child usually has hip pain and refuses to walk. If the fracture is displaced, the leg may appear shortened and externally rotated. Plain films are the best initial study. If plain films are negative, a bone scan or magnetic resonance imaging (MRI) can detect occult fractures.
   C. Classification—The Delbet classification is most commonly used (Fig. 30-1).
      1. Type I—Type I fractures (transepiphyseal fractures [transphyseal separations]) occur more often in younger children. Some 50% are associated with hip dislocations. There is a high incidence of avascular necrosis (AVN), especially with dislocations.
      2. Type II—Type II fractures (transcervical) are the most common, representing 46% of pediatric hip fractures. The risk of AVN is related to the amount of initial displacement.
      3. Type III—Type III fractures (cervicotrochanteric) represent 34% of hip fractures. A good outcome is likely if the fracture is not displaced. AVN is related to both fracture severity and amount of initial displacement.
      4. Type IV—Type IV fractures (intertrochanteric) have the best prognosis. Complications are less common.
   D. Treatment—Hip fractures, particularly displaced ones, require expeditious treatment. In general, in addition to internal fixation, all fractures require cast immobilization for at least 6 weeks if the child is younger than 10 years of age.

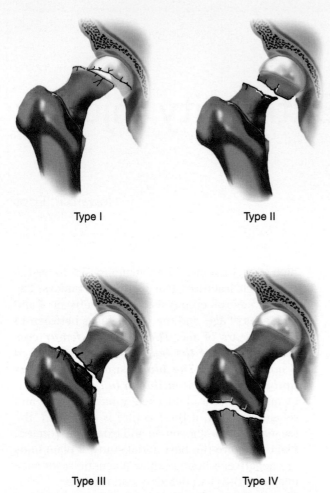

Type I

Type II

Type III

Type IV

<u>FIGURE 30-1</u>   Delbet classification of pediatric hip fractures. Type I, transepiphyseal fracture; Type II, transcervical fracture; Type III, cervicotrochanteric fracture; Type IV, intertrochanteric fracture.

1. Type I fractures—***Type I fractures should undergo a gentle closed reduction and internal fixation***. Fixation is achieved with smooth pins or with cannulated screws in older children. If the child is younger than 2 years of age, reduction and spica cast immobilization without internal fixation is a reasonable treatment for stable fractures. With dislocations, a single attempt at closed reduction is warranted. If unsuccessful, open reduction should be performed from the direction of the dislocation.

2. Type II fractures—Type II fractures require anatomic reduction and stable fixation. A gentle closed reduction may be attempted. If unsuccessful, an open reduction through an anterolateral approach should be performed. Stable fixation is essential. ***Although the physis should be avoided, stable fixation takes precedence over protecting the physis***. Casts

should be applied for 6 to 12 weeks for children who require immobilization.

3. Type III fractures—Type III fractures also require an anatomic reduction and stable fixation. Achieving anatomic reduction requires that an anterolateral open reduction be performed if necessary. The benefit of decompressing the intracapsular hematoma is controversial, but the procedure is advocated by some as a possible means of decreasing the risk of AVN.

4. Type IV fractures—Type IV fractures can usually be treated by closed techniques. Reduction can be achieved under anesthesia or with traction and followed by the application of an abduction spica cast. If the fracture is irreducible or unstable in a cast, internal fixation should be used with a pediatric screw and side plate system. In patients with multiple injuries, Type IV fractures should be treated with open reduction and internal fixation.

E. Complications

1. AVN—AVN is the most common complication, occurring in 6% to 47% of cases. AVN usually occurs during the first 12 to 24 months after injury and is ***related to initial fracture displacement*** with the consequent compromise of blood supply. AVN has also been shown to be associated with increasing age, time to reduction, and quality of reduction. The treatment of AVN of the pediatric hip is controversial but includes restricted weightbearing, bed rest, soft-tissue releases, and containment. There are three types of AVN (Fig. 30-2).

   • Type I involves the whole head. It has the worst prognosis.
   • Type II involves part of the head. The prognosis is fair.
   • Type III occurs from the fracture line to the physis. The prognosis is good.

2. Coxa vara—The incidence of coxa vara after pediatric hip fractures ranges from 14% to 30% but is consistently lower and even absent in series using internal fixation. Coxa vara results from malunion, AVN, inadequate fixation, or partial physeal closure. Observation for 2 years is acceptable because the deformity often remodels with time. If the neck-shaft angle is less than 110° or the child is over 8 years of age, a subtrochanteric valgus osteotomy may be performed.

3. Growth arrest—Growth arrest occurs when AVN is present or when fixation necessitates crossing the physis. Type II and III AVN most often lead to arrest. Leg length measurements and bone age should be followed. Epiphysiodesis

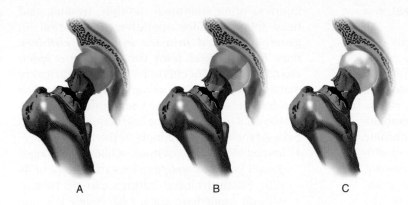

FIGURE 30-2 Patterns of AVN of the pediatric hip. **A.** Total involvement of the capital femoral epiphysis, physis, and metaphysis (Type I). **B.** Anterolateral involvement (Type II). **C.** Metaphyseal involvement (Type III).

or lengthening may be performed if a large leg length discrepancy is anticipated.

4. Nonunion—Nonunion, an infrequent complication, has an incidence of 6% to 10%. An incomplete reduction is often the cause. As soon as it is recognized, nonunion should be treated operatively with subtrochanteric valgus osteotomy with or without bone graft.

F. Special Considerations

1. Pathologic fractures (Fig. 30-3)—Fractures that occur through benign or malignant tumors pose difficult problems. The objective is management of the fracture concurrent with the underlying problem if possible. In some cases, the fracture must heal before tumor management. A guide for management is outlined in Table 30-1.

2. Stress fractures—Stress fractures are rare but can occur in children engaged in activities with cyclic loading. The differential diagnosis includes a slipped capital femoral epiphysis, synovitis, Perthes' disease, avulsion fracture, and neoplasm. Plain films may be negative for several weeks; bone scan and MRI are therefore helpful for early diagnosis. Stress fractures occur in two types: ***tension fractures occur on the superior femoral neck***, whereas ***compression fractures occur on the inferior femoral neck***. Tension fractures are at risk for displacement; therefore, internal fixation is recommended. Compression fractures are more stable and can be managed with either

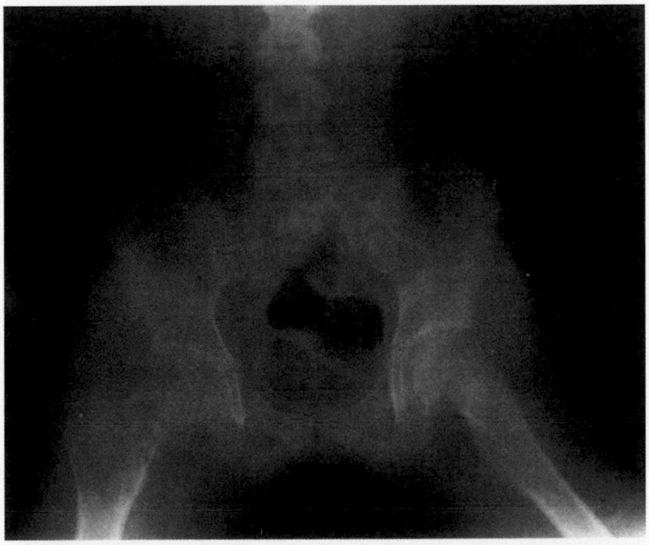

TABLE 30-1

Treatment for Fractures Associated with Tumors and Tumor-like Lesions

Priority for Treatment	*Tumor or Tumor-like Lesion*
Fracture (lesion may heal spontaneously)	Nonossifying fibroma Unicameral bone cyst Eosinophilic granuloma
Fracture—then *lesion* (if necessary)	Unicameral bone cyst Aneurysmal bone cyst Eosinophilic granuloma Nonossifying fibroma Fibrous dysplasia Enchondroma Chondromyxoid fibroma
Fracture and *lesion* (simultaneous)	Angiomas of bone Giant cell tumor Malignant bone tumors
Lesion (fracture may heal with lesional treatment)	Metastatic neuroblastoma Leukemia Selected malignant bone tumors (chemosensitive)

Source: From Green NE, Swiontkowski MF, eds. *Skeletal Trauma in Children.* 2nd ed. Philadelphia, PA: WB Saunders; 1998, with permission.

FIGURE 30-3 Anteroposterior radiograph of the pelvis of a 10-year-old girl shows a radiolucent lesion (aneurysmal bone cyst) of the right proximal femur with a pathologic femoral neck fracture.

restricted weightbearing or a spica cast in a less compliant patient.

3. Slipped capital femoral epiphysis—An unstable acute slipped capital femoral epiphysis presents similarly to a transepiphyseal fracture. Questioning may reveal a history of chronic hip pain, knee pain, or a limp. Radiographs of the hip may demonstrate remodeling of the femoral neck in slips with a chronic component. Stable slips can be stabilized with a cannulated screw inserted percutaneously. Displaced unstable slips should have a gentle reduction by traction or under anesthesia. The femoral head is then stabilized internally in the chronic slip position. Another option is surgical hip dislocation with anatomic restoration of alignment and internal fixation performed by experienced hands.

III. Fractures of the Femoral Shaft
  A. Overview—Femoral shaft fractures, which occur in the region between the lesser trochanter and the supracondylar metaphysis, almost always unite. The challenge is achieving union with acceptable length, alignment, and rotation. Femoral fractures represent 1.6% of all pediatric fractures and 7.6% of all pediatric long-bone fractures. The incidence of child abuse, in children with a femur fracture, approaches 80% in infants younger than walking age, and 30% in children younger than 4 years of age. Young children may sustain femoral fractures with simple falls, whereas older children may be involved in high-energy trauma such as that from motor-vehicle accidents.
  B. Evaluation—Most patients have severe pain and are unable to walk. There may be obvious deformity, swelling, tenderness, and crepitation. Isolated fractures do not cause hypotension. Children with signs of hypovolemia should be carefully evaluated for additional injuries. Plain films are the preferred initial studies and should include the knee and hip to rule out other fractures.
  C. Classification—There is no formal classification system. Descriptors such as *transverse, spiral, oblique, segmental, comminuted, closed,* and *open* are used.
  D. Treatment—The management of pediatric femoral shaft fractures depends on many factors, including age, the mechanism of injury, associated injuries, economic considerations, and psychosocial issues. The goal is to achieve bony union without excessive shortening or malalignment. Current trends attempt to avoid lengthy hospitalization. Fractures with neurovascular injuries, open fractures, multiple trauma, and head injury require operative stabilization. In general, *isolated injuries in young children may be managed with an immediate spica cast*; the injuries of children close to maturity are managed with locked intramedullary nails. For children between 6 and 12 years, there is considerable controversy. All the techniques described have advocates and support in the literature.

1. Immediate spica casting—Children younger than 6 years or weighing less than 60 pounds with isolated closed injuries can be treated with an immediate spica cast. Single leg, one and one half, and double leg spica casts have been reported. If there is more than 2 cm of shortening, some recommend a brief period of skin or skeletal traction before casting. Strict attention to detail is essential for immediate spica casting. Length must be restored, and the cast must be carefully molded to prevent late varus or recurvatum angulation. Radiographic studies are done weekly for the first 2 to 3 weeks to rule out loss of reduction and excessive shortening, which occur in approximately 20% of cases. Loss of reduction may be corrected with cast wedging or cast reapplication. Children who develop unacceptable shortening should be placed in skeletal traction until length is restored and then recasted. The cast is worn for 6 weeks.

2. Traction-delayed spica—Traction with delayed spica cast application yields uniformly good results. The child is placed in skin or skeletal traction for 2 to 3 weeks until the fracture becomes more stable. Radiographs must be checked every few days for excessive shortening or over-distraction. A spica cast is then applied. The technique can present social (and economic) difficulties because of the lengthy hospitalization.

3. Locked intramedullary nail—The injuries of adolescents close to maturity are managed like those of adults: with a rigid locked intramedullary nail. If the capital femoral physis is open, care should be taken to avoid the piriformis fossa when inserting the nail. *Damage to the lateral ascending arteries in the piriformis fossa can cause AVN of the femoral head*; a more anterior or trochanteric starting point is therefore advised. Recently designed pediatric nails avoid the piriformis fossa and the greater trochanteric apophysis. The nail should not violate the distal femoral physis.

4. External fixation—Unilateral external fixation allows early mobilization. The fixator is applied

to the lateral side of the leg; full knee motion must be achieved while in the operating room. The family must be vigilant about pin care because there is a high rate of pin tract infection. Refracture is another complication. A total of 12 weeks may be required before adequate bridging callus is present. Dynamization is important and must be done early.

5. Flexible intramedullary nails—Flexible intramedullary nails (Enders, Nancy) allow early mobilization and therefore avoid the problems of prolonged traction and casting. The nails may be inserted in a retrograde fashion; the starting point is proximal to the distal femoral physis. The nails may also be inserted in an antegrade fashion; the starting point is distal to the greater trochanter. A second operation is necessary to remove the nails after fracture healing. With titanium nails, poor outcomes have been associated with age greater than 11 years, weight greater than 49 kg, and comminution or long oblique fracture patterns. Stainless steel nails had fewer complications than titanium nails in one series.

6. Compression plates—Compression plating is technically simple, convenient for the family, and conducive to early mobilization. It requires large incisions, extensive dissection, and protected weightbearing after insertion. Plate removal is mandatory, and protected weightbearing is continued for 6 weeks.

7. Submuscular bridge plates—Submuscular plating provides all the advantages of compression plating, with less dissection, scarring, blood loss, and more rapid healing. The technique is particularly advantageous for comminuted fractures that are not amenable to treatment with other types of fixation. Achieving an acceptable reduction is critical before applying the plate percutaneously. The plate can then be secured with regular or locking screws, the latter providing greater stability.

E. Complications
1. Leg length discrepancy—*Leg length discrepancy is the most common complication*. It can be secondary to fracture union in a shortened position or limb overgrowth. Overgrowth is poorly understood, but it occurs in children between 2 and 10 years of age during the first 2 years after injury. The amount of overgrowth ranges from 0.5 to 2.5 cm. Leg lengths should be followed for at least 2 years after the union of a pediatric femoral shaft fracture. *Projected shortening discrepancies greater than 6 cm or those with significant deformity can be treated with lengthening and/or deformity correction*. Smaller projected discrepancies without deformity are treated with epiphyseodesis (of the ipsilateral extremity in the case of overgrowth and of the contralateral extremity in the case of shortening).

2. Angular deformity—Angular deformity frequently occurs, and there are several recommendations for acceptable amounts of deformity. Femoral shaft fractures remodel considerably in younger children. Lateral view angulation of $30°$ is acceptable in children younger than 2 years, but the limit decreases to $10°$ in children 11 years and older. In the coronal plane, valgus angulation is better tolerated in general than varus angulation. Anteroposterior (AP) view angulation of $20°$ to $30°$ is acceptable in infants, $15°$ in children younger than 5 years, $10°$ up to 10 years of age, and $5°$ in children 11 years and older.

3. Rotational malunion—Rotational malunion occurs in up to one third of children. There is less remodeling potential than with angular deformities, but up to $30°$ of malrotation is usually well tolerated in children. Derotation osteotomy corrects malunions that require intervention.

4. Neurovascular injuries—Neurovascular injuries are rare, occurring in less than 2% of femoral shaft fractures. Fractures with vascular injuries should be stabilized rapidly, followed by vessel repair. Most nerve injuries associated with the fracture spontaneously recover.

5. Compartment syndrome—compartment syndrome can occur after application of a 90/90 spica cast. Application of the short leg portion of the cast first with subsequent application of traction is believed to be the etiology.

F. Special Considerations
1. Floating-knee injuries—defined by fractures of the femur and the ipsilateral tibia, are usually high-energy injuries. Most authors agree that at least one of the fractures should be managed operatively.

2. Stress fractures—stress fractures of the femoral diaphysis are rare in children. The history of an increase in activity may not be present. Radiographs may be normal, or show periosteal new bone suggestive of a neoplasm. MRI is helpful in making the diagnosis.

IV. Fractures of the Distal Femoral Metaphysis and Epiphysis
A. Overview—The distal femoral physis is the largest and fastest growing in the body. It is responsible for 70% of the femoral length and 37% of the leg length. It grows approximately 1 cm a year,

fusing between 14 and 16 years of age in girls and 16 and 18 years in boys. Because the physis undulates, an accurate reduction is important for preventing physeal bar formation in displaced fractures. Fractures involving the distal femoral physis are relatively uncommon, representing only 7% of all physeal fractures. *Injuries usually result from sports or motor vehicle accidents*. The fracture typically occurs during periods of rapid growth such as the adolescent growth spurt. In children before walking age, there is a strong association between complete fractures and child abuse.

B. Evaluation—The child has an acute onset of pain and is usually unable to walk. The thigh may be angulated or shortened. The knee is tender, with an effusion and ecchymosis. Careful attention to the neurovascular examination is essential for ruling out an associated injury. AP and lateral plain films are the best initial studies. Oblique films may detect a fracture if the initial films are negative. Gentle-stress views or an MRI can be used for difficult cases.

C. Classification—The Salter-Harris classification, although not prognostic, is most commonly used. Salter-Harris Types I and II fractures have a more frequent incidence of growth disturbance. The most important prognostic factors are the magnitude of displacement, age, adequacy of reduction, and severity of trauma.

D. Treatment—*Nondisplaced fractures should be stabilized percutaneously with smooth pins because of the high risk of displacement*. Displaced Salter-Harris Types I and II fractures require reduction and percutaneous fixation. The reduction maneuver is primarily traction with gentle manipulation. Percutaneous fixation is performed with either smooth wires or screws, followed by a cast for 6 weeks with the knee in 10° of flexion. Anatomic reduction is desirable. In children near maturity, up to 5° of varus or valgus angulation is acceptable. In children younger than 10 years, 20° of posterior angulation is acceptable. Displaced Salter-Harris Types III and IV fractures necessitate anatomic reduction with internal fixation by closed or open methods. Fixation is accomplished with screws followed by a cast for 6 weeks. *Pathologic fractures through benign lesions should receive standard fracture care, with management of the neoplasm secondarily after healing*.

E. Complications
1. Leg length discrepancy—Leg length discrepancy is the most common complication (32%). The age at injury is important; discrepancies usually occur with high-energy injuries in younger children. The risk is greater if fracture displacement is greater than 50% of the width of the bone. Treatment options are those that are standard for leg length discrepancy.
2. Angular deformity—Angular deformity (incidence, 24%) occurs most frequently after Salter-Harris Type II fractures. It is usually due to direct physeal injury on the side of the physis opposite the metaphyseal spike. Management may include epiphysiodesis or osteotomy depending on the child's age. The former is performed when a child is close to the end of growth.
3. Physeal bars—Physeal bars can be assessed with tomograms or computed tomograms (CT) to determine the size. *Bars measuring less than 50% of the physeal area can be resected, with fat interposition*. Resection is contraindicated if the patient has fewer than 2 years of growth remaining. *Extensive bars in children near skeletal maturity can be treated with epiphysiodesis of the uninjured leg*.
4. Neurovascular injuries—Neurovascular injuries (incidence, 2%) are rare and usually result from hyperextension injuries. The popliteal artery is injured with anterior displacement, and the peroneal nerve is injured with varus angulation. *Fractures with suspected neurovascular injuries should be reduced emergently with prompt reassessment of vascular status*. If the vascular supply is restored, the patient should be observed for 48 to 72 hours to rule out an intimal tear with thrombosis. If the fracture is irreducible, an open reduction is performed through a posteromedial approach, and the neurovascular structures are directly assessed.
5. Extension contracture of the knee—Extension contracture of the knee rarely follows severe supracondylar femur fractures. Cases failing rehabilitation are managed with Judet quadricepsplasty.

V. Fractures of the Intercondylar Eminence
A. Overview—The intercondylar eminence lies between the anterior horns of the menisci. Fractures of the intercondylar eminence are most common in children between 8 and 14 years of age. Injuries occur after hyperextension of the knee, a fall from a bicycle or motorbike, or a direct blow to the knee.
B. Evaluation—The child typically has pain, an effusion in the knee, and an inability to bear

weight. An aggressive examination should be avoided before radiographic studies to prevent displacement of the fragment. AP and lateral plain films are the best diagnostic studies; the most useful information is obtained from the lateral view. Stress views can be added if an associated physeal or ligamentous injury is suspected.

C. Classification—The Myers and McKeever classification is standard (Fig. 30-4).
  1. Type I—Type I is nondisplaced.
  2. Type II—Type II is one-third to one-half displaced and is hinged.
  3. Type III—Type III is completely displaced.

D. Treatment—For Types I and II fractures, first the hemarthrosis is aspirated. The knee is hyperextended to reduce the fragment, and a long leg cast in 10° to 15° of flexion is worn for 4 to 6 weeks. Irreducible Type II and III fractures may have a meniscus blocking reduction. Reduction is performed open or with arthroscopic assistance. Fragment fixation should be done with absorbable sutures in young children. In older children, nonabsorbable sutures or an intraepiphyseal screw is used.

E. Complications—Loss of knee extension occurs in up to 60% of cases but is rarely a functional problem. Anterior laxity of the knee occurs in 75% of cases, probably as a result of plastic deformation of the anterior cruciate ligament (ACL) before fracture. Patients generally have good outcomes despite residual laxity.

VI. Meniscal Injuries
  A. Overview—The menisci are semilunar cartilaginous cushions in the medial and lateral compartment of the knee. They are completely vascularized at birth. With maturation, the vascular supply to the inner two thirds diminishes. The discoid meniscus is an uncommon congenital anomaly occurring in 3% to 5% of the population. Meniscal tears are rare in prepubescent children unless a discoid meniscus is present. Injuries occur primarily in adolescents.

  B. Evaluation—The child typically complains of activity-related pain, possibly mechanical symptoms. Acutely the child may have an effusion of the knee, but it usually develops over a few hours after injury. There may be joint-line tenderness, or the results of McMurray's test may be positive. Plain films should be done to rule out osteochondritis dissecans or a loose body. MRI is the test of choice.

  C. Classification—Injuries are classified by the anatomy of the tear: radial, flap, longitudinal, horizontal cleavage, and bucket handle.

  D. Associated Injuries—Associated injuries include cruciate ligament tears.

  E. Treatment—In children, some meniscal tears can be managed nonoperatively. Indications for nonoperative management are tears 10 mm or smaller in the outer 30% of the meniscus, radial tears smaller than 3 mm, and stable partial tears. Cast immobilization is required for 6 to 8 weeks. Tears requiring surgical treatment are managed by partial meniscectomy or repair. Repair is considered if the tear is located in the outer 10% to 30% of the meniscus, displaced less than 3 mm, and lacking a complex component.

VII. Ligamentous Injuries of the Knee
  A. Overview—The exact incidence of ligamentous tears in children is unknown, but is thought to be increasing. Studies suggest that roughly 4%

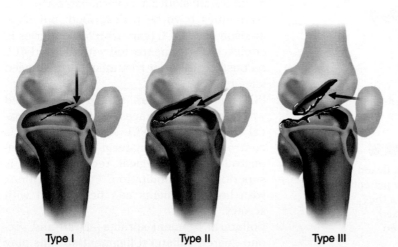

FIGURE 30-4 Myers and McKeever classification of intercondylar eminence fractures. Type I, Nondisplaced. Type II, Displaced with a posterior hinge. Type III, Completely displaced.

Type I   Type II   Type III

of all ACL tears occur in skeletally immature patients. Injuries of the posterior cruciate ligament (PCL) and the collateral ligaments are less common. Both the ACL and the PCL originate from the intercondylar notch. The ACL inserts anterior to the tibial spine, whereas the PCL inserts on the posterior aspect of the tibial epiphysis. The medial collateral ligament (MCL) and lateral collateral ligament (LCL) originate from the distal femoral epiphysis and insert onto the proximal tibia epiphysis and metaphysis and the fibular epiphysis, respectively. ACL tears result from hyperextension, sudden deceleration, or valgus and rotation forces with a planted foot. PCL ruptures result from hyperextension or forceful posterior displacement of the tibia with the foot planted. Ligamentous injuries in young children usually result from multiple trauma.

B. Evaluation—The patient is often unable to walk. The knee usually has a large effusion unless the capsule has been disrupted. There is significant muscle spasm. Lachman's test may be positive with ACL tears, although it is difficult to demonstrate acutely secondary to pain. The best test for acute PCL tears is the quadriceps active test (Fig. 30-5). The collateral ligaments should be palpated at the origins and insertions. Varus and valgus stability should be checked in full extension and 30° of flexion and then compared with the uninjured side. Joint-line tenderness

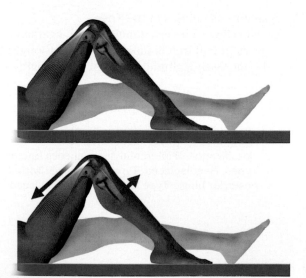

<u>**FIGURE 30-5**</u> Quadriceps active test. The knee is flexed to 90°. Slight resistance is applied to the foot. The patient then contracts the quadriceps muscle, which pulls the tibia anteriorly from its resting, posteriorly subluxed position to a neutral but not an anteriorly displaced position.

may be present if there is a meniscal injury. Plain films are obtained first to rule out a bony avulsion fracture. MRI is the best test for detecting purely ligamentous injuries.

C. Classification
1. First-degree sprain—First-degree sprain involves tenderness without instability.
2. Second-degree sprain—Second-degree sprain involves loss of function without instability.
3. Third-degree sprain—Third-degree sprain involves complete rupture with instability.

D. Associated Injuries—Associated injuries include other ligamentous tears.

E. Treatment
1. ACL tears—Before the management plan is determined, many factors must be considered: the patient's age, skeletal maturity, and the expectations of function after treatment. Studies suggest that children treated nonoperatively have greater difficulty returning to their previous level of function; there is a high incidence of subsequent meniscal injuries, chondral injuries, and episodes of instability. Intra-articular surgical reconstruction necessitates violating the physis, particularly if the surgeon attempts to achieve isometric placement of the graft. Extra-articular reconstruction avoids the physis, but the techniques preclude isometric graft placement. Nonoperative treatment consists of bracing, rehabilitation, and activity limitation. This approach is particularly desirable in younger children and is used as a method to delay surgery until skeletal maturity. Operative intra-articular techniques include reconstruction with hamstrings or the middle third of the patellar tendon. ACL reconstruction using the patellar tendon is done only in adolescents close to maturity to avoid epiphysiodesis. Several extra-articular techniques have been described, but none are isometric. ACL tears with MCL injuries in adolescents can be treated with delayed ACL reconstruction after treatment with a hinged knee brace.
2. PCL tears—PCL tears should be managed with hinged knee braces for 6 weeks. Surgical management of PCL tears in children is controversial. No long-term data exist demonstrating that surgical reconstruction is superior to rehabilitation. PCL disruptions with bony fragments can be secured with screws.
3. Collateral ligament sprains—First- and second-degree collateral ligament sprains may

be treated with hinged knee braces for 1 to 3 weeks. Complete disruptions require 6 weeks in hinged braces. Third-degree sprains combined with ACL injuries should be surgically repaired. Injuries with bony fragments off the tibia or femur may be fixed with screws.

F. Complications—Knee instability, meniscal injuries, and neurovascular injuries are the most common complications of ligamentous injuries of the knee.

G. Special Considerations—Knee dislocations are characterized by extensive ligamentous injury. Usually, both cruciate ligaments are disrupted, and the collateral ligaments may also be involved. The popliteal artery may be damaged. Fortunately, the injury is unusual in children because such trauma is more likely to cause physeal fractures. The child with a knee dislocation should have a careful neurovascular examination followed by emergent reduction. The vascular supply should be closely followed after reduction for 48 to 72 hours. Dislocations in younger children can be managed in a long leg cast for 6 weeks, after the acute swelling has subsided. The injuries of children close to maturity are managed like those of adults: with repair of the collateral ligaments and reconstruction of the cruciate ligaments as indicated.

VIII. Fractures of the Patella
A. Overview—The patella is the largest sesamoid bone. The secondary center of ossification appears between 3 and 6 years of age. There may be up to six ossification centers, which ordinarily coalesce. The bipartite patella is a normal variant (0.2% to 6%) resulting from incomplete coalescence. The line of demarcation is usually superolateral, and fractures may occur through this junction. Pediatric patellar fractures are uncommon because of the high ratio of cartilage to bone, increased patellar mobility, and soft-tissue resilience. Fractures result from a direct blow to the patella or a forceful contraction of the extensor mechanism. Over half of patellar fractures in children occur in motor vehicle accidents.

B. Evaluation—The child has a tender, swollen knee with an effusion. If the fracture is displaced, active knee extension is impossible. Plain films of the knee demonstrate most fractures.

C. Classification—Patellar fractures are classified by the fracture pattern: transverse, longitudinal, or comminuted. The **_sleeve fracture_**

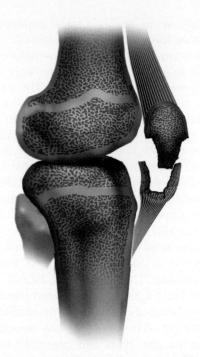

FIGURE 30-6 Sleeve fracture of the patella.

(Fig. 30-6) is another variant; it is defined by a small, visible bony fragment with a large portion of the cartilaginous articular surface attached.

D. Treatment—The objective of treatment is restoration of the extensor mechanism and the articular surface. If there is less than 3 mm of displacement and active knee extension is possible, the child can be immobilized in a cylinder cast for 4 to 6 weeks. Displaced fractures require open reduction and internal fixation. Several techniques have been described for fixation, including a wire loop, tension band wiring, nonabsorbable sutures through drill holes, and screws. Displaced fractures at the margins can be excised.

E. Complications—Most complications result from improper restoration of the normal anatomic relationships. Extensor lag, patella alta, and quadriceps atrophy have been reported.

IX. Patellar Dislocation
A. Overview—Dislocation of the patella is a relatively common injury in children and occurs more frequently in girls. Up to 60% of patients develop recurrent dislocation. The Q angle is the angle subtended by lines from the anterosuperior iliac spine to the center of the patella and from the center of the patella to the tibial tubercle. Patients with recurrent patellar dislocation typically have a larger than normal Q angle. Injuries

usually occur during sports, commonly from a twisting force with the foot planted.

B. Evaluation—Many dislocations reduce spontaneously or with extension of the knee before the child seeks medical attention. The patient, however, can often describe the dislocation. The knee is swollen and diffusely tender around the patella. A large effusion may be present. Ligamentous injuries and physeal fractures should be excluded. Plain radiographs should be obtained to identify possible osteochondral fractures of the patella or the femoral condyles. If an osteochondral fracture is the suspected but only a small ossified fragment is seen, MRI helps demonstrate the actual size.

C. Classification—Injuries are classified by the direction of displacement: lateral, medial, or intra-articular. The majority are lateral.

D. Associated Injuries—Associated injuries include osteochondral fractures of the patella or femur.

E. Treatment—The hemarthrosis should be aspirated for pain relief and inspected for fat droplets. The latter suggest an osteochondral fracture, which may be primarily cartilaginous and not visualized on radiographs. Simple dislocations should be immobilized in a cylinder cast or knee immobilizer for 4 weeks, followed by a rehabilitation program. Osteochondral fragments can be removed with the arthroscope. Particularly large fragments can be repaired open, with either Herbert screws or countersunk minifragment screws.

F. Complications—Recurrent dislocation and instability are the most common complications. Deficiency of the vastus medialis obliquus, patellofemoral dysplasia, and increased Q-angle predispose patients to instability. Aggressive rehabilitation of the vastus medialis obliquus and the quadriceps is the first approach. Several procedures are described for those in whom nonoperative management has failed. Options are lateral retinacular release with or without medial imbrication, semitendinosus tenodesis, medial transfer of the lateral half of the patellar tendon (RouxGoldthwait), or medial transfer of the tibial tubercle (Elmslie-Trillat). The latter is only done when the physis is closed.

G. Special Considerations—Habitual dislocation of the patella is an atraumatic condition characterized by painless dislocation whenever the knee is flexed. Management requires quadriceps lengthening proximal to the patella and lysis of adhesions.

X. Fractures of the Tibial Tubercle

A. Overview—The tibial tubercle, where the patellar tendon inserts, is the most anterior and distal portion of the proximal tibia epiphysis. Active children older than 8 years frequently develop pain in this area, a condition called *Osgood-Schlatter disease.* Superficial microfractures of the cartilage at the insertion of the tendon cause the syndrome. Failure of cartilage deeper to the secondary centers of ossification results in tibial tubercle fractures. Injuries usually result from jumping or a rapid quadriceps contraction against a flexed knee. Adolescents most commonly sustain the fracture.

B. Evaluation—Children have pain, swelling, and tenderness over the tibial tubercle. With undisplaced fractures, there may not be an effusion, and the child is capable of limited active knee extension. Displaced fractures render active knee extension impossible; an effusion is present, and the fragment is often palpable. Plain films, particularly the lateral view, demonstrate the injury.

C. Classification—Ogden has described a classification system, based on the location of the fracture line (Fig. 30-7). In Type I fractures, the fracture line crosses the secondary center of ossification

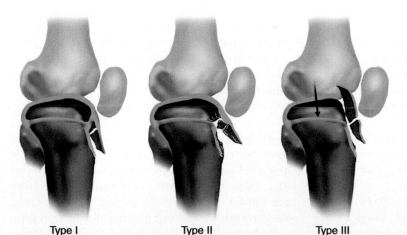

Type I   Type II   Type III

FIGURE 30-7 Classification of tibial tubercle fractures in children. Type I, fracture through the secondary center of ossification; Type II, fracture through the junction of the primary and secondary centers of ossification; Type III, intra-articular fracture.

of the tibial tubercle. The fracture line exits more proximally in Type II fractures, between the centers of ossification for the tibial tubercle and the proximal tibial epiphysis. Type III fractures have intra-articular involvement.

D. Treatment—Nondisplaced Type I fractures can be immobilized in a long leg cast in extension for 4 to 6 weeks. Displaced Type I fractures and Type II and III fractures require open reduction and internal fixation with screws and washers. Postoperative immobilization is used for 4 to 6 weeks.

E. Complications—*Genu recurvatum can occur late after the injury from an anterior growth arrest*. Compartment syndrome can occur due to tearing of the anterior tibial recurrent vessels, which retract into the anterior compartment when torn.

XI. Fractures of the Proximal Tibial Epiphysis

A. Overview—These fractures are uncommon, comprising only 3% of epiphyseal injuries of the lower extremity. The physis is infrequently injured because few ligaments attach to the epiphysis. The proximal tibial epiphysis appears during the first 3 months of life, and the secondary center of ossification of the tibial tubercle appears at 8 years. Ossification does not reach the intercondylar eminence until adolescence. The proximal tibial physis provides 55% of the length of the tibia, 25% of the entire length of the limb, or roughly 0.6 cm per year. The popliteal artery lies close to the epiphysis in the popliteal fossa, becoming tethered as the anterior tibial artery courses into the anterior compartment. The artery is at risk for injury with displaced proximal tibia fractures.

B. Evaluation—The child has pain, swelling, decreased knee range of motion, and sometimes a visible deformity. A careful neurovascular assessment should be performed, especially with displaced fractures. AP and lateral plain films are the recommended initial studies, followed by oblique or stress views if necessary. An arteriogram should be done if a vascular injury is suspected.

C. Classification—The Salter-Harris classification is used.

D. Associated Injuries—Associated injuries include popliteal artery and peroneal nerve injury.

E. Treatment—Salter-Harris Types I and II fractures require closed reduction followed by immobilization for 4 to 6 weeks. Closed reduction and fixation with percutaneous pins or cannulated screws is recommended for Salter-Harris Type III and IV fractures. Displaced fractures with vascular compromise should be urgently reduced and the vascular status reassessed. If the fracture is irreducible or a vascular injury is present, open reduction is mandatory. After reduction, the safest course is to splint the leg in 10° to 20° of flexion; a cast should be applied only when the risk of compartment syndrome has decreased.

F. Complications—Complications include knee instability, leg length discrepancy, arterial injury, and nerve injury. (Peroneal nerve injury is most common.)

XII. Fractures of the Shaft of the Tibia and Fibula

A. Overview—The tibial shaft, defined by the region between the proximal and distal physes, is the third most common long bone fractured in children. Fractures may result from either indirect or direct trauma. Injury may follow a low-energy fall in a young child or higher-energy trauma. Approximately 10% of tibial fractures are open. The four compartments of the leg (anterior, lateral, posterior superficial, and posterior deep) are at risk for developing an acute compartment syndrome.

B. Evaluation—The child may have pain and swelling, but deformity is less common because the fibula is frequently uninjured. Young children may simply stop walking. Point tenderness may be the only physical finding in this group. The skin should be carefully inspected for lacerations, and the neurovascular status of the lower extremity should be documented. Orthogonal plain films are the preferred first studies, although oblique views may be helpful in young children whose initial radiographs reveal no problems. The fracture may be invisible in toddlers and infants. A bone scan may be used if the diagnosis is equivocal.

C. Classification—No formal classification system exists. Injuries are grouped by anatomic location: proximal metaphysis, diaphysis, and distal metaphysis.

D. Treatment
 1. Proximal metaphyseal fractures—Proximal metaphyseal fractures are potentially troublesome because of the poorly understood *complication of late valgus alignment*. There are several theories for the pathogenesis of the valgus deformity (Table 30-2). The deformity occurs within 6 months and is largest 2 years after the injury. After the fracture, any valgus angulation should be corrected before casting. If soft-tissue interposition prevents the correction of valgus malalignment, open reduction is necessary. A long leg cast should be molded into

TABLE 30-2

Theories of the Pathogenesis of Valgus Deformity after Proximal Tibia Fracture in Children

Asymmetric physeal growth

Tethering effect of the fibula

Poor reduction

Soft-tissue interposition

Early weightbearing

Hypertrophic callus

Lateral physeal injury

Dynamic muscle action

varus and worn for 4 to 6 weeks. Alignment is followed with weekly radiographs for the first few weeks; any loss of reduction should be corrected. Some authors also restrict early weightbearing.

2. Closed diaphyseal fractures—Closed diaphyseal fractures can almost always be managed nonoperatively. Angular and rotational deformity should be corrected and a long leg cast applied. If present, associated plastic deformation of the fibula should be corrected to prevent recurrent deformity. Radiographs are obtained weekly for the first few weeks to monitor the reduction, and the cast is wedged if necessary. Acceptable alignment is greater than 50% of fragment apposition, less than 10° of angulation seen on AP and lateral radiographs, less than 20° of rotation, and less than 1 cm of shortening. Isolated fractures of the tibia tend toward varus malalignment. Fractures that fail closed management are stabilized operatively.

3. Open fractures—Open fractures are managed according to the principles of all open fractures. Immobilization can be achieved with a windowed cast in stable low-energy injuries. External fixation, smooth pins, or limited internal fixation are used in fractures with more extensive soft-tissue damage. Soft-tissue coverage should be accomplished within 7 days. Use of subatmospheric pressure dressings can decrease the need for free tissue transfer for coverage.

4. Distal metaphyseal fractures—Distal metaphyseal fractures frequently malalign in recurvatum as a result of impaction of the anterior cortex. After closed reduction, a long leg cast is applied with the foot in plantar flexion to maintain alignment. A shorter cast with the foot in neutral position may be applied later to allow weightbearing for the remainder of fracture healing.

E. Complications

1. Compartment syndrome—Compartment syndrome is a potentially devastating complication that can accompany both closed and open fractures. The complication results from increased pressure in the fascial compartments of the leg, ultimately leading to irreversible nerve and muscle damage if not treated early. A high index of suspicion is essential, particularly in patients who may have difficulty verbalizing their symptoms. *Poorly controlled pain is the earliest sign; it is accompanied by increased discomfort during passive stretch of muscles in the involved compartments*. Splitting the cast and underlying padding may reduce pressures by 50%. *Compartment pressures should be measured and fasciotomies performed if indicated*. A two-incision, four-compartment fasciotomy is recommended; partial fibulectomy has been described as a method of decompressing all four compartments of the leg but can lead to a valgus deformity in children and should not be performed.

2. Delayed union or nonunion—Delayed union or nonunion, defined by failure to heal within 6 months, is unusual. The mean time for healing is 10 weeks in closed fractures and 5 months in open fractures. Severe open injuries are the ones most likely to result in delayed and nonunion. Iliac crest bone grafting is usually successful in healing the nonunion in children.

3. Angular deformity—Angular deformity may result from poor alignment or overgrowth. Valgus deformity from fractures of the proximal tibia metaphysis frequently corrects spontaneously over several years. Observation is recommended. Varus osteotomy performed close to maturity corrects severe valgus deformities that fail to resolve.

4. Rotational deformity—Rotational deformity results from inadequate reduction and does not spontaneously correct. If the deformity exceeds 20°, rotational osteotomy may be necessary.

5. Proximal tibial physeal closure—Proximal tibial physeal closure is a rare complication that causes a genu recurvatum deformity. It occurs gradually over the first few years

after injury and is corrected with an opening wedge osteotomy.

6. Leg length discrepancy—Leg length discrepancy may occur but it is less of a problem than with femur fractures. Overgrowth is usually the cause. Treatment options are those that are standard for leg length discrepancy.

F. Special Considerations

1. Toddler's fractures—Toddler's fractures are isolated, oblique, distal tibia fractures that occur after low-energy trauma in young children. The fall is often unwitnessed; the child may simply stop ambulating. Swelling, deformity, and ecchymosis are usually absent on examination. Point tenderness may be the only sign. The appearance of plain films may be normal. The first evidence of fracture may be periosteal bone formation seen on X-ray film 10 days after injury. A short leg cast for 4 weeks is sufficient treatment.

2. Bicycle spoke injuries—Bicycle spoke injuries occur when the foot of a child riding on the back of a bicycle catches in the wheel. The injury may seem innocuous, but extensive soft-tissue injury may manifest over the first 48 hours. The child should be admitted for bedrest, elevation, and serial examinations of the soft tissues. Surgical debridement may be necessary as the zone of injury demarcates.

3. Stress fractures—Stress fractures occur in children participating in activities to which they are not accustomed. The most frequent sites are the posteromedial and posterolateral aspects of the proximal tibia. Point tenderness is present, and there may be a cortical lucency on radiographs. If plain films are negative, MRI or a bone scan is diagnostic. Activity restriction or casting for 2 to 4 weeks is usually sufficient.

4. Child abuse—Child abuse must always be considered. The tibia is the third most commonly fractured long bone with child abuse. Corner or bucket-handle metaphyseal fractures are pathognomonic for child abuse (Fig. 30-8).

5. Congenital pseudoarthrosis of the tibia— Congenital pseudoarthrosis of the tibia is a rare condition characterized by abnormal bone that is at risk for fracture. The condition is frequently associated with neurofibromatosis. The tibia is usually tapered and has sclerosis and cysts. An anterolateral bow is typical. If the child comes to medical attention before fracture, indefinite bracing is recommended. After the bone has fractured, union is extremely difficult to achieve. Intramedullary fixation with bone graft, vascularized fibula grafts, and resection with bone transport have been reported.

6. Isolated fractures of the fibular diaphysis— Isolated fractures of the fibular diaphysis occur after direct trauma to the leg. Immobilization is all that is necessary for treatment.

7. Proximal tibia–fibular joint dislocations— Proximal tibia–fibular joint dislocations are rare injuries, and over 30% are initially missed. Displacement is anterolateral, posteromedial, or superior. There may be an associated proximal tibia fracture or knee ligament injury. Reduction and immobilization in a cylinder cast is recommended.

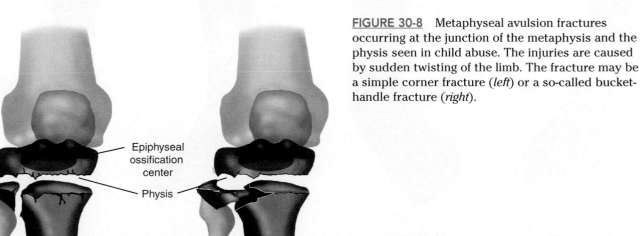

FIGURE 30-8 Metaphyseal avulsion fractures occurring at the junction of the metaphysis and the physis seen in child abuse. The injuries are caused by sudden twisting of the limb. The fracture may be a simple corner fracture (*left*) or a so-called bucket-handle fracture (*right*).

Epiphyseal ossification center

Physis

XIII. Fractures of the Ankle
1. Overview—Approximately 10% to 25% of all physeal fractures occur around the ankle. The deltoid ligament and the three lateral ligaments are less likely to fail than the growth plates. Injuries usually result from indirect forces. The distal tibia physis begins to close at 12 years in girls and 13 years in boys. Closure occurs over 18 months. The physis closes in the central portion earliest, followed by the medial portion, and finally the lateral portion. This progression explains the unique Tillaux and triplane injuries seen in adolescents.
2. Evaluation—The child often has difficulty describing the exact mechanism of injury. The injury is characterized by pain, swelling, tenderness, and sometimes a deformity. AP, lateral, and mortise radiographic views adequately demonstrate most injuries. CT scanning is helpful for precisely delineating complex patterns and intra-articular fractures.
3. Classification—Ankle fractures are usually classified by anatomic pattern or mechanism of injury. The Salter-Harris classification describes the anatomic patterns of injury sufficiently. The Lauge-Hansen mechanism of injury system was developed for adult injuries. Tachdjian and Dias modified this classification for pediatric injuries (Fig. 30-9).
4. Treatment—Ankle fracture treatment depends on the age of the patient and the extent of the injury. Most authors feel that a maximum of 2 mm of intra-articular displacement is acceptable, although anatomic restoration of the joint surface is ideal. The mechanism of injury classification guides the reduction maneuver. Because the injuries involve the physis, forceful repeated attempts at reduction should be avoided. Open reduction follows if closed attempts fail. Immobilization in a short- or long-leg cast depends on fracture stability, the presence or absence of internal fixation, and the reliability of the patient and family.
   - Salter-Harris Type I distal tibia fractures—Salter-Harris Type I distal tibia fractures can be immobilized in a short leg walking cast for 4 to 6 weeks if nondisplaced. ***Malrotation of the foot is frequently overlooked with this injury***. Displaced fractures are reduced and placed in a long leg cast for 3 weeks, followed by a short leg walking cast.
   - Salter-Harris Type II distal tibia fractures—Salter-Harris Type II distal tibia fractures

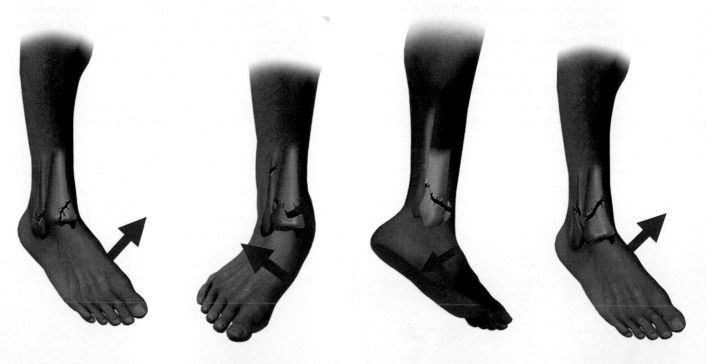

| A. Supination-inversion | B. Pronation-eversion-external rotation | C. Supination-plantar flexion | D. Supination-external rotation |

FIGURE 30-9 Tachdjian-Dias classification of pediatric ankle fractures. **A.** Supination-inversion. **B.** Pronation–eversion–external rotation. **C.** Supination–plantar flexion. **D.** Supination–external rotation.

are the most common type and are usually associated with a fibular fracture. A closed reduction is performed, attempting to achieve less than 5° of varus or valgus angulation. A long leg cast is worn for 2 weeks, followed by a short leg walking cast until union.

- Salter-Harris Type III and IV distal tibia fractures—Salter-Harris Types III and IV distal tibia fractures may be treated by closed means if undisplaced. Fractures that can be reduced to less than 2 mm of displacement may be treated closed as well. Percutaneous fixation with pins or cannulated screws can supplement casting. Irreducible fractures require open reduction and internal fixation.

- Salter-Harris Type V distal tibia fractures—Salter-Harris Type V distal tibia fractures, which are extremely rare, are diagnosed retrospectively. There are no formal recommendations for treatment.

- Tillaux fractures—Tillaux fractures (Fig. 30-10) are Salter-Harris Type III fractures caused by an external rotation force in a child close to maturity. In a small percentage of cases, closed reduction can be achieved by internal rotation of the foot and direct pressure over the fragment. The adequacy of reduction should be confirmed by a CT scan. The 6 weeks of immobilization is divided equally between long and short leg casts. ***Irreducible fractures require open reduction with internal fixation to restore joint congruity.***

- Triplane fractures—Triplane fractures (see Fig. 30-10) are multiplanar, Salter-Harris Type IV injuries also occurring near maturity. The exact anatomic structures are often difficult to visualize; CT scanning helps assess displacement and plan surgery if needed. Less than 2 mm of displacement must be achieved by closed or open means. Open reduction may require two approaches or a transfibular approach. The posteromedial fragment is generally reduced first, followed by the intraarticular fragment.

- Salter-Harris Type I fractures of the distal fibula—Salter-Harris Type I fractures of the distal fibula are common in children. Up to 50% displacement is acceptable. Immobilization in a short leg walking cast or a removable ankle brace for 4 weeks is adequate. The removable brace has been shown to hasten functional recovery and is better tolerated by families.

5. Complications
- Malunion—Malunion occurs if an ankle fracture is inadequately reduced. If there is a

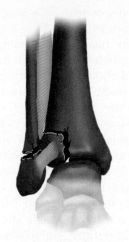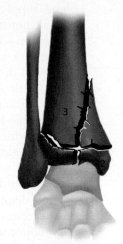

Juvenile Tillaux   Triplane

FIGURE 30-10   Special types of ankle fractures that occur in adolescents include the juvenile Tillaux and Triplane. Note the three fragments involved in the Triplane fracture: *1*, anterolateral physis (Salter-Harris Type III); *2*, remaining physis (Salter-Harris Type IV); *3*, tibial metaphysis.

significant deformity at the end of growth, a supramalleolar osteotomy is performed.

- Growth arrest—Growth arrest is most common with Salter-Harris Types III and IV fractures. For Salter-Harris Type I and II fractures, premature physeal closure may be related to interposition of periosteum. Physeal bars can be resected with fat interposition and combined with a corrective osteotomy.

- Arthritis

XIV. Injuries of the Foot—Foot injuries usually result from direct trauma. In young children, the bones are primarily cartilaginous and therefore pliable and less susceptible to fracture. Ossification is variable in pattern, but progression with growth makes fractures more common with age. The foot consists of 26 bones plus the sesamoids. The talus and calcaneus make up the hindfoot; the navicular, cuneiforms, and cuboid make up the midfoot; and the metatarsals and phalanges make up the forefoot. Over half of the entire length of the foot is achieved by age 2 years, leaving less potential for remodeling with growth.

A. Talus Fractures
1. Overview—Talus fractures usually result from forced dorsiflexion of the foot, sometimes combined with inversion or eversion. The injury is rare in children. The blood supply is precarious as in adults, and AVN may follow displaced fractures. In younger children, the

blood supply is less dependent on a single system, but this changes with growth.

2. Evaluation—The child has pain, swelling, tenderness, and difficulty bearing weight. Radiographs of the foot demonstrate the injury.

3. Classification—Talus fractures can be classified according to Hawkins, as in adults.

4. Treatment—Nondisplaced fractures are treated with a nonweightbearing cast for 6 to 8 weeks, followed by a weightbearing cast for 2 weeks. A closed reduction may be attempted for displaced fractures; up to 5 mm of displacement may be accepted. Otherwise, open reduction with internal fixation is recommended. Postoperative immobilization is similar to that for nondisplaced fractures. All talus fractures should be monitored with periodic radiographs to rule out AVN.

5. Complications—AVN is the most serious complication following a talus fracture. It usually occurs during the first 6 months after injury. Hawkins' sign, a subchondral lucency visualized on plain films, signifies an intact blood supply to the body of the talus. The absence of Hawkins' sign, however, does not indicate AVN in children. Authors therefore recommend MRI to screen for AVN. AVN is difficult to treat. Nonweightbearing in a patellar tendon-bearing articulated orthosis is recommended until revascularization, which may take years, occurs.

6. Special considerations
   • Lateral and medial talar process fractures—Lateral and medial talar process fractures are tender beneath the malleoli on examination. Immobilization with avoidance of weightbearing is recommended.
   • Osteochondral fractures—Osteochondral fractures result from plantar flexion or dorsiflexion combined with inversion. Posteromedial fragments are more common than posterolateral fragments. MRI provides the most information. Undisplaced fragments may be treated in a cast. There are four stages.
     (a) Stage I involves subchondral compression.
     (b) Stage II involves a partially detached fragment.
     (c) Stage III involves a completely detached fragment remaining in its crater fragment.
     (d) Stage IV lesions should be surgically excised with drilling or curettage of the crater.

B. Calcaneus Fractures

1. Overview—The calcaneus is the largest bone in the foot and the earliest to ossify. Fractures are fairly common, but diagnosis is difficult and frequently delayed. Most authors report that the clinical course is benign, particularly in young children.

2. Evaluation—A history of a fall is common. The foot may be swollen and tender. The exact area of tenderness is frequently difficult to locate. The appearance of radiographs is often normal. Initial studies should include lateral, axial, and dorsoplantar views. Intra-articular depression is best judged on the lateral view. If there is a significant intra-articular injury, a CT scan should be performed as well.

3. Classification—Injuries are classified as by Rowe (Table 30-3).

4. Treatment—The majority of calcaneus fractures in children may be treated in a cast. Outcomes are always good for extra-articular fractures. Intra-articular displacement frequently remodels over time, particularly in young children. Weightbearing in the cast depends on the surgeon's preference. Older children and adolescents have less potential for remodeling. Significantly displaced intra-articular fractures should be reduced percutaneously or open and should be stabilized. Weightbearing is usually avoided for at

TABLE 30-3

Calcaneal Fracture Patterns

Type	Description
1	Fracture of the tuberosity
	Fracture of the sustentaculum tali
	Fracture of the anterior process
2	"Beak" fracture
	Avulsion fracture of the insertion of the achilles tendon
3	Oblique fracture in the posterior portion not involving the subtalar joint (corresponds to a metaphyseal fracture of a longitudinal bone)
4	Fracture involving the subtalar region with or without actual articular involvement
5	Central depression with varying degrees of comminution
6	Involvement of the secondary ossification center

Source: From Rowe CR, Sakellandes HT, Freeman AT, et al. *JAMA.* 1963;184:920–923, with permission.

least 6 weeks with displaced intra-articular fractures.

5. Associated injuries—***Lumbar spine injuries*** are associated with calcaneus fractures, particularly after falls from a height. Some recommend a lumbar spine series in all patients with displaced intra-articular fractures.

C. Navicular Injuries—Injury of the navicular is unusual, but a dorsal chip fracture is the most common type. Cast immobilization is sufficient. Stress fractures of the navicular bone, which can occur in adolescents, are a more difficult problem. Immobilization in a nonweightbearing cast for 6 to 8 weeks is recommended. The accessory navicular bone is a normal variant occurring in up to 15% of the population. The fibrocartilaginous junction can fracture, causing medial foot pain. A total of 4 weeks in a short leg cast cures the problem. Surgery should be considered only after conservative measures fail.

D. Injuries of the Tarsometatarsal Joints

1. Overview—Injuries of the tarsometatarsal joints or Lisfranc's joint result from direct or indirect trauma. The injury follows an impact while on tiptoe, heel-to-toe compression, or a fall backward while the foot is fixed. The second tarsometatarsal joint is a true mortise, which provides stability for the other rays.

2. Evaluation—Patients have pain, swelling, and difficulty bearing weight. The involved joints are tender. Plain films are recommended. The oblique view assesses the joints, and the lateral view excludes dorsal dislocation.

3. Classification—Classification is by Hardcastle, as with adults.

4. Treatment—Nondisplaced injuries are managed in a short leg cast. Displaced fractures are reduced closed or open and fixed with threaded pins or screws.

5. Complications—Angular deformity can be a complication.

E. Metatarsal Fractures

1. Overview—Metatarsal fractures are common injuries that result from direct or indirect trauma. Injuries occur most frequently at the metatarsal neck because the diameter is smallest. Children under 5 years most commonly fracture the first metatarsal, usually after a fall from a height. Children over 5 years fracture the fifth metatarsal most often, and sustain the injury most commonly from a fall on a level surface.

2. Evaluation—Patients have pain, swelling, difficulty bearing weight, and tenderness. AP and oblique radiographs allow the clinician to make the diagnosis. The lateral view is essential for excluding plantar flexion of the distal fragment. Fractures of the second, third and fourth metatarsals are frequently associated with additional metatarsal fractures.

3. Classification—There is no specific classification system.

4. Treatment—Most metatarsal fractures heal uneventfully in a short leg weightbearing cast. Lateral angulation or translation does not affect outcome. Plantar displacement should be corrected because metatarsalgia can ensue. If reduction is necessary, finger-trap traction or open reduction is performed. Smooth wires are suitable for fixation if necessary. In cases with significant swelling, the possibility of compartment syndrome should be considered.

5. Special considerations
   • Avulsion fractures—Avulsion fractures of the base of the fifth metatarsal are common. The injury is hypothesized to be secondary to pull of the peroneus brevis or the abductor digiti minimi. Usually, local pain and tenderness occur, but the appearance of radiographs may be normal. The apophysis of the metatarsal, or os vesalianum, is present between 8 and 12 to 15 years. It should not be confused with a fracture. A short leg walking cast for 3 to 6 weeks is curative.
   • Jones fractures—Fractures at the metaphyseal-diaphyseal junction of the fifth metatarsal, or Jones fractures, are problematic. Most represent chronic stress fractures and must be managed more aggressively. Jones fractures may have antecedent pain. Sclerosis of the medullary cavity may be present on radiographs. The best results are with intramedullary screw fixation or open bone grafting.

F. Phalangeal Fractures

1. Overview—Fractures of the phalanges are fairly common in children and usually result from direct trauma. The proximal phalanx is most frequently injured. The majority of these injuries heal without complication.

2. Evaluation—Patients have pain and swelling and may also have a visible deformity. Plain films are sufficient for making the diagnosis.

3. Classification—There is no classification system, although the Salter-Harris system applies to physeal injuries.

4. Treatment—Nondisplaced fractures can be managed with buddy taping and a hard-soled shoe. Displaced fractures can be reduced with traction and then buddy taped. Displaced Salter-Harris fractures of the distal phalanx should be carefully evaluated. ***Often the nail bed is disrupted; thus the fracture is open. Irrigation and debridement, antibiotics, and nail bed repair are necessary.*** A pin is sometimes used to counteract the long flexors pulling the distal fragment into flexion.

G. Special Considerations

1. Lawn-mower injuries—Lawn-mower injuries are severe crush injuries to the lower extremity that are usually grossly contaminated. Aggressive irrigation and debridement must be performed every 2 to 3 days until the wound is clean and all tissue is viable. Antibiotic prophylaxis requires a cephalosporin, aminoglycoside, and penicillin. The challenge is deciding between amputation and salvage, but waiting until the wound has been adequately debrided over a few days is a judicious approach. Salvage requires soft-tissue coverage by a skin graft or free muscle flap. Amputation rates in most series approach 70%.

2. Tendon lacerations—Tendon lacerations usually follow a benign course in children. The Achilles, tibialis anterior, and tibialis posterior tendons should be repaired to prevent secondary deformity. The lesser tendons may be managed by casting in a position that minimizes stress on the injured tendon.

3. Compartment syndrome—Compartment syndrome should be considered in any child with extensive swelling of the foot, particularly after crush injuries. Unrecognized, it causes a clawed foot. One sign of compartment syndrome is pain that worsens with passive stretch of the muscles of the affected compartment. Compartment pressures should be measured and fasciotomies performed if indicated. There are nine compartments in the foot, but all can be reached through two dorsal incisions plus one medial incision.

4. ***Puncture wounds of the foot***—Puncture wounds of the foot occur frequently in active children. The concern is the potential development of cellulitis, osteomyelitis, or septic arthritis. *Staphylococcus aureus* and *Pseudomonas aeruginosa* infections are most common; the latter is most characteristic when the nail has punctured through the sole of a sneaker. Initial management after the injury includes debridement of the skin, irrigation, and tetanus prophylaxis. No data support routine prophylactic antibiotic coverage. If pain does not subside after 2 or 3 days, warm soaks, elevation, and oral antistaphylococcal antibiotic coverage are started. Injuries not responding to this regimen require surgical debridement and intravenous antibiotics. *Pseudomonas* osteomyelitis always requires aggressive surgical debridement and parenteral antibiotics for eradication. Sometimes a piece of shoe is found during wound debridement.

5. Metatarsophalangeal and interphalangeal joint dislocations—Metatarsophalangeal and interphalangeal joint dislocations are rare. Reduction and buddy taping for 3 weeks are adequate.

6. Cuboid and cuneiform fractures—Fractures of the cuboid and cuneiforms are generally treated with cast immobilization.

7. Heel pain—Sever's disease is the most common cause of foot pain in active children. It represents an overuse syndrome of the calcaneal apophysis. Treatment includes heel cups, Achilles stretching, the application of ice, activity modification, and the administration of nonsteroidal antiinflammatory medications.

XV. Traumatic Amputations—Traumatic amputations most often result when children play around trains, farm equipment, and other heavy machinery. Acute surgical amputation is indicated for Type IIIC open fractures with unreconstructible nerve or vessel injuries. The limb should be irrigated and debrided of all devitalized tissue. Care should be taken to preserve as much length as possible. Soft-tissue coverage is performed when the tissue bed is healthy. With amputations around the foot, residual muscle imbalance may necessitate tendon transfers to prevent late deformity. ***Stump overgrowth is a common complication of traumatic amputations. Below-the-knee amputations overgrow more frequently than above the-knee amputations.***

SUGGESTED READINGS

Classic Articles

Burkhart S, Peterson H. Fractures of the proximal tibia epiphysis. *J Bone Joint Surg.* 1979;61A:996–1002.

Cooperman D, Spiegel P, Laros G. Tibial fractures involving the ankle in children: the so-called triplane epiphyseal fracture. *J Bone Joint Surg.* 1978;60A:1040–1046.

Daoud H, O'Farrell T, Cruess R. Quadricepsplasty: the Judet technique and results of six cases. *J Bone Joint Surg.* 1982;64B:194–197.

Dias L, Giegerich C. Fractures of the distal tibial epiphysis in adolescence. *J Bone Joint Surg.* 1983;65A:438–444.

Dias L, Tachdjian M. Physeal injuries of the ankle in children. *Clin Orthop.* 1978;136:230–233.

Ertl J, Barrack R, Alexander A. Triplane fracture of the distal tibial epiphysis. *J Bone Joint Surg.* 1988;70A:967–976.

Grogan D, Carey T, Leffers D. Avulsion fractures of the patella. *J Pediatr Orthop.* 1990;10:721–730.

Kleiger B, Mankin H. Fracture of the lateral portion of the distal tibial epiphysis. *J Bone Joint Surg.* 1964;46A:25–32.

Lombardo S, Harvey J. Fracture of the distal femoral epiphyses. *J Bone Joint Surg.* 1977;59A:742–751.

Riseborough E, Barrett J, Shapiro F. Growth disturbances following distal femoral physeal fracture-separations. *J Bone Joint Surg.* 1983;65A:885–893.

Schmidt T, Weiner D. Calcaneal fractures in children. *Clin Orthop.* 1982;171:150–155.

Spiegel P, Cooperman D, Laros G. Epiphyseal fractures of the distal ends of the tibia and fibula. *J Bone Joint Surg.* 1978;60A:1046–1050.

Sugi M, Cole W. Early plaster treatment for fractures of the femoral shaft in childhood. *J Bone Joint Surg.* 1978;1978 69B:743–745.

Torg J, Pavlov H, Cooley L. Stress fractures of the tarsal navicular. *J Bone Joint Surg.* 1982;64A:700–712.

Wiley J. Tarso-metatarsal joint injuries in children. *J Pediatr Orthop.* 1981;1:255–260.

Recent Articles

Accadbled F, Cassard X, Sales de Gauzy J, et al. Meniscal tears in children and adolescents: results of operative treatment. *J Pediatr Orthop B.* 2007;16:56–60.

Anderson A. Transepiphyseal replacement of the anterior cruciate ligament in skeletally immature patients: a preliminary report. *J Bone Joint Surg.* 2003;85-A:1255–1263.

Arkader A, Friedman J, Warner WC, et al. Complete distal femoral metaphyseal fractures: a harbinger of child abuse before walking age. *J Pediatr Orthop.* 2007;27:751–753.

Arkader A, Warner W, Horn BD, et al. Predicting the outcome of physeal fractures of the distal femur. *J Pediatr Orthop.* 2007;27:703–708.

Boutis K, Willan A, Babyn P, et al. A randomized controlled trial of a removable brace versus casting children with low-risk ankle fractures. *Pediatrics.* 2007;119:e1256–e1263.

Ceroni D, Rosa VD, De Coulon G, et al. Cuboid nutcracker fracture due to horseback riding in children. *J Pediatr Orthop.* 2007;27:557–561.

Dedmond B, Kortesis B, Punger K, et al. Subatmospheric pressure dressings in the temporary treatment of soft tissue injuries associated with type III open tibial shaft fractures in children. *J Pediatr Orthop.* 2006;26:728–732.

Epps H, Molenaar E, O'Connor DP. Immediate single-spica cast for pediatric femoral diaphysis fractures. *J Pediatr Orthop.* 2006;26(4):491–496.

Flynn J, Wong K, Yeh GL, et al. Displaced fractures of the hip in children. Management by early operation and immobilisation in a hip spica cast. *J Bone Joint Surg.* 2002;84B:108–112.

Gaulrapp H, Haus J. Intraarticular stabilization after anterior cruciate ligament tear in children and adolescents: results

6 years after surgery. *Knee Surg Sports Traumatol Arthrosc.* 2006;14:417–424.

Gebhard F, Ellerman A, Hoffmann F, et al. Multicenter-study of operative treatment of intra ligamentous tears of the anterior cruciate ligament in children and adolescents: comparison of four different techniques. *Knee Surg Sports Traumatol Arthrosc.* 2006;14:797–803.

Hedquist D, Bishop J, Hresko T, et al. Locking plate fixation for pediatric femur fractures. *J Pediatr Orthop.* 2008;28:6–9.

Ilharreborde B, Raquillet C, Morel E, et al. Long-term prognosis of Salter-Harris type 2 injuries of the distal femoral physis. *J Pediatr Orthop B.* 2006;15:433–438.

Jarvis J, Davidson D, Letts M, et al. Management of subtrochanteric fractures in skeletally immature adolescents. *J Trauma.* 2006;60:613–619.

Kocher M, Foreman E, Micheli LJ, et al. Laxity and functional outcome after arthroscopic reduction and internal fixation of displaced tibial spine fractures in children. *Arthroscopy.* 2003;19:1085–1090.

Kocher M, Garg S, Micheli LJ, et al. Physeal sparing reconstruction of the anterior cruciate ligament in skeletally immature prepubescent children and adolescents. *J Bone Joint Surg.* 2005;87A:2371–2379.

Lee S, Baek J, Han SB, et al. Stress fractures of the femoral diaphysis in children. *J Pediatr Orthop.* 2005;25(6):734–738.

Moon E, Mehlman C. Risk factors for avascular necrosis after femoral neck fractures in children: 25 Cincinnati cases and meta-analysis of 360 cases. *J Orthop Trauma.* 2006;20:323–329.

Moroz L, Launay F, Kocher MS, et al. Titanium elastic nailing of fractures of the femur in children predictors of complications and poor outcome. *J Bone and Joint Surg.* 2006;88B:1361–1366.

Mubarak S, Frick S, Sink E, et al. Volkmann contracture and compartment syndromes after femur fractures in children treated with 90/90 spica casts. *J Pediatr Orthop.* 2006;26(5):567–572.

Petit C, Lee B, Kasser JR, et al. Operative treatment of intraarticular calcaneal fractures in the pediatric population. *J Pediatr Orthop.* 2007;27:856–862.

Pombo M, Shilt J. The definition and treatment of pediatric subtrochanteric femur fractures with titanium elastic nails. *J Pediatr Orthop.* 2006;26(3):364–370.

Ramseier L, Bhaskar A, Cole WG, et al. Treatment of open femur fractures in children: comparison between external fixator and intramedullary nailing. *J Pediatr Orthop.* 2007;27:748–750.

Rohmiller M, Gaynor T, Pawelek J, et al. Salter-Harris I and II fractures of the distal tibia: does mechanism of injury relate to premature physeal closure? *J Pediatr Orthop.* 2006;26:322–328.

Sabharwal S. Role of Ilizarov external fixator in the management of proximal/distal metadiaphyseal pediatric femur fractures. *J Orthop Trauma.* 2005;19(6):563–569.

Sankar W, Wells L, Sennett BJ, et al. Combined anterior cruciate ligament and medial collateral ligament injures in adolescents. *J Pediatr Orthop.* 2006;26:733–736.

Senaran H, Mason D, De Pellegrin M, et al. Cuboid fractures in preschool children. *J Pediatr Orthop.* 2006;26(6):741–744.

Shrader M, Jacofsky D, Stans AA, et al. Femoral neck fractures in pediatric patients: 30 years experience at a level 1 trauma center. *Clin Orthop.* 2006;454:169–173.

Singer G, Cichocki M, Schalamon J, et al. A study of metatarsal fractures in children. *J Bone Joint Surg Am.* 2008;90:772–776.

Sink E, Hedquist D, Morgan SJ, et al. Results and technique of unstable pediatric femoral fractures treated with submuscular bridge plating. *J Pediatr Orthop.* 2006;26(2):177–181.

Togrul E, Bayram H, Gulsen M, et al. Fractures of the femoral neck in children: long-term follow-up in 62 hip fractures. *Injury.* 2005;36:123–130.

Wall E, Jain V, Vora V, et al. Complications of titanium and stainless steel elastic nail fixation of pediatric femoral fractures. *J Bone Joint Surg.* 2008;90A:1305–1313.

Woods G, O'Connor D. Delayed anterior cruciate ligament reconstruction in adolescents with open physes. *Am J Sports Med.* 2004;32:201–210.

Wright J, Wang E, Owen JL, et al. Treatments for paediatric femoral fractures: a randomised trial. *Lancet.* 2005;365:1153–1158.

Review Articles

Anglen J, Choi L. Treatment options in pediatric femoral shaft fractures. *J Orthop Trauma.* 2005;19:724–733.

Bales C, Guettler J, Moorman C 3rd. Anterior cruciate ligament injuries in children with open physes. *Am J Sports Med.* 2004;32:1978–1985.

Larsen M, Garrett W Jr, DeLee J, et al. Surgical management of anterior cruciate ligament injuries in patients with open physes. *J Am Acad Orthop Surg.* 2006;14:736–744.

Lascombes P, Haumont T, Journeau P. Use and abuse of flexible intramedullary nailing in children and adolescents. *J Pediatr Orthop.* 2006;26:827–834.

Quick T, Eastwood D. Pediatric fractures and dislocations of the hip and pelvis. *Clin Orthop.* 2005;432:87–96.

Ribbans W, Natarajan R, Alavala S. *Pediatric Foot Fractures. Clin Orthop.* 2005;432:107–115.

Schnetzler K, Hoernschemeyer D. The pediatric triplane ankle fracture. *J Am Acad Orthop Surg.* 2007;15:738–747.

Vaquero J, Vidal C, Cubillo A. Intra-articular traumatic disorders of the knee in children and adolescents. *Clin Orthop.* 2005;432:97–106.

Textbooks

Beaty J, Kasser J, eds. *Rockwood and Wilkins' Fractures in Children.* 7th ed. Philadelphia, PA: Lippincott Williams & Wilkins; 2010.

Green N, Swiontkowski M. *Skeletal Trauma in Children.* Vol 3. 3rd ed. Philadelphia, PA: WB Saunders; 2003.

Herring J. *Tachdjian's Pediatric Orthopaedics from the Texas Scottish Rite Hospital for Children.* 3rd ed. Philadelphia, PA: Saunders Elsevier; 2008.

Morrissy R, Weinstein S, eds. *Lovell and Winter's Pediatric Orthopaedics.* Philadelphia, PA: Lippincott Williams & Wilkins; 2006.

Wenger D, Pring M, Rang M. *Rang's Children's Fractures.* 3rd ed. Philadelphia, PA: Lippincott Williams & Wilkins; 2005.

CHAPTER 31

Pediatric Upper Extremity Injuries

Brian E. Grottkau and Umesh S. Metkar

I. Scapular Fractures—Fractures of the body of the scapula in children occur infrequently, result from high-energy trauma, and are often associated with concomitant injuries of the thorax and chest. Treatment is generally nonsurgical (except for open injuries) and consists of an arm sling and range of motion exercises of the shoulder to decrease stiffness.

II. Injuries of the Clavicle and the Sternoclavicular and Acromioclavicular Joints
   A. Clavicle—The clavicle is the first bone to ossify in the human embryo and one of the last to fuse its epiphyses to its diaphysis. The medial epiphysis ossifies at 12 to 19 years of age and fuses at 22 to 25 years of age. The lateral epiphysis fuses to the diaphysis at 19 years of age, is thin and difficult to see on plain radiographs.
      1. Mechanisms of injury—***The clavicle is the most frequently fractured bone in children***. Fractures are generally caused by a direct blow, a fall on the point of the shoulder or outstretched arm or during delivery.
      2. Evaluation
         • Physical examination—In the newborn, the fracture may present only as ***pseudoparalysis of the upper extremity***. This must be distinguished from a brachial plexus palsy. The fracture may not be apparent on plain radiographs until callus appears 1 to 2 weeks after injury. Other findings may include those seen in toddlers and children including crepitation, swelling, point tenderness, decreased shoulder motion, and the head turning away from the fracture.
         • Imaging—Anteroposterior (AP) and 30° cephalic tilt radiographs (serendipity view) can be obtained. If inconclusive, computed tomographic (CT) scan, tomograms or stress views with weights (for suspected lateral fractures) may be helpful.
      3. Associated injuries—Associated injuries are uncommon and are primarily neurovascular. Venous distention, absent pulses or numbness should be evaluated. Concomitant obstetric brachial plexus palsies can occur in the newborn.
      4. Treatment—The primary purpose of the clavicle is to connect the trunk to the shoulder girdle. Because of the excellent healing and remodeling potential in children, open surgical treatment of clavicle fractures is rarely indicated with the exception of open fractures, fractures with severe tenting of the skin that may become open and fractures associated with neurovascular compromise. Parents should be warned about a visible residual bump of healing callus at the fracture site that will likely persist over time. Most fractures require simple immobilization of the shoulder girdle. This can generally be accomplished with a Velpeau sling or shoulder immobilizer in children and adolescents. In neonates, the affected extremity should be bound to the thorax by safety pinning the arm of the onesie to the vest of the onsie or by fashioning a custom immobilizer out of stockinette.
      5. Complications—Cosmetic bump.
      6. Differential diagnoses
         • Congenital pseudoarthrosis of the clavicle usually occurs on the right side except in newborns with *situs inversus*. There will be no history of trauma.
         • Cleidocranial Dysostosis affects the clavicle and other bones of intramembranous ossification including the skull, mandible, and vertebrae.

B. Sternoclavicular Joint—The clavicle articulates medially with the sternum and the first rib. Injuries in this region in children are usually Salter-Harris Types I or II physeal fractures rather than true joint dislocations. Posterior displacement of the medial clavicle can cause impingement on the innominate artery and vein, vagus and phrenic nerves, trachea, esophagus and/or brachial plexus. Anterior displacement is more common.

1. Evaluation
    • Physical examination—A lump or depression at the sternoclavicular joint may be evident with tenderness, possible hoarseness, dyspnea, dysphasia, diminished affected upper extremity pulses or venous engorgement of the extremity.
    • Imaging—On Serendipity view, posteriorly displaced separation will appear more caudad and anterior displacement will appear more cephalad. Because the medial epiphysis may not ossify until 19 years of age, CT scan may be required to adequately visualize the bony anatomy.
2. Treatment—Anterior sternoclavicular injuries generally require only symptomatic treatment with sling and swathe due to excellent remodeling potential. Asymptomatic posteriorly displaced injuries are closed reduced by placing a blanket roll longitudinally between the shoulder blades and placing posteriorly directed pressure on the lateral clavicle or shoulder thereby distracting, while simultaneously grasping the medial clavicle percutaneously with a pointed reduction forceps or towel clip under a general anesthetic. Some advocate having a pediatric or vascular surgeon available in case the displacement is tamponading a vessel. Open reduction is reserved for symptomatic irreducible posteriorly displaced injuries and is rarely required.

C. Acromioclavicular Joint—Injuries of the acromioclavicular joint in children are usually fractures, not dislocations. The coracoclavicular and acromioclavicular ligaments remain attached to the thick periosteal sleeve.

1. Classification (Dameron and Rockwood) (Fig. 31-1)
    • Type I—Mild sprain without periosteal disruption.
    • Type II—Partial disruption of the dorsal periosteal tube with some distal clavicle instability.
    • Type III—Large longitudinal dorsal split in the periosteum with gross instability.
    • Type IV—Similar to Type III; the distal clavicle is displaced posteriorly and buttonholed through the trapezius.
    • Type V—Complete dorsal periosteal split with superior subcutaneous displacement through the deltoid and trapezius.
    • Type VI—Inferior dislocation of the distal clavicle beneath the coracoid.

FIGURE 31-1 Acromioclavicular separation in children (Dameron and Rockwood classification).

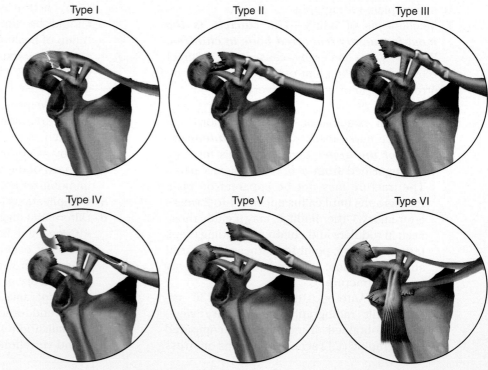

Type I   Type II   Type III

Type IV   Type V   Type VI

2. Evaluation—Serendipity and AP radiographs or a CT scan can be obtained; stress views may be required due to bony overlap on the AP radiograph.

3. Treatment—Closed treatment with sling and swathe for Types I and II. Open reduction is indicated for Types III to VI in adolescents.

III. Injuries of the Humerus and Glenohumeral Joint

A. Glenohumeral Dislocations—Glenohumeral dislocations are uncommon in children but appear to be increasing with increasing sports participation. Treatment is similar to that for adults. The two primary predictors of recurrent dislocation are (a) number of prior dislocations and (b) age at first dislocation. Recurrence in children is very common.

B. Proximal Humerus Fractures—Fractures of the proximal humeral physis occur most commonly in adolescents secondary to high-energy sports participation and a weak perichondrial ring; in newborns, this injury most often results from a complicated delivery or child abuse. The distal fragment normally displaces anteriorly and laterally because of the strong posteromedial periosteum; the proximal fragment flexes, abducts, and externally rotates. Salter I and II fractures and fractures of the proximal humerus metaphysis occur most commonly between 5 and 12 years of age. Pathologic fractures may occur secondary to unicameral bone cysts of the proximal humeral metaphysis.

1. Mechanism of injury—Mechanisms of injury to the proximal humerus include birth trauma (usually Salter I) and falls on an outstretched arm (usually Salter I or II or metaphyseal).

2. Classification
   • Neer and Horwitz classification—based on displacement.
     (a) Grade I—displaced less than 5 mm
     (b) Grade II—displaced at least one-third of the shaft width
     (c) Grade III—displaced at least two-thirds of the shaft width
     (d) Grade IV—displaced more than two-thirds of the shaft width
   • Pathologic fractures—Primarily occur through simple bone cysts of the proximal metaphysis. Active cysts are within 1 cm of the physis and latent cysts are greater than 1 cm from the physis.

3. Evaluation
   • Physical examination—Pseudoparalysis, tenderness, swelling, and pain may be present.
   • Imaging—Fractures with or without displacement are frequently seen on plain radiographs. Because the proximal epiphysis does not ossify until 6 months of age, newborn physeal separations may appear as an abnormal relationship between the scapula and humerus on plain radiographs. Ultrasonography is beneficial in these patients. Pathologic fractures through bone cysts can be confirmed by MRI.

4. Treatment—Most proximal humerus fractures can be treated by closed means. Eighty percent of the longitudinal growth of the humerus comes from the proximal physis resulting in significant remodeling potential. In addition, the large range of motion of the shoulder joint allows for minimal loss of function despite nonanatomic reduction. Acceptable limits of reduction in adolescent proximal humeral fractures include angulation of 35° and bayonet apposition. If the displacement exceeds these recommendations, closed reduction should be attempted. The shoulder should be immobilized in a shoulder immobilizer if stable, in a spica cast in the "salute position," or with percutaneous pinning. Open reduction may be needed in severely displaced fractures and in open fractures. Common impediments to closed reduction include the biceps tendon and periosteum. If no reduction is required, the extremity should be immobilized in a sling and swathe, or stockinette in newborns and infants, as previously described for obstetric clavicle fractures. Minimally displaced pathologic fractures through cysts are initially treated symptomatically with a sling. Latent and active cysts are treated with serial aspiration and steroid injections or bone marrow injection until they resolve. Curettage and bone grafting results in more reliable healing but may lead to growth arrest in active cysts.

5. Complications—Complications include growth arrest, diminished shoulder motion, malunion, recurrence of a cyst, and refracture.

C. Humeral Shaft Fractures—Fractures of the humeral shaft are uncommon. Fractures involving the proximal and distal metaphyses are more common.

1. Incidence—Humeral shaft fractures occur more commonly in infants and toddlers and in adolescents older than 12 years.

2. Mechanism of injury—Pediatric humeral shaft fractures may result from birth trauma, torsional forces (child abuse), direct trauma, falls, or from throwing activities.

3. Evaluation—In newborns or infants, irritability and pseudoparalysis may be the only

indicators of a recent fracture. The only physical finding may be a palpable lump that manifests 7 to 10 days after the initial injury. In a child or toddler, there may be pain, swelling, and an inability to use the extremity. Although most of these fractures result from accidental trauma, other evidence of child abuse should be sought if there is a suspicion of nonaccidental trauma. Fractures of the humeral shaft can also occur through areas of compromised bone strength such as a cyst, nonossifying fibroma or other lesions. De novo spiral fractures of the humerus can occur in adolescent throwing athletes. The fracture is typically long, and the degree of displacement is small due to a thick periosteum.

4. Treatment
   • Infants and children—A shoulder immobilizer, sling and swathe, or hanging arm cast is usually sufficient. Skeletal traction is rarely indicated. All states mandate reporting of suspected child abuse by attending physicians, residents, physician assistants, and nurses.
   • Adolescents—Nonsurgical treatment including functional bracing, hanging arm cast, or coaptation splinting should allow for acceptable healing in the vast majority of cases including fractures resulting from throwing. Open treatment including plating or intramedullary nailing is rarely indicated unless an acceptable closed reduction is not achievable or in multitrauma patients. Frequently, unacceptably angulated and displaced humeral shaft fractures will reduce to an acceptable position over the course of one week as the muscle spasm relaxes secondary to gravity and a sling or coaptation splint.

5. Complications
   • Overgrowth—Mild overgrowth occurs in 80% of humeral shaft fractures in children but is rarely significant.
   • Radial nerve injury—Radial nerve injuries may occur with fractures at the junction of the middle 1/3 and distal 1/3, but are infrequent. Radial nerve dysfunction that is present initially after injury should be observed for recovery on physical examination (likely a stretch injury). Nerve dysfunction that occurs only following attempted closed reduction may prompt consideration for surgical exploration of the radial nerve (possible entrapment). These guidelines remain controversial, however.

IV. Injuries of the Elbow Region (Figs. 31-2 Through 31-10)

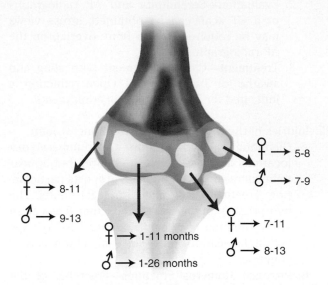

FIGURE 31-2 Age of appearance of the ossification centers around the elbow.

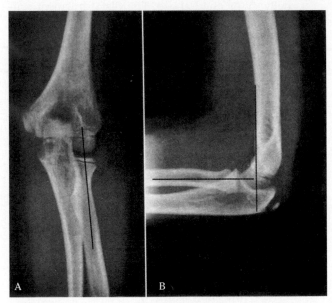

FIGURE 31-3 Radiographic lines for the evaluation of pediatric elbow injuries. A line drawn along the long axis of the proximal radius should bisect the capitellum on both the AP (A) and lateral (B) views. A line drawn along the anterior cortex of the distal humerus on the lateral view (B) (anterior humeral line) should bisect the capitellum. Disruption of these normal radiographic relationships is suggestive of injury. (Reprinted with permission from Brinker MR, Miller MD. *Fundamentals of Orthopaedics*. Philadelphia, PA: WB Saunders, 1999, with permission.)

A. Transphyseal Fractures (Distal Humeral Physeal Separation) (see Fig. 31-6)
   1. Incidence—Transphyseal fractures generally occur in children 3 years old and younger.

2. Mechanism of injury—Transphyseal fractures occur as a result of a fall on an outstretched arm or from birth trauma but may occur secondary to child abuse in up to 50% of children under 2 years of age.

3. Classification (DeLee)
   - Type A—A Salter I fracture occurring before ossification of the lateral condyle epiphysis, usually before age 1 year.

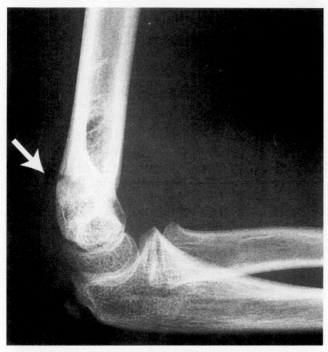

FIGURE 31-4 Posterior fat-pad sign (*arrow*) suggests the presence of an intra-articular effusion and fracture of the elbow. (Reprinted with permission from Brinker MR, Miller MD. *Fundamentals of orthopaedics*. Philadelphia, PA: WB Saunders, 1999, with permission.)

   - Type B—A Salter I or II fracture with a small fleck of lateral metaphysis generally occurring between the ages of 7 months and 3 years.
   - Type C—A fracture that includes a large metaphyseal fragment (Salter II) either medially or laterally, and generally occurring between ages 3 and 7 years.

4. Evaluation
   - Physical examination—This injury should be suspected in any infant with a swollen elbow and irritability. This fracture has a larger surface area than the comparable supracondylar humerus fracture, and so rotation and angulation tend to be less. This injury must be differentiated from an elbow dislocation.
   - Imaging—the proximal radius and ulna are in anatomic relationship with each other but tend to displace posteromedially with lend respect to the distal humerus. ***The key to distinguishing this injury from an elbow dislocation is maintenance of the radial head–capitellar relationship*** (see Fig. 31-5). In children younger than 3 years of age, the capitellum may not be ossified making the diagnosis difficult. An ultrasound, a MRI, or an arthrogram may be required.

5. Treatment—Closed reduction and percutaneous smooth K-wire fixation (see technique for supracondylar humerus fractures) diminishes the occurrence of cubitus varus that has been reported following closed reduction and cast immobilization, especially in patients younger than 2 years of age. The arm should be immobilized in a long arm cast postoperatively. Open reduction is rarely required. Healing normally occurs by 3 weeks.

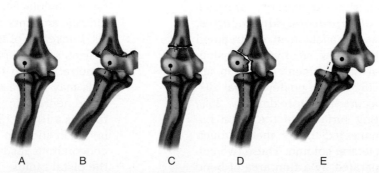

A   B   C   D   E

FIGURE 31-5 Radiocapitellar relationships. **A. *Normal elbow*** in which the long axis of the radius extends into the center of capitellum. **B. *Separation of the entire distal humeral physis (transphyseal fracture)*** in which the radiocapitellar relationship remains intact but the ossification center of the capitellum is posteromedial to the metaphysis of the distal humerus. **C. *Supracondylar fracture*** in which the radiocapitellar relationship is maintained. **D. *Fracture of the lateral condyle*** in which the capitellum is lateral to the long axis of the radius. **E. *Dislocation of the elbow*** in which the long axis of the radius is lateral to the capitellum.

Type A: 0-12 months   Type B: 1-3 years   Type C: 3-7 years

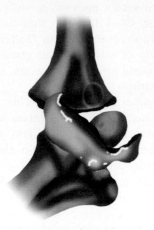 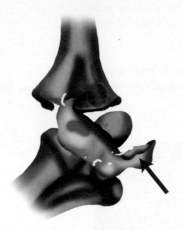 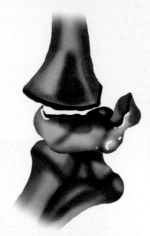

No ossification of   Ossification of the lateral   Ossification of the lateral
the lateral condyle,   condyle, can be SH I   condyle, usually SH II
usually SH I   or SH II with a small   with a large metaphyseal
          metaphyseal fragment   fragment

FIGURE 31-6 Transphyseal fractures of the distal humerus (DeLee classification): Type A, Type B, and Type C fractures.

6. Complications—Neurovascular injuries are less common than in supracondylar humerus fractures. Cubitus varus occurs following closed reduction and long arm cast immobilization and is diminished with percutaneous pin fixation. Avascular necrosis has also been reported.

B. Supracondylar Humerus Fractures (see Fig. 31-5)

1. Incidence—Supracondylar humerus fractures most commonly occur between 3 and 10 years of age. They are responsible for 50% to 70% of elbow fractures in children. They occur more frequently in boys than in girls. Injuries on the left side are more common than on the right.

2. Mechanisms of injury
   • Extension injuries—***Represent approximately 95% of supracondylar fractures.*** They are caused by a fall on an outstretched arm with the elbow in hyperextension. Posteromedial displacement occurs in approximately 75% while posterolateral displacement occurs in approximately 25%. The articulating surfaces of the distal humerus are connected to the shaft through a medial and lateral column. These two columns are separated by a thin area of bone formed anteriorly by the coronoid fossa and posteriorly by the olecranon fossa. This area is vulnerable to fracture when forced into hyperextension with the olecranon acting as a fulcrum.

   • Flexion injuries—Flexion supracondylar fractures are caused by a fall on the posterior aspect of a flexed elbow.

3. Classification (Gartland)
   • Type I—Nondisplaced or minimally displaced
   • Type II—Displaced but with an intact posterior cortical hinge
   • Type III—Completely displaced without cortical contact

4. Evaluation
   • Physical examination—Patients with Type I or II fractures will complain of pain in the elbow especially with attempts at range of motion. Swelling is usually evident but may be minimal. In Type III fractures, there may be an obvious S-shaped deformity with significant amounts of swelling and ecchymosis. Puckering of the anterior skin generally indicates severe displacement with fracture penetration into the subcutaneous tissues. This may evolve into an open fracture. Detailed neurologic examination is required as there is a 10% to 15% incidence of neurologic injury. In addition, there is a 5% incidence of concomitant ipsilateral fracture, usually of the distal radius.

   • Imaging—AP and lateral elbow views should be obtained. The lateral should be obtained in external rotation, as these fractures most frequently are unstable in internal rotation. On the lateral X-ray, the anterior humeral line (a line extending distally from the anterior humeral cortex) should intersect the middle third of the capitellum (see Fig. 31-3). Comparison views of the opposite elbow can also be obtained. Multidetector CT (MDCT) scanning can be obtained in the presence of a positive posterior fat pad sign (see Fig. 31-4), pain with range of motion, and a history of trauma if no fracture is readily identified. The scan can be obtained in a cast with comparable radiation exposure to a standard elbow series (minimal scatter with CT) when the arm is held above the head with the head tilted out of the field in the prone position. The rapidity of the MDCT scanning technique obviates the need for sedation even in the youngest child.

5. Associated injuries
   • Vascular—The brachial artery can be torn or, more commonly, set into spasm in and a Type III extension fracture. In a cold, pale, and pulseless extremity with a displaced supracondylar humerus fracture, initial management should include urgent fracture reduction in order to reconstitute the blood flow to the distal extremity. Preoperative arteriograms are contraindicated because they only delay treatment and do not alter the treatment plan. Capillary refill and pulse oximetry are unreliable in this situation. Doppler and manual palpation of the radial and ulnar arteries should be undertaken. If the ischemia does not resolve with closed reduction, open exploration is required. Brachial artery lacerations should be repaired or bypassed by a pediatric vascular surgeon. Arterial spasm can often be quelled by use of papaverine or 20% lidocaine directly applied to the area of spasm (not injected) under direct visualization.
   • Neurologic—Documentation of a thorough motor and sensory examination of the involved extremity should be undertaken. This evaluation should include anterior interosseous nerve (AIN) function (ability to flex the distal interphalangeal joint of the index finger and the interphalangeal joint of the thumb; remember this is a motor branch so there is no sensory loss). Nerve injuries occur in 7% to 15% of these fractures. *AIN palsy is the most commonly occurring nerve injury with extension-type supracondylar fractures*. Radial nerve injury has been reported more commonly with posteromedially displaced fractures and median nerve injuries with posterolateral

displacement. Ulnar nerve injuries can occur with flexion supracondylar fractures but more commonly occur iatrogenically as a result of medial pin placement.

6. Treatment—There are no standard guidelines for the amount of displacement and angulation acceptable for a supracondylar humerus fracture.
   • Extension injuries
      (a) Type I—These nondisplaced or minimally displaced fractures require long arm casting with the elbow in approximately 90° of flexion for 3 to 4 weeks.
      (b) Type II—There is considerable debate over the proper treatment of these displaced fractures with an intact posterior cortical hinge. These have been traditionally treated with closed reduction and long arm casting. In order to avoid repeat displacement, studies have suggested that elbow flexion of 120° in the cast is necessary. Unfortunately, this may lead to ischemia of the distal forearm and hand because of swelling and may increase the incidence of compartment syndrome. In addition, malunion and cubitus varus are more common in the Type II fractures that are treated with closed reduction and casting. Many surgeons now prefer closed reduction and percutaneous pinning (CRPP) for all displaced supracondylar fractures. The advantage is that the elbow can then be immobilized at 90° of flexion or less which facilitates venous return. This author performs a closed reduction and assesses the vascularity of the distal extremity with the elbow flexed at 120°. If there is evidence of vascular embarrassment in this position, he proceeds to percutaneous pin fixation (see below).
      (c) Type III—CRPP is the current standard of care. Many recent studies suggest that this does not need to be undertaken emergently in a patient with an uncompromised neurovascular status.
         • CRPP technique—The patient is placed under a general anesthetic on a standard operating room table with lead covering the testicles/ovaries, breasts, and thyroid. Two arm boards are placed longitudinally along the operative side of the table. An image intensifier positioned vertically with the large flat collector portion pointing up

from below is brought into the space between the two arm boards and left slightly lower than these. The child is then moved to the edge of the table so that the elbow is centered over the center aspect of the image intensifier collector. A closed reduction is then undertaken first applying longitudinal traction followed by correction of varus or valgus angulation, then rotation. The surgeon's thumb is then placed over the olecranon, and the elbow is flexed and the forearm pronated. Image intensification views are then obtained in the lateral position (externally rotated) and oblique views are obtained to assess the medial and lateral column reduction. Once reduction is obtained, the elbow is assessed for stability in approximately 120° of flexion. If the hand blanches or the pulses are absent, the surgeon proceeds to percutaneous pin fixation. (If acceptable reduction cannot be achieved, the surgeon proceeds to open reduction.) With the elbow in extension, the author then preps and drapes the entire affected upper extremity including the axilla and the deltoid region using split sheets. The image intensifier is draped in as part of the table. The surgeon then repeats closed reduction. Once anatomic reduction is achieved, the surgeon pronates the forearm and tapes the arm to the distal forearm in maximal flexion with sterile Coban wrap. A smooth K-wire (usually 0.062) appropriate for the size of the elbow is inserted under biplanar fluoroscopy from the lateral epicondyle percutaneously across the fracture site and anchored just through the contralateral proximal humeral cortex. A second comparably sized smooth K-wire is then placed parallel to the first approximately 1 cm apart from it in the same manner. The Coban wrap is then released and the elbow is allowed to extend, and true AP and lateral image intensification views are obtained. Assuming that these are satisfactory, the surgeon then externally rotates the elbow and, under real-time fluoroscopy, flexes and extends the elbow to assess for instability. If any motion is present,

the two lateral pins are supplemented with a medial pin placed with the elbow in extension by milking the ulnar nerve posteriorly into the ulnar groove and making a small incision over the medial epicondyle and spreading down to bone with a snap. The stability is then reassessed on the lateral view. The pins are then cut and bent external to the skin for incorporation under a cast or splint. A posterior splint can then be placed for one week or, alternatively, a long arm cast can be placed with the elbow in approximately 70° of flexion to facilitate venous return. This is possible because of the stability achieved with percutaneous pinning. If concerns over swelling exist, the cast can be either univalved down the volar aspect or bivalved. Three to four weeks of immobilization is required, and the pins can be removed in the office setting. No further immobilization is needed. Cross-pinning of the supracondylar fracture (one medial and one lateral) is the most biomechanically stable, followed by two parallel lateral pins, followed by two lateral pins crossing at or near the fracture site. A medial pin places the ulnar nerve at risk either during insertion or postoperatively by chronic tenting of the nerve over the wire with the elbow in flexion. The risk to the ulnar nerve during insertion can be diminished by inserting the pin under direct vision with a small incision or by placing the pin with the elbow in extension as described above.

- Open reduction—Indications for open reduction include open fractures, vascular compromise, or a fracture that cannot be adequately reduced closed. The surgical approach should be based on the surgeon's opinion as to what is obstructing fracture reduction. The approach may be medial, lateral, combined, or anteriorly based. A posterior triceps splitting incision is contraindicated in extension supracondylar fractures.

- Traction—Indications for traction include an inability to reduce or to stabilize a fracture and severe swelling. The advantage is the ability to check vascular status. The disadvantages include difficulty in controlling the position of the child in bed, difficulty of obtaining AP X-ray imaging, difficulty achieving fracture reduction and cost of hospitalization. In general, a manual reduction under general anesthesia will still be required.

- Flexion injuries—Similar principles apply as for extension injuries except that flexion injuries are reduced and stabilized in extension given the greater likelihood of an intact anterior periosteal hinge. Because of the difficulties in achieving an adequate reduction, operative intervention is frequently indicated.

7. Complications
    - Neurologic complications—Most neurologic complications involve a neurapraxia and recover spontaneously over weeks to months. If no improvement is seen 3 months after injury, exploration of the nerve can be considered. The AIN is a branch of the median nerve that provides motor innervation (no sensory) to the flexor pollicis longus (thumb IP joint flexion) and the flexor digitorum profundus to the index finger (index DIP joint flexion). *AIN function should be tested pre-and postreduction as it is the most frequently injured nerve seen in extension-type supracondylar humerus fractures*.
    - Vascular complications
        (a) If the extremity is pulseless, fracture reduction and stabilization are performed emergently. If the radial pulse is not restored by reduction and stabilization, an intraoperative arteriogram or direct exploration should be performed. If the radial pulse is absent but perfusion of the extremity appears normal (pink, pulseless hand) after reduction and stabilization, treatment options are controversial. These options include observation, immediate exploration, and delayed arteriogram.
        (b) Compartment syndrome—Volkmann's ischemic contracture was first described in 1881 as a consequence of the treatment of upper extremity fractures including supracondylar humerus fractures. This debilitating condition was later found to be the sequela of an unrecognized forearm compartment syndrome. Signs and symptoms of compartment syndrome of the forearm include pain out of proportion to the injury, pain with passive digital

extension and lack of active digital extension. Classically the five P's (pain, pallor, pulselessness, paresthesias, and paralysis) have been conveyed as diagnostic criteria; however, most of these occur late in the course of the disease after irreparable damage may have occurred. A high index of suspicion is required to make the diagnosis in a timely manner. Once considered, all circumferential dressings should be split and casts should be completely bivalved including under cast padding. Manometry of the muscle compartments and clinical examination determine the need for emergent fasciotomies of the forearm. In general, a volar compartment fasciotomy alone adequately decompresses both forearm compartments.

- Cubitus varus (gunstock deformity)—A cubitus varus deformity is the result of a malunion of a supracondylar fracture rather than an acquired growth deformity. While this deformity is primarily a cosmetic one, some recent evidence suggests it may present functional issues including the late development of a tardy ulnar nerve palsy. Nonetheless, supracondylar osteotomy for correction of a cubitus varus deformity will primarily result in improved cosmesis rather than improved function over the short term. Initial fracture treatment with CRPP decreases the incidence of cubitus varus.
- Stiffness—Almost all children eventually regain a normal range of motion following supracondylar humerus fracture. If significant stiffness persists beyond 3 weeks after cast removal, physical therapy is indicated. Occasional permanent stiffness may result from fibrosis of the muscles or elbow capsule or heterotopic ossification, especially in markedly displaced fractures.

C. Medial Epicondyle Fractures
1. Incidence—Medial epicondyle fractures generally occur between 9 and 14 years of age. Approximately half of these fractures are associated with an elbow dislocation, which may reduce spontaneously. This may be the origin of the elbow stiffness so commonly seen following this injury.
2. Mechanism of injury—Mechanisms of injury for a medial epicondyle fracture include a direct blow to the medial aspect and the elbow, a valgus stress placed on the elbow and a sudden flexion-pronation muscle contraction

resulting in avulsion. The ulnar collateral ligament of the elbow and the common flexor tendon of the forearm take origin from the medial epicondyle. The flexor-pronator mass serves as a deforming force on the fracture fragment.

3. Evaluation
   • Physical examination—The medial aspect of the elbow will be tender and swollen, and may be ecchymotic. If an elbow dislocation is present, there will be a visible deformity in the sagittal plane. Valgus stressing of the elbow under either anesthesia or sedation in 15° of flexion (in order to eliminate the stabilizing effect of the olecranon) can be undertaken to assess the stability of the medial structures.
   • Imaging—A comparison elbow radiograph of the contralateral side may be needed to determine the normal ossification pattern and for evaluating the position of the medial epicondyle if the apophysis is not readily seen. The medial epicondyle can be easily confused with the multiple ossification centers of the trochlea (the mnemonic is "CRMTOL"). Congruity of the elbow joint on a lateral X-ray should be assessed. Beware of the inability to obtain a true lateral X-ray of the elbow, as this may portend an entrapped medial epicondyle fragment within the joint.
4. Associated injuries—Associated injuries include elbow dislocation, radial neck fracture, olecranon fracture, coronoid process fracture, and ulnar nerve injury secondary to stretching (neurapraxia).
5. Treatment—Current controversy exists regarding the proper treatment of medial epicondyle fractures. This fracture involves an apophysis (a growth plate under tension) not an epiphysis (a growth plate under compression) and so no longitudinal or angular growth disorder occurs as a result. Displacement is tolerated unless the elbow is subject to forceful valgus loading such as during throwing activities or gymnastics. The ulnar collateral ligament remains lax with the elbow in extension if the medial epicondyle is displaced anteriorly. Open reduction is associated with increased stiffness of the elbow. Ogden has recommended ORIF for displacement of more than 5 mm and rotation of 90° or if the elbow is unstable to valgus stress. Absolute indications for open reduction include incarceration of the fragment within the elbow joint, ulnar nerve dysfunction, or demonstration of elbow instability. Long-term studies have demonstrated that isolated medial epicondyles fractures

with 5 to 15 mm of displacement heal well with brief immobilization (2 weeks) in a long arm cast.

6. Differential diagnosis
   • Medial condyle fracture—Medial condyle fractures are uncommon. A medial condyle fracture is an intra-articular fracture that produces an elbow hemarthrosis. A medial epicondyle fracture is extra-articular and rarely produces a hemarthrosis (posterior fat pad sign). The trochlea ossification center appears at 9 years of age. Prior to this age, a medial condylar fracture may be difficult to differentiate from a medial epicondyle fracture. A metaphyseal fragment indicates that the fracture involves the medial condyle.
   • Multiple Ossification Centers of the Trochlea
7. Complications—Complications of medial epicondyle fractures include valgus elbow instability and ulnar neurapraxia.
D. Lateral Condyle Fractures (see Fig. 31-7)
   1. Incidence—Lateral condyle fractures occur in children 5 to 10 years of age.
   2. Mechanism of injury—Lateral condyle fractures result from a fall on an outstretched arm that produces a varus stress on the elbow. Alternatively, a valgus force acting through the radial head can directly impact the lateral condyle fracturing it.
   3. Classification
      • Milch Type I—The fracture extends through the secondary ossification center of the capitellum entering the joint just lateral to the trochlea groove (Salter IV fracture). This is a stable fracture pattern.

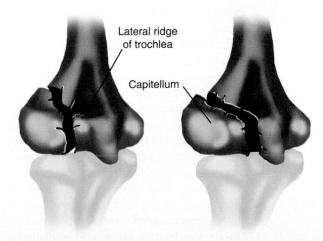

Type I   Type II

FIGURE 31-7 Lateral condylar fracture of the humerus (Milch Classification): Milch Type I and Type II fractures.

- Milch Type II—The fracture extends medial to the trochlea groove (Salter II) resulting in an unstable joint (intact medial articular hinge is key to stability and congruity).
4. Evaluation
   - Physical examination—A swollen elbow that is tender to palpation over the lateral condyle but not tender to careful examination over the medial condyle.
   - Imaging—The AP view of the involved elbow frequently demonstrates a subtle fracture line extending just proximal and parallel to the physis of the capitellum. A lateral X-ray demonstrates a classic subtle metaphyseal fragment that is often missed in minimally displaced fragments. Oblique views of the elbow, arthrograms, and ultrasound may be helpful in identifying minimally displaced fractures. MRI has been utilized, but the need for sedation and the long scan times make this impractical. Recent advances in MDCT technology allow for rapid scanning times (with radiation exposure that is comparable to a standard plain film series of the elbow) to help identify minimally displaced fractures and those at risk for late displacement. It is not recommended for routine use, however.
5. Associated injuries—Associated injuries include elbow dislocation, fracture of the ulnar shaft, and fracture of the medial epicondyle.
6. Treatment—Treatment is based on the degree of displacement. Stable nondisplaced fractures can be treated nonoperatively with long arm casting for 4 to 5 weeks. Weekly follow-up with serial X-ray evaluation needs to be undertaken to assess for displacement until radiographic healing occurs. Unstable minimally displaced fractures and displaced fractures require open reduction and internal fixation. Displaced fractures include those that are displaced 2 mm or more. Open reduction is performed through an anterolateral approach because the blood supply to the lateral humeral condyle arises posteriorly through the soft tissues. Dissection should not be carried out posteriorly to avoid osteonecrosis of the fragment. An anterolateral approach allows direct visualization of the lateral metaphysis, the anterior metaphysis, and the intra-articular surface. Each of these has to be anatomically reduced prior to K-wire fixation. The role of closed reduction and percutaneous pin fixation remains controversial. CRPP can be performed for minimally displaced fractures or nondisplaced fractures if poor compliance with immobilization is anticipated.

7. Complications
   - Nonunion/delayed union—***Lateral condyle fractures in children are associated with a high incidence of nonunion.*** An anatomic reduction with stable internal fixation minimizes the likelihood of nonunion. The intra-articular nature of the fracture and the limited blood supply likely contribute to these complications. It is imperative to closely monitor these fractures until definitive union occurs. The treatment of late-presenting fractures remains controversial. Most recent studies favor surgical treatment for these fractures.
   - Osteonecrosis—The blood supply to the lateral condyle enters posteriorly through the musculature and soft tissue from extra-articular vessels. These must be meticulously preserved during ORIF.
   - Physeal arrest—Physeal arrests are rarely of clinical significance in this patient population.
   - Cubitus varus—This is the most common complication occurring in up to 40% of patients. It rarely necessitates clinical intervention. Parents should understand that there will be a lateral prominence.
   - Lateral spur formation—Lateral spur formation results from operative and nonoperative treatment of these fractures. It presents as an apparent cubitus varus. It does not affect function.
   - Fishtail deformity—The etiology of fishtail deformity of the distal humerus is unknown but likely results from either malunion, osteonecrosis, growth arrest, or some combination of these.
E. Medial condyle fractures (see Figure 31-8)
   1. Incidence—Medial condyle fractures occur most often in children ages 8 to 14 years.
   2. Mechanism of injury—The mechanism of injury is the same as that for medial epicondyle fractures and can include a direct blow, valgus

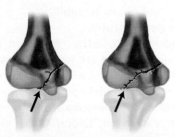

Type I   Type II

FIGURE 31-8 Fracture patterns of medial humeral condyle fractures, as described by Milch.

stress, and a violent flexor-pronator muscle contraction.

3. Classification
   - Milch System—The Milch system is based on the location of the fracture line (see Figure 31-8).
     (a) Type I—Type I is through the apex of the trochlea; it is the more common type.
     (b) Type II—Type II is through the capitulotrochlear groove; it is the less common type.
   - Kilfoyle System—The Kilfoyle system is based on the fracture location and degree of displacement.
     (a) Type I—Type I is a fracture through the medial condyle metaphysis.
     (b) Type II—The fracture extends into the medial condyle physis.
     (c) Type III—Rotation and displacement occur.
4. Evaluation
   - Physical Examination—A displaced medial condyle fracture is intraarticular; unlike the extraarticular medial epicondyle fracture, it produces a hemarthrosis.
   - Imaging—Before the ossification of the trochlea at age 9, this fracture may be difficult to diagnose; arthrography or magnetic resonance imaging (MRI) may be useful.
5. Treatment
   - Long Arm Cast—A long arm cast for 3 to 4 weeks suffices for undisplaced fractures; as with lateral condyle fractures, x-ray studies should be performed every 5 to 7 days (to check for displacement) until evidence of healing is seen.
   - CRPP—CRPP can be attempted for an undisplaced or minimally displaced fracture, but the alignment must be anatomic.
   - ORIF—ORIF with K-wires or bioabsorbable pins is necessary for displaced fractures.
6. Complications—Complications include growth disturbance, avascular necrosis, loss of motion, and elbow instability.

F. Olecranon Fractures
   1. Incidence—Pediatric olecranon fractures are uncommon and are associated with concomitant elbow fractures in up to 50% of cases (most commonly medial epicondyle fractures).
   2. Mechanism—Olecranon fractures result from hyperextension, hyperflexion, shear or a direct blow.
   3. Classification—There is no universally accepted classification system for olecranon fractures in children. Wilkins has classified these based on mechanism of injury.

   - Type A—Flexion injury
   - Type B—Extension injury
     (a) Valgus pattern—Associated with radial neck fracture
     (b) Varus pattern—Associated with dislocation of the radial head and posterior interosseus nerve injury
   - Type C—Shear injury

   4. Associated injuries—Associated elbow fractures occur in 20% to 50% of olecranon fractures and include medial epicondyle, lateral epicondyle and radial neck fracture.
   5. Treatment principles—The most important considerations in treatment include the degree of displacement (3 mm or lesser is considered minimal), whether intra- or extra-articular, and stability. Due to a thick periosteum, most olecranon fractures remain minimally displaced and can be treated with cast immobilization for 3 to 4 weeks. Shear injuries (rare) are usually stable in flexion while flexion fractures occasionally must be treated in extension. Displaced intra-articular fractures may require ORIF with a tension band technique or resorbable pins.

G. Nursemaid's Elbow ("pulled elbow," radial head subluxation)
   1. Incidence—The peak incidence is 1 to 3 years; this injury is rare after age 5 years. It is slightly more common in girls and on the left side.
   2. Mechanism of injury—The injury occurs by traction on the hand when the forearm is pronated and the elbow extended. In this position, the anterior aspect of the annular ligament subluxates over the radial head and interposes itself into the radial head-capitellar articulation (see Fig. 31-9).
   3. Evaluation
      - Physical examination—The child holds the arm at the side with the elbow in minimal flexion with the forearm pronated.
      - Imaging—X-rays are not indicated with a history of traction on a pronated forearm. Radiographs appear normal with no evidence of effusion.
   4. Treatment—Reduction is achieved by simultaneous full flexion of the elbow and full supination of the forearm. The child will protest but will return to normal uninhibited utilization of the extremity within minutes.
   5. Differential diagnosis—Other injuries including septic elbow, radial neck fracture, or other fractures about the elbow may present in a similar manner. Frequently, children present with a pseudoparalysis of the elbow that has lasted for more than a day. They may have undergone prior attempts at reduction of a

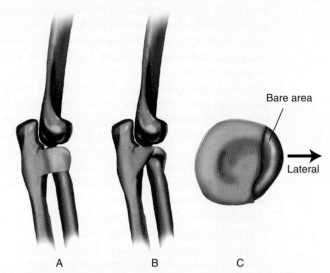

Bare area

Lateral

A   B   C

FIGURE 31-9 A. Normal annular ligament of the elbow. **B.** Nursemaid's elbow with a tear in the distal part of the annular ligament and a portion of the ligament trapped within the radiocapitellar joint. **C.** Axial view of the tear in the annular ligament.

nursemaid's elbow. A repeat attempted reduction is indicated with the appropriate history. These children may not achieve immediate relief and may benefit from 2 weeks of long arm casting with the forearm in supination.

6. Complications—Recurrence is the primary complication. Recurrence can be avoided in most instances with proper education of the family. Recurrent episodes should be treated the same as primary occurrences. Long arm cast immobilization may be necessary in some instances. Some children suffer multiple recurrences secondary to a stretched annular ligament. Proper familial education combined with bone growth will allow a proper bone–ligament relationship over time.

H. Elbow Dislocation (see Fig. 31-5)
1. Incidence—Elbow dislocations are an uncommon occurrence in children. The peak incidence for elbow dislocations is 13 years of age with dislocations occurring more frequently in boys than in girls. Elbow dislocations are rare in young children. ***An apparent elbow dislocation in a young child should raise the possibility of a transphyseal fracture***.
2. Mechanism of injury—Elbow dislocations result from a fall on the supinated, outstretched forearm with the elbow in full extension or mild flexion. The resultant hyperflexion and valgus strain on the elbow results in dislocation. The resultant dislocation is usually posterior or posterolateral but less commonly anterior, medial, lateral, and divergent dislocations can occur.

Divergent dislocations are quite rare resulting in displacement of the radius and ulna in opposite directions.

3. Classification—Wilkins has classified pediatric elbow dislocations based on the direction of displacement with respect to the humerus.
   • Type I—The proximal radial ulnar joint remains intact.
     (a) Posterior
        • Posteromedial
        • Posterolateral
     (b) Anterior
     (c) Medial
     (d) Lateral
   • Type II—The proximal radial ulnar joint is disrupted.
     (a) Divergent
        • Anteroposterior
        • Mediolateral (transverse)
     (b) Radioulnar translocation
4. Evaluation
   • Physical examination—The child presents with a painful, swollen elbow held in flexion and appears S-shaped. The antecubital fossa appears markedly widened because of the distal humerus.
   • Imaging—Plain radiographs demonstrate radioulnar displacement with respect to the distal humerus. The congruency between the capitellum and the radial head and neck is lost differentiating this injury from a transphyseal fracture in the very young. Special attention needs to be paid to associated elbow injuries including a medial epicondyle fracture. The prereduction and postreduction position of the medial epicondyle must be carefully scrutinized.
5. Associated injuries—Elbow dislocations are frequently associated with fractures of the elbow particularly fractures of the medial epicondyle. Proximal radius fractures, cornoid process fractures, olecranon fractures, brachial artery injury, median nerve injury, and brachialis muscle injury can also be associated with an elbow dislocation.
6. Treatment
   • Closed treatment—The acute posterior dislocation can usually be treated closed without the need of a general anesthetic. This is accomplished by providing longitudinal traction with minimal hyperextension of the elbow, supination of the forearm followed by flexion of the elbow. Care must be taken to avoid significant hyperextension in order to avoid further injury to the median nerve or brachial artery. This normally results in

a stable reduction that requires immobilization in a long arm splint for approximately 2 weeks, followed by active and active assisted range of motion. Anterior dislocations generally require a general anesthetic for reduction and are accomplished with longitudinal traction on the flexed elbow with posteriorly directed force applied to the forearm as the elbow is gradually extended.

- Open treatment—Open treatment is primarily indicated for an irreducible elbow dislocation usually caused by a medial epicondyle fracture fragment trapped within the joint, an open elbow injury or a brachial artery injury.

7. Complications
- Stiffness
- Recurrent dislocation—Recurrent dislocation is rare and difficult to treat. It is seen most commonly in late adolescence with posterior and posterior-lateral dislocations. The posterior capsule may fail to firmly reattach to the posterolateral aspect of the humerus owing to a large amount of cartilage in this region.
- Nerve injuries
  (a) Ulnar nerve—The ulnar nerve can be trapped in the joint with a displaced medial epicondyle avulsion fragment. Open reduction and extraction of the medial epicondyle and ulnar nerve normally results in complete recovery.
  (b) Median nerve—Median nerve injuries are less common than ulnar nerve injuries due to elbow dislocations, but have a poorer prognosis for recovery. The nerve can be trapped between the trochlea and olecranon during reduction, can be trapped between the medial epicondyle fracture and the humerus, or can become displaced behind the medial condylar ridge and trapped between the distal humerus and the olecranon as the joint reduces. Median nerve dysfunction following a suspected elbow dislocation should prompt a thorough evaluation for one of these situations.
- Brachial artery injury—The brachial artery is uncommonly injured as a result of a closed elbow dislocation, but is more frequently injured in open dislocations. Vascular repair may be required.

I. Proximal Radius (Head and Neck) Fractures
1. Incidence—Because of the cartilaginous makeup of the radial head, radial neck fractures are much more common in children. Approximately one half of all radial neck fractures are associated with other elbow injuries. The peak incidence for proximal radial fractures is 4 to 14 years of age.
2. Mechanisms of injury—Fractures of the radial head and neck generally result either from a fall onto an outstretched upper extremity with the elbow in extension with a resultant valgus force applied or during the course of an elbow dislocation. A radial neck fracture can also occur in combination with a proximal ulnar fracture as a Monteggia variant.
3. Classification (O'Brien's) (see Fig. 31-10)
- Type I—Angulation is less than 30°.
- Type II—Angulation is 30° to 60°.
- Type III—Angulation is greater than 60°.
4. Evaluation
- Physical examination—The child will present with discomfort over the lateral aspect of the elbow and will demonstrate pain and limited pronation and supination of the forearm. There will be tenderness to palpation over the radial head especially with pronation and supination.
- Imaging—AP and lateral X-rays of the elbow may not demonstrate obvious injury. Frequently, multiple oblique views are needed when a high index of suspicion is present. Alternatively, MDCT can be utilized, as previously described.
5. Associated injuries—Fractures of the proximal ulna, medial epicondyle, lateral condyle,

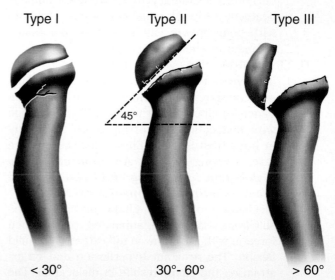

Type I	Type II	Type III
< 30°	30°- 60°	> 60°

FIGURE 31-10 Radial neck fractures in children (O'Brien's classification): Type I, Type II, and Type III fractures.

olecranon or rupture of the medial collateral ligament can be seen with radial neck or head fractures.

6. Treatment—The two primary determinants of treatment are angulation and displacement. Wilkins recommends early motion for angulation less than 30° and translation less than 5 mm, a closed reduction for angulation of 30° to 60° and ORIF for angulation more than 60° or translation more than 5 mm. Ogden considers angulation more than 10° to 15° in a child over 10 years of age as unacceptable because of the limited remodeling potential. Reduction may be achieved with closed manipulation, percutaneous K-wire manipulation, or intramedullary wire manipulation, or through open reduction.

7. Complications—Significant loss of motion occurs in 30% to 50% of children with these injuries. In addition, premature physeal closure, osteonecrosis, cubitus valgus, heterotopic ossification, radioulnar synostosis, and radial head overgrowth have all been described in these fractures.

J. Coronoid Process Fractures

1. Incidence—Coronoid process fractures are quite rare in children and are primarily associated with elbow dislocations. As such, they are frequently accompanied by fractures of the medial epicondyle, proximal radius, lateral condyle, and proximal ulna.

2. Classification (Regan and Morrey's)
   • Type I—Involves the tip of the coronoid process.
   • Type II—Involves less than 50% of the coronoid process.
   • Type III—Involves greater than 50% of the coronoid process.

3. Treatment—These fractures are rarely displaced and are almost always treated closed in children.

V. Injuries of the Radius and Ulna

A. Diaphyseal Forearm Fractures

1. Mechanisms of injury—Normally, the mechanism of injury for a diaphyseal radius and ulna fracture (bone forearm fracture) is a fall on an outstretched upper extremity.

2. Evaluation
   • Physical examination—The forearm demonstrates a subtle or obvious deformation with tenderness at the fracture site. Pronation and supination are limited and cause pain.
   • Imaging—Orthogonal radiographs of the entire forearm including the wrist and elbow must be performed. To assess the proper

rotational alignment of the forearm, the surgeon looks for the bicipital tuberosity to be diagonally opposite the radial styloid and the coronoid to be anterior, diagonally opposite the ulnar styloid, which is posterior.

3. Classification—There is no generally accepted classification system for both bone forearm fractures.
   • These fractures can be divided into three distinct types for descriptive purposes.
   (a) Complete fractures—These fractures frequently demonstrate displacement and are characterized by a complete fracture line through the cortex on all radiographic views.
   (b) Greenstick fractures (Fig. 31-11)—These fractures are characterized by a fracture through only one visualized cortex on each radiographic view. The contralateral cortex remains intact. These fractures have a tendency to displace over time.
   (c) Plastic deformation fractures—These fractures demonstrate no discernible fracture through either cortex on radiographic views but demonstrate angular deformity. These fractures are unique to children. Either bone or both bones can be plastically deformed.

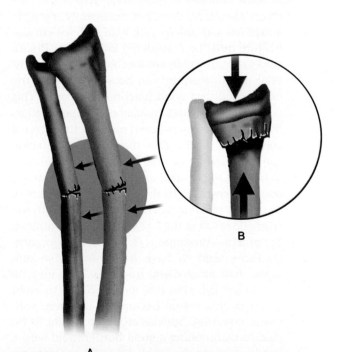

FIGURE 31-11 A. Greenstick fracture of a child's forearm. B. Torus fracture of a child's distal radius. *Arrows* indicate the direction of forces that produce the injury.

- These fractures can also be described based on their location within the bones.
  - (a) Proximal 1/3
  - (b) Middle 1/3
  - (c) Distal 1/3
- These fractures can be described based on their direction of displacement.
  - (a) Apex dorsal
  - (b) Apex volar
  - (c) Apex radial
  - (d) Apex ulnar

4. Associated injuries—Associated injuries include elbow fractures, Monteggia fractures, and Galeazzi fractures. By this reason, it is imperative to visualize the elbow and wrist joints radiologically as part of the forearm evaluation.

5. Limits of acceptable reduction—Much literature has been dedicated to what constitutes an acceptable reduction in a pediatric both bone forearm fracture. Price presented guidelines that included 10° of angulation, 45° of malrotation, complete displacement, and loss of the radial bow to be reasonable limits for an acceptable reduction. The remodeling potential for both bone forearm fractures in children younger than 10 years of age is significant. Angular displacement remodels better than rotational displacement. Malunions following both bone forearm fractures in children are common. Nonetheless, the functional outcome in these children is quite good. Radiologic malunion, therefore, does not necessarily translate into functional deficits. Although each patient and fracture must be considered individually, Price's guidelines are quite reasonable and, frequently, even more deformity can be accepted with the expectation of a good functional outcome. This authors' primary determinant of whether a reduction is satisfactory is based more on the external appearance of the arm than any other factor. Specific attention should be paid to the amount of bowing of the ulna as this is a subcutaneous bone and seems to be the primary determinant of whether a child or parent will be happy with the cosmetic result of the forearm fracture treatment.

6. Treatment—Proximal 1/3 both-bone forearm fractures tend to have a less favorable outcome than more distal fractures. This may be due to the fact that it is more difficult to mold a cast in this region because of the large soft-tissue covering. Special attention needs to be paid to maintaining a good border mold with a good interosseous mold. All of these fractures should be followed at weekly intervals for the first three weeks with AP and lateral X-rays to assure that displacement does not occur.

- Nondisplaced fractures—Nondisplaced both bone forearm fractures should be immobilized in a long arm cast for 5 to 6 weeks depending upon patient age. Middle 1/3 and distal 1/3 fractures can frequently be converted from a long arm cast to a short arm cast at 4 weeks if adequate callus is present.
- Greenstick fractures—Greenstick fractures of the forearm can have a surprisingly significant amount of rotational deformity despite appearing to have minimal angulation. Reduction of these fractures prior to cast immobilization is generally recommended. Reduction is accomplished by the *"rule of thumb."* The *rule of thumb* refers to the maneuver that must be undertaken to achieve adequate fracture reduction. Fractures with apex dorsal angulation have a pronation deformity and so the thumb is moved toward the apex of the fracture to create supination at the fracture site in order to reduce the fracture. Similarly, fractures with apex volar angulation have a supination deformity and so the forearm must be pronated (thumb moved in the direction of the apex of the fracture) in order to correct the deformity and reduce the fracture. Once the reduction is complete, a long arm cast with a good ulnar mold, a good interosseous mold and a good dorsal and volar mold is placed to maintain the correction. Generally, plaster is a better material to use in the acute fracture situation than fiberglass. Plaster allows better molding than fiberglass and is more likely to hold the mold placed by the surgeon .
- Displaced fractures—Most displaced both bone forearm fractures in skeletally immature children can be treated with closed reduction and casting. Reduction can generally be achieved with longitudinal traction, exaggeration of the deformity and correction of the angular and rotational malalignment. The rule of thumb outlined above can be followed for postproduction immobilization. In other words, fractures that were originally apex volar can be casted in slight pronation; those that were originally apex dorsal can be casted in slight supination. More importantly, close attention must be paid to the rotational alignment of the distal fragment with respect to the proximal fragment. These fractures are best stabilized by lining up the bicipital tuberosity opposite to the radial styloid thereby assuring proper rotational alignment. If there is any doubt, the forearm should be placed in the neutral position. These fractures all require

long arm immobilization initially with either a well molded long arm cast, a sugar tong splint, a univalved long arm cast or a bivalved long arm cast. As with all other forearm fractures, these need to be closely scrutinized at weekly intervals for the first three weeks to assure that displacement does not occur.

- Plastic deformation—Recognition of plastic deformation is important in avoiding loss of pronation and supination. When plastic deformation occurs in one forearm bone in conjunction with a displaced fracture in the other, reduction of the plastic deformation must be performed prior to reduction of the displaced fracture. Careful evaluation of the elbow joint for displacement of the radial head must be performed when an isolated plastic deformation of the proximal to mid ulna is encountered.

- Indications for open treatment—The indications for operative treatment of pediatric radius and/or ulnar shaft fractures include an open fracture, an irreducible fracture, a fracture associated with a compartment syndrome or dysvascular extremity, inability to maintain an acceptable reduction or entrapment of nerves or tendons within the fracture site. Skeletal fixation may be accomplished utilizing plates and screws as in adults, intramedullary fixation, or with external fixation. External fixation is generally reserved for forearm fractures associated with significant soft-tissue injuries or burns.

7. Complications
    - Refracture—Refracture occurs in up to 5% of greenstick fractures and open fractures.
    - Loss of reduction—Diaphyseal both bone forearm fractures have a fairly high rate of reduction loss in the weeks following initial reduction. Close scrutiny with weekly X-rays is required. While angular deformities can remodel, rotational deformities do not remodel.
    - Malunion—Frequently malunited forearm fractures do not result in functional deficits for the patient. Corrective osteotomies should not be considered until the functional deficits are clearly identified. Ogden has suggested that angulation of the radius affects forearm rotation more than angulation of the ulna (Fig. 31-12).
    - Cross union—Cross union is a relatively rare complication of both bone forearm fractures but occurs more frequently following surgical intervention, repeat manipulations, and high-energy injuries and in children with head injuries. The results of excision of the synostosis are reportedly not as good in children as they are in adults.
    - Compartment syndrome—Compartment syndrome occurs less frequently in children than in adults. It is more common in open fractures and can be the result of a constricting cast. A high index of suspicion must be maintained following reduction of a both bone forearm fracture.

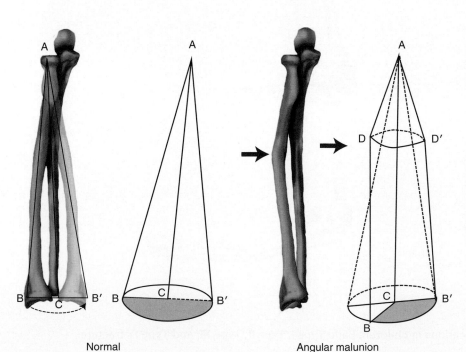

Normal   Angular malunion

FIGURE 31-12 Rotation of the radius on the ulna. Normally, the mechanical triangle of rotation *(ABC)* has an axis from the center of the radial head *(A)* to the ulnar styloid *(C)*. The radial styloid *(B)* rotates around to a pronated position *(B′)*, subtending a semicircular conical base. Angular malunion introduces a frustrum *(D)* into the normal cone of rotation, thereby limiting the area *(stippling)* of the cone base. In this example, residual pronation of the distal radius, caused by angular malunion, restricts full supination.

- Muscle or nerve entrapment—Muscles or peripheral nerves may become entrapped in the fracture site and can lead to residual functional deficits.

B. Monteggia Fracture-Dislocation—A Monteggia fracture-dislocation is a fracture of the ulnar shaft associated with a dislocation of the radial head.

1. Incidence—These injuries have a peak incidence of occurrence between 7 and 10 years of age in children.

2. Classification (Fig. 31-13)
   - Bado has classified these fractures based on the direction of the radial head dislocation. ***The radial head always dislocates in the direction of the apex of the ulnar fracture***.
     - (a) Type I Monteggia fractures demonstrate anterior dislocation of the radial head (70% to 85%).
     - (b) Type II Monteggia fractures demonstrate posterior dislocation of the radial head (5%).
     - (c) Type III Monteggia fractures demonstrate lateral dislocation of the radial head (15% to 25%).
     - (d) Type IV Monteggia fractures involve fractures of both the proximal radius and the ulna with anterior dislocation of the radial head (rare).
   - Letts and coworkers have modified Bado's classification for use in pediatric patients.

They divide these fractures into five types. Letts' Type A, B, and C fractures are similar to Bado Type I fractures.

- (a) Type A fractures demonstrate anterior dislocation of the radial head with apex anterior plastic deformation of the ulna (Bado I).
- (b) Type B fractures demonstrate anterior dislocation of the radial head with a greenstick fracture of the ulna (Bado I).
- (c) Type C fractures demonstrate anterior dislocation of the radial head with a complete fracture of the ulna (Bado I and IV).
- (d) Type D—Type D fractures demonstrate posterior dislocation of the radial head (Bado II).
- (e) Type E—Type E fractures demonstrate lateral dislocation of the radial head (Bado III).

3. Monteggia fracture-dislocation variants—Variants or equivalents of Monteggia fracture-dislocation include an isolated anterior dislocation of the radial head without an ulna fracture, fracture of the ulna with fracture of the radial neck, a fracture of both bones of the forearm with a fracture of the radius proximal to the ulnar fracture and plastic deformation of the ulna with a radial head dislocation. These pediatric variants are addressed in Letts' classification as outlined above.

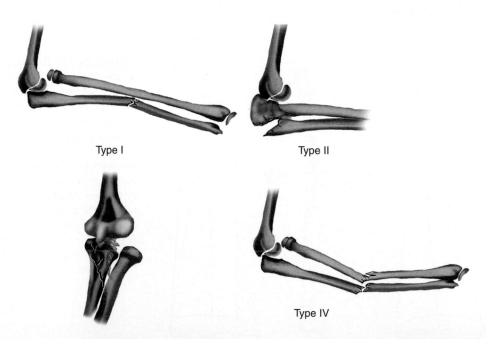

Type I   Type II   Type III   Type IV

FIGURE 31-13 Monteggia fracture-dislocations in children. Bado Type I, Type II, Type III, and Type IV fracture-dislocations.

4. Mechanism of injury (Bado)
   - Type I—There are three theories:
     (a) A fall on an outstretched upper extremity with the hand planted and the forearm pronated results in increased pronation resulting in a fracture of the ulna and subsequent anterior dislocation of the radial head.
     (b) A direct blow to the ulna posteriorly results in an ulna fracture and anterior dislocation of the radial head.
     (c) A fall on an outstretched upper extremity with resultant hyperextension and forceful contracture of the biceps, which dislocates the radial head anteriorly with subsequent fracture of the ulna.
   - Type II—A fall on a flexed elbow.
   - Type III—Most likely results from a varus force applied to a hyperextended elbow.
   - Type IV—Unknown mechanism.
5. Evaluation
   - Physical examination—Children with Monteggia fracture-dislocations present with deformity of the elbow and forearm. There is pain and limitation on active and passive forearm rotation. The dislocated radial head may be palpable as a lump in the position of its dislocation.
   - Imaging—True AP and lateral X-rays of the elbow are critical in the diagnosis of Monteggia fracture-dislocation. The radial head-capitellar alignment must be closely scrutinized by drawing a line down the long axis of the radius and assuring that it passes through the center of the capitellum on each radiographic view, regardless of the amount of elbow flexion (see Fig. 31-3). It is easy to miss a subtle radial head dislocation.
6. Differential diagnosis—Congenital dislocation of the radial head is almost always posterior and bilateral. The radial head is usually enlarged and elliptical in shape.
7. Treatment
   - Closed reduction
     (a) Type I—Reduce the ulna fracture with longitudinal traction and three-point force centered on the apex. The radial head can then be reduced with direct pressure. The reduction is best maintained with elbow flexion to 120° and neutral forearm positioning in a cast.
     (b) Type II—Reduce the ulna fracture with longitudinal traction and three-point force centered on the apex. The radial head can then be reduced with direct pressure. The reduction is best maintained with the elbow in extension and the forearm in neutral position in a cast.
     (c) Type III—Longitudinal traction is placed on the forearm with the elbow in extension and direct pressure is placed over the apex of the radial head and ulna fracture. The reduction is best maintained with the elbow at 90° and the forearm in supination.
8. Complications—There is a high association of ipsilateral extremity fractures in patients with Bado II Monteggia fracture-dislocations. The potential for redislocation of the radial head is high. Therefore, close weekly radiographic follow-up is required to assure that no redisplacement occurs in patients treated with closed reduction.

C. Distal Radius and Ulna Fractures
1. Incidence—Distal radius and ulnar fractures are extremely common injuries in children. These injuries occur throughout childhood but are more likely to occur in adolescents than in younger children.
2. Mechanism of injury—These fractures are normally caused by a fall on an outstretched hand. If the wrist is in extension, the patient will most likely sustain a volarly angulated fracture. If the wrist is in flexion, the patient will most likely sustain a dorsally angulated fracture.
3. Classification—These fractures include buckle (torus) fractures (see Fig. 31-11), growth plate fractures (usually Salter-Harris I or II), metaphyseal fractures, or greenstick fractures.
4. Evaluation
   - Physical examination—In displaced or angulated fractures there may be a visible "dinner fork" deformity. There is discomfort with palpation and range of motion of the wrist.
   - Radiographic evaluation—High-quality AP views and lateral X-rays of the distal radius must be obtained. As with other forearm fractures, visualization of the elbow is also desirable although not absolutely required if the physical examination is indicative of an isolated distal injury.
5. Treatment—Treatment decisions are based on the amount of angulation deemed acceptable for a given patient. Because the motion of the wrist is usually in the same plane as the displacement, significant remodeling can occur even in individuals nearing skeletal maturity. Bayonet apposition is quite acceptable as it usually remodels. In patients 10 years old or younger, up to 40° of sagittal plane angulation and 20° of coronal plane angulation can be accepted. Because distal radius fractures

remodel at rates of up to 10° per year, 10° of angulation can be accepted in patients felt to be within one year of skeletal maturity. As with other forearm fractures, it may be wise to reduce clinically apparent angular deformities so that less frequent reassurance to the parents need to be undertaken during remodelling.

- Torus (buckle) fractures—Recent studies suggest that these fractures can be treated symptomatically in a removable wrist splint. Most surgeons still prefer to treat these in a short arm cast for three weeks. After three weeks, the immobilization is removed and no further X-rays are required.

- Nondisplaced fractures—Nondisplaced complete fractures can be treated in a short arm cast for 5 weeks. If there is pain with pronation and supination at initial presentation, a long arm cast is advisable for the initial 2 to 3 weeks.

- Greenstick fractures—The periosteum is disrupted on the convex side of the fracture and the bone is deformed on the concave side making progression of angulation likely. Angulation can result in a permanent rotational deformity so reduction of these fractures, normally with completion of the fracture on the concave side, is recommended. A well-molded long arm cast should be applied for 5 to 6 weeks.

- Distal metaphyseal fractures—Distal metaphyseal fractures of the forearm rarely occur in a single bone. Generally, the radius demonstrates a complete fracture with either a complete fracture of the ulna, an ulnar styloid fracture, plastic deformation of the ulna, or a greenstick fracture of the ulna. These fractures are treated with closed reduction of the radius. The ulna fracture usually does not require separate attention. Careful molding of the cast is required in order to maintain the reduction. Hyperflexion of the wrist in the cast can precipitate an acute carpal tunnel syndrome and should be avoided. These fractures are generally healed within 4 to 5 weeks.

- Distal physeal fractures—Distal physeal fractures of the radius are common. These can be treated similar to displaced metaphyseal fractures and rapid healing can be expected. Only one attempt at closed reduction under conscious sedation should be made in the emergency room. If the reduction is unsuccessful, subsequent reduction should be done under general anesthetic in the operating room with full muscular relaxation. This avoids secondary trauma to the growth plate with repeated reduction attempts. Repeat closed reductions after 10 to 14 days for progressive malalignment requires forceful manipulation and has an increased risk of growth arrest. Distal physeal fractures of the ulna are uncommon but have a fairly high incidence of growth arrest.

- Indications for operative intervention—Indications for surgery in distal radius and ulna fractures include open fractures, failure to obtain an acceptable closed reduction, compartment syndrome, acute carpal tunnel syndrome that does not improve with closed reduction, ipsilateral upper extremity fracture and recurrent displacement after initial closed reduction. When loss of reduction is appreciated 1 week after initial closed reduction despite a well-molded cast, repeat closed reduction in the operating room can be contemplated. In this situation, percutaneous pin fixation should be considered to avoid further or repeat displacement necessitating a return trip to the operating room. In children approximately 10 years of age with a distal both-bone fracture in which the ulna is a greenstick fracture and the radius is displaced, dorsally translated, and shortened, the radius is often buttonholed by the periosteum and cannot be reduced. In these fractures, it is frequently necessary to make a small dorsal incision and reduce the fragment manually.

6. Complications—Complications are uncommon but include growth arrest, median nerve palsy, refracture and malunion.

D. Galeazzi Fracture—A Galeazzi fracture is a combination of a radial shaft fracture and a dislocation of the distal radioulnar joint. A pediatric variant is a distal radial physeal or metaphyseal fracture with a concomitant distal ulnar physeal fracture.

1. Incidence—This injury is much less common in children than in adults.

2. Mechanism of injury—A fall on an outstretched hand is the usual cause of this fracture.

3. Classification
- Type A—The direction of the fracture line is oblique, from proximal to distal-lateral. This fracture is unstable and usually requires ORIF.
- Type B—The direction of the fracture line is from proximal to distal-medial and is more transverse.

4. Evaluation—Standard AP and lateral views of the wrist should be obtained. If the injury is

not visualized on plain films, a CT scan may be required.

5. Treatment—Reducing the radial fracture usually restores the distal radioulnar joint. ORIF is rarely required but should be undertaken when closed reduction fails.

VI. Carpal Fractures

A. Scaphoid Fractures—In the skeletally immature patient, scaphoid fractures are usually avulsion injuries of the distal pole. They present with snuff box tenderness. They frequently result from a fall on an outstretched hand. They can be treated with a thumb spica cast for 4 to 8 weeks. Midwaist scaphoid fractures in children can result in avascular necrosis or nonunion. If a scaphoid fracture is suspected but not evident on plain X-rays, a CT scan should be obtained.

B. Other Carpal Injuries—Other carpal injuries are uncommon in children. Treatment guidelines for adults for equivalent injuries in children should be followed.

VII. Metacarpal and Phalangeal Fractures—Metacarpal and phalangeal fractures are common after relatively minor trauma. They frequently involve the physis but rarely cause growth disturbance. They heal rapidly. The intact periosteal hinge aids in reduction. The method of treatment for these fractures is similar in adults and children. Injuries that are common in children and unique to children are described here.

A. Boxer's Fracture (Fifth Metacarpal Fracture)

1. Incidence—Boxer's fractures occur in preadolescents and adolescents possessing enough strength to generate the force needed to break this bone.

2. Mechanism of injury—The mechanism of injury is a direct blow with a clenched fist striking a hard object.

3. Treatment—Usually, an ulnar gutter splint or cast for 4 to 6 weeks is sufficient for healing. Reduction and fixation are generally not needed because up to 70° of angulation remodels and causes no loss of function. The only residual deformity is a less prominent knuckle on the involved digit. Rotational malalignment must be corrected, as it will not remodel. If needed, reduction can be accomplished by dorsally directed pressure on the distal fragment while the metacarpophalangeal and proximal interphalangeal joints are in flexion. Redisplacement can occur and so percutaneous pinning is often employed

to stabilize the fracture. The examiner must look for evidence of "fight bites" that may indicate contact with the mouth or teeth of another individual. Appropriate prophylactic antibiotic therapy should be employed in this situation.

B. Fracture of the Thumb Metacarpal

1. Classification

• Type A is a metaphyseal fracture that is usually impacted.

• Type B is a Salter-Harris II fracture that is angulated medially.

• Type C is a Salter-Harris II fracture that is angulated laterally.

• Type D is a Salter-Harris IV fracture that is a true Bennett's fracture-dislocation.

2. Treatment

• Type A—Closed reduction and thumb spica casting.

• Type B and C—Closed reduction and thumb spica casting for most. Occasionally, percutaneous pinning is required.

• Type D—This is an intra-articular fracture that requires ORIF for anatomic reduction of the joint surface.

C. Proximal Phalanx Fractures

1. Mechanism of injury—This fracture usually results from either a fall or from being struck by an object.

2. Classification—Most are usually Salter-Harris II fractures of the base of the proximal phalanx but shaft fractures are also seen.

3. Evaluation

• Physical examination—When the small finger is involved there may be excessive abduction present ("extra octave" fracture). Otherwise pain with palpation and swelling as well as some deformity may be evident.

• Imaging—Good AP, lateral and oblique X-rays should be obtained because these fractures are frequently seen on only one view.

4. Treatment

• Nondisplaced fractures—The finger with the fracture can be buddy taped to the adjacent finger for 3 to 4 weeks until healing occurs.

• Displaced or angulated fractures—The fracture should be reduced by placing a pencil in the web space of the apex of the displacement. This provides an effective means of reducing the proximal metaphyseal fracture. It can then be placed either in a short arm ulnar gutter cast or in a radial gutter cast (depending on the digit involved) for 3 to 4 weeks until the fracture is healed. After cast removal, it is advisable to buddy tape the finger to an adjacent finger for sporting activities for an additional 3 to 4 weeks.

D. Distal Phalanx Fractures (Fig. 31-14)

1. Mechanisms of injury—These usually result from a direct blow (usually from a projectile) and hyperflexion.

2. Classification—A Salter-Harris III fracture with avulsion of the extensor tendon is a true mallet finger. A Salter-Harris I or II fracture can be seen in children and adolescents and often presents as an open fracture with dorsal skin disruption.

3. Treatment

   • Salter-Harris III fracture—These fractures are splinted in minimal hyperextension. Skin necrosis can result if placed in too much hyperextension. ORIF may be required if the extensor tendon fragment cannot be adequately reduced or if the fracture involves a large portion (more than 1/3) of the articular cartilage or is accompanied by volar subluxation of the distal phalanx (incongruous joint).

   • Salter-Harris I or II fracture—An open fracture should always be suspected in these injuries, especially in the presence of visible blood. The same rules that govern other open fractures apply here. The fracture should be irrigated and debrided. The nail should be replaced under the eponychial fold and the joint should be immobilized in mild hyperextension. Prophylactic antibiotics should be administered.

4. Complications—Complications include osteomyelitis, growth arrest, extensor lag, nail growth disturbances, and skin necrosis.

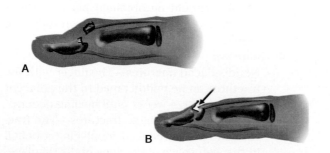

FIGURE 31-14 **A.** Salter Type III fracture of the distal phalanx with avulsion of the extensor tendon insertion; this is a true mallet finger. **B.** Salter Types I or II fracture of the distal phalanx. This is often an open fracture with disruption of the dorsal skin *(arrow)*.

SUGGESTED READINGS

Classic Articles

Bado JL. The Monteggia lesion. *Clin Orthop.* 1967;50:71–86.

Beals RK. The normal carrying angle of elbow: a radiographic study of 422 patients. *Clin Orthop.* 1976;119:194–196.

Bede WB, Lefebure AR, Rosman MA. Fractures of the medial humeral epicondyle in children. *Can J Surg.* 1975;18:137–142.

Bele Tawes AJS. The treatment of malunited anterior Monteggia fractures in children. *J Bone Joint Surg.* 1965;47B:718–723.

Conner AN, Smith MGH. displaced fracture of the lateral humeral condyle in children. *J Bone Joint Surg.* 1970;52B:460–464.

Cullen MC, Roy DR, Giza E, et al. Lateral humeral condyle fractures in children: a report of 47 cases. *J Pediatr Orthop.* 1998;19:14–21.

Davis DR, Green DP. Forearm fractures in children: pitfalls and complications. *Clin Orthop.* 1976;120:172–184.

DeLee JC, Wilkins KE, Rogers LF, et al. Fracture separation of the distal humeral epiphysis. *J Bone Joint Surg.* 1980;62A:46–51.

Flynn JC. Nonunion of slightly displaced fractures of lateral humeral condyle in children: an update. *J Pediatr Orthop.* 1989;9:691-696.

Flynn JC, Matthews JG, Benoit RL. Blind pinning of displaced supracondylar fractures of humerus in children: sixteen year' experience with the long-term follow-up. *J Bone Joint Surg.* 1974;56A:263–272.

Flynn JC, Richards JF. Nonunion of minimally displaced fractures of the lateral condyle of the humerus in children. *J Bone Joint Surg.* 1971;53A:1096–1101.

Flynn JC, Richards JF, Saltzman RT. Prevention and treatment of nonunions of slightly displaced fractures of the lateral humeral condyle in children. *J Bone Joint Surg.* 1975;57A:1087–1092.

Fowles JV, Kassab MT. Displaced supracondylar fractures in children. *J Bone Joint Surg.* 1974;56B:490–500.

France J, Strong M. Deformity and function of in supracondylar fractures of the humerus in children variously treated by closed reduction, splinting, traction and percataenous pinning. *J Pediatr Orthop.* 1992;12:494–498.

Gartland JJ. Management of supracondylar fractures of the humerus in children. *Surg Gynecol Obstet.* 1959;109:145–154.

Holstein A, Lewis GB. Fractures of the humerus with radial nerve paralysis. *J Bone Joint Surg.* 1963;45A:1382–1388.

Hongstrom H, Nilsson BE, Wilner S. Correction with growth following diaphyseal forearm fracture. *Acta Orthop Scand.* 1976;47:299–303.

Jakob R, Fowles JW, Rang M, et al. Observations concerning fractures of the lateral humeral condyle in children. *J Bone Joint Surg.* 1975;57B:432–436.

Josephsson PO, Danielsson LG. Epicondylar elbow fractures in children: 35 year follow-up of 56 unreduced cases. *Acta Orthop Scand.* 1986;57:313–315.

Kilfoyl RM. Fractures of the medial condyle and epicondyle of the elbow in children. *Clinic Orthop.* 1965;41:43–50.

Lascombes P, Prevot J, Ligier JN, et al. Elastic stable intramedullary nailing in forearm shaft fractures in children: 85 cases. *J Pediatr Orthop.* 1990;10:161–171.

Letts M, Locht R, Wiens J. Monteggia fracture-dislocations in children. *J Bone Joint Surg Br.* 1985;67(5):724–727.

Letts M, Rowhani N. Galleazi-equivalent injuries of the wrist in children. *J Pediatr Orthop.* 1993;13:561–566.

Lloyd-Roberts GC, Bucknill TM. Anterior dislocation of the radial head in children: aetiology, natural history and management. *J Bone Joint Surg.* 1977;59B:402–407.

Metaizeau JP, Laseombes P, Lemelle JL, et al. Reduction and fixation of displaced radial neck fractures by closed intramedullary nailing. *J Pediatr Orthop.* 1993;13:355–360.

Mirsky EC, Karas EH, Weiner LS. Lateral condyle fractures in children: evaluation of classification and treatment. *J Orthop Trauma.* 1997;11(2):117–120

Milch H. Fracture of the external humeral condyle. *JAMA.* 1956;160:641–646.

Milch H. Fracture and fracture dislocations of the humeral condyles. *J Trauma.* 1964;4:592–607.

Neer CS, Horwitz BS. Fractures of the proximal humeral epiphyseal plate. *Clin Orthop.* 1965;41:24–31.

Pirone AM, Graham HK, Krajbich JL. Management of displaced extension-type fractures of the humerus in children, *J Bone Joint Surg.* 1988;70A:641–650.

ReganW, Morrey B. Fractures of the cornoid process of the ulna. *J Bone Joint Surg.* 1989;71A:1348–1354.

Ring D, Waters PM. Operative fixation of Monteggia fractures in children. *J Bone Joint Surg.* 1996;78B:734–739.

Rodgers WB, Waters OM, Hall JE. Chronic Monteggia lesions in children: complications and results of reconstruction. *J Bone Joint Surg.* 1996;78A:1322–1329.

Rowe CR. Prognosis in dislocation of the shoulder. *J Bone Joint Surg.* 1956;38A:957–977.

Salter RB, Zalt C. Anatomic investigations of the mechanism of injury and pathologic anatomy of "pulled elbow" in children. *Clinic Orthop.* 1971;77:134–143.

Smith FM. Medial epicondyle injuries. *JAMA.* 1950;142:396–402.

Van der Reis WL, Otsuka NY, Moroz P, et al. Intramedullary nailing versus plate fixation for unstable forearm fractures in children. *J Pediar Orthop.* 1998;18:9–13.

Wiley JJ, Galey JP. Monteggia fractures in children. *J Bone Joint Surg Br.* 1985;67(5):728–731

Woods GW, Tullos HS. Elbow instability and medial epicondyle fractures. *Am J Sports Med.* 1977;5:23–30.

Recent Articles

Chapman V, Grottkau B, Albright M, et al. MDCT of the elbow in pediatric patients with posttraumatic elbow effusions. *AJR Am J Roentgenol.* 2006;187(3):812–817.

Eathiraju S, Mudgal CS, Jupiter JB. Monteggia fracture-dislocations. *Hand Clin.* 2007;23(2):165–177.

Shrader MW. Proximal humerus and humeral shaft fractures in children. *Hand Clin.* 2007;23(4):431–435.

Shrader MW. Pediatric supracondylar fractures and pediatric physeal elbow fractures. *Orthop Clin North Am.* 2008;39(2):163–171.

Storm SW, Williams DP, Khoury J, et al. Elbow deformities after fracture. *Hand Clin.* 2006;22(1):121–129.

Yen YM, Kocher MS. Lateral entry compared with medial and lateral entry pin fixation for completely displaced supracondylar humeral fractures in children. Surgical technique. *J Bone Joint Surg Am.* 2008;90(suppl. 2):20–30.

Review Articles

Kay RM, Skaggs DL.The pediatric Monteggia fracture. *Am J Orthop.* 1998;27(9):606–609.

Minkowitz B, Busch MT. Supracondylar humerus fractures: current trends and controversies. *Orthop Clin North Am.* 1994;25:581–594.

Omid R, Choi PD, Skaggs DL. Supracondylar humeral fractures in children.*J Bone Joint Surg Am.* 2008;90(5):1121–1132.

Otsuka NY, Kasser JR. Supracondylar fractures of the humerus in children. *J Am Acad Orthop Surg.* 1997;5(1):19–26.

Ring D, Jupiter JB, Waters PM. Monteggia fractures in children and adults. *J Am Acad Orthop Surg.* 1998;6:215–224.

Rodríguez-Merchán EC. Pediatric fractures of the forearm. *Clin Orthop Relat Res.* 2005;(432):65–72.

Sullivan JA. Fractures of the lateral condyle of the humerus. *J Am Acad Orthop Surg.* 2006;14(1):58–62.

Wilkins KE. Changes in the management of monteggia fractures. *J Pediatr Orthop.* 2002;22(4):548–554.

Textbooks

Chapman MW. *Chapman's Orthopaedic Surgery.* Philadelphia, PA: Lippincott Williams and Wilkins; 2001.

Herring JA, Rathjen KE, Carter PR. *Upper Extremity Injuries.* 4th ed. Techdjian's Pediatric Orthopedics, Philadelphia, PA: WB Saunders; 2008.

Ogden JA. *Skeletal Injury in the Child.* 3rd ed., New York, NY: Springer; 2000.

Wilkins KE, ed. *Operative Management of Upper Extremity Fractures in Children.* Rosemont, IL: American Academy of Orthopaedic Surgeons; 1994.

CHAPTER 32

Pediatric Spinal and Pelvic Injuries

Scott Rosenfeld

I. Pediatric Spinal Injuries
   A. Epidemiology—Spinal injuries are less common in children than in adults. Patients who are younger than 15 years old account for less than 10% of patients who sustain spinal cord injuries. The most common causes of spinal injury in children are motor-vehicle collisions, falls, and sporting injuries. A very young child with a spinal injury should be evaluated for nonaccidental trauma. Multilevel spinal injuries are common in children.
   B. Differences between Children and Adults with Spine Trauma—Children are not just small adults. There are physiologic and anatomic differences that predispose them to different types of injuries and require different methods for management.
      1. Head size—The pediatric patient's head is disproportionately larger than that of the adult. This raises the fulcrum of motion into a more cephalic position (C2 – C3 in children vs. C5 – C6 in adults) which increases the incidence of upper cervical spine injuries in children. The upper cervical facets in children are also more horizontal, allowing for greater upper cervical motion. During evaluation on a back board, these properties force the cervical spine into greater flexion, which can make radiographic interpretation difficult and may manifest as pseudosubluxation. To accommodate for this a pediatric patient should be evaluated on a pediatric back board with an occipital cutout. Alternatively, a standard back board can be used with supports under the shoulders.
      2. Spine anatomy—The pediatric spine may have open physes and developing ossification centers. This can make evaluation difficult for a physician unaccustomed to viewing pediatric spine radiographs. For instance, the odontoid synchondrosis may be mistaken for a fracture. Furthermore, fractures may occur through these cartilaginous regions, producing distinct pediatric spinal fracture patterns such as vertebral endplate injuries. These fractures may produce only subtle radiographic findings such as disc space widening.
      3. The pediatric spinal column—The pediatric spinal column is more elastic than the spinal cord due to underdeveloped paraspinal musculature and ligaments. The spinal column can tolerate 2 inches of stretch, whereas the spinal cord can only tolerate approximately 0.25 inches of stretch. *This puts the pediatric spine at risk for spinal cord injury without radiographic abnormality (SCIWORA).*
      4. Long-term management—Long-term management of pediatric spinal injury differs from that of adults. The pediatric patient is more likely to recover from neurologic injury due to the greater plasticity of the neural elements. In pediatric spine fractures, physeal injury may result in the development of spinal deformity. Alternatively, growth may allow for remodeling of mild deformities.
   C. Imitators of Pediatric Spine Injuries
      1. Pseudosubluxation (Fig. 32-1)—Pseudosubluxation is a normal physiologic variant in the pediatric cervical spine secondary to the relatively large head size and horizontal upper cervical facets. *On radiographs, it manifests as anterior translation of the cephalic vertebral body relative to the caudad body and is most common at C2 – C3. There may be up to 4 mm and 3 mm of pseudosubluxation at C2 – C3 and C3 – C4, respectively.* It is most commonly seen in children younger than 8 years being evaluated with a supine lateral cervical radiograph taken on a standard back board without shoulder supports or an occipital cut out. The diagnosis is made (true subluxation is

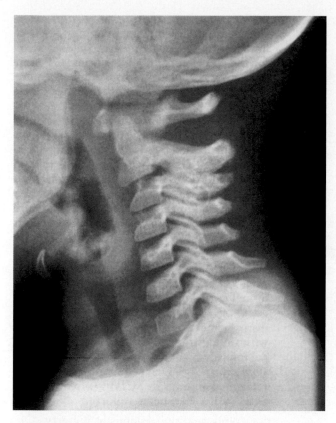

FIGURE 32-1 Pseudosubluxation of C2 on C3. Hypermobility is common in children younger than 8 years. Specific measurement of the movement of the vertebral bodies is unreliable, whereas the relationship with the posterior elements is more consistent. In flexion, the posterior arch of C2 lies in a relatively straight line with C1 and C3. Note the relative horizontal nature of the facet joints, which allows greater mobility. (Reprinted with permission from Capen DA, Haye W. *Comprehensive Management of Spine Trauma*. St Louis, MO: Mosby; 1998.)

ruled out) using the posterior spinolaminar line (Swischuk's line) on the lateral radiograph. This line connects the posterior arches of C1 and C3 and should come within 2 mm of C2.

2. Ossification of the odontoid process—Different stages of ossification of the odontoid process can mimic injuries to this structure. The apical ossification center can mimic an avulsion fracture. The synchondrosis fuses by age 6, but is still visible until age 12 and this may make diagnosis difficult. Persistence of the synchondrosis at the base of the odontoid can mimic fracture. Incomplete ossification of the odontoid process can mimic atlantoaxial instability.

3. Imitators of compression fractures after minor trauma—Eosinophilic granuloma, Mucopolysaccharidoses, Gaucher's disease, Osteogenesis imperfecta, Tuberculosis, tumor.

D. Workup for Pediatric Spine Injury
   1. Clinical examination—Since spinal fractures are often the result of a significant trauma, workup should begin with assessment of the patient: Airway, Breathing, and Circulation. The patient should be transported and assessed on a pediatric back board with an occipital cut out or a standard back board with shoulder supports to accommodate for the relatively large head size. The Primary Survey should include a visual survey and palpation of the head, neck, back, and pelvis. The abdomen should be evaluated for a lap belt sign, which should increase suspicion for an injury of the spine and viscera. A complete neurologic exam should be performed.
   2. Radiographic examination—Patients involved in high-energy trauma should have lateral C-spine, AP pelvis, and AP chest radiographs. Dedicated AP and lateral radiographs should be obtained of any location with tenderness, swelling, or ecchymosis. Any patient with an identified spine fracture should have AP and lateral radiographs of the entire spine as noncontiguous multilevel injuries are common. ***Twenty-four percent of pediatric cervical spine injuries have a second spine injury*** . CT scan and MRI may be used for increased bony and soft-tissue detail. MRI may be used to clear a C-spine in a noncooperative patient.

E. Radiographic Evaluation Specific to the Pediatric Spine
   1. Cervical spine—Powers ratio is used to evaluate the atlanto-occipital junction and should be between 0.7 and 1.0. Normal atlantodental interval may be up to 4.5 mm. At the level of C1, one-third should be taken up by the odontoid, one-third by the spinal cord, and one-third by space available for the cord. Pseudosubluxation up to 4 mm at C2 – C3 is physiologic. Subtle disc height changes may be signs of fracture through vertebral endplates.

F. Developmental Anatomy (Figs. 32-2 and 32-3)—Knowledge of the unique ossification patterns of the pediatric spine is necessary for proper evaluation of an injury.
   1. Atlas (C1)
      • Ossification centers—The atlas has three primary ossification centers. The right and left neural arches are ossified at birth, and the body ossifies at 1 year.
      • Fusion—The atlas body and neural arch synchondroses fuses at 7 years. The spinous process (neural arch) synchondrosis fuses at 3 years.

A   **B**   **C**

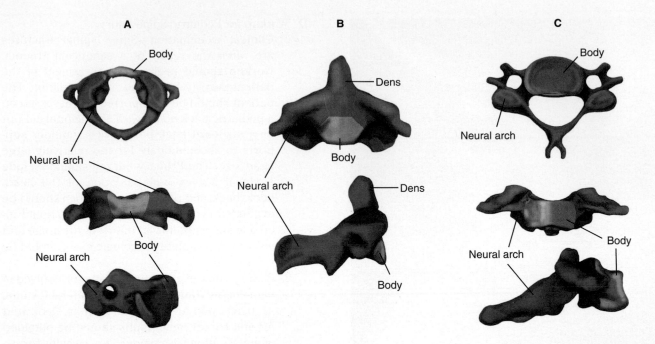

FIGURE 32-2 Ossification centers. **A,** C1. **B,** C2. **C,** Typical of C3-L5.

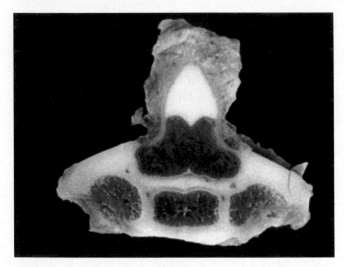

FIGURE 32-3 Morphologic development of the second cervical vertebra at 3 months. The odontoid ossification centers have coalesced. The neurocentral synchondroses separate the centrum from the posterolateral elements. (Reprinted with permission from Ogden JA. In: Ogden JA, ed. *Skeletal Injury in the Child.* 2nd ed. Philadelphia, PA: WB Saunders; 1990.)

2. Axis (C2)
   • Ossification centers—The axis has four primary ossification centers at birth. The two odontoid ossification centers fuse in the midline by the seventh fetal month. The body and the two neural arches are ossified at birth. The secondary ossification center at the tip

of the odontoid appears at 3 years. The inferior epiphyseal ring ossifies at puberty.
   • Fusion—The synchondrosis between the body and the odontoid fuses by 6 years. The fusion line is often visible until age 12. The neural arches fuse to the body by 6 years, and the spinous processes fuse by 3 years. The secondary ossification center at the tip of the odontoid fuses by 25 years, as does the inferior epiphyseal ring ossification center.
3. C3 – C7
   • Ossification centers—Five ossification centers are all present at birth. These are the body, two neural arches, and two transverse processes.
   • Fusion—The transverse processes fuse to the body by age 6. The body and neural arches fuse by age 6. The spinous processes fuse by age 3. Bifid spinous processes appear at puberty and fuse by age 25. The superior and inferior epiphyseal rings fuse by age 25.
4. Thoracic and lumbar spine—Adult characteristics and size are present by age 10 with a similar radiographic examination except for the open epiphyses.
   • Overview—The thoracic and lumbar spine ossify and fuse in a similar manner.
   • Lumbar Ossification Centers—Additional ossification centers are present in the lumbar spine for the mammary processes. They appear during puberty and fuse by age 25.

G. Immobilization Techniques—During initial evaluation, the patient should be immobilized on either a pediatric back board or a standard back board with shoulder supports. Traction should not be used.

1. Rigid immobilization collars—A rigid collar with access to the oropharynx and neck should be used. Rigid collars allow up to 17° of flexion, 19° of extension, 4° of rotation, and 6° of lateral motion. Motion can be decreased to 3° in each direction by supplementing with sandbags and tape.

2. Halo-vest immobilization—Halo-vest immobilization may be used in patients as young as 1 year of age. The thickness of the pediatric skull is variable and therefore pin penetration is a potential complication. CT scan of the skull should be considered to estimate skull thickness at potential pin sites. eight to twelve pins should be placed with torques of only 2 to 4 in-lb. Halo-vest restricts 75% of C1 – C2 motion.

H. SCIWORA—SCIWORA is more common in children than in adults because of the increased elasticity of the vertebral column, shallow facet joints, poorly defined uncinate process, and more proximal fulcrum of cervical motion. The term was coined before MRI was available, and despite having no radiographic abnormality, most will have an MRI abnormality. Approximately 20% to 30% of children with spinal cord injury have SCIWORA. There are two peak incidences:

1. Age 8 to 10 years—Most commonly a proximal injury at the cervicothoracic junction. Neurologic injuries in this group are usually permanent.

2. Adolescents—Most commonly a mid-thoracic injury that may be associated with a visceral injury. Neurologic injuries in this group have a better prognosis for neurologic recovery.

SCIWORA often has delayed onset of neurologic deficit, which may take up to 4 days to manifest. Spine precautions should be maintained until instability is ruled out. Recurrence of neurologic deficit has been reported but it is unclear whether bracing prevents recurrence. Outcome is correlated with MRI findings and severity of neurologic deficit on presentation.

I. Cervical Spine Injuries—Cervical spine fractures account for approximately 1% of pediatric fractures. The incidence is estimated to be 7.41 in 100,000 per year. *There is a 16% mortality rate associated with cervical spine fractures*. Sixty percent of these injuries occur in boys and 27% occur during sporting activities. Other mechanisms of injury include motor-vehicle collisions, falls, and nonaccidental trauma. *Children under age 8 most commonly have upper cervical injuries while older children have lower cervical injuries*. Clinical findings such as facial lacerations and contusion, and palpable posterior cervical defects may be clues to cervical spinal injury.

1. Atlanto-occipital dislocation (Fig. 32-4)

• Incidence—Atlantooccipital dislocation accounted for one-third of deaths from traumatic cervical spine injuries in one series. It is frequently associated with severe spinal cord and brainstem injury causing respiratory arrest. The atlantooccipital joint is a condylar joint that in the pediatric population is almost horizontal and provides little bony stability. Injury mechanism is usually a sudden deceleration causing hyperextension of the occipitocervical junction.

• Evaluation—The Powers ratio can be measured on the lateral cervical spine radiograph. Ratio greater than 1.0 indicates anterior dislocation and a ratio less than 0.7 indicates posterior dislocation.

• Treatment—Associated injuries often include severe head, thoracic, and visceral injuries. Initial cervical stabilization should

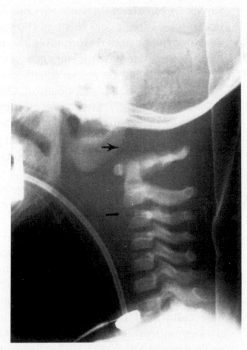

FIGURE 32-4 Atlantooccipital dislocation (*large arrow*). This 3-year-old child was struck by a car. Note the hypopharyngeal soft-tissue swelling, the dislocation of the atlantooccipital joint, and the additional injury at C2 – C3 (*small arrow*). This patient died. (Courtesy Dr. Tim Tyler. Reprinted with permission from Sullivan JA. In: Green NE, Swiontkowski ME, eds. *Skeletal Trauma in Children*. 2nd ed. Vol 3. Philadelphia, PA: WB Saunders; 1998.)

be obtained with a halo vest. Traction is contraindicated. Definitive treatment requires occiput—C2 fusion.

2. C1 – C2 fractures

- C1 and C2 ring fractures—Isolated fracture of the ring of C1 or C2 are rare and are usually caused by axial loading similar to a Jefferson fracture in an adult. Open mouth odontoid views will allow visualization of lateral mass alignment. Neurologic injury is rare because the space available for the cord is preserved. Treatment is with immobilization in either a cervical collar or halo-vest. Distraction should be avoided.

- Traumatic atlantoaxial instability—Acute rupture of the transverse ligament causing C1 – C2 instability occurs in fewer than 10% of pediatric cervical spine injuries. The normal atlantodental interval is 3 mm in adults and 4.5 mm in children; greater than 4.5 mm suggests instability, and reduction in extension with immobilization in a Minerva cast, halo-vest, or cervical orthosis for 8 to 12 weeks is recommended.

- Odontoid fractures—***Odontoid fractures represent up to 75% of cervical spine injuries in children***. In younger children, the fracture usually occurs through the synchondrosis at the base of the odontoid. Neurologic injury is rare. Most displacement occurs anteriorly and should be reduced with extension to obtain at least 50% apposition. Odontoid fractures generally heal uneventfully with 6 to 8 weeks of immobilization in a Minerva cast or halo-vest. Flexion-extension radiographs should be obtained after bony union to assess stability.

3. C3 – C7 fractures and dislocations—Subaxial cervical spine injuries are more common in patients over 8 years of age. Injury types include fracture-dislocations, burst fractures, simple compression fractures, facet dislocations, endplate fractures, and posterior ligamentous injuries. Associated head injuries are common. Treatment should include realigning the spinal canal and immobilization with a halo-vest. Decompression by laminectomy has little role in treatment. Facet dislocations require reduction and halo-vest immobilization. Facet fracture-dislocations are more unstable and more likely to require posterior instrumentation and fusion. Endplate fractures are often associated with neurologic injury and are very unstable but will heal well with appropriate immobilization.

J. Fractures and Dislocations of the Thoracolumbar Spine (Figs. 32-5 and 32-6)

1. Overview—The estimated incidence of thoracolumbar injuries in children is 1/17,000,000. Common mechanisms of injury include motor-vehicle collision, falls, sports injuries, and nonaccidental trauma. Associated injuries are common and may overshadow the spine injury. Most thoracolumbar injuries are around the thoracolumbar junction and are related to a seat-belt injury. The mechanism of injury determines the fracture pattern.

2. Compression fractures—Compression fractures are usually low-energy flexion injuries causing failure of the anterior vertebral body oftentimes at multiple levels. The superior endplate most commonly fails and the posterior cortex and ligamentous complex remain intact. Compression of greater than 50% should be closely evaluated for posterior ligamentous injury. Neurologic injury is rare and these injuries can be managed with activity restriction, physical therapy, and thoracolumbar orthoses.

3. Burst fractures—Burst fractures are rare in the pediatric population. These fractures have a low incidence of neurologic injury, and stable injuries can be managed with thoracolumbar

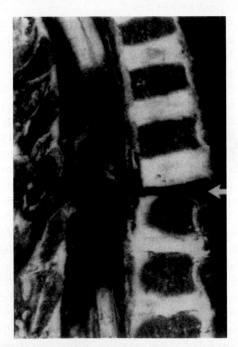

FIGURE 32-5 Fatal thoracic end-plate injury (*arrow*). Note that the hemorrhage in the spinal cord extends several levels above and below the fracture. (Reprinted with permission from Ogden JA. In: Ogden JA, ed. *Skeletal Injury in the Child*. 2nd ed. Philadelphia, PA: WB Saunders; 1990.)

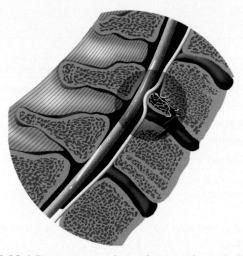

FIGURE 32-6 Posterior epiphyseal injury (*arrow*) (limbus fracture) that may mimic a herniated nucleus pulposus.

orthoses. Anterior vertebral growth may remodel residual kyphosis. If the injury is unstable (posterior element injury) or if there is neurologic injury, posterior spinal instrumentation and fusion is recommended.

4. Limbus fractures (see Fig. 32-6)—Limbus fractures are posterior vertebral epiphyseal fractures, which most commonly occur in the lumbar spine. These injuries may be mistaken for a herniated nucleus pulposus and if symptoms are recalcitrant may be treated with excision of the fragment.

5. Flexion-distraction injuries (lap-belt injuries)—Originally coined by Chance, these injuries occur in the restrained child in a motor-vehicle collision. Three-point harness restrains are not protective from this injury pattern. Patients may have a characteristic abdominal lap belt abrasion and a palpable posterior defect. Associated injuries are common and include small bowel perforation, jejunal transection, and aortic dissection. Paraplegia may be present in up to 30% of these injuries. The spine injury may be bony, soft tissue, or mixed. CT scan with sagittal reconstruction is helpful to detect transverse fractures. Pure bony injuries may be treated with immobilization. Increasing posterior soft-tissue injury results in poor long-term stability and progressive kyphosis, warranting posterior spinal fusion and instrumentation. Patients with multiple injuries should be surgically stabilized as soon as possible.

6. Fracture-dislocations—Thoracolumbar fracture-dislocations are high-energy injuries with a high incidence of neurologic injury and concomitant life-threatening thoracic and abdominal injuries.

Management in the multi-injured patient should include early surgical stabilization with long posterior instrumentation.

K. Complications of Pediatric Spinal Injuries
1. Spinal cord injury—Spinal cord injury is less common in young children than in older children and adults. The overall incidence of spinal cord injury increases 10-fold over age 14. In patients with a spinal injury, children have a higher incidence of spinal cord injury than adults. There is a higher incidence of complete neurologic injury in children than in adults. Death from spinal cord injury occurs more commonly in young children than in older children and adults.
2. Posttraumatic spinal deformity—The pediatric spine has a great propensity for remodeling after injury. Children less than 10 years old with less than 30° of wedging will typically remodel. Increasing deformity in the skeletally mature patient is unlikely to remodel. In addition, factors such as inadequate immobilization, unrecognized posterior ligamentous injury, physeal injury, crankshaft phenomenon, inadequate length of fusion, and spinal cord injury can all contribute to the development of posttraumatic spinal deformity. The prevalence of spinal deformity approaches 100% in children who sustain a spinal cord injury prior to the age of 10 years.

L. Summary (Table 32-1)—The incidence of spinal injuries in children is less than that in adults. However, children with spinal injuries are more likely to have complete neurologic defects. ***Noncontiguous multilevel spinal injuries are common in children, and the identification of one fracture should prompt a physical and radiographic evaluation of the entire spine.*** Children have disproportionately larger heads and should be evaluated on a back board with either an occipital cut out or shoulder supports. Most pediatric spine injuries may be managed with immobilization. Proper halo vest use in children includes the use of multiple (8 to 12) pins placed at lower insertional torque. SCI-WORA is common in children and will usually show changes on MRI. Lap belt injuries are often associated with severe abdominal injuries and general surgeons should be involved early. Traction should be avoided in the treatment of most pediatric spinal injuries.

II. Pediatric Pelvic Injuries
A. Overview—Pelvic fractures comprise only 1% to 2% of all pediatric fractures. They are most commonly associated with high-energy mechanisms such as motor–pedestrian collision, motor-vehicle

TABLE 32-1

Injuries of the Pediatric Spine for Children 8 Years and Under

Injury	Unique Findings	Treatment	Most Common Complication
Atlantooccipital dislocation	Intercondylar distance of over 5 mm	Immobilization and arthrodesis	Neurologic compromise
Atlas fracture	Rare incidence	Immobilization	—
C2 ring fracture	—	Immobilization	—
C1–C2 fractures	Epiphysiolysis of the odontoid	Immobilization	—
C3–C7 fractures	Distraction injury	Immobilization	Spontaneous fusion (common)
Thoracic and lumbar fractures	Apophyseal injuries and multiple level fractures	Treatment is dictated by pathology	Neurologic compromise

collision, and falls. Less commonly pelvic injuries can be sustained in sporting activities. The most important consideration in the evaluation and treatment of a pediatric pelvic fracture is recognition of possible associated life-threatening injuries. The immature pelvic bone has a lower modulus of elasticity and the sacroiliac joint and pubic symphysis have increased elasticity, which allows the pelvis to absorb much greater energy before failure. Therefore, a pediatric pelvic fracture is evidence of a very-high-energy mechanism and should increase suspicion of other injuries. In all, 58% to 87% of pediatric pelvic fractures are associated with injuries to other systems such as genitourinary, neurologic, abdominal, and cardiopulmonary. One series found the pelvic fracture to be the pediatric orthopaedic injury with the greatest number of associated injuries (5.2 concomitant injuries). The mortality rate for pediatric patients with pelvic fractures is 2% to 14% and is most commonly from associated head injuries. Hemorrhage from the pelvic fracture accounts for a very small percentage of deaths. Outcomes are generally associated with the concomitant injuries and once these are addressed, pediatric pelvic fractures usually require minimal treatment and have a good prognosis.

B. Pelvic Ossification Centers—Appreciation of the location and ages of appearance of pelvic ossification centers helps to better understand pediatric pelvic fracture patterns. Apophyseal and physeal cartilage are weaker than ligamentous attachments and are more likely to fracture. This creates different injury patterns in the pediatric pelvis than in the adult pelvis.
1. Primary ossification centers—There are three primary ossification centers: ilium, ischium, and pubis. They are joined at the triradiate

cartilage, which fuses at age 15 to 18 years. The ischium and pubis meet at the inferior pubic rami and fuse at age 6 to 7 years.
2. Secondary ossification centers—There are several secondary ossification centers: iliac crest, ischial apophysis, anterior inferior iliac spine, pubic tubercle, angle of the pubis, ischial spine, and lateral wing of the sacrum. The iliac crest ossification center appears at age 12 to 14 and fuses at 16 to 18 years. The ischial apophysis appears at age 16 and fuses at age 19. The anterior inferior iliac spine appears at age 14 and fuses at age 16.
3. Acetabular secondary ossification centers—Acetabular secondary ossification centers are the os acetabuli, the acetabular epiphysis, and the secondary center of the ischium.

C. Workup
1. Clinical examination—Because pelvic fractures are often the result of a significant trauma, workup should begin with assessment of patient airway, breathing, and circulation. This should be followed by a systems-based evaluation to identify injuries to the head, chest, abdomen, genitourinary tract, and appendicular skeleton. Ecchymosis and crepitus over the iliac crest, pubis, and sacrum as well as hematuria or rectal or vaginal bleeding may be signs of a pelvic fracture.
2. Radiographic examination—Patients involved in high-energy trauma or with clinical signs suspicious of a pelvic injury should have an AP pelvis X-ray. Once the patient is stabilized and life-threatening injuries are treated, Judet view, inlet and outlet views, and a CT scan may be considered. Radiographic evidence of a pelvic fracture should increase the treating team's suspicion of associated injury.

D. Classification of Pediatric Pelvic Fractures—Pediatric pelvic fractures may be classified by concomitant injuries, fracture severity, prognosis, or skeletal maturity.
   1. Quinby and Rang classification addresses prognosis based on soft-tissue injury. It includes uncomplicated fractures, fractures with visceral injuries requiring surgical exploration, and fractures with immediate massive hemorrhage.
   2. Torode and Zieg classification is based on severity and stability of fracture.
      • Avulsion fracture
      • Iliac wing fracture
      • Simple ring fracture
      • Ring disruption—Producing an unstable segment
   3. Silber and Flynn classification is based on skeletal maturity, and it predicts ability of the fracture to remodel without operative intervention.
      • Immature—Open triradiate cartilage
      • Mature—Closed triradiate cartilate
E. Treatment of Pediatric Pelvic Fractures—Life-threatening injuries are the primary focus. The pelvic fracture itself is of low priority in the critical care of the child with multiple traumas and may be addressed after the patient is stabilized. If the patient is hemodynamically unstable and other sources of bleeding have been ruled out, a pelvic binder, sling, or external fixator may be used to stabilize the pelvis and decrease pelvic volume. This may be followed by arteriogram and embolization. Hemodynamic instability due to the pediatric pelvic fracture is much less common than in adults. Definitive management of the pelvic fracture itself is often different from that in adults secondary to the remodeling capacity of the immature pelvis. In general, most pediatric pelvic injuries are treated with protected and progressive weightbearing. However, some studies have suggested specific guidelines for reduction such as (a) articular or triradiate cartilage displacement of greater than 2 mm, (b) pelvic ring disruptions causing more than 2 cm leg length discrepancy, and (c) fractures with more than 1.1 cm of pelvic asymmetry.
F. Avulsion Fractures (Fig. 32-7)—Avulsion fractures are usually of the secondary ossification centers and occur with low-energy mechanisms such as forceful concentric or eccentric contractions of the attached muscles. The ischium (38%), anterior superior iliac spine (32%), and anterior inferior iliac spine (18%) are the most common sites. Treatment involves rest and protected weightbearing. Results are not improved with open reduction and internal fixation.

G. Fractures of the Pubis or Ischium (Fig. 32-8)—*Pubic rami fractures are caused by high-velocity trauma and may have significant associated injuries*. Death occurred in 2% of cases in one series. These fractures represent approximately 38% of pediatric pelvic fractures and are most commonly caused by motor-vehicle collisions or motor-vehicle–pedestrian collisions. Unlike adults, isolated pubic and ischium fractures are seen in pediatric patients secondary to the increased elasticity of the immature pelvis. They are mechanically stable because the pelvic ring is not broken and treatment involves bedrest and progressive weightbearing.
H. Iliac Wing Fractures (Duverney Fracture)—Iliac wing fractures represent approximately 16% of pediatric pelvic fractures. It may occur as an isolated fracture (46%) or in combination with other fractures of the pelvis. The most common etiology is direct lateral compression from a vehicular pedestrian collision (88%). Associated injuries are common and should be sought out. Death occurred in 4% of cases in one series. Displacement is usually mild, and reduction is not necessary as the fractures usually unite without sequelae. Treatment consists of bedrest and progressive weightbearing.
I. Sacral Fractures—Sacral fractures represent approximately 6% of pediatric pelvic fractures. They may be isolated or may occur in combination with anterior pelvic fractures. CT scan can be used to evaluate for sacroiliac subluxation or dislocation. Associated sacral nerve injuries that result in bowel or bladder dysfunction are rare. Treatment consists of progressive weightbearing.
J. Coccygeal Fractures—Coccygeal fractures usually result from direct falls on the buttocks. Associated injuries are rare. Manipulation is unnecessary, and long-term sequelae are rare. Treatment consists of progressive weightbearing.
K. Single Breaks of the Pelvic Ring—In the skeletally immature patient, the mobility of the sacroiliac joint and pubic symphysis and the increased elasticity of bone allow for a single break in the pelvic ring to occur. Single breaks in the pelvic ring can occur as two ipsilateral pubic rami fractures, or fracture or subluxation near the symphysis pubis or near the sacroiliac joint. Given the ability of the immature pelvis to withstand large forces, the presence of these injuries suggests considerable trauma and the likely presence of associated life-threatening injuries.
   1. Ipsilateral pubic rami fractures—Ipsilateral pubic rami fractures represent 8% to 16% of pediatric pelvic fractures. These fractures are usually mechanically stable, but often have

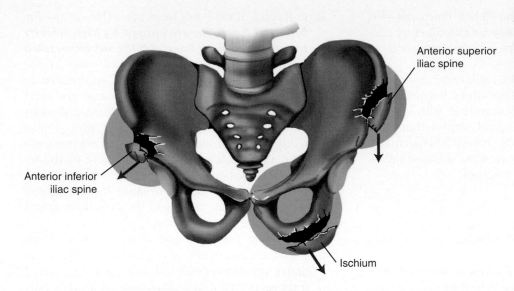

FIGURE 32-7 Avulsion fracture patterns (*arrows*) of the iliac and ischial regions. These fractures occur where secondary ossification centers normally develop.

Anterior superior iliac spine

Anterior inferior iliac spine

Ischium

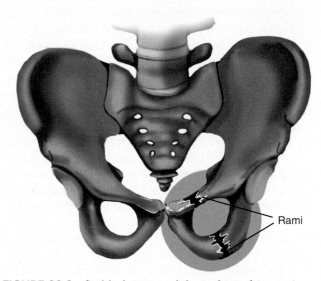

Rami

FIGURE 32-8 Stable fracture of the ischiopubic rami.

major life-threatening associated injuries such as head, genitourinary, abdominal, and cardiovascular injury. The most common mechanism of injury is motor-vehicle–pedestrian. Treatment of the fractures consists of progressive weightbearing.

2. Pubic symphysis fracture or subluxation— Fractures near or subluxation of the pubic symphysis represents approximately 3% of pediatric pelvic injuries. This injury often occurs in combination with a posterior pelvic ring injury. Genitourinary injuries must be ruled out. More than 1 cm difference on lateral compression X-rays may indicate subluxation of the symphysis pubis. One report suggests that diastasis greater than 2.5 cm or rotation greater than 15° implies instability and the need for reduction with traction, external, or internal fixation. Stable fractures may be treated with progressive weightbearing.

3. Sacroiliac joint fracture or subluxation—Sacroiliac joint fracture or subluxation rarely occurs as an isolated injury. It is usually associated with an anterior pelvic fracture or dislocation, which may result in mechanical instability. Apparent sacroiliac joint subluxation may be proven by CT scan to actually be a fracture through subchondral physeal cartilage. Isolated, stable fractures or subluxations should be treated with progressive weightbearing. Unstable fractures may require reduction with internal fixation or a spica cast.

L. Double Breaks of the Pelvic Ring—Double breaks of the pelvic ring are due to high-velocity trauma. They are differentiated from single breaks because of their instability. There is a very high incidence of associated soft-tissue injury and visceral injury.

1. Bilateral fractures of the inferior and superior pubic rami (Straddle fractures)—Straddle fractures are vertical inferior and superior pubic rami fractures on both sides of the pubic symphysis. Alternatively, it may be a unilateral inferior and superior pubic rami fracture with a dislocated pubic symphysis. Both fracture patterns render an unstable floating anterior segment. These injuries are usually caused by a fall while straddling an object or a lateral compression force and are commonly associated with bladder or urethral disruption. Fractures will heal with conservative treatment and remodeling usually corrects displacement. Pelvic sling is contraindicated as it may increase displacement of the floating fragment. Treatment

includes bedrest in the semi-Fowler position followed by progressive weightbearing.

2. Malgaigne fractures (Fig. 32-9)—Malgaigne fractures include all fractures of the posterior arch in combination with fractures or dislocations of the anterior arch. These fractures represent approximately 17% of all pediatric pelvic fractures. Most are the result of motor-vehicle–pedestrian collisions. These unstable fractures are associated with retroperitoneal and intraperitoneal hemorrhage as well as associated injuries. Hemodynamic instability may require a pelvic sling or external fixation to stabilize the fracture and decrease pelvic volume. Initial treatment of the fracture depends on the amount of displacement and may require traction if there is vertical instability or leg length discrepancy. Definitive treatment is usually nonsurgical in skeletally immature patients. Unstable fractures that have failed nonsurgical management and fractures in skeletally mature patients often require open reduction and internal fixation as is often used in adults. Increasing pelvic asymmetry and leg length discrepancy after fracture union has been associated with poorer long-term outcomes.

3. Pelvic crushing and open injuries—Crush injuries cause marked distortion of the pelvis and can be associated with massive hemorrhage. One series of crushed open pelvis injuries reported a mortality rate of 20%. Mobile fragments may lacerate viscera or the arterial tree. Initial treatment should focus on associated injuries and control of pelvic hemorrhage with external fixation and embolization if necessary. Mechanical instability of the pelvic fracture may be addressed with internal or external fixation after the patient is stabilized.

M. Acetabular Fractures—Pediatric acetabular fractures are less common than in adults, representing approximately 9% of pediatric pelvic fractures. Mechanism is similar to that in adults as the force is transmitted through the femoral head to the acetabulum causing fracture and dislocation. High-energy mechanisms often have major associated injuries.

1. Small fragment acetabular fractures associated with hip dislocation—Small fragment acetabular fractures are seen in conjunction with hip dislocations. The majority of pediatric hip dislocations are posterior and may be associated with posterior wall acetabular fractures and anterior capsulolabral avulsions. The goal of treatment is to obtain congruent reduction and prevent recurrent dislocation. CT scan should be performed after reduction of the dislocation to ensure congruency. When a fracture fragment is incarcerated in the reduction causing incongruency, arthrotomy, and open reduction is indicated. Open reduction is often performed from the direction of the dislocation. Postoperative care includes protected weightbearing and hip dislocation precautions for 6 to 8 weeks.

2. Undisplaced stable linear acetabular fractures—Stable linear acetabular fractures are caused by pelvic compression injuries and often occur in association with pelvic fractures. These fractures may be treated nonoperatively with protected weightbearing.

3. Triradiate cartilage fractures (Fig. 32-10)—Triradiate cartilage fractures may result in growth disturbance leading to acetabular dysplasia. Patients younger than age 10 at the time of injury have more remaining growth and are therefore more likely to develop dysplasia. Triradiate cartilage injuries occur as Salter-Harris Types I, II, or V fractures. Types I and II fractures have a favorable prognosis for normal acetabular growth. Crushing Type V injuries have a poor prognosis and often develop a medial osseous bridge, which may result in an acetabular growth deformity. Open reduction should be considered with triradiate cartilage displacement of greater than 2 mm. Nondisplaced injuries are treated with protected weightbearing and early range of motion.

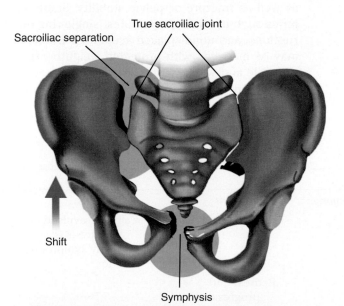

FIGURE 32-9 Unstable Malgaigne fracture of the immature pelvis. The true sacroiliac joint is intact but a chondroosseous separation occurs on the iliac side, mimicking a sacroiliac disruption radiographically.

True sacroiliac joint

Sacroiliac separation

Shift

Symphysis

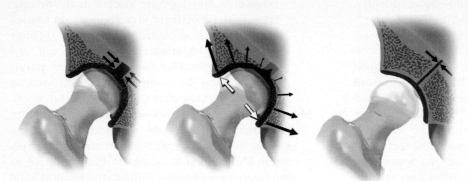

FIGURE 32-10 Triradiate cartilage growth arrest leading to a shallow acetabulum. Dark arrows indicate growth, and white arrows indicate acetabular size.

4. Linear fractures with hip joint instability—Linear fractures with hip instability may cause articular incongruity or injury to the triradiate cartilage. Early management includes restoring acetabular congruity and hip stability. Open reduction should be performed for displacement greater than 2 mm. Late sequelae may include instability, arthrosis, and acetabular dysplasia.

5. Central fracture-dislocation of the hip—Central fracture-dislocation of the hip may cause severe articular injury and may grossly disrupt the triradiate cartilage. These injuries may be associated with severe life-threatening soft-tissue and visceral injuries. Central fractures often have poor outcomes, regardless of treatment modality. Displacement of articular or physeal surfaces greater than 2 mm should be reduced by either closed or open reduction. Open reduction is often associated with heterotopic bone formation. Long-term sequelae include osteonecrosis, acetabular dysplasia, leg length discrepancy, arthrosis, and sciatic nerve injury.

N. Complications of Pelvic Fractures—General complications of pelvic fractures include sacroiliac and pubic symphyseal pain, nonunion, malunion, osteonecrosis, loss of reduction, arthrosis, and sciatic nerve injury. Leg length discrepancy after fracture union has been associated with low-back pain. Triradiate cartilage injury can result in acetabular dysplasia. Open reduction of fractures may result in heterotopic bone formation.

O. Summary (Table 32-2)—*Given the ability of the pediatric pelvis to absorb tremendous energy before failure, the presence of a fracture suggests that the patient has sustained a violent high-energy injury and should alert the treating physician to the possibility of associated life-threatening injuries.* Such injuries should be identified and treated primarily. Once the patient is stabilized, most pediatric pelvic fractures require minimal treatment. The immature pelvis has significant remodeling capacity and treatment decisions should be based on patient age as well as fracture or pelvic stability. Stable injuries such as avulsion fractures, single-ring disruptions, and nondisplaced acetabular fractures may be managed with protected weightbearing. Unstable and widely displaced fractures may require open or closed reduction with or without fixation.

TABLE 32-2

Injuries of the Pediatric Pelvis

Fracture	Type	Associated Injuries	Treatment	Comments
Avulsion	Secondary ossification center injuries	—	Rest and crutches	Callus or avulsed apophysis is rarely symptomatic
Pubis or ischium	Stable high-velocity fracture	Significant	Bedrest and progressive weightbearing	—
Iliac wing (Duverney)	—	Common	Bedrest and progressive weightbearing	—

(Continue)

TABLE 32-2

Injuries of the Pediatric Pelvis (continued)

Fracture	Type	Associated Injuries	Treatment	Comments
Sacrum	—	Possibly combined with an anterior fracture (double break)	Bedrest	There are no reports of associated nerve injuries
Coccyx	—	No associated injuries	No manipulation	Impairment is not prolonged
Single breaks of the pelvic ring	Ipsilateral pubic rami fracture	Common	Bedrest	—
	Fracture near the symphysis pubis	Common	Bucks traction, pelvic sling, or cast immobilization	Lateral compression X-ray films are diagnostic of subluxation
	Fracture near the sacroiliac joint	Common	Avoidance of further displacement	An associated anterior pelvic fracture should be sought
Double breaks of the pelvic ring	Straddle fracture	Bladder or urethral disruption	Bedrest in the semi-Fowler position, avoidance of lateral compression	This is the most dangerous type of pediatric pelvic fracture
	Malgaigne fracture	Common	Bedrest, traction, ORIF or external fixation	—
	Multiple pelvic crushing injuries	Visceral lacerations, arterial tears	Acute injury with external fixation	Survival is rare
Acetabulum	Small-fragment fracture	Hip dislocation	Open reduction if the joint is incongruous	—
	Undisplaced stable linear fracture	Possible involvement of the triradiate cartilage	Bedrest	Acetabular dysplasia may occur
	Linear fracture with hip joint instability	Possible involvement of the triradiate cartilage	Restoration of acetabular congruity	Acetabular dysplasia may occur
	Central fracture-dislocation	Involvement of the triradiate cartilage	Open reduction if reduction is unacceptable after closed treatment	Most patients do poorly

SUGGESTED READINGS

Recent Articles

Galano JG, Vitale MG, Kessler MW, et al. The most frequent traumatic orthopaedic injuries from a national pediatric inpatient population. *J Pediatr Orthop.* 2005;25(1):39–44.

Kay RM, Skaggs DL. Pediatric polytrauma management. *J Pediatr Orthop.* 2006;26(2):268–277.

Kellum E, Creek A, Dawkins R, et al. Age-related patterns of injury in childrens involved in all-terrain vehicle accidents. *J Pediatr Orthop.* 2008;28(8):854–858.

Silber JS, Flynn JM, Katz MA, et al. Role of computed tomography in the classification and management of pediatric pelvic fractures. *J Pediatr Orthop.* 2001;21(2):148–151.

Silber JS, Flynn JM, Koffler KM, et al. Analysis of the cause, classification, and associated injuries of 166 consecutive pediatric pelvic fractures. *J Pediatr Orthop.* 2001;21(4):446–450.

Silber JS, Flynn JM. Changing patterns of pediatric pelvic fractures with skeletal maturation: implications for classification and management. *J Pediatr Orthop.* 2002;22(1):22–26.

Smith W, Shurnas P, Morgan S, et al. Clinical outcomes of unstable pelvic fractures in skeletally immature patients. *J Bone Joint Surg.* 2005;87(11):2423–2431.

Smith WR, Oakley M, Morgan SJ. Pediatric pelvic fractures. *J Pediatr Orthop.* 2004;24(1):130–135.

Vitale MG, Kessler MW, Choe JC, et al. Pelvic fractures in children. *J Pediatr Orthop.* 2005;25(5):581–587.

Review Articles

Holden CP, Holman J, Herman MJ. Pediatric pelvic fractures. *J Am Acad Orthop Surg.* 2007;15(3):172–177.

Reilly CW. Pediatric spine trauma. *J Bone Joint Surg.* 2007;89A:98–107.

Textbooks

Newton PO. Cervical spine injuries in children. In: Beaty JH, Kasser JR, eds. *Rockwood and Wilkens' Fractures in Children.* 6th ed. Philadelphia, PA: Lippincott Williams & Wilkins; 2006.

Warner WC, Hedequist DJ. Cervical spine injuries in children. In: Beaty JH, KasserJR, eds. *Rockwood and Wilkens' Fractures in Children.* 6th ed. Philadelphia, PA: Lippincott Williams & Wilkins; 2006.

Widmann RF. Cervical spine injuries in children. In: Beaty JH, Kasser JR, eds. *Rockwood and Wilkens' Fractures in Children.* 6th ed. Philadelphia, PA: Lippincott Williams & Wilkins; 2006.

INDEX